Textbook of Hemophilia

Edited by

Christine A. Lee
MA, MD, DSc (Med), FRCP, FRCPath
Professor of Haemophilia
Director and Consultant Haematologist
Haemophilia Centre and Haemostasis Unit
The Royal Free Hospital
London
UK

Erik E. Berntorp MD, PhD
Professor of Hemophilia
Lund University;
Director, Department of Coagulation Disorders
Malmö University Hospital
Malmö
Sweden

W. Keith Hoots MD
Professor of Pediatrics
University of Texas M.D. Anderson Cancer Center;
Professor of Pediatrics and Internal Medicine
University of Texas Medical School at Houston;
Medical Director
Gulf States Hemophilia and Thrombophilia Center
Houston, TX
USA

With a foreword by

Louis M. Aledort MD
The Mary Weinfeld Professor of Clinical Research in Hemophilia
Mount Sinai School of Medicine
New York, NY
USA

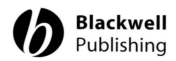

Blackwell
Publishing

First published 2005
Reprinted 2005, 2006

ISBN 10: 1-4051-2769-4
ISBN 13: 978-1-4051-2769-1

Library of Congress Cataloging-in-Publication Data

Textbook of hemophilia / edited by Christine A. Lee, Erik Berntorp,
W. Keith Hoots ; with a foreword by Louis M. Aledort.
     p. ; cm.
   Includes bibliographical references and index.
   ISBN 1-4051-2769-4 (alk. paper)
   1. Hemophilia.
   [DNLM: 1. Hemophilia A—physiopathology.   2. Coagulation Protein
Disorders—physiopathology.   3. Factor IX—physiology.   4. Factor
VIII— physiology.   5. Hemophilia B—physiopathology. WH 325 T355 2005]
I. Lee, Christine A.   II. Berntorp, Erik.   III. Hoots, Keith.
   RC642.T46 2005
   616.1'572—dc22   2004023743

A catalogue record for this title is available from the British Library

Set in Sabon/Frutiger by SNP Best-set Typesetter Ltd, Hong Kong
Printed and bound by Replika Press Pvt. Ltd, India

Commissioning Editor: Maria Khan
Development Editor: Mirjana Misina
Production Controller: Kate Charman

For further information on Blackwell Publishing, visit our website:
http://www.blackwellpublishing.com

The publisher's policy is to use permanent paper from mills that operate a sustainable forestry policy, nd which
has been manufactured from pulp processed using acid-free and elementary chlorine-free practices. urthermore,
the publisher ensures that the text paper and cover board used have met acceptable environmental accreditation
standards.

Contents

CONTENTS

Contributors

Louis M. Aledort MD
The Mary Weinfeld Professor of Clinical Research in Hemophilia, Mount Sinai School of Medicine, New York, NY, USA

Natalya M. Ananyeva PhD
Department of Biochemistry and Molecular Biology, University of Maryland School of Medicine, Rockville, MD, USA

Ekatherine Asatiani MD
Attending Physician, Lombardi Comprehensive Cancer Center, Georgetown University Hospital, Washington, DC, USA

Jan Astermark MD, PhD
Associate Professor, Lund University; Department for Hematology and Coagulation Disorders, Malmö University Hospital, Malmö, Sweden

Trevor W. Barrowcliffe MA, PhD
Head, Division of Haematology, National Institute for Biological Standards and Control, Potters Bar, Hertfordshire, UK

Angelika Batorova MD, PhD
Director of the National Hemophilia Centre, University Hospital, Bratislava, Slovak Republic

Thomas Becker Dr rer nat
Baxter Deutschland GmbH, Unterschleißheim, Germany

Karen Beeton BSc, MPhty, MCSP
Professional Lead, School of Paramedic Sciences, Physiotherapy and Radiography, University of Hertfordshire, Hatfield, UK

H. Marijke van den Berg MD, PhD
Department of Internal Medicine and Paediatrics, van Kreveldkliniek, University Hospital, Utrecht, The Netherlands

Erik E. Berntorp MD, PhD
Professor of Hemophilia, Lund University; Director, Department of Coagulation Disorders, Malmö University Hospital, Malmö, Sweden

Sven Björkman PhD
Adjunct Professor of Applied Pharmacokinetics, Uppsala University, Uppsala, Sweden

Claudia Black MD
World Federation of Haemophilia, Montreal, Quebec, Canada

Victor S. Blanchette MD, FRCP
Professor of Paediatrics, University of Toronto; Chief, Division of Haematology/Oncology, The Hospital for Sick Children, Toronto, Ontario, Canada

Hans H. Brackmann MD
Haemophilia Center Bonn, Institute of Experimental Haematology and Transfusion Medicine, Rheinische Friedrich-Wilhelms University, Bonn, Germany

Simon A. Brown MB, BS, MD, FRCP, MRCPath
Consultant and Honorary Senior Lecturer in Haemophilia and Haemostasis, Haemophilia Centre and Haemostasis Unit, Royal Free Hospital, London, UK

Ulrich Budde MD
Coagulation Laboratory, Hamburg, Germany

Giancarlo Castaman MD
Department of Haematology, San Bortolo Hospital, Vicenza, Italy

Elizabeth Chalmers MB, ChB, MD, MRCP(UK), FRCPath
Consultant Paediatric Haematologist, Royal Hospital for Sick Children, Glasgow, UK

Peter Collins MB, BS, MD, MRCP, FRCPath
Senior Lecturer in Haematology, Department of Haematology, University of Wales College of Medicine, Cardiff, Wales

Donna DiMichele MD
Associate Professor of Pediatrics, Weill Medical College of Cornell University, New York, NY, USA

Alberto Dolce PhD
Researcher, Italian National Institute of Statistics, Rome, Italy

Miguel A. Escobar MD
Assistant Professor of Medicine and Pediatrics, University of Texas Health Sciences Center; Associate Medical Director, Gulf States Hemophilia and Thrombophilia Center, Houston, TX, USA

Bruce L. Evatt MD
National Center for Infectious Diseases, Atlanta, GA, USA

Albert Farrugia PhD
Senior Principal Research Scientist and Head, Blood and Tissues Unit, Office of Devices, Blood and Tissues, Woden, ACT, Australia

Augusto B. Federici MD
Associate Professor of Hematology, Angelo Bianchi Bonomi Hemophilia and Thrombosis Center, University of Milan, Milan, Italy

Kathelijn Fischer MD, PhD
Department of Internal Medicine and Paediatrics, van Kreveldkliniek, University Hospital, Utrecht, The Netherlands

Edith Fressinaud MD, PhD
INSERM U143, Hôpital Bicêtre, Le Kremlin-Bicêtre, France

Paul L.F. Giangrande BSc, MD, FRCP, FRCPath, FRCPCH
Consultant Haematologist, Oxford Haemophilia Centre and Thrombosis Unit, Oxford Radcliffe Hospital, Oxford, UK

Peter M. Green BSc, PhD, MRCPath
Lecturer in Molecular Genetics, Guy's, Kings and St Thomas' School of Medicine, King's College, London, UK

Alessandro Gringeri MD, MSc
Associate Professor of Internal Medicine, Angelo Bianchi Bonomi Hemophilia and Thrombosis Center, University of Milan, Milan, Italy

Nicholas J. Goddard MB, FRCS
Consultant Orthopaedic Surgeon and Honorary Senior Lecturer, Royal Free and University Hospitals School of Medicine, London, UK

Charles R.M. Hay MD, FRCP, FRCPath
Director and Consultant Haematologist, Manchester Haemophilia Comprehensive Care Centre, Manchester Royal Infirmary, Manchester, UK

Ulla Hedner MD, PhD
Professor of Clinical Coagualtion Research, University of Lund, Lund, Sweden

Michael Heim MB, ChB
Professor of Orthopedic Surgery, University of Tel Aviv, Tel Aviv; Deputy Director, Department of Orthopedic Rehabilitation, Chaim Sheba Medical Center, Tel Hashomer, Israel

W. Keith Hoots MD
Professor of Pediatrics, University of Texas M.D. Anderson Cancer Center; Professor of Pediatrics and Internal Medicine, University of Texas Medical School at Houston; Medical Director, Gulf States Hemophilia and Thrombophilia Center, Houston, TX, USA

Jørgen Ingerslev MD, DMSc
Associate Professor of Clinical Biochemistry, University Hospital Aarhus, Aarhus, Denmark

Vytautas Ivaskevicius MD
Institute of Transfusion Medicine and Immunohaematology, DRK Blood Donor Service Baden-Württemberg/Hessen, Johann Wolfgang Goethe University, Frankfurt am Main, Germany

Marc G. Jacquemin MD, PhD
Assistant Professor of Medicine, Center for Molecular and Vascular Biology, University of Leuven, Leuven, Belgium

Rezan Kadir MD, FRCS (Ed), MRCOG
Obstetrician and Gynaecologist, The Royal Free Hospital, London, UK

Walter H.A. Kahr MD, PhD, FRCPC
Assistant Professor of Paediatrics, University of Toronto; Division of Haematology/Oncology, The Hospital for Sick Children, Toronto, Ontario, Canada

Randal J. Kaufman PhD
Professor, University of Michigan Medical School; Investigator, Howard Hughes Medical Institute, University of Michigan, Ann Arbor, MI, USA

Geoffrey Kemball-Cook PhD
Senior Scientist, Haemostasis and Thromobosis, MRC Clinical Sciences Centre, Imperial College Medical School, Hammersmith Hopsital, London, UK

Craig M. Kessler MD
Professor of Medicine, Chief, Division of Hematology and Oncology, Georgetown University Hospital, Washington, DC, USA

Ray F. Kilcoyne MD, FACR
Professor Emeritus, University of Colorado Health Sciences Center, Denver, CO, USA

Peter A. Kouides MD
Associate Professor, University of Rochester School of Medicine, Rochester, NY, USA

Michael Laffan DM, FRCP, FRCPath
Senior Lecturer and Honorary Consultant in Haematology, Imperial College Medical School, Hammersmith Hospital, London, UK

Christine A. Lee MA, MD, DSc (Med), FRCP, FRCPath
Professor of Haemophilia, Director and Consultant Haemotologist, Haemophilia Centre and Haemostasis Unit, The Royal Free Hospital, London, UK

David Lillicrap MD
Professor, Department of Pathology and Molecular Medicine, Richardson Laboratory, Queen's University, Toronto, Ontario, Canada

Rolf Ljung MD
Professor, Department of Pediatrics, Lund University, Malmö University Hospital, Malmö, Sweden

Christopher A. Ludlam PhD, FRCP, FRCPath
Professor of Haematology and Coagulation Medicine, University of Edinburgh; Director, Haemophilia and Thrombosis Centre, Royal Infirmary, Edinburgh, UK

Jeanne M. Lusher MD
Professor of Pediatrics, Children's Hospital of Michigan; Marion I. Barnhart Hemostasis Research Professor, Wayne State University School of Medicine, Detroit, MI, USA

Sylvia v. Mackensen Dr rer hum biol
Medical Psychologist, University Hospital of Hamburg-Eppendorff, Hamburg, Germany

Marilyn J. Manco-Johnson MD
Professor of Pediatrics, University of Colorado Health Sciences Center; Mountain States Regional Hemophilia and Thrombosis Center, The Children's Hospital, Denver, CO, USA

Kenneth G. Mann PhD
Professor and Chair of Biochemistry, University of Vermont, Burlington, VT, USA

Pier M. Mannucci MD
Professor of Medicine, Angelo Bianchi Bonomi Hemophilia and Thrombosis Center, University of Milan, Milan, Italy

Guglielmo Mariani MD
Professor of Hematology, Department of Internal Medicine and Public Health, University of L'Aquila, L'Aquila, Italy

Uri Martinowitz MD
Professor of Hematology, University of Tel Aviv, Tel Aviv; Director, National Hemophilia Center, Chaim Sheba Medical Center, Tel Hashomer, Israel

Dominique Meyer MD
Professor of Hematology, INSERM U143, Hôpital Bicêtre, Le Kremlin-Bicêtre, France

Alec H. Miners BA, MSc, PhD
Visiting Research Fellow, Health Economics Research Group, Brunel University, Uxbridge, UK

Paul E. Monahan MD
Assistant Professor of Pediatrics, University of North Carolina School of Medicine, Chapel Hill, NC, USA

Claude Negrier MD, PhD
Professor of Medicine, University of Lyon, Lyon, France

Johannes Oldenburg MD, PhD
Institute of Transfusion Medicine and Immunohaematology, DRK Blood Donor Service Baden-Württemberg/Hessen, Frankfurt am Main, Germany

Rekha Parameswaran MD
Indiana Hemophilia and Thrombosis Center, Indianapolis, IN, USA

Kathelijne Peerlinck MD, PhD
Center for Molecular and Vascular Biology, University of Leuven, Leuven, Belgium

David J. Perry MD, PhD, FRCP, FRCPath
Senior Lecturer, Haemophilia Centre and Haemostasis Unit, The Royal Free Hospital, London, UK

Holger Pettersson MD, PhD
Professor, Department of Radiology, University Hospital, Lund, Sweden

Flora Peyvandi MD, PhD
Angelo Bianchi Bonomi Hemophilia and Thrombosis Center and Fondazione Luigi Villa, IRCCS Maggiore Hospital, Milan, Italy

Katherine P. Ponder MD
Associate Professor of Medicine, Washington University School of Medicine, St. Louis, MO, USA

Margaret V. Ragni MD, MPH
Professor of Medicine, University of Pittsburg; Director, Hemophilia Center of Western Pennsylvania, Pittsburgh, PA, USA

Francesco Rodeghiero MD
Department of Haematology, San Bortolo Hospital, Vicenza, Italy

E. Carlos Rodriguez-Merchan MD, PhD
Consultant Orthopedic Surgeon, Service of Traumatology and Orthopedics and Hemophilia Center, La Paz University Hospital, Madrid, Spain

Clodagh Ryan MB, BCh, BAO, MRCPI, MRCPath
Lecturer in Haematology, Trinity College Dublin; National Centre for Coagulation Disorders, St James's Hospital, Dublin, Ireland

Evgueni L. Saenko PhD
Associate Professor, Department of Biochemistry and Molecular Biology, University of Maryland School of Medicine, Rockville, MD, USA

Jean-Marie R. Saint-Remy MD, PhD
Associate Professor of Medicine, Center for Molecular and Vascular Biology, University of Leuven, Leuven, Belgium

R. Jude Samulski PhD
Professor of Pharmacology and Director, Gene Therapy Center, University of North Carolina School of Medicine, Chapel Hill, NC, USA

Inge Scharrer MD
Professor, Johann Wolfgang Goethe University, Frankfurt am Main, Germany

Reinhard Schneppenheim PhD, MD
Department of Pediatric Hematology and Oncology, University Hospital of Hamburg-Eppendorf, Hamburg, Germany

Uri Seligsohn MD
Director, Amalia Biron Research Institute of Thrombosis and Hemostasis, Chaim Sheba Medical Center, Tel Hashomer; Sackler School of Medicine, Tel Aviv University, Tel Aviv, Israel

Amy Shapiro MD
Adjunct Professor, Michigan State University; Medical Director, Indiana Hemophilia and Thrombosis Center, Indianapolis, IN, USA

Marta Spreafico PhD
*Angelo Bianchi Bonomi Hemophilia and Thrombosis Center
and Fondazione Luigi Villa, IRCCS Maggiore Hospital, Milan,
Italy*

Alok Srivastava MD, FRACP, FRCPA, FRCP
*Professor of Medicine, Department of Haematology, Christian
Medical College, Vellore, India*

Angela Thomas MB, BS, PhD, FRCPE, FRCPath, FRCPCH
*Consultant Paediatric Haematologist, Royal Hospital for Sick
Children, Edinburgh, UK*

Edward Tuddenham MB, BS, MD, FRCP, FRCPath, FRCPE,
FAC Med Sci
*Professor of Haemostasis, Imperial College Medical School; Head of
Haemostasis and Thrombosis Research, MRC Clinical Sciences
Centre, Hammersmith Hospital, London, UK*

Jane Tuffley MCSP
*Superintendent Physiotherapist, Haemophilia Centre, Royal Free
Hospital, London, UK*

Auro Viswabandya MD, DM
*Lecturer, Department of Haematology, Christian Medical College,
Vellore, India*

Indira Warrier MD
*Professor of Pediatrics, Wayne State University and Children's
Hospital of Michigan, Detroit, MI, USA*

Barry White MD, MSc, MRCPI, MRCPath
*National Haemophilia Director, Ireland; Consultant Haemotologist,
National Centre for Hereditary Coagulation Disorders, St James's
Hospital, Dublin, Ireland*

Gilbert C. White II MD
*John C. Parker Professor of Medicine and Pharmacology, University of
North Carolina School of Medicine; Director, Harold Roberts
Hemophilia Treatment Center, Chapel Hill, NC, USA*

Akira Yoshioka MD, PhD
*Professor and Director, Pediatrics, Nara Medical University, Nara,
Japan*

Kathleen Brummel Ziedins PhD
*Department of Biochemistry, University of Vermont, Burlington,
VT, USA*

Foreword

Little occurred from the earliest descriptions of hemophilia in the Egyptian papyri and the Talmudic understanding of the clinical entity and its genetics until the 1940s. The distinction between factor (F)VIII and FIX deficiency and the recognition that it could be corrected by normal plasma altered the face of hemophilia treatment and initiated the scientific advance that brings us up to the present and is the focus of this book.

The initial aspect of this book focuses on how bleeding disorders are manifested in adults and the use of current laboratory technology available to the clinician to differentiate the various bleeding diatheses. This is augmented by the erudite presentation of how the body maintains balanced hemostasis and how deficiency states alter the homeostasis. Molecular biology has offered us the opportunity to dissect out the individual elements —which ones are primary, how they interact, how when out of control they are modified, and the ways in which thrombin is generated. The advent of genetic engineering has given us the opportunity to understand how both human and animal cells process wild-type FVIII and FIX, as well as B domain-deleted FVIII, such that, currently, recombinant FVIII and FIX products are now in our therapeutic regimen.

FVIII deficiency follows, with initial emphasis on the molecular basis of this most common hemophilia. How it functions in the hemostatic mechanism is defined. The natural history of this deficiency state is elaborated upon, including newer methods of delivering factor replacement. FVIII inhibitors are given a separate section, occurring in both hemophiliacs and normal persons. The multitude of issues related to this challenging entity are approached from the point of view of immunology, predisposing factors, and management of bleeding, as well as eradication.

Hemophilia B (FIX deficiency) is appropriately treated separately, as it differs substantially from FVIII deficiency in prevalence, genetics, and pharmacokinetics, as well as in the newly recognized clinical and immunological implications in patients with inhibitors.

Although we have always recognized that children differ substantially from adults, the field of bleeding disorders is in its naissance regarding the special issues children offer. Newborns and young children and their clinical manifestations and response to therapy, as well as diagnostic issues, are addressed, with recognition of unresolved issues.

Transfusion-transmitted diseases, recognized early regarding hepatitis B, have plagued the treatment of patients with bleeding disorders from the time of the earliest replacement products. The issues of hepatitis, HIV (human immunodeficiency virus), and CJD (Creutzfeldt–Jakob disease) now drive industry, patients, healthcare providers, and patient advocacy organizations. As we understand how to treat, and how much is needed to achieve improved outcomes, there is an ongoing unresolved debate over the margin of safety and efficacy of current human and recombinant products. All these issues are sensitively dealt with, always considering the attendant emotional impact.

One cannot evaluate diagnoses and therapeutic modalities without considering the quality of life, as well as the economic impact of these disorders on the individual, family, and society. This becomes particularly important as we recognize the enormous spectrum of delivery systems throughout the world. As the bulk of patients with these disorders goes with little or no treatment, it is more than appropriate that this work should cover it.

As the most common sequela of inadequate treatment is bleeding into joints, the musculoskeletal system is heavily represented. Pathology and newer diagnostic tools such as MRI (magnetic resonance imaging) to evaluate early joint damage, as well as therapy, are well presented.

One cannot ignore the issue of the impact and importance of the issues surrounding the pregnant woman who may or may not be carrying an affected fetus. Carrier detection, as well as antenatal diagnosis, is suitably covered in this textbook, as advances have made this an important part of the management of bleeding disorders. In this vein, and in the earlier part of this book, one cannot emphasize enough the importance of accuracy in the laboratory for diagnostic purposes and for evaluating the efficacy of biologics and therapy, as well as a need for standardization. We can then all know what and how much factor we are treating with, as well as be able to understand appropriately our failures.

An independent section is devoted to gene therapy. The promise of gene therapy by 2000 has gone unfulfilled. The impediments—sociopolitical and vector challenges, as well as antibody production—have plagued the field. Despite this, investigations and clinical trials are ongoing and we will be kept up to date on this constantly evolving field.

No book on bleeding disorders would be complete if it did not include von Willebrand disease (VWD) and the rare deficiencies. Advances in molecular biology and fractionation technology have made this disease more understandable and treatable. It is the most common bleeding disorder affecting both women and men. A major issue in this and other bleeding disorders is the one surrounding menstruation and pregnancy. The recognition of a bleeding disorder because of menorrhagia is frequently missed but is not overlooked in this text.

Rare bleeding disorders are covered very well. Although uncommon, these clinical problems raise many challenging issues. Most texts give no space to these entities.

It is certainly appropriate and timely that this new book has been carefully put together with an extraordinary array of authors giving a perspective on what we now know, what we yet need to understand, and where therapy is headed. It is relevant to scientists, clinicians, and the many specialist disciplines. Yesterday, today, and tomorrow are all here.

Louis M. Aledort

Overview of hemostasis

Kenneth G. Mann and Kathleen Brummel Ziedins

Laboratory data combined with clinical pathology lead to the conclusion that the physiologically relevant hemostatic mechanism is primarily composed of three procoagulant vitamin K-dependent enzyme complexes [which utilize the proteases factor IXa (FIXa), FXa, and FVIIa] and one anticoagulant vitamin K-dependent complex [1,2] (Figure 1.1). These complexes, which include elements of the "extrinsic" pathway, the FIXa–FVIIIa complex [3], and thrombin–thrombomodulin [4], are each composed of a vitamin K-dependent serine protease, a cofactor protein, and a phospholipid membrane, this last provided by an activated or damaged cell. The membrane-binding properties of the vitamin K-dependent proteins are consequence of the post-translational γ-carboxylation of these macromolecules [5]. The cofactor proteins are either membrane binding (FVa, FVIIIa), recruited from plasma, or intrinsic membrane proteins (tissue factor, thrombomodulin). Each catalyst is 10^3- to 10^6-fold more efficient than the individual serine protease acting on its substrate in solution. Membrane binding, intrinsic to complex assembly, also locates catalysis to the region of vascular damage. Thus, a system selective for regulated, efficient activity presentation provides for a regionally limited, vigorous arrest of hemorrhage.

Additional complexes associated with the "intrinsic" pathway are involved in the surface contact activation of blood [3]. However, the association of the contact-initiating proteins [factor XII (FXXa), prekallikrein, high-molecular weight kininogen] with hemorrhagic disease is uncertain [6].

Of equal importance to the procoagulant processes is regulation of anticoagulation by the stoichiometric and dynamic inhibitory systems. The effectiveness of inhibitory functions is far in excess of the potential procoagulant responses. These inhibitory processes provide activation thresholds, which require presentation of a limiting concentration of tissue factor prior to significant thrombin generation [7]. Antithrombin III (AT-III) [8] and tissue factor pathway inhibitor (TFPI) are the primary stoichiometric inhibitors while the thrombin–thrombomodulin–protein C system [4] is dynamic in its function.

The initiating event in the generation of thrombin involves the binding of membrane-bound tissue factor with plasma FVIIa [9]. The latter is present in blood at ~0.1 nmol/L (~1–2% of the FVII concentration of 10 nmol/L) [10]. Plasma FVIIa does not express proteolytic activity unless it is bound to tissue factor; thus, FVIIa at normal blood level has no significant activity toward either FIX or FX prior to its binding to tissue factor. The inefficient active site of FVIIa permits its escape from inhibition by

the AT-III present in blood. Vascular damage or cytokine-related presentation of the active tissue factor triggers the process by interaction with activated FVIIa, which increases the catalytic efficiency (k_{cat}) of the enzyme and increases the rate of FX activation by four orders of magnitude [11]. This increase is the result of the improvement in catalytic efficiency and the membrane binding of FIX and FX.

The FVIIa–tissue factor complex (extrinsic factor Xase) (Figure 1.2) catalyzes the activation of both FIX and FX, the latter being the more efficient substrate [12]. Thus, the initial product formed is FXa. Feedback cleavage of FIX by membrane-bound FXa enhances the rate of generation of FIXa in a cooperative process with the FVII–tissue factor complex [13].

The initially formed, membrane-bound FXa activates small amounts of prothrombin to thrombin [14]. This initial prothrombin activation provides the thrombin essential to the acceleration of the hemostatic process by serving as the activator for platelets [15], FV [16], and FVIII [17] (Figure 1.1). Once FVIIIa is formed, the FIXa generated by FVIIa–tissue factor complex combines with FVIIIa on the activated platelet membrane to form the "intrinsic factor Xase" (Figure 1.2), which becomes the major activator of FX. The FIXa–FVIIIa complex is 10^6-fold more active as a FX activator and 50 times more efficient than FVIIa–tissue factor in catalyzing FX activation [18,19] (thus, the bulk of FXa is ultimately produced by FIXa–FVIIIa). As the reaction progresses, FXa generation by the more active "intrinsic factor Xase" complex exceeds that of the extrinsic factor Xase [20]. In addition, the "extrinsic factor Xase" is subject to inhibition by the TFPI [21]. As a consequence, most (>90%) FXa is ultimately produced by the FVIIIa–FIXa complex in tissue factor-initiated hemostatic processes. In hemophilia A and hemophilia B, the "intrinsic factor Xase" cannot be assembled, and amplification of FXa generation does not occur [22]. FXa combines with FVa on the activated platelet membrane receptors, and this FVa–FXa "prothrombinase" catalyst (Figure 1.2a) converts prothrombin to thrombin. Prothrombinase is 300 000-fold more active than FXa alone in catalyzing prothrombin activation [23].

The coagulation system is tightly regulated by the inhibition systems. The tissue factor (TF) concentration threshold for reaction initiation is steep and the ultimate amount of thrombin produced is largely regulated by the concentrations of plasma procoagulants and the stoichiometric inhibitors and the constituents of the dynamic inhibition processes [20]. TFPI blocks

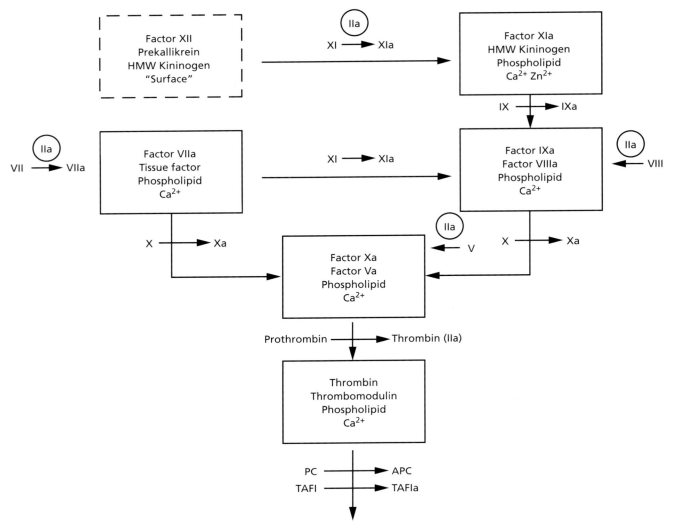

Figure 1.1 A representative map of the various catalysts required to generate the enzymes of the hemostatic system. The outline of the "contact catalyst" of the intrinsic pathway is dashed because of its uncertain contributions to the hemostatic process. The contribution of the contact catalyst to thrombosis is unresolved. The various points at which thrombin catalyzes its own generation by conversion of zymogens and procofactors to the active species required for catalyst formation are illustrated (from Mann KG. *Chest* 2003; **124**: 4–9S, with permission). APC, activated protein C; PC, protein C; TAFI, thrombin activable fibrinolysis inhibitor.

the FVIIa–tissue factor–FXa product complex, thus effectively neutralizing the "extrinsic factor Xase" (Figure 1.2b) [24]. However, TFPI is present at low abundance (~2.5 nmol/L) in blood and can only delay the hemostatic reaction [25]. AT-III, normally present in plasma at twice the concentration (3.2 μmoL) of any potential coagulation enzyme, neutralizes all the procoagulant serine proteases primarily in the uncomplexed state [8].

The dynamic protein C system is activated by thrombin binding to constitutive vascular thrombomodulin (Tm); this complex activates protein C (PC) to its activated species APC (Figure 1.1). APC competes in binding with FXa and FIXa and cleaves FVa and FVIIIa eliminating their respective complexes [16]. The PC system, TFPI, and AT-III cooperate to produce steep tissue factor concentration thresholds, acting like a digital "switch," allowing or blocking thrombin formation [7].

In humans, the zymogen FXI, which is present in plasma and platelets, has been variably associated with hemorrhagic pathology [26]. FXI is a substrate for thrombin (Figure 1.1) and has been invoked in a "revised pathway of coagulation" contributing to FIX activation [27]. The importance of the thrombin activation of FXI is evident only at low tissue factor concentrations [22].

FXII, prekallikrein, and high-molecular-weight kininogen (Figure 1.1) do not appear to be fundamental to the process of hemostasis [28]; the contribution of these contact pathway elements to thrombosis remains an open question and requires further experimentation to resolve this issue.

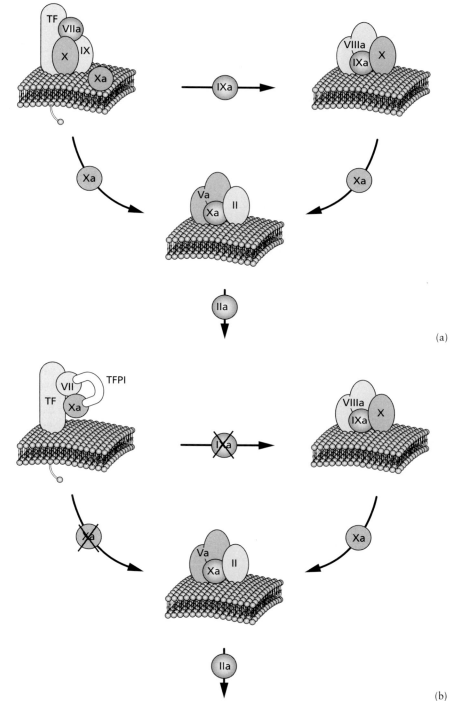

(a)

(b)

Figure 1.2 (a) The factor Xa (FXa) generated by the factor VIIa (FVIIa)–tissue factor complex activates a small amount of thrombin, which activates factor V (FV) and factor VIII (FVIII), leading to the presentation of the intrinsic factor Xase (FIXa–FVIIIa) and prothrombinase (FXa–FVa). At this point in the reaction, FIXa generation is cooperatively catalyzed by membrane-bound FXa and by FVIIa–tissue factor. The thick arrow representing FXa generation by the intrinsic factor Xase illustrates the more efficient Xa generation by this catalyst. (b) The tissue factor pathway inhibitor, (TFPI) interacts with the FVIIa–tissue factor–FXa product complex to block the tissue factor-initiated activation of both FIX and FX, leaving the FIXaβ–FVIIIa complex as the only viable catalyst for FX activation (from Mann KG. *The Dynamics of Hemostasis*. Burlington, VT: Haematologic Technologies, 2002, with permission).

Summary

Advances in genetics, protein chemistry, bioinformatics, physical biochemistry, and cell biology provide arrays of information with respect to normal and pathologic processes leading to hemorrhagic or thrombotic disease. The challenge for the twenty-first century will be to merge mechanism-based, quantitative data with epidemiologic studies and subjective clinical experience associated with the tendency to bleed or thrombose along with the therapeutic management of individuals with thrombotic or hemorrhagic disease. *In vitro* data and clinical experience with individuals with thrombotic and hemorrhagic disease will ultimately provide algorithms which can combine the art of clinical management with the quantitative science available to define the phenotype *vis-à-vis* the outcome of a challenge or the efficacy of an intervention.

References

1 Mann KG, Nesheim ME, Church WR, *et al.* Surface-dependent reactions of the vitamin K-dependent enzyme complexes. *Blood* 1990; **76**: 1–16.

2 Brummel Ziedins K, Orfeo T, Jenny NS, *et al.* Blood coagulation and fibrinolysis. In: Greer JP, Foerster J, Lukens JN, *et al.*, eds. *Wintrobe's Clinical Hematology.* Philadelphia: Lippincott Williams & Wilkins, 2003: 677–774.

3 Davie EW, Ratnoff OD. Waterfall sequence for intrinsic blood clotting. *Science* 1964; **145**: 1310–12.

4 Esmon CT. The protein C pathway. *Chest* 2003; **124**: 26S–32S.

5 Stenflo J. Contributions of Gla and EGF-like domains to the function of vitamin K-dependent coagulation factors. *Crit Rev Eukaryot Gene Expr* 1999; **9**: 59–88.

6 Davie EW. A brief historical review of the waterfall/cascade of blood coagulation. *J Biol Chem* 2003; **278**: 50819–32.

7 van't Veer C, Golden NJ, Kalafatis M, Mann KG. Inhibitory mechanism of the protein C pathway on tissue factor-induced thrombin generation. Synergistic effect in combination with tissue factor pathway inhibitor. *J Biol Chem* 1997; **272**: 7983–94.

8 Olson ST, Bjork I, Shore JD. Kinetic characterization of heparin-catalyzed and uncatalyzed inhibition of blood coagulation proteinases by antithrombin. *Methods Enzymol* 1993; **222**: 525–59.

9 Nemerson Y. Tissue factor and hemostasis. *Blood* 1998; **71**: 1–8.

10 Morrissey JH, Macik BG, Neuenschwander PF, Comp PC. Quantitation of activated factor VII levels in plasma using a tissue factor mutant selectively deficient in promoting factor VII activation. *Blood* 1993; **81**: 734–44.

11 Bom VJ, Bertina RM. The contributions of Ca²⁺, phospholipids and tissue-factor apoprotein to the activation of human blood-coagulation factor X by activated factor VII. *Biochem J* 1990; **265**: 327–36.

12 Osterud B, Rapaport SI. Activation of factor IX by the reaction product of tissue factor and factor VII: additional pathway for initiating blood coagulation. *Proc Natl Acad Sci USA* 1977; **74**: 5260–4.

13 Lawson JH, Mann KG. Cooperative activation of human factor IX by the human extrinsic pathway of blood coagulation. *J Biol Chem* 1991; **266**: 11317–27.

14 Butenas S, DiLorenzo ME, Mann KG. Ultrasensitive fluorogenic substrates for serine proteases. *J Thromb Haemost* 1997; **78**: 1193–1201.

15 Brass LF. Thrombin and platelet activation. *Chest* 2003; **124**: 18S–25S.

16 Mann KG, Kalafatis M. Factor V: a combination of Dr Jekyll and Mr Hyde. *Blood* 2003; **101**: 20–30.

17 Fay PJ. Subunit structure of thrombin-activated human factor VIIIa. *Biochim Biophys Acta* 1988; **952**: 181–90.

18 Mann KG, Krishnaswamy S, Lawson JH. Surface-dependent hemostasis. *Semin Hematol* 1992; **29**: 213–26.

19 Ahmad SS, Rawala-Sheikh R, Walsh PN. Components and assembly of the factor X activating complex. *Semin Thromb Haemost* 1992; **18**: 311–23.

20 Hockin MF, Jones KC, Everse SJ, Mann KG. A model for the stoichiometric regulation of blood coagulation. *J Biol Chem* 2002; **277**: 18322–33.

21 Girard TJ, Warren LA, Novotny WF, *et al.* Functional significance of the Kunitz-type inhibitory domains of lipoprotein-associated coagulation inhibitor. *Nature* 1989; **338**: 518–20.

22 Cawthern KM, van 't Veer C, Lock JB, *et al.* Blood coagulation in hemophilia A and hemophilia C. *Blood* 1998; **91**: 4581–92.

23 Nesheim ME, Taswell JB, Mann KG. The contribution of bovine Factor V and Factor Va to the activity of prothrombinase. *J Biol Chem* 1979; **254**: 10952–62.

24 Baugh RJ, Broze GJ, Jr., Krishnaswamy S. Regulation of extrinsic pathway factor Xa formation by tissue factor pathway inhibitor. *J Biol Chem* 1998; **273**: 4378–86.

25 Novotny WF, Brown SG, Miletich JP, *et al.* Plasma antigen levels of the lipoprotein-associated coagulation inhibitor in patient samples. *Blood* 1991; **78**: 387–93.

26 Seligsohn U. Factor XI deficiency. *J Thromb Haemost* 1993; **70**: 68–71.

27 Gailani D, Broze GJ, Jr. Factor XI activation in a revised model of blood coagulation. *Science* 1991; **253**: 909–12.

28 Colman RW. Contact activation pathway: Inflammatory, fibrinolytic, anticoagulant, antiadhesive and antiangiogenic activities. In: Colman RW, Hirsh J, Marder VJ, *et al.*, eds. *Hemostasis and Thrombosis: Basic Principles & Clinical Practice.* Philadelphia: Lippincott Williams & Wilkins, 2001: 103–21.

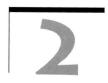

2

Cellular processing of factors VIII and IX

Randal J. Kaufman

Blood coagulation is regulated by the sequential activation of vitamin K-dependent coagulation proteases within the intrinsic and extrinsic pathways. This involves a complex series of reactions that occur as a cascade and culminates in the generation of thrombin to convert soluble fibrinogen into insoluble fibrin. Maintenance of hemostasis relies on the regulated interaction of the vitamin K-dependent proteases, protease cofactors, membrane surfaces and receptors, calcium ions, and protease inhibitors. Three central and fundamental enzyme complexes in the coagulation cascade are the factor Xa (FXa)-generating complex, consisting of factor IXa (FIXa) and the cofactor factor VIIIa (FVIIIa), the FXa-generating complex consisting of factor VIIa (FVIIa) and tissue factor, and the thrombin-generating complex, consisting of FXa and the cofactor factor Va (FVa). The physiologic significance of these pathways is evident from genetic deficiencies that result in bleeding disorders. All the proteins involved in the coagulation cascade require post-translational modifications for appropriate secretion, plasma half-life, and function. The two most common genetic bleeding diseases involving this cascade are hemophilia A and B, which are due to deficiency in coagulation factors VIII and IX respectively. Recombinant DNA technology has provided the ability to produce safe and efficacious preparations of both FVIII and FIX for hemophilia replacement therapy. Gene therapy approaches for these diseases are rapidly approaching and need to consider the requirement for proper post-translational modification in protein secretion and function.

Domain structure of coagulation factors

The domain structures of the vitamin K-dependent coagulation factors FVII, FIX, FX, prothrombin, protein C, and protein S deduced from their cDNA sequences demonstrate they contain common structural features (Figure 2.1). All contain a signal peptide that is required for translocation into the lumen of the endoplasmic reticulum (ER). This is followed by a propeptide that directs vitamin-K dependent γ-carboxylation of the mature polypeptide. Upon transit through the *trans*-Golgi apparatus, the propeptide is cleaved away. The amino terminus of the mature protein contains a γ-carboxyglutamic acid-rich region (Gla) that includes a short α-helical stack of aromatic amino acids. Then there are two epidermal growth factor (EGF)-like domains. In FIX, protein C, and FX, the amino-terminal EGF domain contains β-hydroxyaspartic acid (Hya) at homologous

locations. The next region is the activation peptide (12–52 residues), which is glycosylated on asparagine residues and is released by specific proteolysis accompanying activation. The remainder of the vitamin K-dependent protease comprises the serine protease catalytic triad, which is absent in protein S.

Factor VIII and FV are homologous glycoproteins that serve as cofactors for proteolytic activation of FX and prothrombin respectively. These cofactors act to increase the V_{max} of substrate activation by four orders of magnitude. They have a conserved domain organization of A1–A2–B–A3–C1–C2 [2] (Figure 2.2). The A domains of factors V and VIII are homologous to the A domains of the plasma copper-binding protein ceruloplasmin. Copper has been detected in FVIII and its presence is associated with functional FVIII activity [3]. One mole of reduced Cu(I) was detected in recombinant FVIII and likely resides within a type 1 copper ion binding site within the A1 domain [4]. The C domains are homologous to phospholipid-binding proteins, such as milk-fat globule protein, suggesting a role in phospholipid interaction. Whereas the amino acid sequences in the A and C domains are 40% identical between factors V and VIII, there is only limited homology between the B domains. However, the B domains of both proteins have conserved the addition of a large number of asparagine-linked oligosaccharides as well as a large number of serine/threonine-linked oligosaccharides, suggesting that the carbohydrate has a role in cofactor function.

Factors V and VIII contain a signal peptide that is removed upon translocation into the ER. FV is secreted from hepatocytes as a single-chain polypeptide of 330 kDa. FVIII is processed within the secretory pathway in the cell to yield a heterodimer composed primarily of a heavy chain extending up to 200 kDa (primarily two species from residues 1 to 1313 or 1648, where residue 1 is the amino-terminal amino acid after signal peptide cleavage) in a metal ion-dependent association with an 80-kDa light chain (residues 1649–2332) (Figure 2.3). This association is stabilized by noncovalent interactions between the amino-terminal and carboxy-terminal ends of the factor VIII light chain with the amino terminus of mature von Willebrand factor (VWF). VWF interaction stabilizes FVIII upon secretion from the cell, inhibits factor VIII binding to phospholipids, and increases the half-life of FVIII circulating in plasma [5,6]. The ratio of VWF to FVIII is maintained at 50:1, with an increase or decrease in the plasma VWF level resulting in a corresponding change in the level of FVIII.

Factor V and FVIII circulate in plasma as inactive precursors that are activated through limited proteolysis by either thrombin

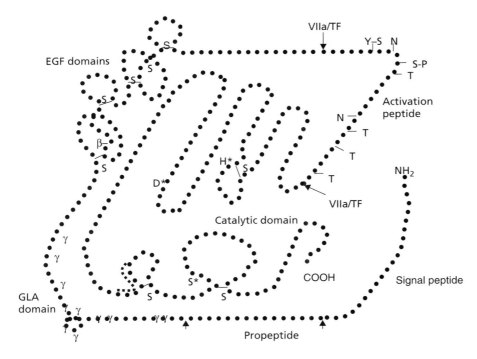

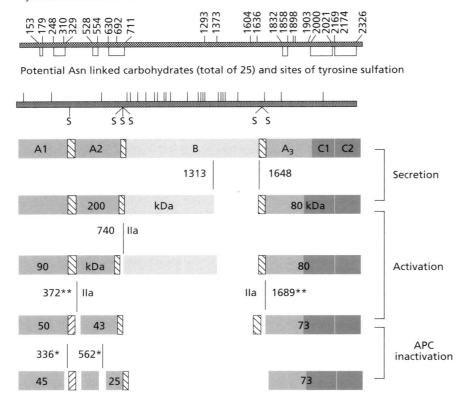

Figure 2.1 Domain structure and processing of factor IX (FIX). FIX is composed of a signal peptide, propeptide, γ-carboxyglutamic acid domain (Gla), epidermal growth factor-like domains (EGF), activation peptide, and serine protease catalytic domain. Short arrows represent intracellular processing sites that cleave away the signal peptide and the propeptide. The long arrows represent the cleavages required for activation by factor VIIa/tissue factor (VIIa/TF) or FXIa. The 35 amino acid activation peptide is indicated. γ represents γ-carboxyglutamic acid and β represents β-hydroxyaspartic acid. The 330–338 loop that interacts with factor VIII is shown by a dashed line. Also indicated are sites of addition of asparagine-linked oligosaccharides (N), serine or threonine-linked oligosaccharides (S and T respectively), tyrosine sulfation (Y-S), and serine phosphorylation (S-P).

Figure 2.2 Domain structure and processing of factor VIII (FVIII). The structural domains of factor VIII are depicted: A1 domain (1–336), A2 domain (372–740), B domain (740–1648), A3 domain (1690–2020) and the C domains (2021–2332). Above, the pairing of disulfide bonds is shown. Below are represented the potential N-linked glycosylation sites (vertical bars up). Three regions (stippled areas) rich in acidic amino acid residues and lying between domains A1 and A2, A2 and B, B and A3 contain sites of tyrosine sulfation(s). Intracellularly, FVIII is cleaved within the B domain after Arg1313 and Arg1648 to generate an approximately 200-kDa peptide and the 80-kDa light chain. The two cleavages required for thrombin activation are indicated (**). The sites for APC cleavage and inactivation are also shown (*).

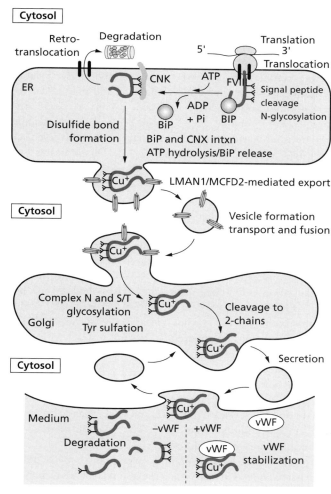

Figure 2.3 Synthesis, processing, and secretion of factor VIII (FVIII) in mammalian cells. The FVIII primary translation product is translocated into the lumen of the ER, where N-linked glycosylation occurs. A fraction of FVIII binds tightly to the protein chaperone BiP and requires ATP hydrolysis for release [43]. A portion of FVIII is retrotranslocated into the cytoplasm and is degraded by the cytosolic 26S proteasome. Another fraction of the molecules interact with the lectins calnexin/calreticulin and then with the protein chaperone complex LMAN1/MCFD2 for transit to the Golgi apparatus. In the Golgi apparatus, additional processing occurs, which includes complex modification of carbohydrate on N-linked sites, addition of carbohydrate to serine and threonine residues, sulfation of tyrosine residues, and cleavage of the protein to the mature heavy and light chains. The presence of VWF in the medium promotes heavy and light chain association and stable accumulation of FVIII in the medium. In the absence of VWF, the individual chains do not associate and are degraded.

or activated factor X (Xa). Thrombin activation of FVIII results in cleavage initially after Arg740 and subsequently after Arg residues 372 and 1689 [7]. Cleavages at both Arg372 and 1689 are required for activation of FVIII procoagulant activity. The cleavage at 1689 releases activated FVIII from VWF, thereby relieving the inhibitory activity of VWF on FVIII, permitting the activated form of FVIII to interact with negatively charged phospholipids. Thrombin-activated FVIII consists of a heterotrimer

of a 50-kDa A1-domain-derived polypeptide, a 43-kDa A2-domain-derived polypeptide, and a 73-kDa-derived light chain fragment [8,9]. Upon thrombin activation, the B domains of both factors V and VIII are released. The amino-terminal sides of the thrombin cleavage sites within factors V and VIII are rich in acidic amino acids and contain the post-translationally modified amino acid, tyrosine sulfate.

Disulfide bond formation

The vitamin K-dependent coagulation factors, exemplified by FIX, have conserved disulfide bonds. Generally, three disulfide bonds occur within each EGF domain, and several disulfide bonds occur within the serine protease catalytic domain. In addition, FIX has a disulfide bond that connects the amino-terminal half with the carboxy-terminal half of the protein so that, after activation, the two portions of the molecule do not dissociate. In factor IX, cysteine residues at 18 and 23 within the Gla domain form a small essential disulfide loop, where mutations at either cysteine residue result in severe hemophilia B.

Factor VIII and FV also have a conserved disulfide bonding pattern in which two disulfide bonds occur within the A1 and A2 domains, whereas only the small disulfide loop is present in their A3 domains. In addition, each C domain in FV and FVIII contains one disulfide bond [10]. There are a number of nondisulfide-bonded cysteine residues within factor VIII; one cysteine residue is not oxidized in each A domain and there are four cysteine residues within the B domain that are also likely not oxidized. Disulfide bond formation occurs in the oxidizing environment of the ER and it is possible that protein chaperones such as protein disulfide isomerase are important to ensure that proper disulfide bond formation and exchange occur prior to exit from the ER.

Asparagine- and serine/threonine-linked glycosylation

Addition of N-linked oligosaccharides to many glycoproteins is an obligatory event for the folding and assembly of newly synthesized polypeptides. The presence of oligosaccharides is often required for the efficient transport of individual glycoproteins through the secretory pathway. In addition, N-linked glycosylation frequently affects the plasma half-life and biological activity of glycoproteins. The consensus site for N-linked glycosylation is Asn–Xxx–Ser/Thr, in which Xxx may be any amino acid except proline. The utilization of a particular consensus site for N-linked oligosaccharide attachment is determined by the structure of the growing polypeptide. As a consequence, proteins expressed in heterologous cells most frequently exhibit occupancy of N-linked sites very similar to that of the native polypeptide.

After addition of the high-mannose-containing oligosaccharide core structure (composed of $glucose_3$-$mannose_9$-N-acetylglucosamine$_2$) to consensus asparagine residues, trimming begins with the removal of the three terminal glucose residues, which is mediated by the action of glucosidases I and II. Glucosidase I removes the terminal α1–3 glucose and glucosidase II subsequently removes the two α1–2 glucose residues. Glucose trimming is required for binding to the protein chaperones calnexin (CNX) and calreticulin (CRT) within the lumen of the ER. Prolonged association with CNX and/or CRT is observed when proteins are unfolded, misfolded, or unable to oligomerize. CNX and CRT bind most avidly to monoglucosylated forms of the N-linked core structure. Removal of the third glucose from the oligosaccharide core structure correlates with release from CNX and CRT and transport to the Golgi apparatus. The selectivity in binding of unfolded glycoproteins to CRT and CNX is mediated by reglucosylation of the deglucosylated N-linked oligosaccharide. This reglucosylation activity is performed by a UDP-glucose:glycoprotein glucosyltransferase (UGT). Only unfolded, mutant, or unassembled proteins are subject to reglucosylation. Reglucosylated proteins rebind CNX and/or CRT and, in this manner, unfolded proteins are retained in the ER through a cycle of CNX/CRT interaction, glucosidase II activity, and UGT activity. Subsequent to glucose trimming in the ER, at least one α1–2-linked mannose is removed by an ER α1–2-mannosidase prior to transport out of the ER.

Upon transit through the Golgi apparatus, a series of additional carbohydrate modifications occur that are separated spatially and temporally and involve the removal of mannose residues by Golgi mannosidases I and II and the addition of N-acetylglucosamine, fucose, galactose, and sialic acid residues. These reactions occur by specific glycosyltransferases that modify the high-mannose carbohydrate to complex forms. Also within the Golgi apparatus, O-linked oligosaccharides are attached to the hydroxyl of serine or threonine residues through an O-glycosidic bond to N-acetylgalactosamine. Serine and threonine residues subject to glycosylation are frequently clustered together and contain an increased frequency of proline residues in the region, especially at positions −1 and +3 relative to the glycosylated residue. Galactose, fucose, and sialic acid are frequently attached to the serine/threonine-linked N-acetylgalactosamine. O-glycosylation occurs in the Golgi complex concomitant with complex processing of N-linked oligosaccharides.

With the development of recombinant factor IX produced in Chinese hamster ovary (CHO) cells for treatment of hemophilia B, a detailed characterization and comparison of the carbohydrate structures was performed between plasma-derived and recombinant-derived factor IX [11]. In both plasma- and recombinant-derived FIX, Asn157 and Asn167 within the activation peptide are fully occupied with complex-type N-glycans [12]. Recombinant FIX contains tetra-antennary, tetrasialylated, core fucosylated glycans at both sites. Plasma-derived FIX contains bi-, tri-, and tetra-antennary, sialylated glycans, with and without fucose. Both molecules have a range of minor structures; however, the glycans present on plasma-derived FIX are

considerably more heterogeneous and diverse. The diversity may be a consequence of the plasma pool.

Both plasma- and recombinant-derived FIX contain a number of O-linked oligosaccharides. In the first FIX EGF domain, serine residues 53 and 61 are uniformly O-glycosylated. The EGF1 domain in both recombinant and plasma-derived FIX contains nonclassical O-linked glycans at Ser53 and Ser61. Ser53 contains Xyl–Xyl–Glc–Ser and Ser61 contains the tetrasaccharide with a terminal sialic acid (NeuAc), NeuAc–Gal–GlcNac–Fuc–Ser61 [13–15]. This indicates that Chinese hamster ovary (CHO) cells (the cells used as a host to produce recombinant FIX) have the enzymatic machinery to produce the structures present on plasma-derived FIX (which is synthesized in human hepatocytes) and that this machinery is not saturated at high expression levels. The carbohydrate structure at Ser61 in FIX contains fucose-linked tetrasaccharide with a terminal sialic acid. Ser61, within the first EGF domain of FIX, has the consensus sequence (C–X–X–G–G–T/S–C) for fucosyl modification of O-linked sugars and is also found in FVII, but not in FX. However, a crystal structure of factor IX demonstrated that both these O-linked modifications reside on the face of the EGF domain that apparently does not interact with other components of the factor Xase complex [16]. In addition to serine-linked oligosaccharide addition in the first EGF domain, both plasma-derived and recombinant-derived factor IX molecules are partially occupied by O-linked glycans at residues Thr159, Thr169, Thr172, and Thr179, as well as at yet unidentified additional sites [12]. The function of these O-linked glycans remains unknown.

Factor V and FVIII contain a large number of N-linked oligosaccharides. Comparison of the N-linked oligosaccharides present on recombinant factor VIII expressed in mammalian cells with human plasma-derived FVIII indicates that both proteins display similar occupancy and complexity at the N-linked sites [17]. However, a detailed analysis demonstrates that differences in the microheterogeneity of oligosaccharides present on human plasma-derived FVIII and recombinant FVIII produced in baby hamster kidney cells do exist [18]. The light chains of FVIIIa and FVa migrate as doublets upon sodium dodecyl sulfate polyacrylamide gel electrophoresis (SDS-PAGE) owing to differences in the complexity of N-linked oligosaccharides present on the light chain [19]. The difference in complexity of the N-linked sugars on the light chain does not affect factor VIII activity. The majority of N-linked oligosaccharides within FVIII and FV occur within the B domain. Recent studies indicate that the N-linked oligosaccharides within the FV and FVIII B domains may be important to interact with the protein chaperone complex LMAN1/MCFD2 for facilitated transport from the ER to the Golgi compartment [20,21] (Figure 2.3). Mutations in either of the subunits of this heterodimeric complex cause combined deficiency of coagulation factors V and VIII [22,23].

Detailed analysis of recombinant factor VIII demonstrated that 3% of the total sugar chains contain a Galα1–3Gal group on some of the outer chains of the bi-, tri-, and tetra-antennary complex-type sugar chains, a group that is absent on factor VIII derived from human plasma. This structure was present in Kogenate (prepared from baby hamster kidney cells) and not in Recombinate (prepared from CHO cells) [18]. The α1–3-galactosyltransferase that produces this structure is expressed in most nonprimate mammalian cells, and primates frequently develop antibodies to this structure. Approximately 1% of immunoglobulin in human plasma is directed toward this moiety, so it is expected that antibodies should be detected. A limited clinical trial did not detect any difference in the efficacy and/or half-life of FVIII that contains the Galα1–3Gal group. Therefore, there is no evidence of detrimental effects of the presence of this structure on recombinant FVIII.

Gamma-carboxylation of glutamic acid residues

The vitamin K-dependent coagulation factors contain the post-translationally modified amino acid γ-carboxyglutamic acid (Gla). The Gla residues are essential for these proteins to attain a calcium-dependent conformation and for their ability to bind phospholipid surfaces, an essential interaction for their function. The precursor of the vitamin K-dependent coagulation factors contains a propeptide that directs γ-carboxylation of up to 12 glutamic acid residues at the amino terminus of the mature protein. The propeptides (residues −18 to −1 in FIX) of these factors share amino acid similarity by conservation of the γ-carboxylase recognition site and the site for cleavage of the propeptide.

The residues that are carboxylated in FIX are glutamic acid residues 7, 8, 15, 17, 20, 21, 26, 27, 30, 33, 36, and 40. Mutations at residues 6, 7, 17, 21, 27, 30, or 33 result in moderate to severe hemophilia B, indicating their functional importance. High-level expression of the vitamin-K dependent plasma proteins in transfected mammalian cells is limited by the ability of the mammalian host cell to efficiently perform γ-carboxylation of amino-terminal glutamic acid residues and also to efficiently cleave the propeptide [24–26]. Analysis of FIX expressed in CHO cells reveals that the protein has a much lower specific activity than the natural human plasma-derived protein. The reduced specific activity is attributed to the limited ability of CHO cells both to cleave the propeptide of FIX and to efficiently perform γ-carboxylation [25,26]. Generally, expression of FIX at levels greater than $1\,\mu g/10^6$ cells/day saturates the activity for most cells studied [24]. Over-expression of the γ-carboxylase does not improve γ-carboxylation of FIX when coexpressed in transfected mammalian cells [25]. These results suggest that the amount of carboxylase protein is not a limiting factor to direct vitamin-K dependent γ-carboxylation in vivo. Several possibilities exist for the inability of the over-expressed γ-carboxylase to improve factor IX carboxylation in vivo. First, the over-expressed γ-carboxylase may be mislocalized within the secretory pathway. It is possible that another protein, such as a protein

chaperone, may be required to utilize a more complex substrate such as FIX as opposed to a small peptide substrate. It is possible that another cofactor, possibly reduced vitamin K, is rate-limiting for FIX carboxylation in vivo. Further information on the mechanism of γ-carboxylation reaction in vivo is required in order to elucidate its rate-limiting step.

Recombinant FIX produced in CHO cells contains 11.8 Gla residues/mole of FIX, compared with plasma-derived FIX, which contains 12 Gla residues/mole. The difference resides in the inefficient carboxylation of residues 36 and 40 within recombinant FIX [27]. In contrast to the first 10 Gla residues in FIX, glutamic acid residues 36 and 40 are not conserved in the other vitamin K-dependent coagulation factors. To date, no functional difference is observed between fully carboxylated FIX and FIX deficient in Gla at residues 36 and 40.

Beta-hydroxylation of aspartic acid and asparagine

Blood coagulation factors IX and X, protein C, and protein S contain the modified amino acid erythro-β-hydroxyaspartic acid in the first EGF domain. In addition, one molecule of β-hydroxyasparagine is found in each of the three carboxy-terminal EGF domains in protein S. Hydroxylation of both aspartic acid and asparagine is catalyzed by aspartyl β-hydroxylase, requires 2-ketoglutarate and Fe^{2+}, and is inhibited by agents that inhibit 2-ketoglutarate-dependent dioxygenases. β-Hydroxylation is unnecessary for high-affinity calcium binding to the first EGF domain [28]. In addition, inhibition of β-hydroxylation of FIX expressed in mammalian cells does not reduce functional activity in FIX [29]. It is interesting that only 0.3 moles/mole of plasma FIX is modified by β-hydroxylation at Asp64 and this same amount of β-hydroxylation occurs in recombinant FIX expressed at high levels in CHO cells [29].

Tyrosine sulfation

Sulfate addition to tyrosine as an O^4-sulfate ester is a common post-translational modification of secretory proteins. The processing occurs in the trans-Golgi apparatus and is mediated by tyrosylprotein sulfotransferase, which utilizes the activated sulfate donor 3′-phosphoadenosine 5′-phosphosulfate (PAPS). This modification occurs on many secretory proteins, including a number of proteins that interact with thrombin, such as hirudin, fibrinogen, heparin cofactor II, α_2-antiplasmin, vitronectin, and bovine FX. In addition, both FV and FVIII contain multiple sites of tyrosine sulfation [30–32]. Tyrosine sulfation can modulate the biological activity, binding affinities, and secretion of specific proteins. For example, tyrosine sulfation at the carboxy terminus of hirudin increases its binding affinity to the anion-binding exosite of thrombin [33].

Recombinant FVIII contains six sites of tyrosine sulfation at residues 346, 718, 719, 723, 1664, and 1680 [30]. All sites are sulfated to near completion, so it does not appear that this modification is inefficient in CHO cells. Site-directed mutagenesis that changes individual or multiple tyrosine residues to the conserved residue phenylalanine allows identification of their role in FVIII function. Tyrosine sulfation at all six sites is required for full FVIII activity. In addition, mutagenesis of Tyr1680 to Phe demonstrates that sulfation at that residue is required for high-affinity interaction with VWF [32,34]. In the absence of tyrosine sulfation at 1680 in FVIII, the affinity for VWF is reduced fivefold. In contrast, mutation at residue Tyr1664 does not affect VWF interaction. The significance of the Tyr1680 sulfation *in vivo* is made evident by the presence of a Tyr1680 → Phe mutation that causes a moderate hemophilia A, likely due to reduced interaction with VWF and decreased plasma half-life [35]. The other sites of tyrosine sulfation within FVIII affect the rate of cleavage by thrombin at the adjacent thrombin cleavage site. It has been suggested that thrombin selectively utilizes the tyrosine sulfate residues adjacent to cleavage sites in factors V and VIII to facilitate interaction and/or cleavage.

Plasma-derived and recombinant-derived FIX are sulfated on Tyr155. Whereas plasma-derived FIX is mostly sulfated, recombinant factor IX is approximately 15% sulfated [11,15]. This is one unusual example in which a sulfated tyrosine occurs adjacent to an occupied N-linked glycosylation site (at asparagine residue 157). Plasma-derived FIX and recombinant FIX differ in their *in vivo* recovery, in that the absolute recovery of plasma-derived FIX is approximately 50% and the recovery of recombinant FIX is approximately 30%. Studies suggest that Tyr sulfation on FIX may be responsible for the difference in the recovery of these two sources of FIX [15]. For example, infusion of recombinant FIX enriched for full sulfation at Tyr155 demonstrates an equivalent recovery to plasma-derived factor IX (approximately 50%). Similarly, removal of the sulfate as well as phosphate from plasma-derived FIX results in a molecule having a recovery similar to recombinant FIX. Finally, administration of recombinant FIX to dogs with hemophilia B and isolation of the circulating FIX yields species that are enriched with tyrosine sulfate compared with the starting material. The sum of these observations suggests that Tyr sulfation at 155 in FIX can influence *in vivo* recovery.

Phosphorylation of serine and threonine residues

Phosphate has been observed in factors V, VIII, and IX, although its significance remains unknown. Plasma-derived FIX is fully phosphorylated at Ser158, whereas recombinant FIX contains no phosphate at this position [15]. The presence or absence of phosphate or sulfate on FIX has no effect on the *in vitro* clotting activity.

Exposure of factors V and VIII to activated platelets results in phosphorylation of serine residues in FV and primarily threonine residues in FVIII [36]. Phosphorylation can occur within both the heavy chains and light chains of FVa and FVIII, possibly within the acid-rich regions. Although the kinase responsible for the phosphorylation remains unknown, it may be related to casein kinase II. Partially phosphorylated FVa is more sensitive to activated protein C (APC) inactivation, suggesting that phosphorylation of these cofactors may downregulate their activity.

Proteolytic processing

The requirement for propeptide processing for FIX function was first made apparent by identification of mutations resulting in hemophilia B that prevent processing of the FIX propeptide. Mutations of the arginine at the P1 or P4 positions inhibit propeptide cleavage and the resultant FIX is secreted into the plasma but is nonfunctional owing to the presence of the propeptide [37,38]. This mutant is unable to bind phospholipid vesicles and may also display reduced γ-carboxylation of glutamic acid residues [38]. It is likely that the presence of the propeptide yields a molecule that is defective in phospholipid interaction owing to an inability to undergo a calcium-dependent conformation in the Gla domain.

Characterization of the amino acid requirements around the propeptide cleavage site indicates that both the P1 and P4 arginine are important for efficient processing mediated by furin/PACE (paired basic amino acid-cleaving enzyme) and/or PACE4 [39,40]. Overexpression of furin in transfected cells as well as in transgenic animals improves the processing ability to yield fully processed proteins [26,41]. Recombinant FIX is produced by coexpression with furin/PACE to ensure complete processing of the propeptide.

Similar to FIX, FVIII proteolytic processing within the B domain after arginine residues 1313 and 1648 can saturate the proteolytic machinery of the cell. Both arginine residues at 1313 and 1648 have consensus sites for furin cleavage. In this case, secretion of heavy chains that extend to residue 1648 and secretion of light chains that extend to 1313 can be detected. In addition, some single-chain FVIII is detected in conditioned medium from transfected mammalian cells and in heparin-treated human plasma [6,42]. However, all analyses to date indicate that these partially processed products of FVIII have identical activity to fully processed FVIII. For example, double mutation of Arg1313 → Ile and Arg1648 → Ile yields a single-chain FVIII molecule with functional activity similar to wild-type FVIII [19].

Summary

Eukaryotic cells contain an extensive machinery to modify polypeptides that transit the secretory compartment. In the case of coagulation factors VIII and IX, a large number of posttranslational modifications occur; many are required for secretion of the polypeptide and others are required for functional activity of the polypeptide. For FIX, cotranslational translocation into the lumen of the ER occurs concomitantly with signal peptide cleavage and addition of core high-mannose oligosaccharides to the polypeptide. In the ER, glucose trimming of the N-linked oligosaccharide core structures, γ-carboxylation of 12 amino-terminal glutamic acid residues, and β-hydroxylation of a portion of molecules on residue Asp64 occurs. Upon transit into the Golgi compartment, additional modifications occur, including (i) complex modification of N-linked oligosaccharides; (ii) tyrosine sulfation at Tyr155; (iii) Ser/Thr glycosylation at residues Ser61 and Ser53 as well as several Thr residues within the activation peptide; and (iv) cleavage of the propeptide. In addition, FIX isolated from human plasma is phosphorylated at Ser158 within the activation peptide. A majority of the modifications within FIX occur within the activation peptide and may regulate activation of FIX. Appropriate γ-carboxylation and propeptide cleavage are essential for functional secretion and activity of secreted FIX. Both of these activities are easily saturated upon expression of FIX in heterologous cells. The large number of other modifications likely also affects FIX activity by mechanisms that are not yet understood.

In the case of FVIII, the primary translation product is also modified by signal peptide cleavage and core high-mannose oligosaccharide addition upon translocation into the lumen of the ER. Within the ER, FVIII requires trimming of glucose residues on the core N-linked glycans for transport to the Golgi compartment. In the Golgi compartment, additional modifications occur, including (i) tyrosine sulfation of six residues that are required for efficient activation by thrombin and for high-affinity VWF interaction; (ii) extensive addition of oligosaccharides to many Ser/Thr residues within the B domain; (iii) complex modification of N-linked glycans; and (iv) cleavage of single-chain factor VIII to its heavy and light chain species. To date, there do not appear to be any specific post-translational modifications that significantly limit secretion and/or functional activity of FVIII compared with the essential processes of γ-carboxylation and propeptide cleavage in FIX. Further studies are required to elucidate the effect of factor VIII and FIX expression in different cell types in order to identify the importance that subtle differences in post-translational modifications may have on their secretion, *in vivo* half-life, and function. These considerations will be important when considering different cells and tissues as targets for gene therapy.

References

1 Davie EW. Biochemical and molecular aspects of the coagulation cascade. *Thromb Haemost* 1995; **74**: 1–6.

2 Toole JJ, Knopf JL, Wozney JM, *et al.* Molecular cloning of a cDNA encoding human antihemophilic factor. *Nature* 1984; **312**: 342–7.

3 Bihoreau N, Pin S, de Kersabiec AM, *et al.* Copper-atom identification in the active and inactive forms of plasma-derived FVIII and recombinant FVIII-delta II. *Eur J Biochem* 1994; **222**: 41–8.

4 Tagliavacca L, Moon N, Dunham WR, Kaufman RJ. Identification and functional requirement of Cu(II) and its ligands within coagulation factor VIII. *J Biol Chem* 1997; **272**: 27428–34.

5 Weiss HJ, Sussman II Hoyer LW. Stabilization of factor VIII in plasma by the von Willebrand factor. Studies on posttransfusion and dissociated factor VIII and in patients with von Willebrand's disease. *J Clin Invest* 1977; **60**: 390–404.

6 Kaufman RJ, Wasley LC, Dorner AJ. Synthesis, processing, and secretion of recombinant human factor VIII expressed in mammalian cells. *J Biol Chem* 1988; **263**: 6352–62.

7 Eaton D, Rodriguez H, Vehar GA. Proteolytic processing of human factor VIII. Correlation of specific cleavages by thrombin, factor Xa, and activated protein C with activation and inactivation of factor VIII coagulant activity. *Biochemistry* 1986; **25**: 505–12.

8 Lollar P, Parker CG. Subunit structure of thrombin-activated porcine factor VIII. *Biochemistry* 1987; **28**: 666–74.

9 Fay PJ, Haidaris PJ, Smudzin TM. Human factor VIII$_a$ subunit structure. *J Biol Chem* 1991; **266**: 8957–62.

10 McMullen BA, Fujikawa K, Davie EW, *et al.* Locations of disulfide bonds and free cysteines in the heavy and light chains of recombinant human factor VIII (antihemophilic factor A). *Protein Sci* 1995; **4**: 740–6.

11 White GC, Beebe A, Nielsen B. Recombinant factor IX. *Thromb Haemost* 1997; **78**: 261–5.

12 Bond MD, Huberty MC, Jankowski MA, *et al.* Identification of O-glycosylation, sulfation and phosphorylation sites in the activation peptide of human plasma factor IX. *Blood* 1994; **84**: 531a.

13 Hase S, Nishimura H, Kawabata S, *et al.* The structure of (xylose)2glucose-O-serine 53 found in the first epidermal growth factor-like domain of bovine blood clotting factor IX. *J Biol Chem* 1990; **265**: 1858–61.

14 Harris RJ, van Halbeek H, Glushka J, *et al.* Identification and structural analysis of the tetrasaccharide NeuAc alpha(2–6)Gal beta(1–4)GlcNAc beta(1–3)Fuc alpha 1–O-linked to serine 61 of human factor IX. *Biochemistry* 1993; **32**: 6539–47.

15 Bond MD, Jankowski MA, Huberty MC, *et al.* Structural analysis of recombinant human factor IX. *Blood* 1994; **84**: 194a.

16 Brandstetter H, Bauer M, Huber R, *et al.* X-ray structure of clotting factor IXa: active site and module structure related to Xase activity and hemophilia B. *Proc Natl Acad Sci USA* 1995; **92**: 9796–800.

17 Kaufman RJ, Wasley LC, Dorner AJ. Synthesis processing and secretion of factor VIII expressed in mammalian cells. *J Biol Chem* 1988; **263**: 6352–62.

18 Hironaka T, Furukawa K, Esmon PC, *et al.* Comparative study of the sugar chains of factor VIII purified from human plasma and from the culture media of recombinant baby hamster kidney cells. *J Biol Chem* 1992; **267**: 8012–20.

19 Pittman DD, Tomkinson KN, Kaufman RJ. Post-translational requirements for functional factor V and factor VIII secretion in mammalian cells. *J Biol Chem* 1994; **269**: 17329–37.

20 Moussalli M, Pipe SW, Hauri HP, *et al.* Mannose-dependent endoplasmic reticulum (ER)-Golgi intermediate compartment-53-mediated ER to Golgi trafficking of coagulation factors V and VIII. *J Biol Chem* 1999; **274**: 32539–42.

21 Cunningham MA, Pipe SW, Zhang B, *et al.* LMAN1 is a molecular chaperone for the secretion of coagulation factor VIII. *J Thromb Haemost* 2003; **1**: 2360–7.

22 Nichols WC, Seligsohn U, Zivelin A, *et al.* Mutations in the ER-Golgi intermediate compartment protein ERGIC-53 cause combined deficiency of coagulation factors V and VIII. *Cell* 1998; **93**: 61–70.

23 Zhang B, Cunningham MA, Nicols WC, *et al.* Bleeding due to disruption of a cargo-specific ER-to-golgi transport complex. *Nat Gen* 2003; **34**: 220–25.

24 Wasley LC, Rehemtulla A, Bristol JA, Kaufman RJ. PACE/furin processes the vitamin K-dependent pro-factor IX precursor within the secretory pathway. *J Biol Chem* 1993; **268**: 8458–65.

25 Kaufman RJ, Wasley LC, Furie BC, *et al.* Expression, purification, and characterization of recombinant gamma-carboxylated factor IX synthesized in Chinese hamster ovary cells. *J Biol Chem* 1986; **261**: 9622–8.

26 Rehemtulla A, Roth DA, Wasley LC, *et al.* In vitro and in vivo functional characterization of bovine vitamin K-dependent gamma-carboxylase expressed in Chinese hamster ovary cells. *Proc Natl Acad Sci USA* 1993; **90**: 4611–15.

27 Gillis S, Furie BC, Furie B, *et al.* gamma-Carboxyglutamic acids 36 and 40 do not contribute to human factor IX function. *Protein Sci* 1997; **6**: 185–96.

28 Sunnerhagen MS, Persson E, Dahlqvist I, *et al.* The effect of aspartate hydroxylation on calcium binding to epidermal growth factor-like modules in coagulation factors IX and X. *J Biol Chem* 1993; **268**: 23339–44.

29 Derian CK, VanDusen W, Przysiecki CT, *et al.* Inhibitors of 2-ketoglutarate-dependent dioxygenase block aspartyl beta-hydroxylation of recombinant human factor IX in several mammalian expression systems. *J Biol Chem* 1989; **264**: 6615–18.

30 Pittman DD, Wang JH, Kaufman RJ. Identification and functional importance of tyrosine-sulfate residues within recombinant factor VIII. *Biochemistry* 1992; **31**: 3315–23.

31 Pittman DD, Tomkinson KN, Michnick D, *et al.* Post-translational sulfation of factor V is required for efficient thrombin cleavage and activation and for full procoagulant activity. *Biochemistry* 1994; **33**: 6952–9.

32 Michnick DA, Pittman DD, Wise RJ, Kaufman RJ. Identification of individual tyrosine sulfation sites within factor VIII required for optimal activity and efficient thrombin cleavage. *J Biol Chem* 1994; **269**: 20095–102.

33 Rydel TJ, Ravichandran KG, Tulinsky A, *et al.* The structure of a complex of recombinant hirudin and human alpha- thrombin. *Science* 1990; **249**: 277–80.

34 Leyte A, van Schijndel HB, Niehrs C, *et al.* Sulfation of Tyr 1680 of human blood coagulation factor VIII is essential for the interaction of factor VIII with von Willebrand factor. *J Biol Chem* 1991; **266**: 740–6.

35 Higuchi M, Wong C, Kochhan L, *et al.* Characterization of mutations in factor VIII gene by direct sequencing of amplified genomic DNA. *Genomics* 1990; **6**: 65–71.

36 Rand MD, Kalafatis M, Mann KG. Platelet coagulation factor Va: the major secretory platelet phosphoprotein. *Blood* 1994; **83**: 2180–90.

37 Bentley AK, Rees DJ, Rizza C, Brownlee GG. Defective propeptide processing of blood clotting factor IX caused by mutation of arginine to glutamine at position -4. *Cell* 1986; **45**: 343–8.

38 Diuguid DL, Rabiet MJ, Furie BC, *et al.* Molecular basis of hemophilia B: a defective enzyme due to an unprocessed propeptide is caused by a point mutation in the factor IX precursor. *Proc Natl Acad Sci USA* 1986; **83**: 5803–7.

39 Rehemtulla A, Kaufman RJ. Preferred sequence requirements for cleavage of pro-vWF by propeptide processing enzymes. *Blood* 1992; **9**: 2349–55.

40 Rehemtulla A, Barr PJ, Rhodes CJ, Kaufman RJ. PACE4 is a member of the mammalian propeptidase family that has overlapping but not identical substrate specificity to PACE. *Biochemistry* 1993; **32**: 11586–90.

41 Drews R, Paleyanda RK, Lee TK, *et al.* Alteration of the posttranslational capacity of the mammary gland. *Proc Natl Acad Sci USA* 1995; **92**: 10462–6.

42 Ganz PR, Tackaberry ES, Palmer DS, Rock G. Human factor VIII from heparinized plasma. Purification and characterization of a single-chain form. *Eur J Biochem* 1988; **170**: 521–8.

43 Swaroop M, Moussalli M, Pipe SW, Kaufman RJ. Mutagenesis of a potential immunoglobulin-binding protein-binding site enhances secretion of coagulation factor VIII. *J Biol Chem* 1997; **272**: 24121–4.

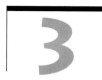

Work-up of a bleeding adult

Barry White and Clodagh Ryan

The assessment of a bleeding patient requires a detailed medical history, physical examination, and appropriate laboratory investigations.

The clinical history

Bleeding disorders can present with a range of clinical symptoms, including easy bruising, mucosal and musculoskeletal bleeding, and excessive blood loss following trauma or surgery. An accurate medical history to assess bleeding disorders can be difficult. It is influenced by differences in exposure to hemostatic challenges, a patient's perception of his or her bleeding tendency, and ability to recall distant events. Surveys of healthy control subjects report excessive nosebleeds in 5–39%, gingival bleeding in 7–51%, bruising in 12–24%, bleeding after dental extraction in 1–13%, postoperative bleeding in 1.4–6%, and menorrhagia in 23–44% [1,2,3].

Easy bruising and skin bleeding

A history of easy bruising commonly attracts attention, but it is often not associated with a bleeding disorder. Purpura simplex or simple easy bruising is commonly seen in females, usually confined to the limbs, and may be associated with menses. Senile purpura, due to the decreased elasticity of blood vessels and subcutaneous fat, is seen in older individuals. Psychogenic purpura is characterized by repeated bruising, especially in areas easily accessible to the patient, and may be quite extensive and slow to resolve. Other conditions associated with bruising are Cushing syndrome and amyloidosis [4].

Bleeding disorders may also present with easy or spontaneous bruising. Multiple bruises, especially larger than 2–3 cm or occurring spontaneously or in unusual sites such as the trunk, should alert the clinician to the possibility of an underlying hemostatic disorder. Patients should also be questioned about prolonged bleeding (greater than 15 min) from superficial cuts, particularly if it required medical attention. Vascular and platelet abnormalities cause immediate bleeding while delayed bleeding or rebleeding is more classically associated with a coagulation factor deficiency. Persistent bleeding from the umbilical stump is seen in 80% of untreated neonates with factor XIII deficiency [5].

Mucosal bleeding

Mucosal bleeding, such as epistaxis, gingival bleeding, and menorrhagia, is common in the general population, and careful questioning is required to determine if it is pathological. Epistaxis is common, particularly in children, with a reported incidence of 5–39% in healthy control subjects [1,2]. However, epistaxis occurring more frequently with age rather than resolving, or requiring medical intervention, such as packing or cauterization, in the absence of a local anatomic abnormality, suggests an underlying bleeding disorder. Spontaneous gingival bleeding, in the absence of poor dental hygiene, is seen in primary hemostatic disorders, particularly thrombocytopenia.

Menorrhagia accounts for 12% of all gynecology referrals [6]. It may be due to local or systemic disorders, but a specific cause is identified in less than 50% of women [7]. Recent studies suggest that 10–15% of patients with unexplained menorrhagia have an inherited bleeding disorder [8]. The presence of menorrhagia, especially dating from menarche, occurs in 60% of patients with von Willebrand's disease (VWD), and 8% of these patients require surgical intervention to control the bleeding [9,10].

The subjective diagnosis of menorrhagia is often inaccurate, and the need for objective measurements of menstrual blood loss is well documented [11,12]. The presence of flooding, excessive menstrual blood loss since menarche, or iron deficiency anemia despite adequate iron supplementation, or the need for surgical intervention to control bleeding are all consistent with an objective diagnosis of menorrhagia and may be indicative of an underlying bleeding disorder. Menorrhagia is defined as menstrual loss in excess of 80 mL per cycle and the gold standard for its assessment involves the measurement of menstrual loss using the alkaline hematin method. However, this method is time-consuming, involves specialized laboratory techniques and is inconvenient for the patient. The pictorial blood assessment chart (PBAC), with a score of more than 100 taken as equivalent to a menstrual loss of more than 80 mL, has a sensitivity of 86% and a specificity of 89% in comparison with the alkaline hematin method [13].

The patient's obstetric history can also be informative in the assessment of a bleeding disorder. While the majority of ante- and postpartum hemorrhages are related to obstetric complications, hemostatic disorders may also be responsible for hemorrhage, especially in the postpartum period. Factor VIII (FVIII) and von Willebrand factor (VWF) levels tend to increase from

12 weeks' gestation and frequently normalize in type 1 VWD and less commonly in type 2 VWD. However, the levels may fall precipitously after parturition, resulting in postpartum hemorrhage (PPH), particularly delayed PPH. The clinical significance of VWD during pregnancy is highlighted by the requirement for red cell concentrate (RCC) transfusion in 7% of patients at the time of parturition, particularly if the VWD is previously undiagnosed [14,15]. Severe FXIII deficiency and hereditary dysfibrinogenemis are associated with recurrent miscarriages, in addition to excess bleeding. Acquired inhibitors to FVIII may occasionally complicate pregnancy and are characterized by extensive soft-tissue bleeding [16].

Bleeding following trauma or surgery

Inherited or acquired bleeding disorders may present with unexplained excessive bleeding at the time of dental extractions, surgery, or trauma. The loss of deciduous teeth and dental extractions, particularly of molars and premolars, are often the first hemostatic challenges experienced by patients. The clinical history should seek to determine the severity and duration of bleeding following dental extractions and the need to return to the dentist for packing, resuturing, or packed red blood cell (PRBC) transfusion. Similarly, the severity and duration of bleeding post surgery or trauma, and the requirement for PRBC transfusion or need to return to the operating theater to stop the bleeding should also be assessed. FXIII deficiency, Ehlers–Danlos syndrome and disorders of fibrinogen are associated with both delayed wound healing and excess bleeding. The absence of excessive bleeding at the time of dental extractions, surgery, or trauma, particularly if the patient has experienced repeated hemostatic challenges, makes the diagnosis of an underlying inherited bleeding disorder unlikely.

Spontaneous bleeding

A history of spontaneous bleeding, especially involving the central nervous or musculoskeletal system, always warrants further investigation. Spontaneous hemarthrosis and intramuscular hematomas are characteristic of severe deficiencies of factors I, VIII, IX, X, and XIII and VWF. Patients with acquired antibodies to FVIII frequently develop extensive soft-tissue bleeding.

Systemic illnesses causing or exacerbating bleeding disorders

A variety of systemic disorders may result in bleeding complications. Uremia impairs platelet function, and end-stage liver disease is associated with a range of hemostatic abnormalities, including thrombocytopenia, coagulation factor deficiencies, and hyperfibrinolysis. Acquired inhibitors to coagulation factors and VWF may be seen in autoimmune disorders and malignancies. Bone marrow failure can present with bleeding due to thrombocytopenia. Disseminated intravascular coagulation (DIC) is most frequently associated with sepsis and may cause

Table 3.1 Conditions that can cause disseminated intravascular coagulation.

Infections
Bacteria
Viruses
Fungi
Protozoa
Neoplasia
Solid tumors
Leukemia, particularly acute promyelocytic leukemia
Obstetric complications
Abruptio placentae
Amniotic fluid embolism
Toxemia of pregnancy
Retained dead fetus syndrome
Tissue damage
Trauma (in particular, CNS injury)
Crush injuries
Hemolytic transfusion reaction
Rhabdomyolysis
Miscellaneous
Shock
Giant hemangioma (Kasabach–Merritt syndrome)
Aortic aneurysm
Near drowning

bleeding due to thrombocytopenia, hypofibrinoginemia, or other coagulation factor deficiencies (Table 3.1). Amyloidosis has been associated with bleeding secondary to defective primary hemostasis due to amyloid deposition in vessels, and acquired factor X (FX) deficiency caused by adsorption of the FX protein by amyloid fibrils [4]. IgM paraproteinemias may cause bleeding complications due to either bone marrow failure or paraprotein-induced defective fibrin polymerization.

Medications

A detailed drug history must always be obtained, asking about use of both prescription and nonprescription medications. Anticoagulants such as warfarin, heparin, and thrombolytic agents, and anti-platelet agents are associated with a clearly defined bleeding risk. Antibiotics may result in decreased synthesis of vitamin K-dependent factors, owing to an overgrowth of gut flora with resultant decrease in vitamin K absorption. A wide range of medications have been implicated in the development of immune-mediated thrombocytopenia. Homeopathic medication should be closely examined as certain agents, such as Chinese black tree fungus, can cause qualitative platelet abnormalities [17].

Table 3.2 Congenital bleeding disorders.

Autosomal dominant disorders
von Willebrand disease
May–Hegglin anomaly

Autosomal recessive disorders
Bernard–Soulier syndrome
Glanzmann's thromboesthenia
Gray platelet syndrome
Deficiencies of factor V, VII, X, XI, XIII
Type 3 von Willebrand disease

Sex-linked recessive disorders
Factor VIII deficiency
Factor IX deficiency
Wiskott–Aldrich syndrome

Table 3.3 Causes of thrombocytopenia.

Congenital thrombocytopenia

Inherited thrombocytopenia
  Bernard–Soulier syndrome
  Wiskott–Aldrich syndrome
  May–Hegglin anomaly
  von Willebrand's disease
  Gray platelet syndrome
  Alport syndrome

Maternal factors
  Maternal autoimmune thrombocytopenia
  Neonatal alloimmune thrombocytopenia
  Intrauterine infections

Acquired thrombocytopenia

Decreased production
  Bone marrow failure or infiltration
  Megaloblastic anemia

Decreased lifespan
  Idiopathic autoimmune thrombocytopenia
  Drug-induced thrombocytopenia
  Autoimmune disease
  Infections, including HIV
  Post transfusion
  Disseminated intravascular coagulation
  Microangiopathic anemia

Hypersplenism

Family history

Inherited coagulation factor deficiencies and certain qualitative platelet disorders follow distinct inheritance patterns, as outlined in Table 3.2. The more severe disorders, such as severe hemophilia (FVIII or FIX deficiency), usually present in the first few years of life. However, milder bleeding disorders may not present until later in life after exposure to a hemostatic challenge. While a family history is important, its usefulness is frequently compromised by the lack of accurate clinical details in family members and the fact that a spontaneous mutation is responsible for hemophilia in one-third of patients.

Clinical examination

The pattern of bruising, along with the characteristics of the lesions, can help differentiate certain conditions, as outlined previously. Cutaneous and mucosal petechiae are typically seen with thrombocytopenia, when the platelet count is less than 10×10^9/L. Cutaneous telangiectasia is seen with increasing age, liver disease, estrogen therapy and vasculitic syndromes, while mucosal and visceral telangiectasia is characteristic of Osler–Weber–Rendu syndrome (hereditary hemorrhagic telangiectasia).

Ehlers–Danlos syndrome is characterized by tissue-paper skin and hyperextensible joints, while platelet storage pool defects such as Chediak–Higashi syndrome and Hermansky–Pudlak syndrome are associated with oculocutaneous albinism. Eczema is frequently seen in patients with Wiskott–Aldrich syndrome. Spontaneous hemarthrosis is usually confined to patients with severe coagulation factor deficiencies, and these patients may present acutely with a swollen, painful joint or have the characteristic changes of hemophilic arthropathy secondary to recurrent bleeds.

Laboratory assessment of a bleeding patient

The laboratory investigations involve a two-step process, beginning with initial screening tests and followed by more specific investigations as indicated. The initial tests should include a complete blood count (CBC) and peripheral blood smear, prothrombin time, activated partial thromboplastin time, thrombin clotting time, fibrinogen, platelet function tests and von Willebrand's screen. Subsequent investigations will depend on the initial investigations and/or the clinical history (e.g., unexplained bleeding from the umbilical stump raises the possibility of FXIII deficiency). The investigation of a patient with a family history of a bleeding disorder will be directed by the nature of the bleeding disorder within the family.

Full blood count and blood film

An automated CBC, along with examination of the peripheral blood smear (to maintain consistency), is essential. One can readily identify quantitative abnormalities, with thrombocytopenia defined as a platelet count less than 150×10^9/L. The causes of thrombocytopenia are outlined in Table 3.3. It is important to ensure that this is not a spurious result caused by blood clots in the sample or platelet agglutination.

Pseudothrombocytopenia, caused by platelet clumping, is observed in 1 in 1000 subjects [18] and is due to an autoantibody to a neoepitope on glycoprotein IIb/IIIa, exposed by the EDTA (ethylenediaminetetraacetic acid) anticoagulant used for routine full blood counts [19]. It is not clinically significant and careful examination of the blood film demonstrates platelet clumping. Many inherited thrombocytopathies have characteristic findings on examination of the blood film. Giant platelets are seen in Bernard–Soulier and gray platelet syndromes, Döhle-like bodies are usually seen in granulocytes in the May–Hegglin anomaly, and microthrombocytes are seen in Wiskott–Aldrich syndrome. While these findings are not unique to these conditions, when correlated with the clinical history and examination, they help guide the clinician in further investigations.

Prothrombin time

The prothrombin time (PT) evaluates the overall efficiency of the coagulation factors of the common and extrinsic pathways — factors V, VII, X, prothrombin and fibrinogen [20]. It will therefore be prolonged with an inherited or acquired deficiency of one or more of these factors. Acquired deficiencies are caused by oral anticoagulation, liver disease, vitamin K deficiency and DIC. The PT may also be prolonged by the development of an inhibitor directed against the clotting factors or a component of the PT reaction.

The test measures the clotting time of plasma following the addition of tissue factor (thromboplastin) and calcium to hypocalcemic plasma. The tissue factor activates FX in the presence of FVII, thereby activating the extrinsic system. The concentration and properties of the thromboplastin and the type of instrumentation influence the result. The PT of normal plasma is usually 12–15 s, but each laboratory must determine its own reference range, using its own method, reagent, and instrument. Each thromboplastin preparation has a different sensitivity to coagulation factor deficiencies and defects, in particular the defect caused by oral anticoagulation. The sensitivity is quantified by its unique international sensitivity index (ISI), which is derived by comparing its prothombotic potential against a standard with an ISI of 1.0. The higher the ISI, the less sensitive the reagent is to deficiencies of vitamin-K dependent factors. The international normalized ratio (INR) was developed to allow monitoring of anticoagulation with warfarin and reduce interlaboratory variability. The INR is calculated as a ratio of the patient's PT to the geometric mean of normal control subjects, which is then raised to the ISI as an exponential power.

The relationship between the PT and the degree of factor deficiency is not linear as the PT prolongs exponentially at lower factor concentrations.

Activated partial thromboplastin time

The activated partial thromboplastin time (aPPT) evaluates the efficiency of the common and intrinsic coagulation pathway — factors VIII, IX, X, XI, XII, and V, prothrombin, fibrinogen, and the contact factors kallikrein and high-molecular-weight kinogen. The aPTT will be prolonged with a deficiency of any of these factors, which may be inherited or acquired, as in disseminated intravascular anticoagulation. A prolonged aPTT is also seen in the presence of an inhibitor directed against any of these clotting factors or a component of the aPTT reaction, such as a lupus anticoagulant.

The aPTT measures the clotting time of plasma following the activation of contact factors without added tissue thromboplastin. A number of aPPT reagents are available, and their concentration and properties, along with different instrumentation used, all contribute to interlaboratory variability. A reference range must be established for each laboratory based on the reagent, method, and instrumentation used in that laboratory. When choosing a reagent for the aPTT, it is important to establish that the activator–phospholipid combination is sensitive to deficiencies of factors VIII:C, IX, and XI at concentrations of 0.35–0.4 IU/mL, as reagents that fail to detect reductions of this degree are too insensitive for routine use [21].

The prolongation of the aPTT is significantly enhanced by deficiencies of contact factors kallikrein and high-molecular-weight kinogen using a shortened incubation time. Factor XII deficiency also causes a prolonged aPTT but is not associated with a bleeding tendency.

Correction studies

Correction studies, also known as "mixing" studies, are useful in the investigation of unexplained prolongation of the PT or aPTT. When the patient's plasma is mixed with normal plasma, a correction suggests a factor deficiency, while a failure to correct suggests the presence of an inhibitor. The optimum calculation for assessing correction has not been universally determined. However, if the prolongation is due to a deficiency of a clotting factor, the PT or aPTT of the mixture should result in a correction of at least 50% [21].

Thrombin clotting time

The thrombin clotting time (TCT) [also known as the thrombin time (TT)] measures the clotting time of citrated plasma following the addition of exogenous thrombin. It reflects the action of thrombin on fibrinogen with the formation of fibrin and is influenced by the inhibitory factors such as fibrin degradation products and heparin. The TCT will be prolonged in inherited or acquired defects of fibrinogen, which can be quantitative or qualitative. It may also be prolonged by heparin, paraproteinemias, and hypoalbuminemia.

Heparin causes a prolonged TCT and this is commonly seen in clinical practice when blood is procured from an indwelling heparinized intravenous line. Reptilase is not inhibited by heparin. Therefore, the reptilase time (which uses reptilase instead of thrombin) will be within normal limits if the prolonged TCT is caused by heparin.

Fibrinogen

In defects of fibrinogen, there is usually prolongation of PT, aPTT, and TCT. There are a number of methods available to measure fibrinogen. Qualitative fibrinogen levels should be measured by determining the amount of clottable fibrinogen, using a functional assay, and the amount of fibrinogen protein as determined by immunological methods [22]. In afibrinogenemia, there is decreased or absent fibrinogen activity and antigen (type I), while dysfibrinogenemia is characterized by decreased fibrinogen activity and normal or moderately reduced antigen level (type II).

Bleeding time

The bleeding time is defined as the time taken for a standardized skin incision to stop bleeding and is designed to measure primary hemostasis. It is influenced by platelet number and function, VWF, and the constriction of the microvasculature. However, the reproducibility of the bleeding time is impaired by a number of operator-dependent factors, such as the depth of the puncture wound and the length of the incision, and it has a sensitivity of less than 60% for VWD [23].

Platelet function tests and the PFA 100

Investigations to assess platelet function include platelet aggregation studies, immunophenotyping, assessment of platelet nucleotides, and electron microscopy. The principle of the aggregometry test is that the light absorbance of platelet-rich plasma falls as platelets aggregate. The pattern of aggregation is assessed in response to the addition of various agonists at different concentrations. The agonists used routinely include collagen, adenosine diphosphate (ADP), arachidonic acid, ristocetin, and epinephrine, and result in characteristic patterns in various platelet disorders.

The PFA 100 (Dade Behring) is an *in vitro* system for measuring platelet-VWF function. Studies have shown this system to be sensitive to platelet adherence and aggregation abnormalities, and it is dependent on normal VWF, glycoprotein Ib and glycoprotein IIb/IIIa but not on plasma fibrinogen or fibrin generation. The PFA-100 system may reflect VWF function better than the bleeding time but it is not sensitive to vascular collagen disorders [23]. Furthermore, the utility of the PFA-100 as a screening test is limited by the fact that it may be normal in patients with VWD and platelet function defects [24].

Diagnosis of von Willebrand disease

Investigations required to diagnose von Willebrand disease include VWF antigen, VWF functional activity (ristocetin cofactor), factor VIII:C, RIPA (ristocetin-induced platelet aggregation) and multimeric analysis. Plasma VWF antigen levels are usually measured by ELISA (enzyme-linked immuno-

Table 3.4 Current classification of von Willebrand disease.

Type	Description
1	Partial quantitative deficiency of VWF
2	Qualitative deficiency of VWF
2A	Decreased platelet-dependent VWF function with lack of HMWM
2B	Increased affinity for platelet GPIb
2M	Decreased platelet-dependent VWF function with normal multimeric analysis
2N	Decreased VWF affinity for FVIII
3	Complete deficiency of VWF

VWF, von Willebrand factor; HMWM, high-molecular-weight multimers; FVIII, factor VIII.

sorbent assay) assays. The VWF ristocetin cofactor is the standard functional assay and measures the ability of VWF to bind glycoprotein Ib in the presence of ristocetin. Alternative functional assays for VWF include an ELISA and collagen-binding assay. However, these assays, especially the ELISA, may be normal in some patients with type 2 VWD. Patients with type 2B VWD have increased sensitivity to ristocetin-induced platelet aggregation (Table 3.4). Environmental factors such as age, menstruation, estrogen therapy, and stress all increase VWF levels and should be considered in the interpretation of the results. The baseline variation in VWF may necessitate repeated testing before a diagnosis can be made. The mean VWF levels in blood group O individuals are 25–30% lower than those in non-O individuals. However, there is no clear evidence that blood group specific ranges improve the ability to predict the risk of bleeding [25].

Further investigations

As outlined above, the screening tests usually dictate the subsequent direction of more specialized investigations. Specific clotting factor assays are available to clarify the diagnosis further, and allow the appropriate management of the patient with a bleeding history. One-stage bioassays are usually employed to measure the clotting factors of the intrinsic and extrinsic pathways.

The general principle of the one-stage bioassay is that if a test sample and reference are assayed in a range of dilutions, and the clotting times are plotted against the plasma concentration on double log paper; the result, in the absence of an inhibitor, will generate two parallel straight lines. The horizontal distance between the two lines represents the difference in potency of the factor assayed. If the test line is to the right of the standard, it contains less of the factor than the standard; if it is to the left it contains more [21].

Functional FVII activity is frequently measured using a one-stage prothrombin-based assay. However, the source of thromboplastin can have a significant effect upon the FVII functional assays, and for these reasons a series of different thromboplastins are often used when investigating patients with suspected FVII deficiency [26].

The diagnosis of platelet storage pool disorders requires the measurement of platelet nucleotides or an assessment of dense body function. Assays based on firefly bioluminescence are used to measure platelet nucleotides. The enzyme luciferase produces light proportional to the concentration of adenosine triphosphate (ATP), and the light can be quantified in a luminometer. The ADP can be measured indirectly by conversion to ATP. Alternatively, the total platelet ATP and ADP may be measured by high-performance liquid chromatography. In storage pool disorders, the ratio of ATP to ADP is 8:1 rather than 2:1, owing to the loss of ADP in the storage granules.

The diagnosis of Glanzmann's thrombasthenia (GpIIb/IIIa deficiency), and Bernard–Soulier syndrome (GpIb deficiency) can be confirmed by immunophenotyping using monoclonal antibodies specific to glycoprotein complexes IIb/IIIa and Ib respectively.

Factor XIII (FXIII) does not cause prolongation of PT, aPTT or TT. FXIII levels should be measured in the presence of a family history suggestive of a severe autosomal recessive bleeding disorder or a personal history of excess bleeding, especially umbilical cord bleeding or spontaneous intracranial hemorrhage in childhood.

Disorders of the fibrinolytic system may rarely be associated with excess bleeding and these include deficiencies of α_2-antiplasmin and plasminogen activator inhibitor-1 (PAI). The measurement of these factors should be considered in patients with excess bleeding, particularly if all other investigations are normal.

Conclusion

A systematic approach must be adopted when assessing a patient with a bleeding history. While the clinical setting often dictates the urgency of the investigations, a comprehensive history and examination must not be omitted, as this often provides the clinician with essential information and allows one to determine the most appropriate investigations.

References

1 Mauser Bunschoten EP, van Houweligen JC, Sjamsoedin Visser EJ, et al. Bleeding symptoms in carriers of haemophilia A and B. Thromb Haemost 1988; 59: 349–52.

2 Sramek A, Eikenboom JC, Briet E, et al. Usefulness of patient interview in bleeding disorders. Arch Intern Med 1995; 155: 1409–15.

3 Nosek-Cenkowska B, Cheang MS, Pizzi NJ, et al. Bleeding/bruising symptomatology in children with and without bleeding disorders. Thromb Haemost 1991; 65: 237–41.

4 Furie B, Voo L, McAdam K, Furie BC. Mechanisms of factor X deficiency in systemic amyloidosis. N Eng J Med 1981; 304: 827–30.

5 Anwar R, Miloszewski KJ. Factor XIII deficiency. Br J Haematol 1999; 107: 468–84.

6 Bradlow J, Coulter A, Brooks P. Patterns of Referral. Oxford: Health Services Research Unit, 1992.

7 Rees M. Menorrhagia. BMJ 1987; 294: 759–62.

8 Kadir R, Economides DL, Sabin CA, et al. Frequency of inherited bleeding disorders in women with menorrhagia. Lancet 1998; 351: 485–9.

9 Kadir R, Economides DL, Sabin CA, et al. Assessment of menstrual blood loss and gynaecological problems in patients with inherited bleeding disorders. Haemophilia 1999; 5: 40–8.

10 Kouides PA, Phatak PD, Burkart P, et al. Gynaecological and obstetrical morbidity in women with Type I von Willebrand Disease. Results of a patient survey. Haemophilia 2000; 6: 643–8.

11 Fraser IS, McCarron G, Markham R. A preliminary study of factors influencing perception of menstrual blood loss volume. Am J Obstet Gynecol 1984; 149: 788–93.

12 Haynes PJ, Hodgson H, Anderson ABM, Turnbull AC. Measurement of menstrual blood loss in patients complaining of menorrhagia. Br J Obstet Gynaecol 1977; 84: 763–8.

13 Hallberg L, Nilsson L. Determination of menstrual blood loss. Scand J Clin Lab Invest 1964; 16: 244–8.

14 Kadir RA, Lee CA, Sabin CA, et al. Pregnancy in women with von Willebrand's disease or FXI deficiency. Br J Obstet Gynaecol 1998; 105: 314–21.

15 Greer IA, Lowe GD, Walker JJ, Forbes CD. Haemorrhagic problems in obstetrics and gynaecology in patients with congenital coagulopathies. Br J Obstet Gynaecol 1991; 98: 909–18.

16 Michiels JJ. Acquired haemophilia A in women postpartum: clinical manifestations, diagnosis and treatment. Clin Appl Thromb Haemost 2000; 6: 82–6.

17 George JN, Shattil SJ. The clinical importance of acquired abnormalities of platelet function. N Engl J Med 1991; 324: 27–39.

18 Garcia Suarez J, Calero MA, Ricard MP, et al. EDTA-dependent pseudothrombocytopenia in ambulatory patients: clinical characteristics and role of new automated cell counting in its detection. Am J Haematol 1992; 39: 146–7.

19 Fiorin F, Steffan A, Pradella P, et al. IgG platelet antibodies in EDTA dependent pseudothrombocytopenia bind to platelet membrane glycoprotein Ib. Am J Clin Pathol 1998; 110: 178–83.

20 Quick AJ. Quick on Quick's test. N Engl J Med 1973; 288: 1079.

21 Laffan MA, Manning RA. Investigation of haemostasis. In: Lewis SM, Bain B, Bates I, eds. Practical Haematology, 9th edn. London: Churchill Livingstone 2001: 339–91.

22 Roberts HR, Stinchcombe T, Gabriel DA. The dysfibrinoginaemias. Br J Haematol 2001; 114: 249–57.

23 Fressinaud E, Veyradier A, Trauchaud F, et al. Screening for von Willebrand's disease with a new analyser using high shear stress: a study of 60 cases. Blood 1998; 91: 1325–33.

24 Burgess C, Credland P, Khair K, et al. An evaluation of the usefulness of the PFA-100 device in 100 children referred for investigation of potential haemostatic disorders. Haemophilia 2000; Abstract B247.

25 Nitu-Whalley IC, Lee CA, Brown SA, et al. The role of the platelet function analyser (PFA-100) in the characterisation of patients with von Willebrand's disease and its relationship with von Willebrand factor and the ABO blood group. Haemophilia 2003; 9: 298–302.

26 Poggio M, Tripodi A, Mariani G, Mannucci PM. Factor VII clotting assays: influence of different thromboplastins and factor VII deficient plasmas. Thromb Haemost 1991; 65: 160–4.

4 Molecular basis of hemophilia A

Geoffrey Kemball-Cook and Edward Tuddenham

Introduction

It is now 20 years since the factor VIII (FVIII) protein was first purified [1], leading to the subsequent cloning of the gene [2]. Detection of causative mutations in the FVIII gene (*F8*) was initially slow and laborious, but recent years have seen great advances both in the technology for detection of variations in *F8*, and in our understanding of the relationship between FVIII structure and the dysfunction of the hemophilic cofactor in coagulation. However, comprehensive mutation detection [often now performed by polymerase chain reaction (PCR) and direct sequencing of all exons] is still a considerable undertaking in many centers, and there are still many questions to answer as to how FVIIIa (the thrombin-activated form of FVIII) interacts with phospholipid membranes and promotes the activity of activated factor IX (FIXa) so enormously in the activation of factor X (FX). FVIII function is briefly described below; however, for details of current thinking on the functional aspects of FVIII, readers may look to Chapter 5 of this volume.

Structure and function of the FVIII gene (*F8*) and protein

F8 gene

The human factor VIII gene was cloned between 1982 and 1984 by Jane Gitschier and collaborators [2] and simultaneously by Toole *et al.* [3]. At the time, the gene was the largest described (186 kb), and is still one of the largest. Mapping positioned the FVIII gene in the most distal band (Xq28) of the long arm of the X chromosome [4,5]. As shown in Figure 4.1, the gene contains 26 exons, 24 of which vary in length from 69 to 262 base pairs (bp); the remaining much larger exons, 14 and 26, contain 3106 and 1958 bp respectively. However, the large majority of exon 26 is 3′ untranslated sequence, so that exon 14 bears by far the largest exonic coding sequence, largely that of the B domain (see below). The spliced FVIII mRNA is approximately 9 kb in length and predicts a precursor protein of 2351 amino acids.

Structure and function of FVIII

(For a detailed treatment of FVIII function in coagulation see Chapter 5). After removal of a secretory leader sequence, FVIII has a mature sequence of 2332 amino acids with the domain structure A1–*a1*–A2-*a2*–B–*a3*–A3–C1–C2 [6]: Figure 4.1 shows the relationship between the domains and the cDNA exons. FVIII circulates in plasma complexed noncovalently with von Willebrand factor, which acts as a plasma carrier, apparently protecting it from proteolysis and rapid clearance.

The domain structure of FVIII is very similar to that of coagulation factor V (FV) [7], although the B domains are unrelated in sequence and FV lacks the short acidic *a1*, *a2*, and *a3* sequences. The A domains of FVIII and FV are homologous to ceruloplasmin and hephaestin (which have the domain structure A1–A2–A3) [7], and homology of the FVIII and FV C domains has been noted with slime mold discoidin I [6], milk-fat globule membrane protein [8], and a receptor tyrosine kinase found in breast carcinoma cells [9]. There is no significant homology between the B domain of FVIII and any other protein sequence in the human genome; however, the B domains of FVIII and FV share the characteristic that they are large and very heavily N-glycosylated, a factor that may be crucial in their intracellular folding and processing (see Chapter 2).

Factor VIII is highly sensitive to proteolytic processing after secretion, and only a small fraction of circulating FVIII is in the single-chain form: the majority consists of heavy chains of variable length (consisting of the A1 and A2 domains together with variable lengths of B domain) linked noncovalently to light chains consisting of the A3, C1 and C2 domains [6]. Expression of active recombinant FVIII lacking the entire length of the B domain has confirmed that this domain is unnecessary for coagulation activity [10]: a cleavage after R740 (probably by thrombin) during coagulation serves to remove it.

The function of FVIII is to accelerate the activation of FX by FIXa on a suitable phospholipid surface, thus amplifying the clotting stimulus many-fold, and specific proteolytic cleavages between the domains both activate and inactivate the cofactor (see Chapter 5). It is clear that the active form (FVIIIa) consists of a heterotrimer of A1–*a1*, A2–*a2*, and A3–C1–C2 chains, and that either spontaneous dissociation of A2–*a2* or proteolysis of FVIIIa by APC results in loss of its function.

Three-dimensional structural analysis of FVIII is so far relatively limited, and there is no high-resolution structure of the protein either before or after proteolytic activation. In 1997, a homology model of the FVIII A domains was constructed, based on the crystal structure of ceruloplasmin [11], suggesting a triangular arrangement of the A domains with extensive interdomain contacts. This was combined with electron microscopy of

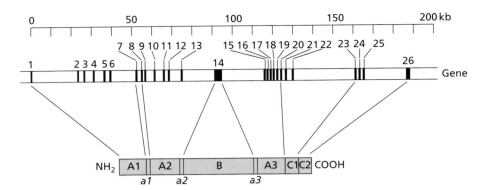

Figure 4.1 Linear representation of the *F8* gene, showing (above) the 26 exons and (below) the domain organization of the protein based on amino acid homology comparisons.

FVIII on a phospholipid (PL) monolayer to yield a low-resolution structure for the whole FVIII on a PL surface [12]. This suggested that the interaction with PL was via the C domains, while the A-domain trimer was held above the surface.

The first X-ray crystallography data were published in 1999, when a structure for the C2 domain was determined [13], suggesting that interaction between C2 and the PL surface could be mediated via insertion of hydrophobic amino acid loops. From this structure, a homology model of the FVIII C1 domain was also generated [14], and additional electron microscopy studies yielded (with these C-domain structures) a medium-resolution structure for the five domains of FVIII bound to the membrane surface. This model demonstrated that the C2 domain was indeed the membrane contact, and numerous VWF-binding regions were arranged, in a patch on one face of the FVIII molecule. A docked model of FVIII with the crystal structure of FIXa was also constructed, which satisfied many previously described biochemical criteria [15], with the A2 and A3 domains arranged so as to contact specific FVIII-binding areas in FIXa.

Notwithstanding the studies described above, the detail of how FVIIIa accelerates the action of FIXa remains to be elucidated. However, the availability of the structures and models described above has permitted the analysis of the "molecular pathology" of a number of hemophilic mutations.

F8 gene defects found in hemophilia A

F8 gene defects associated with hemophilia A may be divided for convenience into several categories: (i) gross gene rearrangements; (ii) insertions or deletions of genetic sequence of a size varying from one base pair up to the entire gene; and (iii) single DNA base substitutions resulting in either amino acid replacement ("missense"), premature peptide chain termination ("nonsense" or stop mutations) or mRNA splicing defects. These classes are described briefly below.

The online hemophilia A mutation database (europium.csc.mrc.ac.uk) now lists over 1800 individual reports of *F8* variants from all over the world, including all insertion/deletions and single-base DNA replacements, whether directly submitted to the database or derived from journal reports. All classes of defects can result in severe disease. However, the single most clinically important defect is a gene rearrangement (an inversion) involving *F8* intron 22 (see below), which results in approximately 50% of all severe disease cases worldwide. Inversions are omitted from the database as they are almost entirely identical both genetically and by phenotype, and therefore highly redundant. For full details of the other categories readers should consult the database. A summary of mutations listed in the online database is given in Table 4.1.

Gene rearrangements

As noted above, gross gene rearrangements of FVIII consist almost entirely of a unique inversion whose mechanism was described in 1993 [16,17] and which is now known to be responsible for approximately 50% of all cases of severe hemophilia A. Prior to these studies, PCR amplification of all 26 *F8* exons detected mutations in only about 50% of cases of severe hemophilia [18]. However, RT-PCR of *F8* mRNA from most of the remaining severe cases showed that no amplification was possible between exons 22 and 23, suggesting a rearrangement within the *F8* gene in this region [19].

Unusually, the intron separating exons 22 and 23 (IVS22) contains a CpG island associated with two additional transcripts, originally termed *F8A* [20] and *F8B* [21]. *F8B* is a transcript of 2.5 kb and is transcribed in the same direction as the *F8* gene, using a private exon plus *F8* exons 23–26. *F8A* is transcribed in the opposite direction to the *F8* gene: furthermore, two additional copies of *F8A* were found approximately 300 and 400 kb telomeric to the *F8* gene [20]. Thus, the large majority of the "missing" cases of severe hemophilia were explained by homologous recombination between the 9.5-kb intronic sequence (now termed *int22h-1*) and one of the two extragenic homologs of this sequence (*int22h-2* and *int22h-3*). The recombination occurs during the meiotic division of spermatogenesis, resulting in a large inversion and translocation of the gene sequence including exons 1–22 away from exons 23–26 (Figure 4.2a and b). Of these two common types of intron 22 inversion, the distal homolog is responsible for the majority of the severe hemophilia A inversion cases, while crossover with the proximal copy results in a further minority of cases [22].

Table 4.1 Summary of *F8* mutations in the online database subdivided by type. "Severe–mild" indicates that the clinical bleeding phenotype of a group of unrelated patients with this mutation ranges between these extremes.

Hemophilia A mutations (excluding inversions)		Clinical severity where known				Inhibitor status where known	
		Severe	Moderate	Mild	Severe–mild	Positive	Negative
Total individual reports (includes repeat reports)	1839						
Total unique mutations	943						
Unique point mutations	615	230	80	146	20	63	365
Missense	462	136	75	146	20	37	312
Stop	100	87	2	0	0	25	49
Splice	62	37	6	10	0	1	40
Unique insertions	57	51	3	1	0	15	28
Unique deletions	272	249	11	2	0	67	145
Small (< 50 bp)	152	141	6	2	0	24	92
Large (> 50 bp)	120	108	5	0	0	43	53

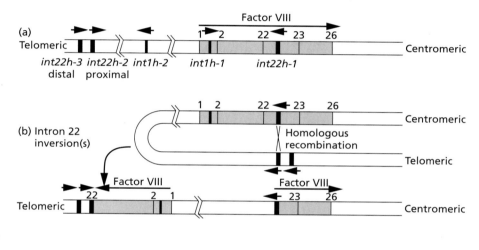

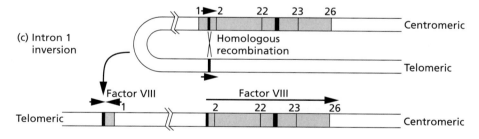

Figure 4.2 Simplified representation of the gene inversion mechanisms resulting in severe hemophilia A, involving sequences in introns 1 and 22 of the *F8* gene. Recombination between homologous sequences in intron 22 and ~400 kb telomeric to the gene leads to separation of exons 1–22 from exons 23–26, with the former sequence inverted and relocated to the site of the telomeric homologous sequence (a and b); alternatively, recombination between the intron 1 sequence and its telomeric homolog results in relocation and inversion of exon 1 (a and c).

Most laboratories now carry out initial screening for the intron 22 inversion in all cases of severe hemophilia A. Southern blotting provides a relatively laborious screening method, while in some centers detection is performed more conveniently by a long-range PCR method [23].

Recently, following prolonged searches for causative mutations in the residual 5% (approximately) of severely affected hemophiliacs with no known defect, a different inversion was found, resulting from recombination between a 1.0 kb sequence in intron 1 (*int1h-1*) and a homologous sequence *int1h-2* ap-

proximately 140 kb 5' to *F8* [24]. Recombination of these sequences results in separation of the *F8* promoter–exon 1 sequence from the remainder of the *F8* gene (Figure 4.2a and c): this inversion may account for approximately 2–5% of severe hemophilia A cases.

Anti-FVIII inhibitor development is a significant complication in hemophilia A: 21% of intron 22 inversion cases have demonstrated inhibitors [25], a rate higher than the average across all mutations but lower than that in cases caused by large deletions or nonsense mutations (see below).

Table 4.2 Hemophilia A – summary of unique mutations reported.

Exon	Point mutations			Deletions		Insertions
	Missense*	Nonsense (stop)	Splicing†	Small	Large	
1	14	1	4	2	n.a.	0
2	5	1	5	6	n.a.	2
3	24	0	3	4	n.a.	0
4	24	5	2	1	n.a.	1
5	11	1	7	3	n.a.	1
6	6	0	3	4	n.a.	2
7	32	4	0	6	n.a.	0
8	21	4	1	8	n.a.	1
9	22	3	1	5	n.a.	1
10	10	1	0	4	n.a.	0
11	27	1	3	1	n.a.	1
12	20	5	2	0	n.a.	1
13	23	3	2	4	n.a.	1
14	37	39	3	63	n.a.	31
15	13	1	4	2	n.a.	0
16	18	4	2	5	n.a.	0
17	24	3	1	5	n.a.	4
18	26	4	1	3	n.a.	3
19	14	1	5	3	n.a.	1
20	5	1	0	0	n.a.	1
21	5	4	0	0	n.a.	1
22	16	5	5	3	n.a.	1
23	25	1	4	6	n.a.	0
24	10	3	3	3	n.a.	2
25	11	2	1	4	n.a.	2
26	19	3	0	7	n.a.	0
Total	462	100	62	152	120	57
Total point mutations	615					
Total unique mutations	943					

*Including nine missense mutations which are also predicted to affect splice junctions.
†In the case of intronic substitutions, splice mutations are referred to the preceding exon.
n.a., not applicable.

Single-base substitutions in the *F8* gene

Substitution of single bases in *F8* exons may result in amino acid substitutions ("missense" variants) or the introduction of stop codons causing premature peptide chain truncation ("nonsense" variants). In addition, single-base substitution at mRNA splicing sites (at the intron–exon boundaries) can result in splice variants, which may or may not also include an amino acid alteration.

As of October 2003, there were over 1400 individual reports of single-base substitutions in the hemophilia A database, with over 600 *unique* variants listed: the actual reports are far too numerous to show here (even condensed to one line per unique mutation), and readers may access the database directly for phenotypic information. This includes FVIII clotting activity and circulating antigen levels, clinical severity, anti-FVIII inhibitor status, and journal reference (where published) for each report. Some overall analysis, however, is presented here.

The unique single-base variants are made up of 462 unique missense mutations (i.e., resulting in an amino acid substitution), 100 unique stop mutations, and 62 unique splice variants. The distribution by exon is given in Table 4.2. Exon 14 is approximately 10 times larger than the average size of the other exons and has a much higher burden of causative mutations generally. Missense mutations are actually very poorly represented per kilobase of coding sequence, reflecting the dispensability of the B domain for functional activity.

Table 4.1 gives some stratification of unique single-base mutations by clinical severity and anti-FVIII inhibitor status. While missense mutations and splice variants are associated with all disease severities, stop mutations (as expected) result almost exclusively in severe disease (87 of 89 cases).

In 427 single-base cases in which inhibitor status is known, 63 are reported as inhibitor positive (15%, broadly in accord with published studies on inhibitor incidence) with 44 (71%) of these associated with severe disease. Stop mutations result in a much higher proportion of cases with positive inhibitor status (25 of 74, 34%) in comparison with the missense mutation group, in which only 11% (37 of 349) are inhibitor positive, or the splice variant group, in which only 1 of 40 cases had inhibitor development. This extremely low incidence is unexplained. Remarkably, of the 25 unique stop mutations associated with the generation of anti-FVIII antibodies *in vivo*, only three are found in the first 13 exons, and none at all in exons 1–8. The reasons for this highly skewed distribution of inhibitor-positive cases relative to the position of the stop mutation in the FVIII mRNA are unknown, although various hypotheses have been formulated [25,26] (see also Chapters 9–11).

Although the large majority (420 of 615) of unique single-base mutations have been reported only once, with over 1400 individual missense reports in the database it is obvious that many other single-base mutations occur in multiple reports (24 unique mutations have been reported independently on 10 occasions or more, with six of those reported independently over 25 times). This suggests some enhanced predisposition to replication errors at the local chromatin level, whether caused by the well-known CpG dinucleotide effect (13/24 have CG → TG), by specific sequence motifs (e.g., "runs" or repetitions of a particular base), or by other local factors.

Frequently, both the clinical phenotype and FVIII activity measurement are highly variable within the cases for a single mutation. For example, the mutation Arg1997 → Trp has been reported 26 times, with clinical severity varying from severe to mild, and FVIII activity from <1% to 5% of normal plasma values. The variability in these multiple reports suggests that additional factors besides the defined disorder in the *F8* gene influence FVIII levels. It is now well known that mutations in at least two genes coding for proteins involved in glycoprotein trafficking in the ER and Golgi apparatus can result in reductions in the secreted levels of both FVIII and FV, resulting in the rare disorder of combined FVIII + FV deficiency [27,28]. However, it is probable that there are additional unknown factors, both genetic and environmental.

Given three-dimensional structural information about normal FVIII and its domains [11–15], it is possible to make interpretations as to the cause of hemophilia at the level of protein structure. The large group of missense mutations in the database might be expected to provide a fertile area for analysis, correlating FVIII function with protein structure, and increasing our understanding of "molecular pathology" in hemophilic mutation cases. However, in order to make interpretations about either FVIII function in plasma, or the ability of a variant molecule to be secreted, it is necessary to know circulating FVIII antigen levels as well as activity levels.

Thus, a hemophilic missense mutation associated with a plasma activity of, for example, 5% of normal may result either from a functionally normal molecule that is poorly secreted or unstable and thus circulates at the level of 5% (often termed "CRM-negative") or from a dysfunctional molecule present at a normal 100% antigen level ("CRM-positive"). In the absence of a FVIII antigen measurement, the analysis of these two possibil-ities at the level of protein structure will be entirely different, since in the former case one seeks to explain the effect of the amino acid substitution on secretion or stability in plasma, while in the latter the substitution will affect the procoagulant function of the variant protein.

Unfortunately, data on FVIII antigen level (in addition to FVIII activity) are available for only a minority of the unique missense reports (152 of 462, 33%) despite the availability of commercial ELISA kits. In addition, for two-thirds of this group of 152 cases, FVIII activity and antigen levels are in reasonable agreement, indicating that the hemophilic mutations result in defective secretion or instability of an otherwise functionally active cofactor. Since we understand the mechanisms of protein folding, chaperoning, secretion, and clearance so poorly, it is extremely difficult to make mechanistic explanations of why these amino acid changes result in low plasma levels in this group. Possibilities include mutations abolishing existing cysteine residues known to be involved in disulfide bridge formation, introducing new cysteine residues which may promote novel illegitimate disulfide bond formation, or mutations at or near site(s) of binding to VWF, which may result in defective association with the plasma carrier for FVIII.

In the remaining 50 or so cases in which activity and antigen are both known, FVIII antigen levels are essentially normal (or only mildly reduced) while activity levels are grossly reduced or even undetectable. This indicates that the mutation causes hemophilia by generation of a functionally inactive molecule that circulates normally. This smaller class of missense mutations gives strong clues as to which amino acids are crucial for functional interactions in this enormous molecule, and several groups have attempted to interpret CRM-positive mutations in terms of structure–function relationships [11,29–32].

Rationalization of the effects of some of these missense mutations is fairly simple: for example, modifications of proteolytic sites known to be required for FVIII activation (Arg372 → Cys/His, Ser373 → Pro/Leu, Arg1689 → Cys) all result in normal circulating FVIII protein levels with functional activity in the range 12% or below. Other mutations would be expected to have their effect by modifying interaction with one of the ligands of FVIII (e.g., VWF, factor IXa, phospholipid membrane) resulting in reduced functional activity. For example, three mutations with very low FVIII activity and normal antigen levels are associated with N-glycosylation variants. Ile566 → Thr leads to a new glycosylation (Asn564) at a FIXa binding site; Met1772 → Thr predicts a new N-glycosylation at Asn1770, also close to a FIXa-binding region; and, unexpectedly, loss of an N-glycosylation site at Asn582 resulting from the Ser584 → Arg mutation also results in a dysfunctional protein.

Mutations impacting the stability of the heterotrimeric form of activated FVIII (FVIIIa) may give rise to hemophilic consequences. There are now examples of these [33,34]. A number of mutations that are widely separated in the linear sequence of FVIII (and which have similar laboratory assay phenotypes) cluster at the interdomain interfaces: mutation of these residues at the interfaces leads to enhanced dissociation of the A2 domain from A1 and A3 and thus reduced FVIII activity (see Plate 1, facing p. 212).

It is a reasonable assumption that approximately two-thirds of all hemophilic missense mutations will cause the phenotype by defective FVIII secretion or stability while the remaining one-third generate a dysfunctional molecule. However, only performance of FVIII antigen assays allows assignment of a particular mutation into the appropriate category of molecular pathology: in the absence of these data, sophisticated analyses of inter-species residue conservation or structural modeling may be misleading.

Sequence insertions and deletions

The hemophilia A mutation database lists both *F8* insertions and the more numerous deletions. *F8* deletions are divided for convenience into large (>50 bp) and small (<50 bp).

Sequence insertions

There are 103 individual reports of insertions associated with hemophilia A; however, these are composed of just 57 unique insertion events, the vast majority of which are very short (less than 10 bp), with a very small number of larger insertions such as LINE elements [35] or Alu repeats [36]. Most of the repetitious reports consist of insertions of an additional adenine base at the site of a run of adenines; for example, there are no fewer than 20 separate unrelated cases of insertion of an A into a run of eight As at codons 1439–1441, and a further 12 cases of insertion of A into a run of nine As at codons 1191–1194. Runs of As in the *F8* cDNA are relatively common, and these insertions (and small deletions, see below) result from DNA polymerase slippage during replication.

Although the vast majority of insertions cause frameshifts resulting in severe hemophilia (Table 4.1), a small number of "A-run" insertion cases are associated with low but measurable FVIII activity levels and only moderate (or even mild) clinical severity. This probably results from a small percentage of normal mRNA molecules being produced by "corrective" slippage errors on the mutant template during transcription.

Of the 57 unique insertions, 43 have inhibitor status reported, with 35% of cases inhibitor positive (Table 4.1) — a very similar percentage to that found in single-base stop mutations (see above), as may be expected.

Sequence deletions

Small deletions subgroup (<50 bp)

There are 211 individual small deletion reports in the database, composed of 152 unique small deletions, of which 47% (71/152) are of single bases. As with small insertions (see above) almost all the multiple reports are of deletions of a single A in a run of As: for example, there are 35 separate reports of an A

deletion in a run of nine As at codons 1191–1194, which is also a hotspot for single-base insertions (see above).

Small deletions generally cause frameshifts and are almost all associated with severe disease: however, as with small insertions, there are a small number of moderate or mild cases, often associated with "A-runs" but also with in-frame deletions. Overall inhibitor development is lower than expected, at 21% of all unique cases with known status, compared with values of around 30% for insertion frameshifts and nonsense point mutations.

Large deletions subgroup (>50 bp)

There are 120 individual reports in the database, probably comprising close to that number of unique large deletions (detection methods are fairly imprecise so it is difficult to compare different reports where the deleted sequence may be simply given as "10 kb" or "exons 1–5"): the deletions range from just a few hundreds of bases up to more than 210 kb deleting the entire gene, and are responsible for about 5% of severe hemophilia A cases.

Large deletions in the *F8* gene almost invariably give rise to clinically severe disease with no measurable FVIII activity or antigen. Unexpectedly, however, there are four independent reports of clinically moderate disease (two quoting low but measurable FVIII activity levels, one also a normal FVIII antigen level), all associated with exon-skipping deletions toward the C-terminus of the FVIII protein, involving exon 22 [37], exons 23–24 [38,39], and exon 25 [40]. Remarkably, significant or even normal secretion of hypoactive FVIII lacking C-terminal amino acid sequences may occur in these cases, alleviating the clinical severity.

There is a very high level of inhibitor development (45%) in this subgroup of cases (43/96) — far higher than that found for the small deletion subgroup (21%): clearly, there is a relationship between the size of deletion and the likelihood of inhibitor development. Grouping all deletions yields an overall inhibitor development rate of 32% (67 of 212, Table 4.1), similar to both the insertion group (35%) and the nonsense mutation group (34%).

Concluding remarks

After about 20 years of mutation hunting in hemophilia, the technology of detection has reached the point where, in large centers with substantial cohorts of patients, causative mutations can be found in around 95% of cases (or more). The remaining small percentage of undetermined genetic causes may suggest that there are unknown gene rearrangements still to be found, or that there are other causes outside the *F8* gene: however, there remains an understandable impetus for afflicted families to have their mutation defined for prenatal diagnosis.

Rather surprising, considering the number of years over which mutations have been accumulating in the database, is the fact that novel mutations continue to be added at an undiminished pace, and there are several large centers which have not as yet submitted their own mutation lists. The number of missense mutations causing clinical disease as a fraction of the length of the FVIII primary sequence currently stands at just over 20% (462 of 2232). How many more disease-causing mutations exist within this remarkable protein is yet to be determined.

References

1 Rotblat F, Goodall AH, O'Brien DP, *et al.* Monoclonal antibodies to human procoagulant factor VIII. *J Lab Clin Med* 1983; **101**: 736–46.

2 Gitschier J, Wood WI, Goralka TM, *et al.* Characterization of the human factor VIII gene. *Nature* 1984; **312**: 326–30.

3 Toole JJ, Knopf JL, Wozney JM, *et al.* Molecular cloning of a cDNA encoding human antihemophilic factor. *Nature* 1984; **312**: 342–7.

4 Poustka A, Dietrich A, Langenstein G, *et al.* Physical map of human Xq27-qter: localizing the region of the fragile X mutation. *Proc Natl Acad Sci USA* 1991; **88**: 8302–6.

5 Freije D, Schlessinger D. A 1.6-Mb contig of yeast artificial chromosomes around the human factor VIII gene reveals three regions homologous to probes for the DXS115 locus and two for the DXYS64 locus. *Am J Hum Genet* 1992; **51**: 66–80.

6 Vehar GA, Keyt B, Eaton D, *et al.* Structure of human factor VIII. *Nature* 1984; **312**: 337–42.

7 Kane WH, Davie EW. Cloning of a cDNA coding for human factor V, a blood coagulation factor homologous to factor VIII and ceruloplasmin. *Proc Natl Acad Sci USA* 1986; **83**: 6800–4.

8 Stubbs JD, Lekutis C, Singer KL, *et al.* cDNA cloning of a mouse mammary epithelial cell surface protein reveals the existence of epidermal growth factor-like domains linked to factor VIII-like sequences. *Proc Natl Acad Sci USA* 1990; **87**: 8417–21.

9 Johnson JD, Edman JC, Rutter WJ. A receptor tyrosine kinase found in breast carcinoma cells has an extracellular discoidin I-like domain [published erratum in *Proc Natl Acad Sci USA* 1993; **90**: 10891]. *Proc Natl Acad Sci USA* 1993; **90**: 5677–81.

10 Eaton D, Rodriguez H, Vehar GA. Proteolytic processing of human factor VIII. Correlation of specific cleavages by thrombin, factor Xa, and activated protein C with activation and inactivation of factor VIII coagulant activity. *Biochemistry* 1986; **25**: 505–12.

11 Pemberton S, Lindley P, Zaitsev V, *et al.* A molecular model for the triplicated A domains of human factor VIII based on the crystal structure of human ceruloplasmin. *Blood* 1997; **89**: 2413–21.

12 Stoylova SS, Lenting PJ, Kemball-Cook G, Holzenburg A. Electron crystallography of human blood coagulation factor VIII bound to phospholipid monolayers. *J Biol Chem* 1999; **274**: 36573–8.

13 Pratt KP, Shen BW, Takeshima K, *et al.* Structure of the C2 domain of human factor VIII at 1.5 A resolution. *Nature* 1999; **402**: 439–42.

14 Knobe KE, Villoutreix BO, Tengborn LI, *et al.* Factor VIII inhibitors in two families with mild haemophilia A: structural analysis of the mutations. *Hemostasis* 2000; **30**: 268–79.

15 Stoilova-McPhie S, Villoutreix BO, Mertens K, *et al.* Three-dimensional structure of membrane-bound coagulation factor VIII: modelling of the factor VIII heterodimer within a three-dimensional density map derived by electron crystallography. *Blood* 2002; **99**: 1215–23.

16 Naylor JA, Brinke A, Hassock S, *et al.* Characteristic mRNA abnormality found in half the patients with severe haemophilia A is due to large DNA inversions. *Hum Mol Genet* 1993; **2**: 1773–8.

17 Lakich D, Kazazian HH Jr, Antonarakis SE, Gitschier J. Inversions disrupting the factor VIII gene are a common cause of severe haemophilia A. *Nature Genet* 1993; **5**: 236–41.

18 Higuchi M, Kazazian HH Jr, Kasch L, *et al.* Molecular characterization of severe hemophilia A suggests that about half the mutations are not within the coding regions and splice junctions of the factor VIII gene. *Proc Natl Acad Sci USA* 1991; **88**: 7405–9.

19 Naylor JA, Green PM, Rizza CR, Giannelli F. Factor VIII gene explains all cases of haemophilia A. *Lancet* 1992; **340**: 1066–7.

20 Levinson B, Kenwrick S, Lakich D, *et al.* A transcribed gene in an intron of the human factor VIII gene. *Genomics* 1990; **7**: 1–11.

21 Levinson B, Kenwrick S, Gamel P, *et al.* Evidence for a third transcript from the human factor VIII gene. *Genomics* 1992; **14**: 585–9.

22 Antonarakis SE, Rossiter JP, Young M, *et al.* Factor VIII gene inversions in severe haemophilia A: results of an international consortium study. *Blood* 1995; **86**: 2206–12.

23 Liu Q, Nozari G, Sommer SS. Single tube polymerase chain reaction for rapid diagnosis of the inversion hotspot of mutation in hemophilia A. *Blood* 1998; **92**: 1458–9 [correction in Liu Q, Sommer SS. Subcycling-PCR for multiplex long-distance amplification of regions with high and low GC content: application to the inversion hotspot in the factor VIII gene. *BioTechniques* 1998; **25**: 1022–8].

24 Bagnall RD, Waseem N, Green PM, Giannelli F. Recurrent inversion breaking intron 1 of the factor VIII gene is a frequent cause of severe hemophilia A. *Blood* 2002; **99**: 168–74.

25 Oldenburg J, Tuddenham, EGD. Genetic basis of inhibitor development in severe haemophilia A and B. In: *Comprehensive Management of Haemophilia Patients with Inhibitors.* Rodriguez-Merchan EC, Lee CA, eds. Blackwell Science, Oxford, 2003.

26 Goodeve AC, Peake IR. The molecular basis of hemophilia A: genotype–phenotype relationships and inhibitor development. *Semin Thromb Haemost* 2003; **29**: 23–30.

27 Neerman-Arbez M, Johnson KM, Morris MA, *et al.* Molecular analysis of the *ERGIC-53* gene in 35 families with combined factor V-factor VIII deficiency. *Blood* 1999; **93**: 2253–60.

28 Zhang B, Cunningham MA, Nichols WC, *et al.* Bleeding due to disruption of a cargo-specific ER-to-Golgi transport complex. *Nat Genet* 2003; **34**: 220–5.

29 Morichika S, Shima M, Kamisue S, *et al.* Factor VIII gene analysis in Japanese CRM-positive and CRM-reduced haemophilia A patients by single-strand conformation polymorphism. *Br J Haematol* 1997; **98**: 901–6.

30 Liu M, Murphy ME, Thompson AR. A domain mutations in 65 haemophilia A families and molecular modelling of dysfunctional factor VIII proteins. *Br J Haematol* 1998; **103**: 1051–60.

31 Liu ML, Shen BW, Nakaya S, *et al.* Hemophilic factor VIII C1- and C2-domain missense mutations and their modeling to the 1.5-angstrom human C2-domain crystal structure. *Blood* 2000; **96**: 979–87.

32 Liu ML, Nakaya S, Thompson AR. Non-inversion factor VIII mutations in 80 hemophilia A families including 24 with alloimmune responses. *Thromb Haemost* 2002; **87**: 273–6.

33 Pipe SW, Saenko EL, Eickhorst AN, *et al.* Hemophilia A mutations associated with 1-stage/2-stage activity discrepancy disrupt protein-protein interactions within the triplicated A domains of thrombin-activated factor VIIIa. *Blood* 2001; **97**: 685–91.

34 Hakeos WH, Miao H, Sirachainan N, *et al.* Hemophilia A mutations within the factor VIII A2-A3 subunit interface destabilize factor VIIIa and cause one-stage/two-stage activity discrepancy. *Thromb Haemost* 2002; **88**: 781–7.

35 Kazazian HH Jr, Wong C, Youssoufian H, *et al.* Haemophilia A resulting from de novo insertion of L1 sequences represents a novel mechanism for mutation in man. *Nature* 1988; **332**: 164–6.

36 Sukarova E, Dimovski AJ, Tchacarova P, *et al.* An *Alu* insert as the cause of a severe form of hemophilia A. *Acta Haematol* 2001; **106**: 126–9.

37 Youssoufian H, Antonarakis SE, Aronis S, *et al.* Characterization of five partial deletions of the factor VIII gene. *Proc Natl Acad Sci USA* 1987; **84**: 3772–6.

38 Wehnert M, Herrmann FH, Wulff K. Partial deletions of factor VIII gene as molecular diagnostic markers in haemophilia. *Dis Markers* 1989; **7**: 113–7.

39 Lavergne JM, Bahnak BR, Vidaud M, *et al.* A directed search for mutations in hemophilia A using restriction enzyme analysis and denaturing gradient gel electrophoresis. A study of seven exons in the factor VIII gene of 170 cases. *Nouv Rev Fr Hematol* 1992; **34**: 85–91.

40 Gau JP, Hsu HC, Chau WK, Ho CH. A novel splicing acceptor mutation of the factor VIII gene producing skipping of exon 25. *Ann Hematol* 2003; **82**: 175–7. [Erratum in: *Ann Hematol* 2003; **82**: 378].

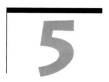

5

Hemophilia A: role of factor VIII in coagulation

Evgueni L. Saenko and Natalya M. Ananyeva

Normal human hemostasis is provided by two functioning co-agulation pathways — the extrinsic, tissue factor (TF)/activated factor VII-dependent pathway and the intrinsic, factor VIII (FVIII)-dependent pathway. While initiation of blood coagulation is ascribed to the extrinsic pathway, in which small quantities of activated factors IX (FIXa) and X (FXa) are generated, the intrinsic pathway dramatically amplifies the coagulation events triggered by the TF-dependent pathway. The life-threatening coagulation disorder hemophilia A is caused by a genetic or acquired deficiency in FVIII or by structural defects affecting its function.

In the intrinsic pathway, activated FVIII (FVIIIa) functions as a cofactor for the serine protease, FIXa, increasing its catalytic activity by several orders of magnitude. This membrane-bound complex (Xase complex) then activates FX to FXa [1]. In turn, FXa participates in a similar complex for conversion of pro-thrombin into thrombin, the key enzyme of the coagulation cascade. Assembly of the Xase complex requires a phospholipid (PL) surface, which is classically provided by activated platelets. A major role of the PL surface is to concentrate components of the Xase complex and limit their interactions from three- to two-dimensional space, i.e. from in plasma volume to on the cell surface. This results in a dramatic acceleration of FXa generation due to a decrease in the Michaelis constant (K_m) for FX [2] and to an increase in the catalytic constant of the reaction (k_{cat}) [3].

The FVIII molecule (~300 kDa, 2332 amino acid residues) consists of three homologous A domains, two homologous C domains, and the unique B domain (A1–A2–B–A3–C1–C2). Prior to its secretion into plasma, FVIII is processed to a series of metal ion-linked heterodimers produced by cleavage at the B–A3 junction and by a number of additional cleavages within the B domain. These cleavages generate the heavy chain (HCh) consisting of the A1 (1–336), A2 (373–719), and B domains (741–1648), and the light chain (LCh) composed of the domains A3 (1690–2019), C1 (2020–2172), and C2 (2173–2332). The C-terminal portions of the A1 domain (amino acids 337–372) and the A2 domain (amino acids 720–740) and N-terminal portion of the A3 domain (amino acids 1649–1689) contain a high proportion of negatively charged residues and are called acidic regions, *a1*, *a2* and *a3*, respectively (Figure 5.1).

Immediately after release into the circulation, FVIII forms a tight noncovalent complex with von Willebrand factor (VWF), with a dissociation constant (K_d) of approximately 0.4 nmol/L [4]. Complex formation with VWF is required for maintaining the normal FVIII level in plasma since it prevents premature assembly of the Xase complex prior to activation of FVIII and protects FVIII from inactivation by activated protein C (APC), FIXa, and FXa.

Direct FVIII interaction with VWF is mediated by LCh with contributions from the *a3* peptide (residues 1649–1689) and regions within the C2 and C1 domains [5]. The *a3* peptide represents the major binding site. Additionally, as demonstrated by the use of conformationally sensitive anti-C2 monoclonal antibodies (MAbs), *a3* is required for maintaining the C2 domain in a conformation optimal for the C2 binding to VWF [4]. Involvement of the C2 region 2303–2332 in binding to VWF was initially suggested from synthetic peptide studies [6]. A deeper insight has been gained through resolution of the X-ray structure of the human C2 domain, which revealed the existence of hydrophobic "feet" formed by the side-chains of Met2199/Phe2200 and Leu2251/Leu2252 [7]. Mutational analysis confirmed that these residues are important contributors in FVIII interaction with both VWF and the PL surface [8]. Involvement of the C1 domain in binding to VWF was first demonstrated by the finding that mutations of three C1 residues (Ile2098, Ser2119, and Arg2150) result in hemophilia A with a direct or indirect effect on VWF binding [9]. According to the latest three-dimensional structure of membrane-bound FVIII, the *a3*, C2 and C1 regions are arranged closely in space to form a "patch" for interaction either with VWF or with the PL surface [10]. HCh does not interact with VWF directly but is required for the maximal affinity of the FVIII/VWF interaction, as evidenced by a 10-fold higher affinity of the whole FVIII molecule for VWF in comparison with its isolated LCh [4].

Factor VIII activation

Activation of FVIII by limited proteolysis at the site of a coagulation event is required for FVIII to exert its cofactor function in the Xase complex; nonactivated FVIII shows no detectable cofactor activity. The major physiological activators of FVIII are thrombin and FXa; both proteases cleave the FVIII molecule within HCh at Arg372 between the A1 and A2 domains and at Arg740 between the A2 and B domains and also within LCh at Arg1689. In heterotrimeric activated FVIII (FVIIIa), the A1 and A3 domains retain the metal ion-mediated interaction, and the relatively stable A1/A3–C1–C2 dimer is weakly associated with the A2 subunit through electrostatic interactions (Figure 5.1).

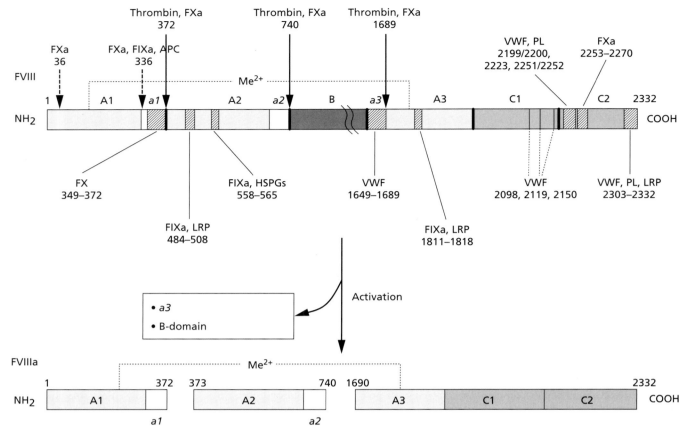

Figure 5.1 FVIII structure and regions involved in its major functional interactions. Non-activated FVIII is shown as a multidomain structure, in which the A1 and A3 subunits are noncovalently linked via a metal ion-mediated interaction (dotted line) and three A domains are flanked by acidic regions *a1*, *a2*, and *a3*. The regions of FVIII involved in binding to VWF, PL, FIXa, FX, FXa, LRP, and heparan sulfate proteogly-cans (HSPGs) are shown as hatched boxes. Solid and dotted arrows point to the activating and inactivating cleavage sites respectively. Activation of FVIII leads to release of the B domain and *a3*; in activated FVIII heterotrimer, the A1 and A3 domains retain the metal ion-mediated interaction, and the stable A1/A3–C1–C2 dimer is weakly associated with the A2 subunit through electrostatic interactions.

Factor VIII sites responsible for binding of these activators have been assigned to the C2 domain of LCh. FXa-binding site was discovered with the use of a mouse anti-C2 MAb ESH8, which inhibited both FVIII activation and FVIII proteolytic cleavage by FXa. FXa-binding site was mapped to the C2 residues 2253–2270 based on the ability of overlapping synthetic peptides covering this region to inhibit interaction of FVIII and its C2 domain with anhydro-FXa, a catalytically inactive derivative of FXa [11]. The site responsible for thrombin-catalyzed cleavage at Arg1689 in LCh has been assigned to the C2 domain of FVIII because the isolated C2 domain was able to bind to anhydro-thrombin, a catalytically inactive derivative of thrombin, and inhibit thrombin-catalyzed cleavage at Arg1689 [12].

Cleavage at Arg1689 results in removal of *a3*, which is a critical requirement for the release of FVIIIa from VWF since the *a3* region bears the major VWF-binding site. Removal of *a3* leads to a 10-fold decrease in the association rate constant and a 160-fold increase in the dissociation rate constant of interaction of FVIIIa with VWF in comparison with nonactivated FVIII [4]. This results in a 1600-fold decrease in FVIIIa affinity for VWF,

allowing FVIIIa to effectively bind to a PL surface and to FIXa during assembly of the Xase complex. In addition, removal of *a3* imposes a conformational change within the C2 domain that facilitates dissociation of FVIII from VWF. This conformational change was suggested from a reduced affinity of thrombin-cleaved LCh (compared with intact LCh) for a conformationally sensitive anti-C2 MAb NMC-VIII/5 [4]. Another MAb, ESH8, has a discontinuous epitope composed of two distinct but spatially close regions of C2. This endows ESH8 with the ability to "lock" the C2 conformation and in this way to prevent any conformational changes. The FVIIIa affinity for VWF in the presence of ESH8 [13] was 20-fold higher than in the absence of MAb [4], thus confirming that removal of *a3* upon activation of FVIII induces a conformational change within the C2 domain, which is required for complete release of FVIIIa from VWF.

Activated heterotrimeric FVIII is highly unstable owing to spontaneous dissociation of the A2 subunit as well as to proteolytic inactivation of FVIIIa by APC, FIXa and FXa. A rapid loss of the A2 subunit occurs because it is weakly associated with the A1/A3–C1–C2 dimer via low-affinity electrostatic interactions, and the loss of A2 is concomitant with the loss of FVIII activity [1]. Proteolytic cleavages by FXa may be both activating and inactivating due to multiple cleavage sites for FXa within the FVIII molecule. In addition to cleavage sites identical to those for thrombin, FXa cleaves the FVIII molecule at Arg1721 within the A3 domain of LCh and at Lys36 and Arg336 within the A1 domain of HCh. While cleavages at Arg1721 and Arg1689 lead to similar activation of FVIII, FXa-mediated cleavages within the A1 domain are associated with proteolytic inactivation of FVIIIa. Owing to these inactivation-related cleavages, the peak activity of FXa-activated FVIIIa is significantly (approximately twofold) lower than that of thrombin-activated FVIIIa [14]. Indeed, in the presence of thrombin, inactivation of FVIIIa is determined primarily by loss of the A2 subunit, whereas in the presence of FXa both loss of the A2 subunit and proteolysis of A1 contribute to inactivation. The specific mechanism of FVIIIa inactivation by cleavage at Arg336 has been confirmed by demonstration that the C-terminal region 336–372 of the A1 subunit is critical for optimal orientation of the A2 subunit in FVIIIa relative to the active site of FIXa [15]. Inactivation of FVIIIa by cleavage at Lys36 has been attributed to a complete loss of affinity of truncated A1 (37–336) for the A2 subunit. This suggests that both N- and C-termini of the A1 subunit are required for maintaining functional interaction of A1 with A2 [16]. The C-terminal FXa cleavage site at Arg336 within the A1 domain coincides with the inactivation-related cleavage site for APC [17] and for FIXa [18]. Additional cleavage sites for APC and FIXa are at Arg562 and Arg1719 respectively.

Thus, activation of FVIII by thrombin or FXa are both physiologically critical events, although not coinciding in time. In the presence of VWF, thrombin-mediated activation of FVIII is more effective because vWF protects FVIII from FXa inactivating cleavages. However, rapid inactivation of thrombin by antithrombin III, along with generation of increasing concentrations of FXa by the intrinsic Xase, makes the contribution of FXa into FVIII activation at later stages more significant, if not dominant. Owing to multiple cleavage sites, subsequent proteolytic attack of FVIIIa by generated FXa would inactivate the cofactor and in this way limit further FXa generation by a self-dampening mechanism.

Interaction of activated FVIII with components of the Xase complex

The cofactor activity of FVIIIa in the assembled intrinsic Xase complex is provided by three essential interactions of FVIIIa: binding to the PL membrane, the enzyme FIXa, and the substrate FX [19]. Conditions favorable for FVIIIa association with cell membrane PL at the site of coagulation are created upon the activation-induced conformational change within the C2 domain that occurs with FVIIIa release from VWF. This results in a 10-fold increase in FVIIIa affinity for PL membranes (K_d ~ 0.4–1.1 nmol/L), approaching the plasma concentration of FVIII (approximately 1 nmol/L) [20].

It was initially believed that high-affinity interaction between FVIII and cell membrane PL is provided by the region 2303–2332 of the C2 domain of LCh. This was based on the ability of synthetic peptides encompassing this region to inhibit FVIII/PL binding [6]. Recent resolution of the 1.5-Å X-ray structure of the human FVIII C2 domain [7] and direct analysis of FVIII/PL binding obtained by electron crystallography [10] have prompted revision of this concept. Analysis of the X-ray structure revealed the presence of three hydrophobic "feet" formed by the side-chains of Met2199/Phe2200, Val2223, and Leu 2251/Leu2252, which were suggested to penetrate the membrane bilayer [7]. Direct analysis of FVIII/PL binding by electron crystallography, which permitted the resolution of five functional domains of FVIII (A1, A2, A3, C1, and C2) on a PL surface, strongly supports the contribution of these three loops in forming the PL-interacting region [10]. This analysis also revealed the presence of a fourth loop formed by residues Trp2313–His2315, which lies within the sequence 2303–2332, earlier implicated in PL binding [6]. Predictions based on the X-ray structure of the C2 domain and electron crystallography studies of FVIII were confirmed by demonstration that Ala mutations of the residues comprising the hydrophobic "feet" Met2199/Phe2200 and Leu 2251/Leu2252 dramatically reduced the affinity of FVIII for PL [8].

In the Xase complex, FVIIIa interacts with and serves as a cofactor for FIXa, a trypsin-like vitamin K-dependent serine protease that catalyzes conversion of FX into FXa (Figure 5.2). In the absence of the cofactor, FIXa displays a very low catalytic activity. Unlike other coagulation factors, full activity of FIXa is achieved in the presence of both the cofactor FVIIIa and the substrate FX. The low intrinsic activity of FIXa is possibly related to a set of surface-exposed structural elements in proximity to the active site of FIXa. Six loops (residues 199–204, 223–229, 235–245, 256–268, 312–322, and 340–347) are involved in the formation of a large substrate-binding groove of FIXa [21,22]. In the absence of the cofactor, the loops maintain a conformation that restricts the interaction of FIXa with its substrates. Physiologic activation of FIXa is postulated to occur as a cooperative two-step conformational rearrangement of the loops: binding of the cofactor FVIIIa releases their inactive conformation and in this way creates satisfactory conditions for subsequent FX binding to the active site cleft. These conformational changes within the active site of FIXa were detected using active site-labeled FIXa, in which a fluorescent label functions as a "reporter group" so that the increase in fluorescence anisotropy reflects the extent of modulation of the FIXa active site imposed by FVIIIa [23]. The major result of interaction of FVIIIa with FIXa is a dramatic (by several orders of magnitude) increase of the catalytic activity of FIXa [2].

The high-affinity interaction between FVIIIa and FIXa is conferred by the LCh of FVIII, which contains a FIXa-binding site (K_d ~ 15 nmol/L) formed by the A3 domain residues 1811–1818 [24]. The complementary region on FIXa molecules lies within its light chain, and experimental data suggest EGF2 to be critical for the binding to FVIIIa. Another, low-affinity FIX-binding site

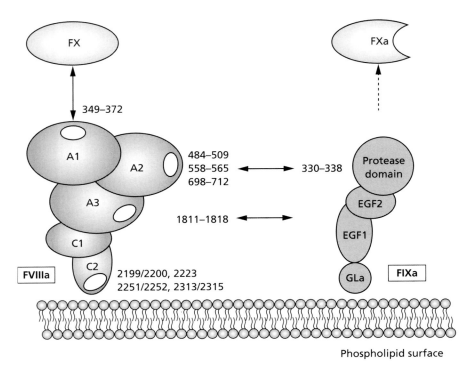

Figure 5.2 Interactions of FVIIIa within the intrinsic Xase complex. The Xase complex is composed of the serine protease FIXa, the cofactor FVIIIa and the substrate FX and is assembled on a PL surface in a Ca²⁺-dependent manner. FIXa is a disulfide-linked, two-chain molecule with a light chain consisting of a N-terminal γ-carboxyglutamic acid (Gla)-rich domain (residues 1–40) and two epidermal growth factor (EGF)-like domains (residues 47–84 and 85–127), and a heavy chain (residues 181–415) containing the serine protease domain. The PL bilayer binds to the C2 domain of FVIIIa and the Gla domain of FIXa. In addition to the indicated hydrophobic "feet", spatially close basic residues Arg2215, Arg2220, Lys2227, and Lys2249 stabilize FVIII binding to PL by electrostatic interactions. Multiple sites provide FVIIIa/FIXa interaction: the FVIII A3 domain interacts with FIXa light chain with high affinity; the low-affinity interaction between the FVIII A2 subunit and the protease domain of FIXa defines the cofactor activity of FVIIIa; the A2 region 558–565 interacts with FIXa helix 330–338.

($K_d \sim 300$ nmol/L), is located within the A2 domain of the HCh and is formed by residues 558–565 [25], 484–509 [26], and 698–712. The A2 sites interact with the catalytic domain of FIXa; specifically, the region 558–565 of FVIIIa interacts with the helix 330–338 within this domain [27]. Despite low affinity, interaction of A2 with FIXa defines the cofactor activity of FVIIIa. As demonstrated by fluorescence anisotropy studies, the A2 domain represents the portion of FVIIIa that modulates the FIXa active site and in this way amplifies the enzymatic activity of FIXa 100-fold [28]. It is noteworthy that the functionally important A2 sites become exposed only upon activation-induced cleavage at Arg1689 within the LCh, leading to a threefold increase in FVIIIa activity [29]. This suggests that removal of *a3* is required for providing a closer contact between A2 and the corresponding region(s) of the FIXa protease domain in proximity to its active site. The maximal modulation of the FIXa active site requires cleavage between A1 and A2 at position 372 in addition to removal of *a3* [30]. Interestingly, addition of FX contributes to a further marked increase in anisotropy, indicating that FX also contributes to correct orientation of the FIXa active site in the assembled Xase complex [28].

Involvement of both A2 and the LCh sites in FVIIIa interaction with FIXa stabilizes FVIIIa within the Xase complex where FIXa serves as a bridge linking the A2 subunit and A1/A3–C1–C2 heterodimer. Accordingly, this significantly reduces the rate of FVIIIa inactivation owing to spontaneous dissociation of the A2 subunit [1]. This stabilizing effect of FIXa increases in the presence of the PL surface and FX.

In addition to stabilizing FVIII, FIXa modulates its activity by irreversible inactivation of FVIIIa via the proteolytic mechanism. Prolonged interaction of FVIIIa with FIXa results in a loss of FVIIIa activity owing to proteolytic cleavage within the A1 subunit at Arg336. Thus, by virtue of its capacity to modulate FVIIIa activity, FIXa regulates the catalytic efficiency of the Xase complex.

The FVIII site involved in interaction with FX has been localized to the *a1* residues 349–372 [31].

Clearance of FVIII

Removal of FVIII from the circulation represents the final event in the FVIII life cycle (Figure 5.3). FVIII catabolism is mediated by low-density lipoprotein receptor-related protein (LRP), a multiligand hepatic receptor that belongs to the low-density lipoprotein (LDL) receptor superfamily of endocytic receptors [32]. Discernment of the involvement of LRP in FVIII turnover was based on the following findings: FVIII is able to bind to purified LRP (K_d 60 nmol/L [33]; K_d 116 nmol/L [34]); it is efficiently internalized and degraded by various LRP-expressing cell lines; and that FVIII half-life in the circulation in a mouse model is significantly prolonged by blocking LRP by its classical antagonist, a 39-kDa receptor-associated protein (RAP) [34,32]. The physiologic role of LRP in regulating plasma levels of FVIII *in vivo* has been confirmed in cre/loxP-mediated conditional LRP-deficient mice (MX1cre⁺LRPflox/flox) in which inactivation of the LRP gene led to an approximately twofold increase in plasma FVIII level compared with that in control mice [35]. In clearance experiments, MX1cre⁺LRPflox/flox mice displayed a 1.5-fold prolongation of FVIII mean residence time. Additionally, adenovirus-mediated overexpression of the receptor antagonist RAP in normal mice resulted in a 3.5-fold increase in plasma FVIII

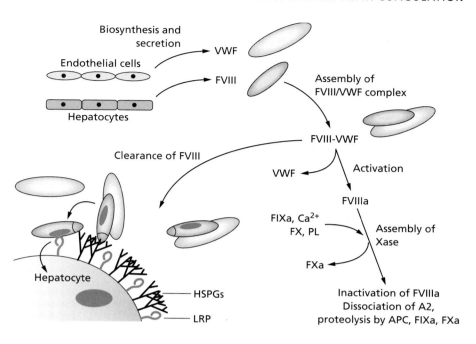

Figure 5.3 The life cycle of FVIII. FVIII is synthesized by various cell types, predominantly by hepatocytes, and is secreted upon post-translational processing. In circulation, it forms a tight complex with VWF secreted by vascular endothelial cells. FVIII acquires its cofactor activity upon activation by thrombin or FXa at the site of a coagulation event and subsequently participates in the assembly of the Xase complex, which activates FX, thereby leading to a burst of thrombin generation. FVIIIa is rapidly inactivated by both enzymatic proteolysis and dissociation of the A2 subunit. Removal of FVIII from the circulation occurs via initial interaction of FVIII/VWF complex with heparan sulfate proteoglycans (HSPGs), which concentrate the complex on the cell surface and present it to a clearance receptor LRP (and possibly to other members of LDL receptor superfamily), followed by LRP-mediated catabolism of FVIII.

level, thus confirming that the regulation of plasma FVIII *in vivo* is indeed mediated by a RAP-sensitive LRP receptor.

LRP-mediated clearance of FVIII from its complex with VWF is facilitated by cell-surface heparan sulfate proteoglycans (HSPGs), one of the major glycoprotein components of the extracellular matrix [36]. Simultaneous blocking of these two receptors led to a greater prolongation of FVIII half-life in mice (5.5-fold) than did the blocking of LRP alone (3.3-fold).

Interaction of FVIII with LRP involves multiple (at least three) FVIII binding sites: within the A2 domain of HCh [34] and within the C2 and A3 domains of LCh [33,37]. The A2 domain LRP-binding site has been mapped to the region 484–509 [34]. One LRP-interactive region within LCh has been ascribed to the C2 domain, based on the observation that an anti-C2 domain MAb ESH4 inhibited a high-affinity binding of the FVIII LCh to LRP. The C2 site likely overlaps with the site responsible for FVIII binding to VWF, since the same antibody inhibited FVIII binding to VWF [33]. An additional LRP-binding site within LCh has been localized to the A3 domain residues Glu1811–Lys1818 based on (i) competition studies using synthetic peptides and (ii) the inhibitory effect of a recombinant antibody fragment that specifically binds to the FVIII sequence Glu1811–Lys1818 [37]. The role of this sequence in LRP binding was further confirmed by a reduced affinity of a chimeric FVIII, in which region Glu1811–Lys1818 was replaced with the corresponding sequence of factor V.

In the circulation, where FVIII is normally present in a complex with VWF, both LRP binding sites located within the LCh of FVIII are likely to be blocked by VWF. Indeed, the C2 site seems to be directly involved in binding to VWF, since the antibody ESH4 inhibits LCh binding both to the LRP and to VWF [33]. The A3 site (residues 1811–1818) contains the same structural elements that contribute to interaction of FVIII with FIXa, and FIXa binding to this site is inhibited by VWF [24]. This implies that VWF would also inhibit binding of LRP to the region 1811–1818. Thus, in most situations, FVIII catabolism is likely to be mediated by the LRP binding site located within the A2 domain.

Why does FVIII deficiency lead to hemophilia?

While both coagulation pathways generate FXa, hemophilia is associated specifically with impairment of the intrinsic, FVIII-dependent pathway. This implies that the functioning of the extrinsic pathway alone is insufficient for maintaining hemostasis. It has been hypothesized that tissue factor pathway inhibitor shuts off the TF-dependent pathway before it can generate enough FXa to support the formation of hemostatic amounts of thrombin. In the intrinsic pathway, as detailed above, FVIIIa increases the catalytic activity of FIXa by several orders of magnitude. This results in approximately 50-fold more efficient conversion of FX into FXa by the intrinsic pathway in comparison with the extrinsic pathway [38]. Thus, the role of the intrinsic pathway is to generate large amounts of FXa and in this way to provide efficient spatial propagation of the clotting process initiated by the TF-dependent pathway. This role is supported by real-time monitoring of spatial clot growth from TF-bearing cell monolayers; in hemophilic plasma there is specific retardation of clot growth during the propagation phase but not the initiation phase [39].

Additional elucidation of the role of the intrinsic pathway in coagulation has been suggested by the cell-based model of coagulation [40]. This model takes into consideration that generation of FXa by the extrinsic and intrinsic pathways occurs on diverse phospholipid surfaces; specifically, it can occur on the surface of TF-bearing cells or, alternatively, on the surface of activated platelets in close proximity to activated factor V, a component of the prothrombinase complex. While FXa generated through the extrinsic pathway will be rapidly inactivated by antithrombin III or tissue factor pathway inhibitor, FXa generated by the intrinsic pathway will be immediately incorporated in the prothrombinase complex. This will trigger a burst of thrombin generation. Thus, in addition to *insufficient amounts* of generated FXa, in hemophilia there is *a specific failure of platelet-surface FX activation*. This leads to a failure of platelet-surface thrombin generation and results in impairment of hemostasis.

References

1 Fay PJ. Regulation of factor VIIIa in the intrinsic factor Xase. *Thromb Haemost* 1999; **82**: 193–200.

2 van Dieijen G, Tans G, Rosing J, Hemker HC. The role of phospholipid and factor VIII$_a$ in the activation of bovine factor X. *J Biol Chem* 1981; **256**: 3433–42.

3 Gilbert GE, Arena AA. Activation of the factor VIIIa-factor IXa enzyme complex of blood coagulation by membranes containing phosphatidyl-L-serine. *J Biol Chem* 1996; **271**: 11120–5.

4 Saenko EL, Scandella D. The acidic region of the light chain and the C2 domain together form a high affinity binding site for von Willebrand factor. *J Biol Chem* 1997; **272**: 18007–14.

5 Saenko EL, Ananyeva NM, Tuddenham EG, Kemball-Cook G. Factor VIII – novel insights into form and function. *Br J Haematol* 2002; **119**: 323–331.

6 Foster PA, Fulcher CA, Houghten RA, Zimmerman TS. Synthetic factor VIII peptides with amino acid sequences contained within the C2 domain of factor VIII inhibit factor VIII binding to phosphatidylserine. *Blood* 1990; **75**: 1999–2004.

7 Pratt KP, Shen BW, Takeshima K, *et al.* Structure of the C2 domain of human factor VIII at 1.5 A resolution. *Nature* 1999; **402**: 439–42.

8 Gilbert GE, Kaufman RJ, Arena AA, *et al.* Four hydrophobic amino acids of the factor VIII C2 domain are constituents of both the membrane-binding and von Willebrand factor-binding motifs. *J Biol Chem* 2002; **277**: 6374–81.

9 Jacquemin M, Lavend'homme R, Benhida A, *et al.* A novel cause of mild/moderate hemophilia A: mutations scattered in the factor VIII C1 domain reduce factor VIII binding to von Willebrand factor. *Blood* 2000; **96**: 958–65.

10 Stoilova-McPhie S, Villoutreix BO, Mertens K, *et al.* Three-dimensional structure of membrane-bound coagulation factor VIII: modeling of the factor VIII heterodimer within a three-dimensional density map derived by electron crystallography. *Blood* 2002; **99**: 1215–23.

11 Nogami K, Shima M, Hosokawa K, *et al.* Role of factor VIII C2 domain in factor VIII binding to factor Xa. *J Biol Chem* 1999; **274**: 31000–7.

12 Nogami K, Shima M, Hosokawa K, *et al.* Factor VIII C2 domain contains the thrombin-binding site responsible for thrombin-catalyzed cleavage at Arg^{1689}. *J Biol Chem* 2000; **275**: 25774–80.

13 Saenko EL, Shima M, Gilbert GE, Scandella D. Slowed release of thrombin-cleaved factor VIII from von Willebrand factor by a mon-

14 Neuenschwander PF, Jesty J. Thrombin-activated and factor Xa-activated human factor VIII: differences in cofactor activity and decay rate. *Arch Biochem Biophys* 1992; **296**: 426–34.

15 Koszelak R, Rosenblum ME, Schmidt K, *et al.* Cofactor activities of factor VIIIa and A2 subunit following cleavage of A1 subunit at Arg336. *J Biol Chem* 2002; **277**: 11664–9.

16 Nogami K, Wakabayashi H, Schmidt K, Fay PJ. Altered interactions between the A1 and A2 subunits of factor VIIIa following cleavage of A1 subunit by factor Xa. *J Biol Chem* 2003; **278**: 1634–41.

17 Fay PJ, Smudzin TM, Walker FJ. Activated protein C-catalyzed inactivation of human factor VIII and factor VIII$_a$. Identification of cleavage sites and correlation of proteolysis with cofactor activity. *J Biol Chem* 1991; **266**: 20139–45.

18 Lamphear BJ, Fay PJ. Proteolytic interactions of factor IXa with human factor VIII and factor VIIIa. *Blood* 1992; **80**: 3120–6.

19 Mertens K, Celie PH, Kolkman JA, Lenting PJ. Factor VIII-factor IX interactions: molecular sites involved in enzyme-cofactor complex assembly. *Thromb Haemost* 1999; **82**: 209–17.

20 Saenko EL, Scandella D, Yakhyaev AV, Greco N. Activation of factor VIII by thrombin increases its affinity for binding to synthetic phospholipid membranes and activated platelets. *J Biol Chem* 1998; **273**: 27918–26.

21 Kolkman JA, Christophe OD, Lenting PJ, Mertens K. Surface loop 199–204 in blood coagulation factor IX is a cofactor-dependent site involved in macromolecular substrate interaction. *J Biol Chem* 1999; **274**: 29087–93.

22 Sichler K, Kopetzki E, Huber R, *et al.* Physiological fIXa activation involves a cooperative conformational rearrangement of the 99-loop. *J Biol Chem* 2003; **278**: 4121–6.

23 Mutucumarana VP, Duffy EJ, Lollar P, Johnson AE. The active site of factor IXa is located far above the membrane surface and its conformation is altered upon association with factor VIIIa. A fluorescence study. *J Biol Chem* 1992; **267**: 17012–21.

24 Lenting PJ, van de Loo J-WHP, Donath M-JSH, *et al.* The sequence Glu1811-Lys1818 of human blood coagulation factor VIII comprises a binding site for activated factor IX. *J Biol Chem* 1996; **271**: 1935–40.

25 Fay PJ, Beattie T, Huggins CF, Regan LM. Factor VIIIa A2 subunit residues 558–565 represent a factor IXa interactive site. *J Biol Chem* 1994; **269**: 20522–7.

26 Fay PJ, Scandella D. Human inhibitor antibodies specific for the factor VIII A2 domain disrupt the interaction between the subunit and factor IXa. *J Biol Chem* 1999; **274**: 29826–30.

27 Bajaj SP, Schmidt AE, Mathur A, *et al.* Factor IXa:factor VIIIa interaction. Helix 330–338 of factor IXa interacts with residues 558–565 and spatially adjacent regions of the a2 subunit of factor VIIIa. *J Biol Chem* 2001; **276**: 16302–9.

28 Fay PJ, Koshibu K. The A2 subunit of factor VIIIa modulates the active site of factor IXa. *J Biol Chem* 1998; **273**: 19049–54.

29 Regan LM, Fay PJ. Cleavage of factor VIII light chain is required for maximal generation of factor VIIIa activity. *J Biol Chem* 1995; **270**: 8546–52.

30 Fay PJ, Mastri M, Koszelak ME, Wakabayashi H. Cleavage of factor VIII heavy chain is required for the functional interaction of A2 subunit with factor IXA. *J Biol Chem* 2001; **276**: 12434–9.

31 Lapan KA, Fay PJ. Interaction of the A1 subunit of factor VIIIa and the serine protease domain of factor X identified by zero-length cross-linking. *Thromb Haemost* 1998; **80**: 418–22.

32 Ananyeva N, Kouiavskaia D, Shima M, Saenko E. Catabolism of the coagulation factor VIII. Can we prolong lifetime of fVIII in circulation? *Trends Cardiovasc Med* 2001; **11**: 252–7.

oclonal and a human antibody is a novel mechanism for factor VIII inhibition. *J Biol Chem* 1996; **271**: 27424–31.

33 Lenting P, Neels JG, van den Berg BM, *et al.* The light chain of factor VIII comprises a binding site for low density lipoprotein receptor-related protein. *J Biol Chem* 1999; **274**: 23734–9.

34 Saenko EL, Yakhyaev AV, Mikhailenko I, *et al.* Role of the low density lipoprotein-related protein receptor in mediation of factor VIII catabolism. *J Biol Chem* 1999; **274**: 37685–92.

35 Bovenschen N, Herz J, Grimbergen JM, *et al.* Elevated plasma factor VIII in a mouse model of low-density lipoprotein receptor-related protein deficiency. *Blood* 2003; **101**: 3933–9.

36 Sarafanov AG, Ananyeva NM, Shima M, Saenko EL. Cell surface heparan sulfate proteoglycans participate in factor VIII catabolism mediated by low density lipoprotein receptor-related protein. *J Biol Chem* 2001; **276**: 11970–9.

37 Bovenschen N, Boertjes RC, van Stempvoort G, *et al.* Low density lipoprotein receptor-related protein and factor IXa share structural requirements for binding to the A3 domain of coagulation factor VIII. *J Biol Chem* 2003; **278**: 9370–7.

38 Mann KG. Biochemistry and physiology of blood coagulation. *Thromb Haemost* 1999; **82**: 165–74.

39 Ovanesov MV, Lopatina EG, Saenko EL, *et al.* Effect of factor VIII on tissue factor-initiated spatial clot growth. *Thromb Haemost* 2003; **89**: 235–42.

40 Hoffman M, Monroe DM, III. The action of high-dose factor VIIa (FVIIa) in a cell-based model of hemostasis. *Semin Hematol* 2001; **38**: 6–9.

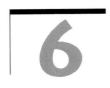

Natural history of inhibitor development in children with severe hemophilia A treated with factor VIII products

Jeanne M. Lusher

Although factor (F) VIII antibodies develop in 25–30% of children with severe hemophilia A following treatment with FVIII-containing products, many factors determine *which* individuals develop inhibitors and when they do so. Factors influencing the development of FVIII inhibitors include patient factors, as well as treatment factors (Table 6.1) [1,2].

Although occasional prospective, long-term studies of inhibitor development were carried out earlier [3], most were designed and conducted beginning in the late 1980s, when high-purity, virally inactivated products and recombinant (r) products were developed for clinical use [4–10]. These multicenter studies included inhibitor assays conducted at specified intervals after each individual's first exposure to a new FVIII product. While patient and treatment factors varied in these observational studies, certain important facts became apparent:

- Most inhibitors occur in persons with severe hemophilia A (those with baseline levels of FVIII < 0.01 U/mL).
- Most develop after relatively few exposure days (ED) to FVIII (median 9–11 ED).
- Most occur in early childhood.
- Inhibitors are more likely to occur in persons of African descent.
- Inhibitors are more likely to occur in patients whose hemophilic brother(s) have inhibitors.
- Some inhibitor patients are "high responders", having a brisk anamnestic response to FVIII, while others are "low responders", with inhibitor concentrations never exceeding a few Bethesda units (BU).
- Some inhibitors (usually low titer) disappear over time, despite continued episodic ("on-demand") treatment with FVIII.

What determines whether or not a person with hemophilia A will develop an inhibitor?

Perhaps the single most important determinant of inhibitor development is the individual's FVIII gene defect. Large deletions, premature termination (stop) codons and nonsense mutations are associated with a higher incidence of inhibitor formation [11–14]. These mutations cause failure to synthesize FVIII; thus, it appears that the individual's immune system recognizes in-fused FVIII as a foreign protein [12]. In large part because affected members of a hemophilic kindred have the same FVIII gene defect, the hemophilic brother(s) of an individual with a FVIII inhibitor are at greater risk of developing an inhibitor [13]. In each of several studies, it has been shown that persons of African descent are more likely to develop an inhibitor than are Caucasians [1,4,6,7,9]. While the reason for this is not clear, it may reflect differences in HLA type, or the influence of other modifying genes. Thus, in looking at the "natural history" of inhibitor development in people with severe hemophilia A following initiation of treatment with FVIII, one must critically look at the demographics of the study population.

Other possible risk factors

As not all individuals with severe hemophilia A who have the same underlying gene defect develop inhibitors, and neither do all hemophilic brothers of an individual with an inhibitor, it has been postulated that other factors may have an influential role. These may include other immunologic challenges occurring at the same time as a FVIII infusion, such as an intercurrent infection, immunization, or an inflammatory response to a hemorrhage. Additionally, others have postulated that frequent large doses of FVIII, as given for major surgery, or for a severe bleeding episode such as an intracranial hemorrhage or retroperitoneal hemorrhage, may predispose an individual to develop an inhibitor.

Some have noted the development of an inhibitor soon after changing the patient from one type of FVIII product to another, and felt that the change of product was causally related to the patient's inhibitor development. It should be noted, however, that there is no convincing body of evidence that any of the above "possible risk factors" play a determining role in inhibitor development.

Only rarely has a particular *product* resulted in an increased incidence of inhibitors. This did happen with each of two intermediate-purity, plasma-derived concentrates (used in Belgium, the Netherlands, and Germany). Both antigenic products had undergone solvent/detergent treatment plus pasteurization [15,16]. The combination of solvent/detergent treatment plus pasteurization was then shown to modify the FVIII molecule, resulting in heightened antigenicity of the C2 domain [17]

Table 6.1 Factors influencing the development of FVIII inhibitors. (Modified from Yee and Lee [2].)

Patient factors
Gene defect causing hemophilia
Family history of inhibitors
Ethnicity (African descent doubles the risk)
Immunologic response characteristics
Other immunologic challenges at the time of FVIII infusion (e.g., infections, vaccinations)

Treatment factors
Rarely, a particularly antigenic FVIII product
Number of exposures to FVIII
Pattern of exposures
Effects of exposure to several different products (?)

Table 6.2 Definition of incidence and prevalence in the context of inhibitors.

Incidence refers to the percentage of individuals who develop an inhibitor over a specified period of time

Prevalence refers to the percentage of individuals who have an inhibitor at a certain point in time

As new products have been developed and introduced over the past 16 years or so [plasma-derived products of higher purity and with improved methods of viral attenuation, as well as recombinant (r) FVIII concentrates], many expressed concern that each new product might prove to be more antigenic, resulting in a higher incidence of inhibitor development. Fortunately, this has not proven to be the case.

The prospective, multicenter studies conducted in the late 1980s with plasma-derived products of higher purity (and virally attenuated with pasteurization or solvent/detergent treatment) were designed primarily as hepatitis (and HIV) safety trials, and were thus short-term (approximately 6 months) studies [8]. While these studies were done on previously untreated patients (PUPs), inhibitor development may have been missed due to infrequent inhibitor assays (generally every 6 months) and the relatively short-term periods of observation. Nonetheless, the higher than expected percentage of PUPs developing inhibitors (24%, most of which were high titer) in one of these short-term hepatitis safety trials (with a monoclonal antibody-purified FVIII concentrate [8]) led to a greater concern.

Following the development of the first two rFVIII preparations, Kogenate™ (Bayer Corp., Berkeley, CA, USA) and Recombinate™ (Baxter-Hyland, Glendale, CA, USA), in the late 1980s, prospective trials in PUPS and previously treated patients (PTPs) with severe hemophilia A yielded significantly more information. These trials were longer in duration, and inhibitor assays were done more frequently (every 3 months in the PUP trials, and more often if an inhibitor was suspected clinically). Inhibitor assays (Bethesda method) were performed centrally. Interestingly, the incidence of inhibitor development with these two rFVIII products was quite similar, with 28 and 30.5% of PUPs, respectively, developing inhibitors over the study period of 5 years or 100 ED to rFVIII [6,7]. While this at first seemed higher than expected, when compared with the inhibitor incidence (52%) in a cohort of prospectively followed German patients with severe hemophilia A treated primarily with intermediate purity plasma-derived products [3], 28–32% did not seem alarmingly high. In the Ehrenforth et al. trial, the median number of ED until inhibitor development was 11.7 days, which was notably similar to that found in the two rFVIII trials. Furthermore, in each of the rPUP trials, many of the inhibitors were low titer and some of these were transient, disappearing despite continued episodic (as necessary) treatment with rFVIII. (Such transient inhibitors, which were often detected only once, or a few times, may well have been missed in older, cross-sectional or even long-term determinations of inhibitor frequency in which inhibitors were looked for much less often.) As a result of these transient inhibitors, plus others which disappeared with immune tolerance induction (ITI) with rFVIII, the *prevalence* of inhibitors at the end of each of these two trials was considerably lower than the *incidence* of inhibitor development [6,7] (Tables 6.2 and 6.3).

More recently, newer rFVIII products were developed, such as B-domain deleted (BDD) rFVIII (Wyeth's ReFacto™) [9] and products produced without addition of albumin as a stabilizer and without the use of any human or animal materials in the culture media (for example, Bayer's Kogenate™ FS, Baxter's Advate™) [10]. These have also undergone carefully designed multicenter prospective studies in PUPs and PTPs. While not all of these studies are complete, there is no evidence to date that any of these so-called second- and third-generation rFVIII products are more antigenic that earlier plasma-derived or recombinant FVIII concentrates.

The PUP study with BDD rFVIII (ReFacto™), which began in 1994, was very similar in design to the PUP studies with the two original full-length rFVIII products, Kogenate™ and Recombinate™. All subjects had severe hemophilia A, and Bethesda inhibitor assays were done every 3 months in one of two central laboratories (one for North American and one for European samples). Any sample testing positive (≥0.6 BU) by the standard Bethesda assay was retested using the Nijmegen modification [18]. As in the Kogenate™ and Recombinate™ PUP trials, all of the samples obtained at 3-month intervals for inhibitor testing were also tested for FVIII antibodies by ELISA [9]. Of the 101 severely affected PUPs enrolled and treated in the ReFacto™ trial, 32 (32%) developed inhibitors during the 5-year course of the study (27 September 1994 to 31 August 1999), after a median of 12 ED (range 3–609). The median age at the time of first infusion for the 32 PUPs who developed inhibitors was 8 months (range

Table 6.3 Rate of high-responder inhibitors in patients with severe hemophilia A. (Modified from Scharrer *et al.* [4].)

Study	Product	Period	$n < 2\%$ FVIII activity	Inhibitors (total) (%)	Inhibitors (>10 BU) (%)	Inhibitors (>5 BU) (%)	Ref.
Lusher *et al.* (2003)	ReFacto™	1994–99	101	32	12	16	9
Gruppo *et al.* (1998)	Recombinate™	1990–97	72	32	11	13	7
Lusher *et al.* (2004)	Kogenate™	1989–96	64	38	16	23	6
Lusher *et al.* (1991)	Monoclate™	1986–89	25	24	16	20	8
Ehrenforth *et al.* (1992)	Various (mainly plasma-derived concentrates, intermediate purity)	1976–91	27	52	41	44	3
Addiego *et al.* (1993)	Cryoprecipitate and low-purity products	1975–85	89	28	21	24	21
de Biasi *et al.* (1994)	Various concentrates	1975–92	48	22	17	19	20

Table 6.4 Inhibitor incidence and prevalence in the previously untreated patient cohort from the BDD rFVIII (ReFacto) trial. (Reprinted with permission from Lusher *et al.* [9]).

	October 1996 ($n = 87$)	July 1998 ($n = 101$)	February 2001 ($n = 101$)
Number of patients who developed an inhibitor	17	30	32
Median (mean) exposure days*	9 (16)	25 (70)	70 (146)
Median exposure days until inhibitor detection	11	12	12
Inhibitor incidence (%)	20	30	32
Peak titer ≥10 BU, n (%)	5 (29)	11 (37)	12 (38)
Peak titer ≥5 BU, n (%)	2 (12)	5 (17)	4 (13)
Peak titer, <5 BU, n (%)	10 (59)	14 (47)	17 (52)
Inhibitor incidence after 20 exposure days† (%)	1	5	6
Inhibitor prevalence‡ (%)	10	15	8

*Exposure days up to the time of inhibitor development in all patients.

†Seventy-five percent of patients had inhibitor detected before 16 exposure days.

‡Includes only patients whose inhibitors did not disappear (<0.6 BU/mL) with "on-demand" therapy for acute bleeding episodes, with a regimen of regular prophylaxis, or with immune tolerance therapy, regardless of study withdrawal.

<1–33 months), while the median age at the time of inhibitor detection was 16 months (range 1–62 months). Half (16) were high-titer inhibitors (≥5 BU) while the other half of the persistent antibodies were low titer, never reaching 5 BU. Eight of the 16 low-titer inhibitor patients underwent ITI; this was successful in 75% of them. Nine of 14 with high-titer inhibitors who underwent ITI had a good response during the study period. In 9 of 10 patients who did not undergo an ITI regimen (most were low-titer inhibitor patients), spontaneous disappearance of inhibitors occurred during episodic treatment with BDD rFVIII. Thus, at the end of the study, only 8 of the 101 PUPs had inhibitors (prevalence at that time, 8%) [9]. Three of three black patients in the cohort developed inhibitors as did two out of two Hispanic patients. Thus, the incidence and types of inhibitors (low or high) and number of ED until inhibitor development seen in the ReFacto™ trial were very similar to those seen in the clinical trials with the full-length recombinant and plasma-derived FVIII concentrates (Table 6.4).

One observation made in each of the PUP studies (regardless of product received) has been that persons of African descent with severe hemophilia A are much more likely to develop an FVIII inhibitor than are persons of other racial groups [1,4,6,7,9,19,20].

Thus, in reviewing published papers or data from presentations or abstracts concerning inhibitor development in persons with hemophilia A (particularly when comparing one cohort with another), one must carefully scrutinize the demographics of the cohort being described. Do all of the study subjects have severe hemophilia A, or can one at least stratify a subgroup of those within the study group who have severe hemophilia A? What percentage of study subjects are of African descent, and what percentage have a close relative with an inhibitor? If all members of the study cohort have been genotyped, what percentage have FVIII gene defects that have been associated with a high likelihood of inhibitor development?

Despite some heterogeneity in these variables, it is interesting to note that the cumulative incidence of inhibitor development is very similar, being approximately 30% in most of the recent prospective studies in PUPs with severe hemophilia A, regardless of the demographics of the study populations, and regardless of the product used for treatment [4]. A comprehensive 1999 paper by Scharrer *et al.* [4] compared the incidence of inhibitor development in severe hemophilia A patients treated with recombinant or plasma-derived FVIII products, and concluded that the data did *not* suggest a greater inhibitor risk with recombinant products than with products sourced from plasma. Their findings also demonstrated that the "most clinically relevant inhibitors" (those with peak inhibitor titers of >10 BU) occurred in 10–20% of individuals with severe hemophilia A in nearly all published studies [4]. It is noteworthy that this range (10–20%) was reported (and often quoted) as the inhibitor prevalence in older retrospective studies in which inhibitor testing was done less frequently, suggesting that many low-titer and transient inhibitors were missed.

It is also noteworthy that a relatively recent study from the UK reported a much lower incidence of inhibitors. Among 37 PUPs treated exclusively with a dry heat-treated, intermediate-purity British product (8Y, BioProducts Laboratories, Elstree, UK), only one patient developed an inhibitor (low titer, transient) during a 10-year study period (1985–95), ranging from 40 to 700 FVIII ED [2]. Otherwise, the majority of prospective studies conducted in severe hemophilia A subjects in which inhibitor assays are performed at least every 3 months over a 4- to 5-year period (or 100 ED) have shown a cumulative inhibitor incidence of ~30%.

In view of all these observations, what *is* the natural history of inhibitor development (and often "disappearance") in individuals with severe hemophilia A who are treated with FVIII products? If we look at a cohort of PUPs with severe hemophilia A, we would not expect to see any of them develop an inhibitor prior to treatment with a FVIII-containing product (such as a blood transfusion, fresh-frozen plasma, cryoprecipitate, intermediate-purity, or very high-purity plasma-derived FVIII concentrate or rFVIII). Once treatment with a FVIII-containing product is initiated, which on average is at approximately 8 months of age, one would expect that approximately 25–30% of the individuals in the cohort would develop an inhibitor after a median of 10–12 ED. (This is assuming that individuals are being checked for inhibitors at 3-month intervals.) Roughly one-third to one-half of these inhibitors will be low titer (generally defined as <5 BU, although it should be noted that some studies used a definition of <10 BU). Some of the low-titer inhibitors will be "transient", being detected on only one, a few, or several time points, despite continued episodic ("on demand") treatment with FVIII. An occasional high-titer inhibitor may also be transient.

Individuals with higher titer, clinically problematic inhibitors, or even some with low-titer inhibitors, often undergo an ITI regimen in an attempt to eradicate the inhibitor. Most ITI regimens consist of frequent infusions of higher doses of FVIII. Dosage and dosing intervals vary considerably, depending on the patient's current and historic maximum inhibitor titer, availability (including affordability) of product, and the experience and preference of the treating physician. (An ongoing multicenter, multinational study is aimed at answering some of the questions concerning the optimal protocol for ITI.) Not only before embarking on a prospective study of ITI, but whenever considering an ITI regimen for a particular patient, the patient and/or his family should be educated concerning all that is involved, including the possible need for a central venous access device, and all possible risks as well as potential benefits. In the author's experience, 75–80% of patients with severe hemophilia A with a persistent, clinically problematic inhibitor will have an excellent response to ITI, i.e., no measurable inhibitor and normal or near-normal half-life of FVIII within a few to several months (generally " 12 months). However, the family, as well as the medical staff, must be committed to a long period of frequent infusions and frequent visits to the hemophilia treatment center.

Since some inhibitors are, by their very nature, transient, and since other inhibitors respond well to an ITI regimen, a typical cohort of patients with severe hemophilia A will ultimately have an inhibitor prevalence of approximately 10%.

Transient inhibitors seldom recur. Recurrence is also rare among patients who have had an excellent response to ITI. However, many of these young patients, once tolerized, are continued on a prophylactic regimen, with a standard dose of FVIII being given two or three times a week, or as often as every other day. Thus, they may in fact be continuing on ITI under another name (prophylaxis).

While most inhibitors develop early in life (in fact, most are first noted in children under 10 years of age), some occur later. While most develop before 50 ED, there is probably no age or number of ED at which an individual is completely safe from developing an inhibitor. So, in looking at a cohort of patients, even a few of those who have not developed an inhibitor during childhood may still develop one later.

References

1 Lusher JM. Natural history of inhibitors in severe haemophilia A and B: incidence and prevalence. In: Rodriguez-Merchan ED, Lee CA, eds. *Inhibitors in Patients with Haemophilia*. Blackwell Science: Oxford, 2002: 3–8.

2 Yee TT, Lee CA. Incidence and prevalence of inhibitors and type of blood product in haemophilia A. In: Rodriguez-Merchan EC, Lee CA, eds. *Inhibitors in Patients with Haemophilia*. Blackwell Science: Oxford, 2002: 14–20.

3 Ehrenforth S, Kreuz W, Scharrer I, *et al.* Incidence of development of factor VIII and factor IX inhibitors in hemophiliacs. *Lancet* 1992; 339: 594–8.

4 Scharrer I, Bray GL, Neutzling O. Incidence of inhibitors in haemophilia A patients: a review of recent studies of recombinant and plasma-derived factor VIII concentrates. *Haemophilia* 1999; **5**: 145–54.

5 Lusher JM. Inhibitors in young boys with haemophilia. *Baillière's Best Prac Res Clin Haematol* 2000; **13**: 457–8.

6 Lusher JM, Abildgaard C, Arkin S, *et al.* Human recombinant DNA-derived antihemophilic factor in the treatment of previously untreated patients with hemophilia A: final report on a hallmark clinical investigation. *J Thromb Haemost* 2004 (in press).

7 Gruppo R, Chen H, Schroth P, Bray GL. Safety and immunogenicity of recombinant factor VIII (Recombinate) in previously untreated patients (PUPs). A 7.3 year update. Abstract no. 291, XXIII Congress of the WFH, The Hague. *Haemophilia* 1998; **4**: 228.

8 Lusher JM. Viral safety and inhibitor development associated with monoclonal antibody-purified FVIIIc. *Ann Hematol* 1991; **63**: 138–41.

9 Lusher JM, Lee CA, Kessler CM, Bedrosian CL. The safety and efficacy of B-domain deleted recombinant factor VIII concentrate in patients with severe haemophilia A. *Haemophilia* 2003; **9**: 38–49.

10 Ewenstein B, Collins P, Shapiro A, Tarantino M, *et al.* Global evaluation of Advate rAHF-PFM, an advanced category antihemophilic factor prepared using a plasma/albumin-free method. *Blood* 2003; **102**: 52a, abstract 172.

11 Schwaab R, Brackmann HH, Seehafer J *et al.* Haemophilia A: mutation type determines risk of inhibitor formation. *Thromb Haemost* 1995; **74**: 1402–6.

12 Tuddenham EGD, McVey JH. The genetic basis of inhibitor development in haemophilia A. *Haemophilia* 1998; **4**: 543–5.

13 Astermark J, Berntorp E, White GC, Kroner BL, and the MIBS Study Group. The Malmö International Brother Study (MIBS): further support for genetic predisposition to inhibitor development. *Haemophilia* 2001; **7**: 267–72.

14 Oldenburg J, Tuddenham E. Genetic basis of inhibitor development in severe haemophilia A and B. In: Rodriguez-Merchan EC, Lee CA, eds. *Inhibitors in Patients with Haemophilia.* Blackwell Science: Oxford, 2002: 21–6.

15 Rosendaal FR, Nieuwenhuis HK, van den Berg HM, *et al.* A sudden increase in factor VIII inhibitor development in multitransfused hemophilia A patients in The Netherlands. *Blood* 1993; **81**: 2180–6.

16 Peerlinck K, Arnout J, Gilles JG, *et al.* Factor VIII inhibitors in previously treated haemophilia A patients with a double virus-inactivated plasma derived factor VIII concentrate. *Thromb Haemost* 1997; **77**: 80–6.

17 Laub R, di Giambattista M, Fondu P, *et al.* Restricted epitope specificity of factor VIII inhibitors which appeared in previously treated hemophiliacs after infusion with OCTAVI DS plus. Abstract no. OC-2409, ISTH Congress, Florence. *Thromb Haemost* 1997 (Suppl.): 590.

18 Verbrugen B, Novakova I, Wessels H, *et al.* The Nijmegen modification of the Bethesda assay for factor VIII inhibitors: improved specificity and reliability. *Thromb Haemost* 1995; **73**: 247–51.

19 Rothschild C, Laurian Y, Satre EP, *et al.* Inhibitor incidence in French previously untreated patients (PUPs) with severe haemophilia A receiving recombinant factor VIII. One-year additional exposure to rFVIII. Abstract no. 285, XXIII Congress of the WFH, The Hague. *Haemophilia* 1998; **4**: 227.

20 Addiego JE, Kasper CK, Abildgaard CF, *et al.* Frequency of inhibitor development in haemophiliacs treated with low-purity factor VIII. *Lancet* 1993; **342**: 462–4.

7 Prophylaxis

H. Marijke van den Berg and Kathelijn Fischer

Introduction

The prevention of bleedings in hemophilia by prophylactic therapy has now been advocated for almost half a century. It started with the observation that the clinical phenotype of patients with moderate hemophilia was very different from severe hemophilia [1]. Patients with moderate hemophilia with factors VIII/IX of >0.01–0.05 IU/L bleed only after trauma and have a fairly normal life expectancy, while patients with severe hemophilia (factor VIII/IX < 0.01 IU/mL) have spontaneous severe muscle and joint bleedings and early crippling from hemophilic arthropathy, with a life expectancy of only 20 years. Because of this observation, it seemed logical, in patients with severe hemophilia, to increase the level of clotting factor activity above 1%.

Professor Inga Marie Nilsson from Malmö, Sweden, was the first to start prophylactic treatment with cryoprecipitate in boys with severe hemophilia A [1]. The patients first started on prophylactic therapy were those with frequent bleedings. Observation of those boys demonstrated that their number of bleeds decreased and that they lost fewer days from school or work. This Swedish initiative was repeated in the Netherlands: Professor Van Creveld undertook a similar experiment on two boys with severe bleeding and also demonstrated that it was possible to reduce the number and the severity of bleedings [2]. Once clotting factor concentrates became more available, the group of patients that received prophylaxis was extended. Also, studies became available that investigated the dose and frequency of the administered clotting factors necessary to prevent patients from bleeding [3,4]. The patients who initially received prophylaxis had already experienced joint bleeding and in effect received what has become known as "secondary" prophylaxis since it was initiated after the development of primary joint dysfunction from recurrent hemarthroses. The data on this first group of patients showed that it was possible to prevent bleedings, but joint function deteriorated further. Therefore, it was concluded that, in order to preserve joint function completely, all joint bleeds should be prevented. So, in subsequent years, prophylaxis was started earlier, before the occurrence of joint damage (primary prophylaxis) [1,5–9,10].

During the last few decades, more European countries have initiated long-term prophylactic therapy. The German experience has been reported by Schramm [11] and by Brackmann *et al.* [12]. In their first study, a comparison was made between 70 patients treated on demand and 17 treated with prophylaxis. It was shown that patients on prophylaxis had fewer joint bleeds (9.1 versus 14.3 per year). However, the age range of the patients on prophylaxis was very broad (4–36 years), making a comparison of outcome difficult. In the second study [12], the clinical and radiologic assessments of pediatric patients followed from 1978 to 1989 were presented. An individualized regimen was used: after receiving prophylaxis during childhood, many patients were switched to on-demand treatment in adulthood without important changes in their bleeding pattern. With this regimen, 58% of patients had radiological scores of zero (see Chapter 32 for discussion of the Pettersson score). Over the 12-year period, clinical scores improved slightly, but radiologic scores remained stable.

In the UK, prophylactic therapy was started on a small scale during the 1970s and has since been prescribed for an increasing number of children with severe hemophilia. Liesner *et al.* [13] performed a study on 27 boys with severe hemophilia whose mean age was 8.5 years and who had started with prophylaxis at a mean age of 6.2 years. Follow-up was short, with a mean of 30 months, but a reduction in bleeds, clinical problems, and hospital admissions was clearly demonstrated.

Manco-Johnson *et al.* [14] published a detailed report on 13 patients with severe hemophilia who started prophylaxis at a mean age of 6.9 years (range 2–12.5 years). Most boys already had target joints before they started prophylaxis. Joint disease which was already present on X-rays at the start of prophylaxis did not return to normal. The development of arthropathy was also evaluated in a later German study. Stringent prophylactic therapy was started in boys aged 3–6 years with severe hemophilia who had normal baseline clinical and radiologic scores. Prophylaxis was begun after a median of six joint bleeds. After 3 years of follow-up, they had abnormal joints despite their prophylactic regimen [15]. The authors emphasized that prophylaxis should be started before the occurrence of joint damage because secondary prophylaxis was ineffective in reversing the radiologic findings. This eventually led to the definition of primary prophylaxis: regular continuous treatment commences before the age of 2 years or after the occurrence of the first joint bleed [16].

The optimal treatment regimen for prophylaxis

The half-life of clotting factor concentrates is short: for factor VIII it is about 8 h in children and about 12 h in adults. By contrast, the mean half-life for factor IX is about 24 h [17]. As a consequence, prophylactic administration is most effective when given frequently. Carlsson et al. [18] calculated that daily prophylactic infusions would reduce factor VIII use by 82%. In addition, efficiency could further be improved by taking the patient's individual pharmacokinetic profile into account [19]. In theory, daily prophylactic infusions would be most cost-effective. In practice, however, the lifelong need for frequent intravenous injections, especially with prophylactic treatment, imposes a heavy burden on the patient and his family [20,21]; hence, very few patients take daily prophylaxis.

Prophylactic therapy is typically given in a dose of 25–40 IU/kg three times per week. This dosing is predicated on the original Swedish protocol, which targeted a preinfusion level of >1% in order to mimic the clinical phenotype of moderate hemophilia (high-dose regimen). In contrast, in the Netherlands, prophylactic dosages are adjusted according to bleeding pattern and aimed at preventing spontaneous joint bleeds. Trough levels are not taken into account. Commonly, this strategy is associated with a relatively low clotting factor consumption (intermediate-dose regimen).

Both Sweden and the Netherlands have followed their cohorts of patients with severe hemophilia longitudinally in using a comparable strategy for follow-up. Therefore, the long-term outcome of these cohorts gives information on the extent to which bleeding and arthropathy can be prevented with these two regimens. Although in both countries prophylaxis has been intensified over the decades, the difference in their treatment regimens remains considerable. All patients born between 1970 and 1990 were included in a retrospective study comparing the regimens of the Malmö and the Van Creveld Kliniek (n = 128). No selection of patients was made. Only the country of birth determined treatment regimen [22]. Patients were divided, according to age, into two groups. For patients born in the 1970s, twice-weekly prophylaxis was started earlier in the intermediate-dose group. This changed in the 1980s (Table 7.1). Radiologic evaluation of the Swedish cohort was performed 5 years earlier than in the case of the Dutch cohort. Patients treated with the high-dose regimen had fewer joint bleeds per year. When long-term orthopedic outcomes were compared, the eldest Swedish group had a total Pettersson mean score of 4 points, compared with 10 points for the Dutch cohort; however, this difference was not statistically different (Table 7.2). This same trend could be seen for the youngest group; although both groups had a mean total score of zero, the proportion of patients with a zero score was 100% for the Swedish patients and 54% for the Dutch cohort. The largest differences were the clotting factor consumption per kilogram per year. In all age groups, this was at least twice as high for the Swedish patients (Table 7.2). It can be concluded that both prophylactic regimens have demonstrated that they are able to prevent arthropathy to a large extent. Further follow-up of both cohorts, preferably at the same points in time, needs to be performed in order to compare cost efficacy of the regimens. The youngest groups in particular are very interesting as most of these patients received primary prophylaxis. Apart from the Pettersson score and MRI, the clinical status requires further evaluation with validated functional methods.

When to start prophylaxis

As the preceding discussion indicates, the timing of the initiation of prophylaxis is an important issue: the long-term experience of the Swedish group has shown that early prophylaxis can prevent joint damage [1,5–9]. In addition, it has been shown that late prophylaxis may decrease, but does not stop, further deterioration of damaged joints [23].

Recently, it has been suggested that prophylactic treatment should be individualized according to patient characteristics [24–26]. One of the arguments in favor of an individualized approach is the large variability of bleeding patterns in patients with severe hemophilia, as reflected also by the age at first joint bleed, ranging in several studies from 0.2 to 5.8 years

Table 7.1 Comparison of patient characteristics, treatment history, and long-term orthopedic outcome according to year of birth and prophylactic treatment strategy between the high-dose regimen of Sweden and the intermediate-dose regimen of the Netherlands.

	Patients born 1970–79			Patients born 1980–89		
	Intermediate dose (the Netherlands) (n = 44)	High dose (Sweden) (n = 24)	P-value	Intermediate dose (the Netherlands) (n = 42)	High dose (Sweden) (n = 18)	P-value
Age at evaluation (years)	22.7 (20.4–25.3)	17.2 (15.2–20.4)	<0.01	13.5 (10.6–15.7)	9.0 (6.3–13.5)	<0.01
Age at start of prophylaxis 2×/week (year)	5.5 (4.2–8.7)	12.1 (9.5–13.6)	<0.01	4.7 (3.7–6.2)	2.1 (1.2–4.6)	<0.01
Joint bleeds/year (n)*	2.5 (1–5.7)	0.5 (0.2–1.8)	<0.01	3.7 (1.7–5)	0.2 (0–0.3)	<0.01
Patients without joint bleeds (%)*	5	25		10	50	
Clinical score (maximum 90)	2 (0–5)	0 (0–4)	0.45	0 (0–2)	0 (0–0)	<0.01
Pettersson score (maximum 78)	10 (3.5–17.5)	4 (0–15)	0.75	0 (0–5)	0	<0.01

*Values are medians (interquartile ranges).

Table 7.2 Treatment received in the last 3 years before evaluation (last Pettersson score), according to year of birth and treatment strategy for the high-dose Swedish regimen and the intermediate-dose Dutch regimen.

	Patients born 1970–79			Patients born 1980–89		
	Intermediate dose ($n = 44$)	High dose ($n = 24$)	P-value	Intermediate dose ($n = 42$)	High dose ($n = 18$)	P-value
On full prophylaxis (> 45 weeks/year) (%)	82	100	0.22	100	100	
Frequency of prophylaxis (n/week)	3 (2–3)	3 (2–3)	0.68	3 (2.5–3)	3.3 (3–3.5)	<0.01
Dose of prophylaxis (IU/kg/week)	35 (24–44)	82 (57–90)	<0.01	40 (33–49)	89 (78–107)	<0.01
Annual clotting factor use (IU/kg/year)	1466 (1039–1926)	4301 (3034–4726)	<0.01	2126 (1743–2755)	4616 (4105–5571)	<0.01

Values are medians (interquartile ranges) or percentages.

[25,27,28]. It has been suggested that arthropathy is best prevented if prophylaxis is started before the second [15] or third [25] joint bleed, but the benefits of starting before the first joint bleed have not been established. It has been shown that patients on prophylaxis still experience joint bleeds [5,13,15,23,29]. Thus, starting prophylaxis before the first joint bleed postpones its occurrence, but joint bleeds are not completely prevented. An advantage of later start of prophylaxis is that it is more likely to prevent the use of central venous catheters [30]. This advantage is counterbalanced by data of Petrini et al., which support an early start to prophylaxis [8,9]. In two cohorts of seven boys with severe hemophilia, it was demonstrated that the children who started prophylaxis at a mean age of 3 years had a better outcome than the boys who started at a mean age of 5 years. The dosing and frequencies of administration in both groups were the same and the total dose was approximately 3000 IU/kg/year. An update of the total Swedish cohort was performed recently [26]. In an analysis of 121 patients with severe hemophilia, it was demonstrated that age at start of prophylaxis was an independent predictor for the development of arthropathy, but dose and interval of prophylaxis at the start of prophylactic treatment were not [24].

Prophylaxis versus on-demand therapy — issues of cost-effectiveness

Until now, three large studies have prospectively compared prophylaxis with on-demand treatment, two in children [23,29] and one in adults [31]. A large prospective multicenter study on 477 patients with severe hemophilia has been reported by Aledort et al. [23]. All patients were younger than 25 years and were followed for a period of 5 years. Orthopedic examinations were performed annually and the radiologic score was measured at study entry and exit. The major determinants for joint outcome

were the number of joint bleeds and whether a patient had received prophylaxis for more than 45 weeks per year. A multicenter US study by Smith et al. [29] described 96 patients with a follow-up of 2 years. Both studies reported fewer bleeding episodes and approximately 200% higher clotting factor consumption for patients treated with prophylaxis. For adults with severe hemophilia, Szucs et al. [32] reported a lower number of joint bleeds, but also a lower (<100%) increase of clotting factor consumption. The period of follow-up in this study was 6 months and the number of weeks on prophylaxis per year was not described. No differentiation between primary and secondary prophylaxis was made. Thus, the difference in bleeding episodes may be underestimated and the difference in clotting factor consumption between both treatment strategies may have been overestimated because prophylaxis was prescribed to patients with more severe bleeding patterns.

When comparing the effects of prophylaxis in pediatric studies with those in adult studies, the differential clotting factor consumption between prophylaxis and on-demand regimens appears to decrease with age. The trend of decreasing clotting factor consumption with age for patients on prophylaxis has been reported previously [5,33]. By contrast, for on-demand treatment clotting factor consumption appears to increase with age. This may be due to greater bleeding from worsening arthropathy, as was suggested in the economic analysis of the study by Aledort et al. [34]. However, because prophylaxis offers distinct and substantial clinical (and probably also psychologic) benefits, this treatment strategy may be warranted on medical rather than economic grounds. A similar cost–utility study has been performed in the UK [35]. In their study design, the authors compared hypothetical cohorts of 100 individuals with severe hemophilia or severe von Willebrand's disease. Although they calculated a significant difference between prophylactic and on-demand therapy, they stated that prophylaxis was cost-effective compared with treatment on demand in some scenarios. They recommended more research to assess the relationship between treatment modalities and the respective clotting factor use and the resultant health-related quality of life.

Recently, a comparison was made between Norwegian patients treated on demand and Swedish patients treated with prophylaxis [36]. One hundred and fifty-six patients with severe hemophilia were studied, including 61 Norwegian patients treated with on-demand therapy and 95 Swedish patients treated with prophylaxis. The number of surgical procedures performed for arthropathy was substantially higher in patients treated on demand than in those on prophylaxis: patients on prophylactic therapy had a 50% lower probability of undergoing a major surgical procedure. In addition, days lost from school or work for hemophilia-related causes was higher. The median annual clotting factor consumption was 780 IU/kg/year for on-demand therapy and 3024 IU/kg/year for patients on prophylaxis.

Another study comparing on-demand versus prophylaxis examined cohorts from France and the Netherlands born between 1970 and 1980 and followed consecutively for 20 years [37]. In this study, an "intention to treat" model was utilized; the prevailing treatment strategies in the two countries determined whether patients received either on-demand or prophylactic therapy. Both cohorts were on early home treatment and had free access to clotting factor concentrates. The average annual clotting factor consumption was 1612 IU/kg for the cohort of patients treated on demand compared with 1488 IU/kg for the cohort of patients treated initially with intermediate prophylaxis. However, the orthopedic outcome for the French patients who received the on-demand strategy was significantly worse, with a mean total Pettersson score of 16 compared with 7 in the prophylaxis group (Figure 7.1). In addition, 55% of the

French patients needed rehabilitative orthopedic surgery compared with only 20% of the Dutch patients. To determine the differential clotting factor consumption from childhood to adulthood, data from a nonselected subgroup of both cohorts were analyzed (Figure 7.2). In the first decade, there was clearly a higher clotting factor consumption in the on-demand group than in prophylaxis cohort studies. However, this disappeared during subsequent decades of adult follow-up.

It is worth conjecturing that patients treated on demand will likely require even more treatment in the years to come because of their longer lifespan. With modern treatment, patients with severe hemophilia have a normal life expectancy. It can therefore be hypothesized that prophylaxis may become more cost-effective, with less burden for the patient, as patients treated exclusively by on-demand regimens survive more years with extensive hemarthropathy, requiring frequent infusions of clotting factor concentrates.

Future issues in prophylaxis

Both the high costs of prophylaxis and the lack of randomized controlled trials comparing prophylaxis with on-demand therapy have been important reasons for its limited introduction. Two randomized controlled trials comparing intensive on-demand therapy and primary prophylaxis are currently under way: one in the USA by Manco-Johnson and Blanchette [38] and one in Italy by Gringeri [39]. It has to be determined whether or not the results of these trials will favor prophylaxis. Especially in children, clotting factor consumption for prophylaxis is expected to be 2–3 times higher than with on-demand therapy. The beneficial effects of prophylaxis for both clotting factor consumption and prevention of hemophilic arthropathy are to be

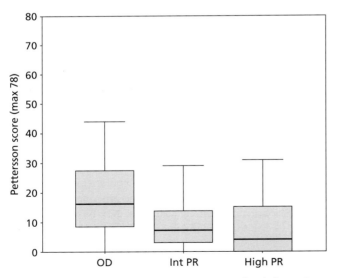

Figure 7.1 Long-term orthopedic outcome estimated with the total Pettersson score in the French cohort treated on demand (OD) compared with the Dutch cohort treated with intermediate-dose prophylaxis (Int PR) and the Swedish cohort treated with high-dose prophylaxis (High PR) [43].

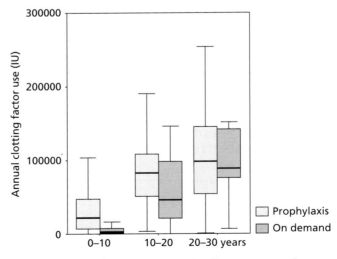

Figure 7.2 Clotting factor consumption for all treatment years for patients treated on demand (OD) versus intermediate-dose prophylaxis (Int PR).

expected only after a minimum of 20 years. It can be anticipated that after 6 years of follow-up, as has been hypothesized in these trials, there may be a small difference in clinical and radiologic outcome in favor of prophylaxis, but at a higher cost for clotting factor consumption and a higher burden of frequent venous access. When health-related quality-of-life measurements are taken into account, they may also be lower for children receiving early prophylaxis, owing to the morbidity associated with frequent venous punctures. The potential exists that this could create a misleading view that prophylaxis is not preferable to on-demand therapy – although better clinical outcome over time would likely supersede any rash preliminary conclusion.

An option for making prophylactic therapy affordable for more patients may be to prescribe primary prophylaxis for young children with a dose and frequency intended to prevent all bleeds and then to stop prophylaxis in adulthood. This was proposed previously in 1992, with one group suggesting that prophylaxis be a standard of treatment until age 18 only [12]. No follow-up reports from this group of treaters have been forthcoming to date. Recently, data from a cohort study of 49 patients with severe hemophilia suggested that 22% of patients treated exclusively with prophylaxis could change to on-demand therapy in adulthood without compromising their "normal" clinical outcome [40]. Apparently, these patients were all treated with early prophylaxis but were characterized by a milder bleeding pattern than the patients who continued prophylaxis. However, the long-term effects of discontinuing prophylaxis in patients with milder bleeding patterns need to be assessed, preferably in a prospective study, before this becomes standard therapy. It is a very challenging option and would permit primary prophylaxis to become an obtainable goal for a much larger group of children in societies where economic constraints have thus far precluded use of "universal" prophylaxis.

Implementation of prophylaxis — comparison of the USA/Canada and Europe

Although advised by both the Medical and Scientific Advisory Council (MASAC) of the National Hemophilia Foundation (NHF) in the USA and the World Federation of Hemophilia (WFH) in 1994, the worldwide introduction of prophylaxis has been slow. Recently, two surveys have been performed on the introduction of prophylaxis, one by Dr Ljung through the European Pediatric Network and one by Dr Blanchette in Canada and the USA [16,41]. In the European survey, full prophylaxis was defined as at least twice a week for >45 weeks per year. For North America, only once-a-week prevention infusions were required to qualify as "prophylaxis". Hence, the number of patients on complete prophylaxis in the USA/Canada survey may be overestimated. The European survey included 1583 patients up to 18 years of age, treated in 20 hemophilia centers. Thirty-nine percent of these patients received primary prophylaxis, 40% secondary prophylaxis, and 19% were still treated by on-demand therapy (the remaining 2% of the patients did not yet receive treatment). The USA/Canadian survey, conducted in 2002 and including 1667 boys up to 18 years of age with severe hemophilia A, reported 47% of hemophilic boys in the USA and 77% of boys living in Canada to be receiving prophylaxis.

A very important issue for the future is how will physicians decide whether to use prophylaxis in children less than 5 years old. The physicians in the USA/Canada survey reported about 30% full prophylaxis (at least twice a week) for this age group. Similar data from the European cohort are not yet available. However, a different attitude could be detected in the willingness to participate in a randomized controlled trial comparing prophylaxis with on-demand therapy. From the doctors treating hemophilia that responded in the USA and Canada, 62% were willing to participate in such a trial, while this was not the case in Europe. The physicians of the European Paediatric Network were all in favor of starting early prophylaxis, and stated that this was the treatment they were planning to give to their future children. By contrast, in the US and Canada, 38% of the hemophilia centers reported that they would start primary prophylaxis and 66% of the centers were still in favor of secondary prophylaxis.

Interestingly, studies on escalating-dose regimens, which start with prophylaxis once weekly and increase the frequency of infusions according to bleeding pattern, are currently under way in both Canada and the USA [38,42].

Controversies in prophylaxis

The introduction of prophylaxis on a large scale has been hampered mainly by the high cost of treatment, with limited data on long-term outcome cost-effectiveness. Because the results of prophylaxis are only visible after long-term follow-up, evidence for the benefits of prophylaxis determined by randomized controlled trials (RCTs) is lacking. Another reason to be reluctant to start prophylaxis in very young children has been the alleged risk of inhibitor development. The reported incidence of inhibitor development varies from 10% to 50%. However, from the cohorts with a long-term follow-up on prophylaxis, the incidence of *persistent* inhibitor varied between 15% and 20% [22]. This suggests that the frequency of inhibitor development in children started early on prophylaxis is lower than for the children receiving on-demand therapy, although this requires confirmation from prospective studies. It can be hypothesized that, by giving frequent therapy, some low-responder inhibitors disappear before they become clinically important.

Another problem with the early start of prophylaxis is the difficulty of venous access in young children. The use of central venous catheters is associated with side-effects, especially the occurrence of infections. The reported incidence of infections varies between 0.23 and 1.8 per 1000 patient-days [43,44]. However, a very important benefit of the implantation of a central catheter is often forgotten: the feasibility of early home treatment by the parents. In the cohort of the Van Creveld Kliniek, home treatment was started almost 2 years earlier in the patients with a central catheter (mean age of 2.8 years versus a mean of 4.5 years in the children without a central catheter). This has made coping with hemophilia much easier for the parents.

Concluding remarks

Although it has been proven that early prophylactic therapy can prevent bleeding and arthropathy, it is currently attainable only for a small proportion of children with severe hemophilia. Products are now safe and inhibitor development does not appear to be increased in patients on prophylaxis. However, the high costs are the main reason for its slow introduction. Because the beneficial effects of early prophylaxis are much higher than for secondary prophylaxis, this should be the treatment of choice for young children. Once these children have reached adulthood, with normal joints and muscles, they may be able to continue with on-demand therapy thereafter.

References

1 Nilsson IM, Blomback M, Ahlberg A. Our experience in Sweden with prophylaxis on haemophilia. *Bibl Haematol* 1970; **34**: 111–24.
2 Van Creveld S. Prophylaxis of joint hemorrhages in hemophilia. *Acta Haematol* 1969; **41**: 206–14.
3 Schimpf K, Fischer B, Rothmann P. A controlled study of treating haemophilia A on an out-patient basis [author's transl.]. *Dtsch Med Wochenschr* 1976; **101**: 141–8.
4 Aronstam A, Kirk PJ, McHardy J, et al. Twice weekly prophylactic therapy in haemophilia A. *J Clin Pathol* 1977; **30**: 65–7.
5 Lofqvist T, Nilsson IM, Berntorp E, Pettersson H. Haemophilia prophylaxis in young patients—a long-term follow-up. *J Intern Med* 1997; **241**: 395–400.
6 Nilsson IM, Berntorp E, Lofqvist T, Pettersson H. Twenty-five years' experience of prophylactic treatment in severe haemophilia A and B. *J Intern Med* 1992; **232**: 25–32.
7 Nilsson IM. Experience with prophylaxis in Sweden. *Semin Hematol* 1993; **30**: 16–19.
8 Petrini P, Lindvall N, Egberg N, Blomback M. Prophylaxis with factor concentrates in preventing hemophilic arthropathy. *Am J Pediatr Hematol Oncol* 1991; **13**: 280–7.
9 Petrini P. What factors should influence the dosage and interval of prophylactic treatments in patients with severe haemophila A and B? *Haemophilia* 2001; **7**: 99–104.
10 Liesner RJ. Prophylaxis in haemophilic children. *Blood Coagul Fibrinolysis* 1997; **8** (Suppl. 1): S7–10.
11 Schramm W. Experience with prophylaxis in Germany. *Semin Hematol* 1993; **30**: 12–15.
12 Brackmann HH, Eickhoff HJ, Oldenburg J, Hammerstein U. Long-term therapy and on-demand treatment of children and adolescents with severe haemophilia A: 12 years of experience. *Hemostasis* 1992; **22**: 251–8.
13 Liesner RJ, Khair K, Hann IM. The impact of prophylactic treatment on children with severe haemophilia. *Br J Haematol* 1996; **92**: 973–8.
14 Manco-Johnson MJ, Nuss R, Geraghty S, Funk S, Kilcoyne R. Results of secondary prophylaxis in children with severe hemophilia. *Am J Hematol* 1994; **47**: 113–17.
15 Kreuz W, Escuriola-Ettingshausen C, Funk M, et al. When should prophylactic treatment in patients with haemophilia A and B start? The German experience. *Haemophilia* 1998; **4**: 413–17.
16 Ljung R, Aronis-Vournas S, Kurnik-Auberger K, et al. Treatment of children with haemophilia in Europe: a survey of 20 centres in 16 countries. *Haemophilia* 2000; **6**: 619–24.
17 Matucci M, Messori A, Donati-Cori G, et al. Kinetic evaluation of four Factor VIII concentrates by model-independent methods. *Scand J Haematol* 1985; **34**: 22–8.
18 Carlsson M, Berntorp E, Bjorkman S, Lindvall K. Pharmacokinetic dosing in prophylactic treatment of hemophilia A. *Eur J Haematol* 1993; **51**: 247–52.
19 Berntorp E, Bjorkman S.
20 Steinglass P. Psychosocial issues related to prophylactic therapy for severe hemophilia. *Semin Hematol* 1994; **31**: 19–25.
21 Miller R, Sabin CA, Goldman E, et al. Coping styles in families with haemophilia. *Psychol Health Med* 2000; **5**: 3–12.
22 Fischer K, Astermark J, van der Bom JG, et al. Prophylactic treatment for severe haemophilia: comparison of an intermediate-dose to a high-dose regimen. *Haemophilia* 2002; **8**: 753–60.
23 Aledort LM, Haschemeyer R, Pettersson H. A longitudinal study of orthopaedic outcomes for severe factor VIII-deficient hemophiliacs. The Orthopaedic Outcome study. *J Intern Med* 1994; **236**: 391–9.
24 Astermark J, Petrini P, Tengborn L, et al. Primary prophylaxis in severe haemophilia should be started at an early age but can be individualized. *Br J Haematol* 1999; **105**: 1109–13.
25 Fischer K, van Hout BA, van der Bom JG, et al. Association between joint bleeds and Pettersson scores in severe haemophilia. *Acta Radiol* 2002; **43**: 528–32.
26 Petrini P. What factors should influence the dosage and interval of prophylactic treatment in patients with severe haemophilia A and B? *Haemophilia* 2001; **7**: 99–102.
27 Pollmann H, Linnenbecker S. The frequency of joint bleedings in early childhood in patients with severe haemophilia. *WFH* 1996; **17**: PAGE.
28 Fischer K, van der Bom JG, Mauser-Bunschoten EP, et al. The effects of postponing prophylactic treatment on long-term outcome in patients with severe haemophilia. *Blood* 2002; **99**: 2337–41.
29 Smith PS, Teutsch SM, Shaffer PA, et al. Episodic versus prophylactic infusions for hemophilia A: a cost-effectiveness analysis. *J Pediatr* 1996; **129**: 424–31.
30 Berntorp E, Bjorkman S. The pharmacokinetics of clotting factor therapy. *Haemophilia* 2003; **9**: 353–9.
31 Szucs TD, Offner A, Schramm W. Socioeconomic impact of haemophilia care: results of a pilot study. *Haemophilia* 1996; **2**: 000.
32 Royal S, Schramm W, Berntorp E, et al. Quality-of-life differences between prophylactic and on-demand factor replacement therapy in European haemophilia patients. *Haemophilia* 2002; **8**: 44–50.
33 Britten AF. Prophylaxis in hemophilia. *Bibl Haematol* 1970; **34**: 104–110.
34 Bohn RL, Avorn J, Glynn RJ, et al. Prophylactic use of factor VIII: an economic evaluation. *Thromb Haemost* 1998; **79**: 932–7.
35 Miners AH, Sabin CA, Tolley KH, Lee CA. Cost-utility analysis of primary prophylaxis versus treatment on-demand for individuals with severe haemophilia. *Pharmacoeconomics* 2002; **20**: 759–74.
36 Steen CK, Hojgard S, Glomstein A, et al. On-demand vs. prophylactic treatment for severe haemophilia in Norway and Sweden: differences in treatment characteristics and outcome. *Haemophilia* 2003; **9**: 555–66.
37 Fischer K, van der Bom JG, Molho P, et al. Prophylactic versus on-demand treatment strategies for severe haemophilia: a comparison of costs and long-term outcome. *Haemophilia* 2002; **8**: 745–52.

38 Manco-Johnson MJ, Blanchette VS. North American prophylaxis studies for persons with severe haemophilia: background, rationale and design. *Haemophilia* 2003; **9**: 44–8.

39 Gringeri A. Prospective controlled studies on prophylaxis: an Italian approach. *Haemophilia* 2003; **9**: 38–42.

40 Fischer K, van der Bom JG, Prejs R, *et al.* Discontinuation of prophylactic therapy in severe haemophilia: incidence and effects on outcome. *Haemophilia* 2001; **7**: 544–50.

41 Blanchette VS, McCready M, Achonu C, *et al.* A survey of factor prophylaxis in boys with haemophilia followed in North American haemophilia treatment centres. *Haemophilia* 2003; **9**: 19–26.

42 Berntorp E, Astermark J, Bjorkman S, *et al.* Consensus perspectives on prophylactic therapy for haemophilia: summary statement. *Haemophilia* 2003; **9**: 1–4.

43 Liesner RJ, Vora AJ, Hann IM, Lilleymann JS. Use of central venous catheters in children with severe congenital coagulopathy. *Br J Haematol* 1995; **91**: 203–7.

44 Ljung R, van den BM, Petrini P, *et al.* Port-A-Cath usage in children with haemophilia: experience of 53 cases. *Acta Paediatr* 1998; **87**: 1051–4.

45 Fischer K, Van Den BM. Proclinical and economical issues. *Haemophilia* 2003; **9**: 376–81.

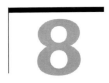

Continuous infusion of coagulation products in hemophilia

Uri Martinowitz and Angelika Batorova

Introduction

Continuous infusion (CI) of coagulation factors at a rate corresponding to their pharmacokinetic elimination was suggested by Brinkhous as early as 1954 [1]. The first report of therapeutic CI of factor VIII (FVIII), employing cryoprecipitate and glycine-precipitated concentrate, was published almost 20 years later [2], and the mathematical model for such treatment was developed shortly afterwards [3]. The model demonstrated that CI reduced overall FVIII requirement by 30% by eliminating the unnecessary peaks of FVIII that commonly accompany treatment by intermittent bolus injection (BI). Despite the demonstrated benefit of CI of FVIII in initial reports [4], this mode of therapy has not been widely used. Reasons for this include a lack of information about the stability of concentrates after reconstitution, the frequent development of thrombophlebitis at the site of infusion, concern regarding bacterial contamination (with risk of bacterial overgrowth in the reconstituted concentrate retained for hours in the container at room temperature), and a lack of data and guidelines on dosing and dose adjustment. These limitations inspired extensive research in the early 1990s [5,6]. Since then, CI has been incorporated into standard hemophilia care practice in many hemophilia centers worldwide.

Pharmacokinetic rationale for continuous infusion regimen

The idea of administering coagulation factors by CI was conceived by Brinkhous [1] and was supported by the theoretical work of Hermens [3], who developed a mathematical model of different modes of administration of FVIII and FIX. The dose needed to keep the plasma level above a desired hemostatic minimum increases linearly with the interval between injections. The total dose, which is minimized when FVIII is infused continuously, is 7% higher when FVIII is given every 2 h and 120% higher if given at 24-h intervals. McMillan *et al.* [2], who observed that the plasma level of FVIII remained steady after 12 h of constant infusion of the glycine-precipitated concentrate, concluded that CI could also ensure a steady minimum FVIII level during surgery. Hathaway *et al.* [4] found that, using CI, minimum FVIII levels were higher than when the same daily amount of FVIII was administered by conventional bolus therapy. In both cases, the authors suggested a dosage regimen for FVIII by CI based on the observation that the infusion rate of 2 IU/kg/h produces a plasma FVIII level of around 0.5 IU/mL.

The differences between CI and intermittent BI are demonstrated schematically in Figure 8.1. The area under the curve (AUC) that corresponds to the total amount of FVIII required when injections are administered every 12 h (BI q 12h) is approximately 30% greater than the AUC that results from CI (adjusted dose). However, when FVIII is infused at a constant rate, higher than expected levels are observed (fixed-rate CI), which is caused by a gradual decrease in the clearance after a steady hemostatic factor level has been achieved [6]. The reason for the reduced clearance observed during CI of FVIII, FIX, von Willebrand factor, and, although inconsistently, recombinant FVIIa (rFVIIa) is still not clear. However, this phenomenon provides a potential for additional saving of factor concentrates by permitting downward adjustment of the rate of infusion proportionate to the decreasing clearance. This was the rationale for the guidelines for the adjusted-dose continuous infusion of coagulation factors introduced by Martinowitz *et al.* in 1992 [5].

Essentials for continuous infusion of coagulation factors

Stability of concentrates and mode of continuous administration

The current mode of CI, using portable minipumps or syringe pumps to deliver concentrated factors, developed from studies that showed that most currently available concentrates, either plasma derived (pdFVIII/IX) or recombinant (rFVIII/IX), remain stable after reconstitution and storage at room temperature for several days, and sometimes even for weeks [5,7–10]. This allows the exchange of infusion bags at intervals of 1–3 days [5], making current CI protocols much more convenient than in the past, when large volumes of diluted factors meant that the infusate bag had to be changed every 8–12 h because of very low stability of first-generation concentrates [2]. However, reconstitution volumes higher than those recommended by the manufacturer may also cause loss of activity of some newer, high-purity FVIII products as well as of porcine FVIII [11,12]. Despite this, several hemophilia centers have perfected infusion strategies that use FVIII/FIX concentrates diluted in saline (final factor concentration 5–10 IU/mL) without diminishing the effect of therapy [13,14].

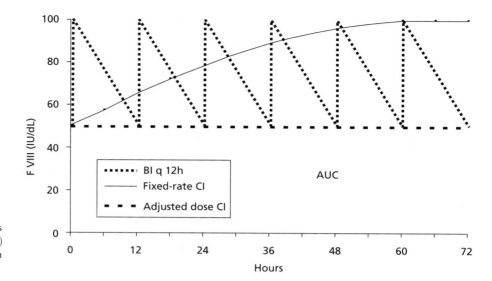

Figure 8.1 Factor VIII levels obtained during replacement with intermittent bolus injections (BI) and continuous infusion (CI) of fixed or adjusted doses. From ref. 6, with permission.

The type of infusion set used for CI may also affect the stability of reconstituted concentrates to some extent, probably as a result of initial adsorption of factor to the wall of the container and tubing. However, reports in the literature on the influence of polyvinylchloride, polyethylene, and polypropylene material on factor activity are contradictory [10,12]. In view of these observations it is advisable to test/assay the stability of each concentrate type and its compatibility with the particular infusion set to be used before initiating CI.

Risk of contamination

The risk of contamination and bacterial overgrowth during prolonged incubation of concentrate in the pump reservoir has been extensively studied. Experiments in which a variety of bacterial agents are inoculated into reconstituted concentrates support the microbiological safety of CI, proving that FVIII and FIX concentrates are a poor growth medium for most bacterial strains [8,9,15]. Studies employing simulated CI with minipumps failed to find any microbial contamination of the infusion sets used for up to 6–7 days [8,15], and the bacterial safety of CI is also confirmed by a recent clinical trial showing negative cultures in all 62 infusion sets tested after the end of 24–72 h of CI treatment [16]. To date, no clinical report has indicated an increased incidence of infectious complications after CI, even in settings employing central venous catheters. Nevertheless, in these cases, CI should be used with extreme caution. The preparation/filling of the containers and syringes for CI should be done under sterile conditions, e.g., under laminar air flow.

Thrombophlebitis

Thrombophlebitis at the site of venous access is a frequent adverse event of CI of undiluted FVIII concentrates, probably because of their high osmolarity [2]. This complication can be avoided by adding small amounts of heparin (2–5 U/mL) to the concentrate [5,6]. Such minor amounts of unfractionated and low-molecular weight heparin (LMWH) neither influence the stability of the reconstituted FVIII and FIX [7–10] nor affect *in vivo* hemostasis achieved by CI. However, the addition of unfractionated heparin to rFVIIa leads to immediate loss of activity of 20–30%, and the addition of LMWH to rFVIIa causes aggregate formation without the loss of activity [17]. Although some centers still add LMWH to rFVIIa without diminishing the efficacy of CI, the most widely adopted method of preventing local phlebitis during CI of rFVIIa is the parallel infusion of saline (10–20 mL/h) through a three-way connector [10,18,19].

Guidelines for adjusted-dose continuous infusion and treatment protocols

The dosing of factor replacement is based on both the clinical experience of the treating hematologist and specific pharmacologic calculations that take into account the basic pharmacokinetics of clotting factors, such as *in vivo* recovery and biological half-life. Using intermittent BI regimens, unnecessary high peaks are achieved after the administration of the concentrate and the levels drop to a trough before the next dose. Sometimes, trough levels are below the hemostatic minimum, thus exposing the patient to the risk of bleeding. The main goal of CI is to maintain a steady-state level of the coagulation factor in circulation, eliminating the peaks as well as the trough levels, which may fall below the minimum hemostatic level. A secondary, but no less important, goal of CI is to reduce the amount of factor required for the maintenance of desired hemostatic levels.

Adjusted-dose continuous infusion

This employs pharmacokinetic dosing and takes advantage of decreasing clearance of coagulation factor during CI. The simple protocol for this method is based on the following set of principles [5]:

1 Pharmacokinetic evaluation (PK) prior to a planned CI is recommended but not mandatory. PK testing, according to the guidelines of the International Society for Thrombosis and Hemostasis [20], is based on a bolus administration of approximately 50 IU/kg of factor and measurement of factor levels before infusion and then at nine postinfusion time points over the following 36–50 h. A model-independent method of determining the PK parameters is utilized [21]. The most important PK parameter for calculating the ideal rate of continuous infusion is the clearance.

2 The loading dose is calculated using *in vivo* recovery (IU/dL per IU/kg). A dose is selected that will raise the level to the desired minimum level appropriate for the specific bleeding manifestation or surgical procedure requiring hemostatic replacement therapy.

3 CI is initiated immediately following bolus administration of the loading dose. The initial rate is calculated using the clearance obtained in the preprocedure PK evaluation according to the following steady-state equation:

Rate of infusion (IU/kg/h) = clearance (mL/kg/h) ×
    desired level (IU/mL)

4 From the second day, the CI maintenance dose is adjusted using the same equation according to actual clearance, which is calculated from the daily factor level measurements.

5 Acceptable target minimum FVIII levels for major surgery are >0.5 IU/mL and >0.3 IU/mL for the first and second postoperative week respectively.

In the absence of pharmacokinetic evaluation or, in particular, in emergency situations, the initial maintenance dose may be calculated using the mean of a hemophilia population-based clearance, which is approximately 3.5 mL/kg/h for FVIII and 4.5 mL/kg/h for FIX [5,13]. However, one has to be aware of possible inter-individual variations in clearance, which may be influenced by age, body weight, laboratory assay employed, and even the type of factor concentrate used [22,23]. In addition, perioperative hemostatic demands may further increase factor consumption [5,13,24] beyond that expected. In order to prevent an unexpected drop in the factor level, it is advisable to check factor activity, or at least the activated partial thromboplastin time (aPTT), 8–12 h after the start of CI, and to increase the rate if necessary.

In most patients who require treatment for more than 1 week, a significant decrease in FVIII clearance is observed during the first 5–6 days of CI, followed by a plateau at a significantly lower level than that observed in the first days postoperatively [5,16,25]. This allows one to reduce the maintenance dose progressively and results in a significant sparing of concentrate.

Preoperative PK evaluation is recommended whether replacement is planned via intermittent BI or CI, as it may reveal the variation in clearance and half-life of the clotting factor in particular patients, thereby increasing the safety and efficacy of any intensive factor therapy. In fact, the PK is even more useful for treatment with BI than with CI, as in CI the clearance calculated from the PK is used only on the first day, whereas the half-life has to be considered all the time during BI therapy. PK evaluation may also alert one to an unsuspected low-titer inhibitor that may be undetectable by conventional inhibitor testing methods.

Fixed-rate continuous infusion

Some authors, aiming at maintenance FVIII/IX levels of >0.6 IU/mL, or even 1.0 IU/mL for the first few postoperative days, have shown that this may be achieved with a fixed rate of FVIII and FIX of 3–4 IU/kg/h and ≥4 IU/kg/h respectively, on average [14,24,26]. However, these levels are higher than those required to achieve satisfactory postoperative hemostasis; further, during fixed-rate CI, the levels would be expected to rise gradually over the first 4–6 days owing to the decrease in clearance, which may result in unnecessarily high factor consumption using this dosing mode of CI unless appropriate adjustments are made daily, as described above.

Clinical experience and indications for continuous infusion

Currently, the indications for continuous infusion of coagulation factors in hemophilia A and B are conditions that require the maintenance of efficient hemostatic factor levels for a prolonged period (longer than 3 days). Such situations include the treatment of major bleeds, minor and major surgical procedures, management of bleeding in some patients with low-titer or low-affinity inhibitors, and, rarely, short- and/or long-term prophylaxis.

Continuous infusion of FVIII

Continuous infusion has been proved to be safe and hemostatically effective for all indications mentioned above using either pdFVIII or rFVIII concentrates [5,14,16,26,27]. CI has been used also in home therapy settings for large bleeds requiring the maintenance of adequate and sustained FVIII levels over several days [28]. A prospective controlled study of CI and BI for major surgery, comparing protocols that were similar in terms of surgical technique and postoperative target minimum levels, demonstrated that efficacy and safety were better with CI than with BI: minimum factor levels were significantly higher (nadir 0.44 ± 0.06 IU/mL vs. 0.31 ± 0.09 IU/mL, respectively, in the first postoperative week), blood loss, as measured by a decrease in hemoglobin level, was lower (15.6 ± 12.1 vs. 30.1 ± 21.3 g/L; $P < 0.05$), and fewer patients required a blood transfusion (12% vs. 39%; $P < 0.01$) in the CI group (Table 8.1). The clearance of FVIII decreased over 6 days of CI from initial rates of 3.89 ± 0.86 mL/kg/h to a plateau at a minimum of 2.1 ± 0.54 mL/kg/h ($P < 0.01$) [16]. No bleeding complications occurred in the CI group, while in the BI group three patients (17%) developed major bleeding when the FVIII level dropped

Table 8.1 Continuous infusion versus intermittent injections of factor VIII in severe hemophilia A patients undergoing major surgery.

	Bolus injections	Continuous infusion	P
Number (patients/operations)	18/18	22/25	
Age (years)	24 ± 14	26 ± 14	NS
Body weight (kg)	6 ± 17	58 ± 25	NS
Treatment period (days)	13 ± 1	13 ± 1	NS
Factor consumption — first week (IU/kg)	493 ± 81	342 ± 69	≤0.01
Total factor consumption (IU/kg)	733 ± 126	467 ± 104	≤0.01
Factor VIII levels* — first week (IU/mL)	0.43 ± 0.09	0.54 ± 0.09	≤0.01
Nadir of FVIII — first week (IU/mL)	0.31 ± 0.09	0.44 ± 0.06	≤0.01
Major bleeding complications	3/18	0/25	NS
Postoperative drop in hemoglobin (g/L)	30.1 ± 21.3	15.6 ± 12.1	≤0.01
Patients requiring blood transfusion	7/18	3/25	≤0.01

*Constant levels in CI and trough levels in BI.
Values expressed as mean ± SD.
NS, not significant.

below 0.3 IU/mL because of either an unexpectedly low FVIII half-life or a missed bolus injection. These complications were not observed in the CI group. An additional advantage of CI is the convenience of monitoring; there is no need for exact timing of blood sampling as is required for assessing trough levels with intermittent or BI (before/after the bolus dose): samples for monitoring factor levels can be taken at any time from individuals undergoing CI.

Economic benefit of continuous infusion of FVIII

Elimination of the unnecessary peaks associated with BI as a result of having to keep trough levels above hemostatic minimum as well as the progressive decrease in clearance that occurs during CI have the effect of reducing the total amount of factor concentrate required. Indeed, a reduction in factor requirements in the region of 19–35% has been found in both prospective and retrospective studies comparing subjects receiving CI with historical control subjects receiving BI [5,24,25]. In one prospective controlled study whose aim was to compare factor requirements in patients undergoing major surgical procedures treated with adjusted-dose CI or intermittent injections using a similar treatment protocol, FVIII consumption was 36% lower in the CI group (total dose of FVIII for 13 days 467 ± 104 IU/kg vs. 733 ± 126 IU/kg, $P < 0.01$). The dose reduction could have been even greater (70%) if the targeted minimum levels had been the same in both groups; however, the factor levels in the CI group were at all times higher than the troughs in the BI group [16].

Some studies which have failed to demonstrate an economic benefit of CI utilized "fixed" rather than "adjusted" dose CI, or compared mean or different targeted minimum levels (0.6–1.0 IU/mL with CI vs. 0.5 IU/mL with BI) [26,29]. In the study of Tagariello *et al.* [26], which compared fixed-rate CI for surgery with historical control subjects treated with BI, the cost

benefit of CI was that no additional FVIII injections were needed in the CI group, whereas 31% of patients treated with BI required extra boluses. The requirement for additional FVIII infusions may be explained by variations in factor VIII pharmacokinetics. Applying the previously presented preoperative PK evaluation model to this study indicates that the half-life was "10 h in 36% of 25 patients tested [16]. This probably resulted in troughs lower than expected when bolus injections were administered at 12-h intervals, the dosing strategy traditionally employed in postoperative BI regimens.

Optimal minimum postoperative levels are still not well defined, and prospective randomized studies are needed to evaluate this issue. However, such studies are not very feasible. Srivastava *et al.* [30] targeted maximum cost-effectiveness of postoperative factor replacement when they used a low-dose CI protocol aimed at maintaining levels at 0.3 IU/mL for the first 3–5 postoperative days. In spite of low FVIII levels (0.48 ± 0.26 IU/mL and 0.31 ± 0.18 IU/mL on postoperative days 1–2 and 3–4 respectively), only delayed minor bleedings were observed in 4 of 19 (21%) surgical procedures. Lower FVIII levels in the early postoperative period, resulting in the formation of initial fragile clots, may explain the delayed postoperative bleeding. Unfortunately, the experience of Srivastava *et al.* is not universally applicable as most of their patients were asthenic Indians, who may have a lower risk of postoperative bleeding owing to a lower soft-tissue mass, perhaps creating a lower hemostatic demand at the surgical wound site.

Continuous infusion of factor IX

The longer half-life of factor IX makes it less attractive for CI as greater benefit compared with BI is achieved with products of short half-life. Despite this, data are accumulating concerning successful FIX replacement by CI [10,13,31]. The steady-state infusion rates of FIX vary widely (1.74–7.33 IU/kg/h), reflecting a wide range of rates of FIX clearance (2.45–9.65 mL/kg) [22] in the hemophilia B population. In some individuals the clearance may even be higher, up to 11.4 mL/kg/h [10]. Plasma-derived and recombinant FIX have different pharmacokinetics. Poon *et al.* [32] observed *in vivo* recovery of 1.05 ± 0.26 IU/dL/IU/kg and 0.77 ± 0.19 IU/dL/IU/kg for pdFIX and rFIX, respectively, with no significant difference in half-life. For high-risk surgery, Menart *et al.* [33] proposed the installation of an initial rate of continuous infusion of 4 IU/kg/h when recovery is >1.3 IU/dL/IU/kg and 7 IU/kg/h when recovery is <0.7 IU/dL/IU/kg. However, it is important to emphasize that clearance, and not recovery, is the parameter that determines the rate of infusion.

Like *in vivo* recovery, the clearance of pdFIX may also differ significantly from that of rFIX in the CI setting (4.25 mL/kg/h vs. 7.71 mL/kg/h respectively) [23]. Therefore, PK evaluation prior to CI of FIX is recommended whenever possible [13], in order to determine the clearance and to choose the dosing accordingly.

Continuous infusion in the treatment of hemophilia with inhibitor

Continuous infusion of human FVIII

Continuous infusion of human FVIII may be used for the treatment of bleeding in some inhibitor patients with low-titer or low-affinity inhibitor. It has been suggested that the measured factor level does not accurately reflect the *in vivo* situation: the theory is that, during the time that elapses between sampling and performance of the laboratory test, the antibody continues to neutralize the residual factor in the test tube, thereby underestimating the *in vivo* functional factor level. Hence, a hemostatic level may be achieved in the circulation even when the inhibitor titer suggests that the CI infusion rate is inadequate to produce a measurable *in vivo* level. The fact that the aPTT following initiation of CI in such patients is markedly reduced despite undetectable levels of FVIII by assay supports this assumption [34].

Continuous infusion of porcine FVIII

This has been shown to be effective in patients with either congenital or acquired hemophilia with inhibitors. However, the required maintenance doses are usually higher than those in noninhibitor patients. In a retrospective multicenter study using median infusion rate of porcine FVIII of 17.2 IU/kg/h (range 2.6–26 IU/kg/h) in 29 bleeding episodes, the overall clinical efficacy reported was 96%. The high rate of anamnestic response (anti-human 77%, anti-porcine 88%) observed did not affect clinical efficacy [12]. An additional advantage of CI of porcine FVIII is the lower drop of platelet counts as compared with bolus therapy.

Continuous infusion for induction of immune tolerance

Immune tolerance has been induced successfully with CI in patients with a low-titer inhibitor [6]. However, this method failed to induce sustained immune tolerance in high responders [35]. Recently, CI of high-dose FVIII has been introduced as a part of modified Malmö–Heidelberg protocol for inhibitor eradication in acquired hemophilia [36].

Continuous infusion of recombinant FVIIa

In view of the very short half-life of rFVIIa (1.5–2.7 h), the concomitant increased risk that injections will be delayed or missed, and the very high cost of rVIIa in the context of higher saving potential with CI in products with a short half-life, the use of rFVIIa in CI appears to be a logical and attractive approach. CI of rFVIIa has been used successfully in inhibitor patients with classical and acquired hemophilia [18,19,37–39]. The pharmacokinetic evaluation of rFVIIa is less commonly used for initial dosing of rFVIIa CI, mostly owing to its very high cost and frequent use in an emergency set-up. Owing to wide variations of clearance observed in CI settings (32–138 mL/kg/h) [18,19] for the purpose of safety, a clearance of 60–80 mL/kg/h can be used to calculate the initial dosing using the steady-state equation. The dose can then be recalculated after 3–4 half-lives (6–8 h) according to the actual FVII:C level commonly used to monitor the treatment efficacy. Increasing clinical experience over the years has shown that rFVIIa levels required for efficient hemostasis exceed 10 IU/mL, which had been claimed by earlier preclinical and clinical studies to be a hemostatic minimum [39]. However, the optimal target level and maintenance dose of FVIIa still remain to be defined. The overall clinical efficacy of CI of rFVIIa of 91–92% was reported in major bleeds and surgery with maintenance doses of 17–20 μg/kg/h, resulting in FVII:C levels of 13–70 IU/mL [19,37]. Lower efficacy of CI of rFVIIa for dental extractions and oral bleeding was observed in one study using the doses of 17–18 μg/kg/h, but neither fibrin glue nor antifibrinolytic mouthwash had been used in these cases [37].

Recently, plasma levels of rFVIIa as high as 50 IU/mL and high CI maintenance doses of 50 μg/kg/h have been suggested [40] and the clinical efficacy of such a high maintenance dose CI for major surgery was demonstrated [41,42]. On the other hand, Santagostino *et al.* [19] found no benefit of high-dose regimens (40–50 μg/kg/h) over maintenance doses of 15–20 μg/kg/h. Even though these high-dose regimens confer a very high cost even when administered by CI, there can still be an improved standard of care by avoiding the inconvenience and mistakes arising from frequent intermittent injections.

However, in view of recent understanding of the mechanism of action of rFVIIa, emphasizing the need for high levels of rFVIIa to induce a high and fast thrombin burst, resulting in the formation of a clot resistant to fibrinolysis via the activation of thrombin-activatable fibrinolysis inhibitor (TAFI) [40], it is possible that administration of the product via BI is more advantageous than via CI. Further studies are required to determine if this is the case.

Continuous infusion for long-term prophylaxis

Based on the theoretical calculations, Carlsson *et al.* [43] demonstrated a remarkable cost saving of CI compared with the standard prophylactic protocol (theoretical reduction from 275 000 IU/year to only 22 000 IU/year for maintenance of FVIII above 1 IU/mL). However, there are still several unresolved questions regarding the feasibility of CI for long-term prophylaxis, including patient compliance and inconvenience, which limits some daily activities, as well as the suitability and safety of currently available delivery systems for long-term delivery. CI was used for prolonged periods of 6–24 months in three patients after partial resection of a giant pseudotumor, in whom bleeding from the pseudotumor occurred when the FVIII level dropped below 10–20% (U. Martinowitz and M. Heim, unpublished).

Complications of continuous infusion

Factor replacement with continuous infusion has been proved to be an effective, safe, convenient, and cost-effective treatment for various hemostatic challenges in hemophilia. The main theoretical complications of CI, instability of concentrates, bacterial contamination during CI, local phlebitis, and pump failure, can be prevented by scrupulous planning before initiation. This should include PK evaluation, the use of concentrates with an acceptable stability, preparation of infusion sets under sterile conditions, addition of a minor amount of heparin into the reconstituted concentrate, or use of the parallel infusion of saline to prevent phlebitis, as well as careful selection of a reliable infusion device [44].

Recently, concerns have been raised regarding the possible role of CI in the development of inhibitors. Over the years several new-onset inhibitor cases have been described, most of them after CI for surgery using recombinant or high-purity FVIII concentrates, with a major proportion of moderate/mild hemophiliacs in this group of patients [45–49]. Whether there is truly an increase in the incidence of inhibitors cannot be determined in view of the large numbers, as at least 100 hemophilia treatment centers worldwide appear to use continuous infusion for intensive factor replacement [50]. The pattern of exposure typical in CI with leaking of FVIII into the subcutaneous tissue may theoretically play a role in inhibitor development. Changes in the concentrate structure resulting from a long incubation may also play a role. However, recent wide use of CI coincides with increasing use of rFVIII and increased inhibitor surveillance; in addition, other confounding variables, such as major surgery, a large amount of factor given over a short period, particularly in

patients with mild/moderate hemophilia [48,51,52], or the occasional switch to a new type of product for CI [45,47,48], may also predispose to increased inhibitor occurrence. Further prospective studies are required to evaluate inhibitor development after surgery and treatment with either CI or BI.

References

1 Brinkhous KM. Hemophilia. *Bull NY Acad Med* 1954; **30**: 325.
2 McMillan CW, Webster WP, Roberts HR, Blythe WB. Continuous intravenous infusion of factor VIII in classic haemophilia. *Br J Haematol* 1970; **18**: 659–67.
3 Hermens WTH. Dose calculation of human factor VIII and factor IX concentrates for infusion therapy. In: Brinkhous KM, Hemker HC, eds. *Handbook of Hemophilia*, part II. New York: American Elsevier Publishing, 1975; 569–89.
4 Hathaway WE, Christian MJ, Clarke SL, Hasiba U. Comparison of continuous and intermittent factor VIII concentrate therapy in hemophilia A. *Am J Hematol* 1984; **17**: 85–8.
5 Martinowitz U, Schulman S, Gitel S, *et al.* Adjusted dose continuous infusion of factor VIII in patients with haemophilia A. *Br J Haematol* 1992; **82**: 729–34.
6 Martinowitz U, Schulman S. Continuous infusion of coagulation products. *Int J Pediatr Hematol/Oncol* 1994; **1**: 471–8.
7 Schulman S, Gitel S, Martinowitz U. Stability of factor VIII concentrates after reconstitution. *Am J Hematol* 1994; **45**: 217–23.
8 Schulman S, Varon D, Keller N, *et al.* Monoclonal purified F VIII for continuous infusion: Stability, microbiological safety and clinical experience. *Thromb Haemost* 1994; **72**: 403–7.
9 Thomas KB, Urbancik W, Turecek PL, *et al.* Continuous infusion of FVIII and FIX concentrates: *in vitro* analysis of clinically relevant parameters. *Haemophilia* 1999; **5**: 17–25.
10 Chowdary P, Dasani H, Jones JA, *et al.* Recombinant factor IX (BeneFix) by adjusted continuous infusion: a study of stability, sterility and clinical experience. *Haemophilia* 2001; **7**: 140–5.
11 DiMichelle DM, Lasak ME, Miller CH. *In vitro* factor VIII recovery during the delivery of ultrapure factor VIII concentrate by continuous infusion. *Am J Hematol* 1996; **51**: 99–103.
12 O'Gorman P, DiMichelle DM, Kasper CK, et al. Continuous infusion of porcine factor VIII in patients with haemophilia A and high responding inhibitors: stability and clinical experience. *Haemophilia* 2001; **7**: 537–43.
13 Hoots WK, Leissinger C, Stabler S, *et al.* Continuous infusion of a plasma derived factor IX concentrate (Mononine®) in haemophilia B. *Haemophilia* 2003; **9**: 164–72.
14 Dingli D, Gastineau DA, Gilchrist GS, *et al.* Continuous factor VIII infusion therapy in patients with haemophilia A undergoing surgical procedures with plasma- derived or recombinant factor VIII concentrates. *Haemophilia* 2002; **8**: 629–34.
15 Belgaumi AF, Patrick CC, Deitcher SR. Stability and sterility of a recombinant factor VIII concentrate prepared for continuous infusion administration. *Am J Hematol* 1999; **62**: 13–18.
16 Batorova A, Martinowitz U. Intermittent injections vs. continuous infusion of factor VIII in haemophilia patient undergoing major surgery. *Br J Haematol* 2000; **110**: 715–20.
17 Bonde C, Bech Jensen M. Continuous infusion of recombinant activated factor VII: stability in infusion pump system. *Blood Coagul Fibrinolysis*; 1998; **9**: 103–5.
18 Schulman S for the rFVIIa–CI group. Continuous infusion of recom-

binant factor VIIa in haemophilic patients with inhibitor: safety, monitoring, and cost effectiveness. *Semin Thromb Haemost* 2000; **26**: 421–4.

19 Santagostino E, Morfini M, Rocino A, *et al*. Relationship between factor VII activity and clinical efficacy of recombinant factor VIIa given by continuous infusion to patients with factor VIII inhibitors. *Thromb Haemost* 2001; **86**: 954–8.

20 Morfini M, Lee M, Messori A. The design and analysis of half-life and recovery studies for factor VIII and factor IX. *Thromb Haemost* 1991; **66**: 384–6.

21 Matucci M, Messori A, Donati-Cosi G, *et al*. Kinetic evaluation of four factor concentrates by model independent methods. *Scand J Haematol* 1985; **34**: 22–8.

22 Björkman S, Carlsson M. The pharmacokinetics of factor VIII and factor IX: methodology, pitfalls and applications. *Haemophilia* 1997; **3**: 1–8.

23 Hermans C, Brown S, Harrington C, *et al*. Differences in clearance of plasma-derived versus recombinant factor VIII and IX during continuous infusion. *Thromb Haemost* 2001; July (Suppl.): OC1746.

24 Hay CRM, Doughty HI, Savidge GF. Continuous infusion FVIII for surgery and major bleeding. *Blood Coagul Fibrinolysis* 1996; **7**: 15–9.

25 Rochat C, McFadyen ML, Schwyzer R, *et al*. Continuous infusion of intermediate-purity factor VIII in haemophilia A patients undergoing elective surgery. *Haemophilia* 1999; **5**: 181–6.

26 Tagariello G, Davoli PG, Gajo GB, *et al*. Safety and efficacy of high-purity concentrates in haemophiliac patients undergoing surgery by continuous infusion. *Haemophilia* 1999; **5**: 426–30.

27 Schulman S, Roussel-Robert V, Stieltjes N, *et al*. A retrospective evaluation of the use of B-domain deleted recombinant Factor VIII (Refacto) administered by continuous infusion during surgical procedures. *J Thromb Haemost* 2003; July (Suppl.): P1641.

28 Varon D, Schulman S, Beshari D, Martinowitz U. Home therapy with continuous infusion of factor VIII after minor surgery or serious haemorrhage. *Haemophilia* 1996; **2**: 207–10.

29 Lethagen S, Berntorp E. Octonativ–M as continuous infusion in connection with invasive procedures. *Haemophilia* 2000; **6**: 353–4.

30 Srivastava A, Mathews B, Lee V, *et al*. Continuous infusion of low doses of factors for post-operative hemostasis in haemophilia. *Thromb Haemost* 2001; July (Suppl.): Abstract P2569.

31 Schulman S, Gitel S, Zivelin A, *et al*. The feasibility of using concentrates containing factor IX for continuous infusion. *Haemophilia* 1995; **1**: 103–10.

32 Poon M-CH, Lillicrap D, Hensman C, *et al*. Recombinant factor IX recovery and inhibitor safety: a Canadian post-licensure surveillance study. *Thromb Haemost* 2002; **7**: 431–5.

33 Menart C, Petit CY, Attali O, *et al*. Efficacy and safety of Mononine during five surgical procedures in three haemophilic patients. *Am J Hematol* 1998; **58**: 110–6.

34 Martinowitz U, Schulman S. Continuous infusion of factor concentrates: review of use in haemophilia A and demonstration of safety and efficacy in haemophilia B. *Acta Haematol* 1995; **92**: 35–42.

35 Berntorp E. Regimens of factor VIII administration—continuous vs. bolus. *Haematologica* 2000; **85**: 69–71.

36 Huth-Kühne A, Ehrenfort S, Scharrer I, Zimmermann R. A new treatment option for patients with acquired haemophilia A. The modified Malmö–Heidelberg protocol. *Thromb Haemost* 2001; July (Suppl.): CD3364.

37 Mauser-Bunschoten EP, Koopman MMW, Goede-Bolder ADE *et al*. Efficacy of recombinant factor VIIa administered by continuous infusion to haemophilia patients with inhibitor. *Haemophilia* 2002; **8**: 649–56.

38 Baudo F, Gaidano GL, Carloni MT, *et al*. Recombinant activated Factor VII (rFVIIa) for the treatment of bleeding secondary to acquired factor VIII inhibitor. *J Thromb Haemost* 2003; July (Suppl.): P0596.

39 Schulman S, Bench Jensen M, Varon D, *et al*. Feasibility of using recombinant factor VIIa in continuous infusion. *Thromb Haemost* 1996; **75**: 432–6.

40 Hedner U. Treatment of patients with factor VIII and factor IX inhibitors with special focus on the use of recombinant factor VIIa. *Thromb Haemost* 1999; **26**: 102–8.

41 Ludlam C, Smith M, Gringeri A, Savidge G. Pharmacokinetics of rFVIIa. *Haemophilia* 2002; **8**: 574.

42 Tagariello G, Bisson R, Radossi P, *et al*. Contemporary total hip and knee replacement in patients with haemophilia and high titre of inhibitors to FVIII using recombinant FVIIa (NovoSeven) by continuous infusion. *J Thromb Haemost* 2003; July (Suppl.): P1146b.

43 Carlsson M, Berntorp E, Björkman S, Lindvall K. Pharmacokinetic dosing in prophylactic treatment of haemophilia A. *Eur J Haematol* 1993; **51**: 247–52.

44 Martinowitz U, Schulman S. Review of pumps for continuous infusion of coagulation factor concentrate: what are the options? *Blood Coagul Fibrinolysis* 1996; **7**: 27–33.

45 Batorova A, Martinowitz U, Porubska M, Filova A, Mistrik M. Recombinant factor VIII – Kogenate in previously treated patients. *Haemophilia* 1998; **4**: 187.

46 Baglin T, Beacham E. Is a change of factor VIII product a risk factor for the development of a factor VIII inhibitor? *Thromb Haemost* 1998; **80**: 1036–7.

47 Yee TT, Lee CA. Is a change of Factor VIII product a risk factor for the development of a factor VIII Inhibitor? *Thromb Haemost* 1999; **81**: 852.

48 Sharathkumar A, Lillicrap D, Blanchette S, *et al*. Intensive exposure to factor VIII is a risk factor for inhibitor development in mild haemophilia A. *J Thromb Haemost* 2003; **1**: 1228–36.

49 Von Auer C, Oldenburg J, Auerswald G, *et al*. The development of inhibitors directed against factor VIII after continuous infusion of factor VIII concentrates in patients with haemophilia A. *J Thromb Haemost* 2003; July (Suppl.): P1623.

50 Schulman S. Continuous infusion. *Haemophilia* 2003; **9**: 368–75.

51 Rothschild C, Laurian Y, Satre EP, *et al*. French previously untreated patients with severe haemophilia A after exposure to recombinant factor VIII: incidence of inhibitor and evaluation of immune tolerance. *Thromb Haemost* 1998; **80**: 779–83.

52 Hay CRM, Ludlam CA, Colvin BT, *et al*. on behalf of the UK Haemophilia Centre Directors Organisation, and Berntorp E, Mauser-Bunschoten EP, Fijnvandraat K, *et al*. Factor VIII inhibitors in mild and moderate-severity haemophilia A. *Thromb Haemost* 1998; **79**: 762–6.

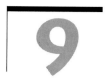

9 Inhibitors to factor VIII — immunology

Jean-Marie R. Saint-Remy and Marc G. Jacquemin

The immune response toward factor VIII (FVIII) presents several characteristics that make it unique. Antibodies to FVIII are made by healthy individuals, by patients suffering from hemophilia A, and by patients affected by some autoimmune diseases. FVIII is an autoantigen in the first and third of these situations. In the second instance, FVIII is administered intravenously and on a recurrent basis. The diverse characteristics make it essential to consider the immune response to FVIII from a general point of view, and not just as a peculiar response occurring in only a proportion of patients with hemophilia A.

A detailed evaluation of FVIII inhibitors has proven difficult because of the large diversity of the humoral response. Antibodies that do not interfere with FVIII activity make it difficult to establish a link between epitope specificity and the mechanism of FVIII inactivation. Moreover, anti-idiotypic antibodies that neutralize FVIII inhibitors have been described. To circumvent these difficulties, human monoclonal antibodies directed against FVIII and representative of patients' pathogenic antibodies have been produced by either immortalization of B lymphocytes or phage display technology. Immortalization of B lymphocytes can provide antibodies that carry both heavy and light chains representing the patient's repertoire. Phage display technology makes use of random association between heavy and light chains.

The purpose of this chapter is to review our current understanding of the homeostasis of the anti-FVIII response, to summarize information recently gathered from animal models, and to update data obtained from relevant clinical observations.

Homeostasis of the anti-FVIII immune response

The production of antibodies to FVIII, analogous to the immune response to any soluble glycoprotein, depends on the interaction between specific B and T lymphocytes. There are, however, two exceptions. As FVIII is administered i.v., it can activate B cells directly, resulting in the production of antibodies without contribution of T cells. The second circumstance in which T cells might not be required occurs when memory B cells are reactivated (see below).

The repertoire of T cells is established primarily in the thymus (see ref. 1 for a review). The role of the latter is threefold: (i) to eliminate T cells that do not recognize MHC class I or class II determinants, a process through which CD4/CD8(–) T cells mature into CD8$^+$ or CD4$^+$ respectively; (ii) to eliminate T cells that recognize with high affinity the complex of self epitopes and MHC determinants; and (iii) to select a population of regulatory T cells expressing CD25.

For a number of reasons, it is unrealistic to expect that such a selection will eliminate all T cells with the capacity to react with FVIII. First, the T-cell repertoire is of such a magnitude that it contains diversity sufficient to react to any possible T-cell epitope. Second, the processing of an antigen results in the presentation of only a few T-cell epitopes, selected in the late endosome for best fit within MHC class II determinants. Third, the selection process in the thymus removes only high-affinity T cells, and here, as is well demonstrated, T cells with intermediate activity are maintained and sent to the periphery. Fourth, the T-cell receptor, once thought to be tightly specific for sequences, does in fact react with multiple conformations of peptides presented by MHC class II determinants; one T cell can therefore recognize a large number of different sequences with more or less affinity, depending on the peptide itself, the MHC determinant, and the T-cell receptor (TCR) avidity. The practical consequence of this is that the use of short peptides to screen for T-cell reactivity will undoubtedly identify FVIII-specific T cells in healthy individuals. This has been confirmed experimentally. On the other hand, the T-cell repertoire is relatively fixed over time.

By contrast, the B-cell repertoire is continuously replenished over the lifespan [2]. Random rearrangement of the B-cell receptor (BCR) in the bone marrow generates cells with the potential of reacting with FVIII. The majority of autoreactive B cells are eliminated before entering the periphery. However, B cells use a number of mechanisms by which they can further diversify in the periphery. Germline-encoded antibodies are polyspecific, and it has been estimated that any single antibody molecule could recognize up to 10^6 different epitopes. The primary interaction between B cells and antigen depends on physicochemical interactions in which the primary influence is minimizing energy requirements, and not recognition of specific sequences. A possible exception to this will be described below for anti-FVIII antibodies toward the C2 domain. Antibodies of different genetic origin can therefore bind to the same epitope and acquire affinity by adopting a number of different chemical strategies: attractions via van der Waals forces, creation of hydrogen bonds, and establishment of disulfide bridges are examples. This is rendered possible by somatic hypermutation, which is a property of B cells. It involves the random introduction of mutations in antibody hypervariable regions, followed by affinity-driven selection.

All conditions are therefore assembled for an immune response to FVIII to emerge: specific T and B cells are present. However, the mechanisms by which the immune response is kept under control, i.e., without emergence of inhibitor antibodies, are many: specific cells maintained in a state of anergy or unresponsiveness, the presence of anti-idiotypic antibodies, and regulatory T cells are but a few of these mechanisms. However, subtle alterations in this equilibrium can rapidly lead to the production of antibodies.

Lessons from animal models

Significant progress in our understanding of how anti-FVIII murine antibodies are elicited has been made since the mouse hemophilia A model became available. Strains with target disruption of exons 16 or 17 mimic the situation of severe hemophilia A patients and have been used to study the conditions under which antibodies are generated.

Injection of physiologic quantities of human rFVIII by the intravenous route elicits a strong antibody response, with T-cell activation observed after only 3 days [3]. The characteristics of the antibody response match those observed in patients with inhibitors, namely long-term persistence of significant antibody titers, dependence on costimulatory signals, and resistance to suppression of established responses [4]. Specific CD4+ T cells belong to both the Th1 and Th2 subsets, with production of IgG1 and IgG2a antibodies. Interferon gamma (IFN-γ) and interleukin 10 (IL-10) dominate the cytokine pattern. An additional insight gleaned from FVIII immunization in hemophilia A mice is that von Willebrand factor (VWF) may somehow affect the immunogenicity of FVIII, both by reducing the overall antibody response toward FVIII and by modifying the profile of antibody specificity [5]. These results must be interpreted with caution, however, since human FVIII was used for these experiments. There is evidence that the immunogenicity of mouse FVIII in such a model could be different, both qualitatively and quantitatively [6].

Clinical observations

Characterization of anti-FVIII antibodies

Physicochemical characteristics

Antibody specificity

Mapping B-cell epitopes on FVIII has been the subject of many studies. It is clear that any part of FVIII that is exposed to the surface in the native or activated form of the molecule, or when FVIII is associated with VWF or phospholipids (PL), constitutes a potential binding site for antibodies. The characteristics of the B-cell repertoire described above strongly suggest that this is the case, and this has been confirmed by experimental evidence [7].

The presence of antibodies to FVIII is often confused with the presence of inhibitor antibodies, which constitute only a subset of antibodies with functional properties related essentially to the epitope they recognize. Whether or not noninhibitory antibodies can alter other parameters of the FVIII physiology is not entirely clear (see below, Mechanisms of FVIII inactivation). Our limited experience with a human monoclonal antibody partially neutralizing FVIII activity showed no effect on clearance (unpublished observations).

It is traditional to describe the B-cell epitopes on FVIII as organized in clusters. This characterization as a "cluster" must be interpreted cautiously because of the imprecision of the analysis made from polyclonal antibodies, which, in the best cases, were affinity purified [8]. However, this term makes sense insofar as antibodies of diverse genetic origin tend to recognize closely related epitopes by adopting converging strategies. Further, inhibitor antibodies often recognize parts of functional epitopes on FVIII, and not the entire area involved in FVIII functional interaction. The best example of this is provided by antibodies inhibiting the binding of FVIII to VWF; the latter has numerous points of interaction with FVIII, located over the entire FVIII light chain [9].

To date, clusters of B-cell epitopes have been identified primarily on the C2 and A2 domains, located in between residues 2181–2243 and 2248–2312 for the C2 domain, and 484–508 for the AZ domain, respectively [10]. However, in the case of the C2 epitopes, it is known that the three-dimensional conformation is important for full antibody recognition, as shown by the importance of the disulfide bridge within this domain. Additional clusters of B-cell epitopes have been described on the A3 (residues 1778–1823; [11]) and C1 (circa 2150; [12]) domains, the frequency of which is unclear. An intriguing finding is that antibodies recognizing the acidic regions *a1* and *a3* (and possibly *a2*) are likely to be more frequent than previously thought, although the mechanism by which they inhibit the function of FVIII is less well understood (see below and ref. 13). Immortalization of B lymphocytes as well as phage display will continue to provide information on antibodies directed to the A2, A3, C1, and C2 domains, and will help to determine the repertoire of immunoglobulin genes coding for anti-FVIII antibodies [14].

Interestingly, the long quest toward the mapping of B-cell epitopes of FVIII has resulted in significant advances in our understanding of the function of FVIII and, indirectly, of its three-dimensional structure. Through the application of crystallization techniques, the entire conformation of FVIII will hopefully be elucidated. On the other hand, the availability of monoclonal antibodies derived from patients' repertoire makes it feasible to analyze the dynamics of the antibody interaction with FVIII as well as the mechanisms by which inhibitor antibodies are formed and regulated (see below). The first of such characterized human monoclonal antibodies, BO2C11, recognizes the FVIII C2 domain and inhibits FVIII binding to both phospholipids and VWF [15]. The antigenic determinant recognized by BO2C11 was determined by the crystallographic study of BO2C11 Fab fragments bound to recombinant C2 domain

[16]. BO2C11 makes direct contacts with most hydrophobic and basic residues predicted to mediate FVIII binding to phospholipids, which is consistent with its inhibitory activity.

Antibody isotype and genetic origin

The anti-FVIII antibody response recruits all subclasses of IgG, but the IgG4 isotype is somewhat over-represented [17], considering that IgG4 accounts for only 3% of the total IgG concentration in plasma. There is no clear explanation for this finding. The isotype switch from IgM to IgG4 depends on the presence of IL-4 and/or IL-13, the very cytokines involved in the production of IgE antibodies. Yet IgE antibodies against FVIII are not observed, in contrast to what is occasionally observed in the case of FIX inhibitors. IgG4 is associated with long-term exposure to antigens [18], a situation that characterizes hemophilia A patients with long-standing inhibitors. Interestingly, IgG4 is considered to be functionally monovalent owing to the limited flexibility of its hinge region. However, this does not seem to lower avidity, as can be observed with human monoclonal antibodies.

Recent data on the genetic origin of anti-FVIII antibodies show that antibodies toward the C2 domain belong to two distinct antibody subfamilies: in the first instance, antibodies of the DP5 subfamily are prominent among antibodies recognizing the PL binding site of FVIII. Convergent data have been obtained by two independent approaches, i.e., the study of human VH repertoire by phage display [19] and the derivatization of monoclonal antibodies from memory B cells of patients with inhibitors [15]. The reason why the DP5 family is recruited may be related to the unusual characteristics of the CDR3 of such antibodies, which carry a number of negatively charged residues able to interact with positive charges constitutive of the phospholipid binding site of FVIII. A second family of antibodies to C2 has been identified (DP84), although it remains unclear why DP84 antibodies are over-represented. Preliminary data on inhibitory antibodies to the A2 domain show less convincing evidence of restricted genetic origin [20]. More data about the natural repertoire of memory B cells from phage display analysis are needed to clarify this phenomenon.

Functional properties

Kinetics of FVIII inactivation

One usually distinguishes two types of inhibitor antibodies: type 1 antibodies completely inhibit FVIII procoagulant activity following second-order kinetics, while type 2 antibodies follow more complex kinetics and cannot inhibit FVIII completely [21]. The reason for such a difference is not known. It may be related to different mechanisms of FVIII inactivation (see below) and/or to differences in affinity, although it is possible that interaction with VWF plays a role. Indeed, Gawryl and Hoyer [22] reported that, for most type 2 inhibitors, FVIII inactivation was partial only when the antibody was in presence of VWF. The later ob-

servation that antibodies to the A3 and C2 domains competed with VWF for binding to FVIII provided an explanation for the effect of VWF on inhibitor kinetics. It is noteworthy that antibodies competing with VWF and with a sufficiently high affinity for FVIII can inactivate FVIII completely (type I inhibitor), albeit following a complex kinetics because binding to FVIII requires the preliminary dissociation of the FVIII–VWF complex [15]. Alternatively, VWF can be required for inhibitor activity. In such a case, it is likely that antibodies reduce the rate of dissociation of FVIIIa from VWF [23].

In contrast, rare antibodies only partially inhibit FVIII even in the absence of VWF [22]. The human monoclonal antibody LE2E9, which was derived from a patient with mild hemophilia A with inhibitor, recognizes the FVIII C1 domain and inhibits only 85% FVIII activity in the absence of VWF. The mechanism of action of this antibody is still under investigation, but its high affinity ($K_d = 0.5 \times 10^{-9}$ mol/L) indicates that, when it is present in excess over FVIII, all FVIII molecules must be complexed to the antibody [24]. Antibodies such as LE2E9 probably, therefore, reduce the cofactor activity of the FVIII molecule in the X-ase complex. An additional possibility is that type 2 antibodies recognize epitopes at a distance from a functional FVIII site, inducing a conformational change in the functional site sufficient to partly inhibit the function of FVIII. However, it should be kept in mind that a type 1 or type 2 activity is attributed to polyclonal antibody populations and that the kinetics of FVIII interaction therefore represents an average evaluation.

Whatever the precise reason for this difference, the distinction between type 1 and type 2 inhibitors remains useful. Thus, type 1 inhibitors are most often observed in severe hemophilia A patients who respond to FVIII infusions by producing high antibody titers. In contrast, type 2 inhibitors are observed preferentially in mild or moderate hemophilia A patients, in previously untreated patients (PUPs) mounting a transitory response to FVIII infusion, and in patients producing antibodies toward FVIII molecules altered by preparation procedures [25,26]. This distinction is also relevant for the bleeding phenotype and response to treatment. Type 2 inhibitor patients usually present with skin and soft tissue bleeding rather than the joint and intra-organ bleeding observed in patients with type 1 inhibitors. In addition, eradication of the inhibitor, either spontaneously or as the result of infusion with high doses of FVIII, is readily achieved in patients with type 2 inhibitors, whereas type 1 inhibitor patients are far less responsive [27].

Mechanisms of FVIII inactivation

The FVIII molecule is characterized by its plasticity, which is brought about both by its requirements for proteolytic cleavage for activation and inactivation and by binding to a number of other proteins to either protect itself (VWF) or to exert its cofactor activity (phospholipids, FIXa, FX). These characteristics also make it vulnerable to inactivation by specific antibody binding.

One usually distinguishes two main categories of inhibitor antibodies. In the first case, antibodies bind to or within short distance of a site of FVIII that is involved in its function. It is worth noting that almost all possibilities have been illustrated by the study of mouse or human anti-FVIII antibodies. Thus, antibodies have been observed that inhibit the binding of FVIII to PL, to VWF [28], to FIXa [11,29], and to FX [30]. There is also evidence that antibodies are formed to FVIII acidic regions [13], thereby interfering with thrombin cleavage. On the other hand, binding to FVIII sites involved in inactivation, essentially by FXa or activated protein C (APC), have also been described [31], although the clinical relevance of such antibodies is less well understood.

In addition to this generic steric hindrance mechanism, antibodies can be formed to epitopes that are accessible only when the molecule is either bound to VWF or activated. Such antibodies are much more difficult to distinguish from polyclonal antibody populations, making it difficult to determine either their prevalence and/or their clinical relevance [23].

Recently, antibodies with catalytic activity to FVIII have been described, demonstrating a strong correlation between such an activity and the titer of inhibitor antibodies [32]. Their presence is detectable in ~ 50% of hemophilia A patients with inhibitors [33]. Highly purified preparations of polyclonal anti-FVIII antibodies exert this catalytic activity when contaminating enzymes are excluded. Studies are ongoing (i) to determine whether monoclonal antibodies can also cleave FVIII, (ii) to identify the precise cleavage sites on FVIII, and (iii) to demonstrate their clinical relevance.

Notably, the majority of anti-FVIII antibodies do not interfere with FVIII function, as evaluated by current assay systems [7]. However, it is not yet clear whether or not such "nonfunctional" antibodies have a pathophysiologic role. It has been suggested that such antibodies could increase the clearance rate of FVIII from the circulation [34], perhaps thereby increasing the uptake of FVIII–immunoglobulin complexes by phagocytic cells of the reticuloendothelial system. Now that the mechanisms by which FVIII is cleared from the circulation have begun to be deciphered, it is easier to evaluate whether or not some antibodies can reduce the clearance by binding to the low-density lipoprotein receptor-related protein (LRP) or heparan sulfate FVIII binding sites. So far, the difficulty has been that, in humans, the above described interactions have been identified using antibodies prepared from patients, namely polyclonal antibodies exhibiting different specificities and affinities. The described effects are therefore the result of many interactions. A more thorough understanding of interactions between FVIII and human antibodies may be provided by the production of human monoclonal antibodies, as well as through studies carried out in the FVIII–/– mouse model.

Factor VIII-specific T cells

Several clinical observations indicate that FVIII-specific T cells support the development of the humoral response to FVIII. In some patients with an established humoral response to FVIII,

HIV infection leads to a decline in FVIII inhibitor as well as T-cell counts [35]. A large proportion of anti-FVIII antibodies belong to the IgG4 subclass [17]. This pinpoints a role for T cells in the development of the humoral response to FVIII since isotype switching is T-cell dependent. Lastly, hypermutations have been consistently detected in the genes coding for the variable part of cloned anti-FVIII antibodies either by immortalization of peripheral blood lymphocytes from patients with an inhibitor [14] or by phage display technology [16]. This indicates that B cells secreting anti-FVIII antibodies undergo affinity maturation processes that require specific T-cell help [36].

Factor VIII-specific T cells have been identified in the peripheral blood of hemophilia A patients with inhibitor using T-cell proliferation assays with native FVIII [37]. The epitope(s) recognized by such T cells have been mapped using synthetic peptides covering the entire FVIII molecule [38]. In severe hemophilia A patients, FVIII-specific T cells recognizing a large array of peptides scattered over the entire FVIII molecule have been detected. T cells proliferating in response to such peptides have also been identified in hemophilia A patients without an inhibitor and in healthy individuals. Only minor qualitative or quantitative differences have been identified between FVIII-specific T cells isolated from healthy individuals and T cells isolated from hemophilia A patients with or without inhibitor.

However, clear-cut differences between normal individuals and hemophilia A patients with an inhibitor have been observed when FVIII-specific T cells were examined at the clonal level. FVIII-specific T-cell lines were expanded and cloned using dendritic cells and FVIII-specific lymphoblastoid cells loaded with native FVIII. Under these experimental conditions, successful isolation of FVIII-specific T-cell lines was reported when blood from a hemophilia A patient with inhibitor was used but not when blood of normal individuals was used (ref. 39 and Renaud Lavend'homme, personal communication). The epitope specificity of the few T-cell lines characterized so far is also much more restricted than that observed when peptides are used to stimulate CD4+ T cells isolated from blood of hemophilia A patients or from normal individuals [39].

Such seemingly discrepant observations reiterate what was observed from animal studies and clinical observations in other fields such as autoimmune diseases (see above, Homeostasis of the anti-FVIII immune response). Two populations of FVIII-specific T cells coexist in the periphery. One population is detectable in normal individuals and in hemophilia A patients irrespective of inhibitor status and is demonstrable only when the entire FVIII-specific T-cell repertoire is screened through the use of peptides. A second population of bona fide pathogenic T cells is present only in patients with inhibitor antibodies.

Perspectives

Many questions remain concerning the immune response to FVIII. However, it is clearly worth pursuing these types of investigations. Beyond the primary goal, which is to provide new methods to prevent and/or suppress the production of inhibitors in patients, more broadly applicable information will undoubtedly be gathered.

The anti-FVIII immune response represents the only known situation in which allo- and autoimmune responses are observed concurrently and in which patients at risk can be followed longitudinally. This offers the possibility of studying the way in which tolerance is established in central and peripheral organs. With the help of suitable animal models and experiments carried out at the clonal level (including transgenic animals), there is little doubt that mechanisms leading to anti-FVIII immune responses will be progressively unraveled.

References

1 Walker LS, Abbas AK. The enemy within: keeping self-reactive T cells at bay in the periphery. *Nature Rev Immunol* 2002; **2**: 11–19.

2 McHeyzer-Williams M. B cell as effectors. *Cur Opin Immunol* 2003; **15**: 354–61.

3 Qian J, Collins M, Sharpe AH, Hoyer LW. Prevention and treatment of factor VIII inhibitors in murine hemophilia A. *Blood* 2000; **95**: 1324–9.

4 Reipert BM, Ahmad RU, Turecek PL, Schwarz HP. Characterization of antibodies induced by human Factor VIII in a murine knockout model of hemophilia. *Thromb Haemost* 2000; **84**: 826–32.

5 Behrmann M, Fasold H, Pasi J, et al. Von Willebrand factor modulates factor VIII immunogenicity: comparative study of different plasma-derived and recombinant factor VIII concentrates in a hemophilia A mouse model. *Thromb Haemost* 2002; **88**: 2221–9.

6 Doering C, Parker ET, Healey JF, et al. Expression and characterization of recombinant murine factor VIII. *Thromb Haemost* 2002; **88**: 450–8.

7 Gilles JGG, Arnout J, Vermylen J, Saint-Remy JMR. Anti-Factor VIII antibodies of haemophiliac patients are directed primarily towards non-functional determinants and do not exhibit isotypic restriction. *Blood* 1993; **82**: 2452–61.

8 Scandella DH. Properties of anti-factor VIII antibodies in haemophilia A patients. *Semin Thromb Haemost* 2000; **26**: 137–42.

9 Jacquemin MG, Lavend'homme R, Benhida A, et al. A novel cause of mild/moderate hemophilia A: mutations scattered in the Factor VIII C1 domain reduce Factor VIII binding to von Willebrand factor. *Blood* 2000; **96**: 958–65.

10 Saenko EL, Scandella D. A mechanism for inhibition of factor VIII binding to phospholipid by von Willebrand factor. *J Biol Chem* 1995; **270**: 13826–33.

11 Fijnvandraat K, Celie PHN, Turenhout EAM, et al. A human alloantibody interferes with binding of factor IXa to the factor VIII light chain. *Blood* 1998; **91**: 2347–52.

12 Jacquemin MG, Benhida A, Peerlinck K, et al. A human antibody directed to the factor VIII C1 domain inhibits factor VIII cofactor activity and binding to von Willebrand factor. *Blood* 2000; **95**: 156–65.

13 Raut S, Villard S, Gribble S, et al. Anti-heavy chain monoclonal antibodies directed to the acidic regions of the factor VIII molecule inhibit the binding of factor VIII to phospholipids and von Willebrand factor. *Thromb Haemost* 2003; **90**: 385–97.

14 van den Brink EN, Bril WS, Turenhout EA, et al. Two classes of germline genes both derived from the V(H)1 family direct the forma-

tion of human antibodies that recognize distinct antigenic sites in the C2 domain of factor VIII. *Blood* 2002; **99**: 2828–34.

15 Jacquemin MG, Desqueper BG, Benhida A, et al. Mechanism and kinetics of factor VIII inactivation: study with an IgG4 monoclonal antibody derived from a hemophilia A patient with inhibitor. *Blood* 1998; **92**: 496–506.

16 Spiegel PC Jr, Jacquemin M, Saint-Remy JMR, et al. Structure of a Factor VIII C2 domain:IgG4k Fab complex: Identification of an inhibitory antibody epitope on the surface of Factor VIII. *Blood* 2001; **98**: 13–19.

17 Andersen BR, Terry WD. Gamma G4-globulin antibody causing inhibition of clotting Factor VIII. *Nature* 1968; **217**: 174–5.

18 Aalberse RC, Schuurman J. IgG4 breaking the rules. *Immunology* 2002; **105**: 9–19.

19 van Den Brink EN, Turenhout EA, Davies J, et al. Human antibodies with specificity for the C2 domain of factor VIII are derived from VH1 germline genes. *Blood* 2000; **95**: 558–63.

20 Voorberg J, van den Brink EN. Phage display technology: a tool to explore the diversity of inhibitors to blood coagulation factor VIII. *Semin Thromb Hemostasis* 2000; **26**: 143–50.

21 Biggs R, Austen DE, Denson KW, et al. The mode of action of antibodies which destroy factor VIII. II. Antibodies which give complex concentration graphs. *Br J Haematol* 1972; **23**: 137–55.

22 Gawryl M, Hoyer L. Inactivation of factor VIII coagulant activity by two different types of human antibodies. *Blood* 1982; **60**: 1103–8.

23 Gilles JG, Lavend'homme R, Peerlinck K, et al. Some factor VIII (FVIII) inhibitors recognise a FVIII epitope(s) that is present only on FVIII–vWF complexes. *Thromb Haemost* 1999; **82**: 40–5.

24 Singh I, Smith A, Vanzieleghem B, et al. Antithrombotic effects of controlled inhibition of factor VIII with a partially inhibitory human monoclonal antibody in a murine vena cava thrombosis model. *Blood* 2002; **99**: 3235–40.

25 Laub R, Di Giambattista M, Fondu P, et al. Inhibitors in German hemophilia A patients treated with a double virus inactivated factor VIII concentrate bind to the C2 domain of FVIII light chain. *Thromb Haemost* 1999; **81**: 39–44.

26 Peerlinck K, Arnout J, DiGiambattista M, et al. Factor VIII inhibitors in previously treated haemophilia A patients with a double virus-inactivated plasma derived factor VIII concentrate. *Thromb Haemost* 1997; **77**: 80–86.

27 Mariani G, Siragusa S, Kroner BL. Immune tolerance induction in hemophilia A: a review. *Semin Thromb Hemostasis* 2003; **29**: 69–76.

28 Scandella D, Gilbert GE, Shima M, et al. Some factor VIII inhibitor antibodies recognize a common epitope corresponding to C2 domain amino acids 2248 through 2312, which overlap a phospholipid-binding site. *Blood* 1995; **86**: 1811–9.

29 Zhong DG, Saenko EL, Shima M, et al. Some human inhibitor antibodies interfere with factor VIII binding to factor IX. *Blood* 1998; **92**: 136–42.

30 Nogami K, Shima M, Nishiya K, et al. Human factor VIII inhibitor alloantibodies with a C2 epitope inhibit factor Xa-catalyzed factor VIII activation: a new anti-factor VIII inhibitory mechanism. *Thromb Haemost* 2002; **87**: 459–65.

31 Nogami K, Shima M, Giddings JC, et al. Circulating factor VIII immune complexes in patients with type 2 acquired hemophilia A and protection from activated protein C-mediated proteolysis. *Blood* 2001; **97**: 669–77.

32 Lacroix-Desmazes S, Moreau A, Sooryanarayana, et al. Catalytic activity of antibodies against factor VIII in patients with hemophilia A. *Nature Med* 1999; **5**: 1044–7.

33 Lacroix-Desmazes S, Horn MP, Bayry J, et al. High prevalence of antibodies with proteolytic activity to Factor VIII in hemophilia A pa-

tients with Factor VIII inhibitors. *New Engl J Med* 2002; **346**: 662–7.

34 Dazzi F, Tison T, Vianello F, *et al.* High incidence of anti-FVIII antibodies against non-coagulant epitopes in haemophilia A patients: a possible role for the half-life of transfused FVIII. *Br J Haematol* 1996; **93**: 688–93.

35 Bray GL, Kroner BL, Arkin S, *et al.* Loss of high-responder inhibitors in patients with severe hemophilia-A and human immunodeficiency virus type-1 infection — a report from the Multi-Center Hemophilia Cohort Study. *Am J Hematol* 1993; **42**: 375–9.

36 Rajewsky K. Clonal selection and learning in the antibody system. *Nature* 1996; **381**: 751–8.

37 Singer ST, Addiego JE, Reason DC, Lucas AH. T lymphocyte proliferative responses induced by recombinant factor VIII in hemophilia A patients with inhibitors. *Thromb Haemost* 1996; **76**: 17–22.

38 Reding MT, Wu H, Krampf M, *et al.* Sensitization of CD4+ T cells to coagulation factor VIII: response in congenital and acquired hemophilia patients and in healthy subjects. *Thromb Haemost* 2000; **84**: 643–52.

39 Jacquemin MG, Vantomme V, Buhot C, Lavend'homme R, Burny W, Demotte N *et al.* A single mutation Arg2150His regulates the T cell specificity for the factor VIII C1 domain: a molecular mechanism responsible for the higher incidence of inhibitor in mild/moderate hemophilia A patients with mutations in the C1 domain. *Blood* 2003; **101**: 1351–8.

10 Inhibitors to factor VIII — molecular basis

Johannes Oldenburg and Edward Tuddenham

Introduction

Observations in the mid-1970s and 1980s showed that the risk of inhibitor formation is influenced by the degree of severity, the history of inhibitors in family relatives, and ethnicity/race, implying an important role of patient genetics in inhibitor formation (Figure 10.1). Molecular candidates for a genetic predisposition to inhibitor development are mutation within the FVIII gene [1] and genes involved in the immune response such as the major histocompatibility complex (MHC) class I and II loci [2,3]. In hemophilia A, inhibitor formation is a common phenomenon, affecting about one-third of severe hemophilia A patients [4,5].

Although the presentation of a novel or immunologically altered FVIII antigen to the patient's immune system has been identified as the main cause of inhibitor development, the pathogenesis is only partly understood. Why do only some patients with severe molecular defects develop an inhibitor and others do not? What is protecting the latter group against inhibitor formation? Which mechanisms determine the antibody epitopes on the surface of the FVIII protein and what makes an inhibitor become high titer, low titer, or transient? This chapter will address the genetic factors that may contribute to the pathogenesis of inhibitor formation.

Factor VIII genotype and risk of inhibitor development

An overview of the risk of inhibitor formation with respect to the underlying FVIII gene mutation types is shown in Table 10.1 and Figure 10.2. In general, these stratify into two main groups. One group is composed of severe molecular defects — called null mutations because they do not make any FVIII protein. Patients in this group have large deletions, nonsense mutations, and intron 22 inversions and exhibit high inhibitor prevalence, with a range of 21–88%. The second group consists of individuals with missense and splice-site mutations, which result in loss of function but not complete absence of the FVIII protein, and exhibits an inhibitor prevalence of less than 10%. Individuals with small deletions/insertions exhibit only a moderate risk for inhibitor formation (for detailed discussion see below).

Most of these mutation types can be further subdivided according to their risk of inhibitor formation. Data taken from the HAMSTeRS (Haemophilia A Mutation, Structure, Test and Re-

source Site) mutation register (http://europium.csc.mrc.ac.uk) [6] and also data from the Bonn Centre (Table 10.1) show that patients with *large deletions*, affecting more than one domain of the FVIII protein, are at the highest risk (about 88%) for developing an inhibitor, which is about three times the risk of single-domain deletions. *Nonsense mutations* on the light chain double the risk of inhibitor formation relative to those on the heavy chain, although the predicted truncated proteins are logically shorter in patients with stop codons in the heavy chain. At present, no explanation for this observation exists. A further high-risk mutation type in hemophilia A is the *intron -22 inversion*, with an inhibitor prevalence of about 21%. This mutation is the most common cause of severe hemophilia A, especially in the subgroup of patients who develop an inhibitor, with up to 60% of such patients demonstrating the mutation [7].

Within the group of low-risk mutations, the mutation type of *small deletions/insertions* is of special interest because it shows an unexpectedly low risk of inhibitor formation in hemophilia A. From the nature of the mutation type — most of the small deletions/insertions lead to a frameshift with a subsequent stop codon — a relatively high inhibitor risk similar to the nonsense mutations would be expected. One reason for this discrepancy may be found in the interesting observation of Young *et al.* [8]. They reported an endogenous restoration of the reading frame by polymerase errors during DNA replication/RNA transcription in patients with small deletion/insertion mutations that were located at stretches of adenines. The resulting small amounts of endogenous FVIII protein evidently protect against inhibitor development [9]. Since the two A runs in the B domain represent mutation hotspots, the high proportion of such small deletions/insertions lowers the overall inhibitor prevalence in this mutation type.

Missense mutations represent the most frequent mutation type, accounting for 15% of mutations in severe hemophilia A [10] and for almost all mutations in the nonsevere hemophiliacs [6]. These patients synthesize some endogenous, although nonfunctional, protein that is sufficient to induce immune tolerance in most patients. Consequently, the inhibitor prevalence in this mutation type is as low as 5%. However, for patients with missense mutations in the C1 and C2 domains, the risk of inhibitor formation is threefold higher (10% vs. 3%) than for missense mutations in other regions, suggesting that this part of the FVIII molecule is especially immunogenic. This assumption is supported by several publications [11–14].

From these data it can be hypothesized that the C1/C2

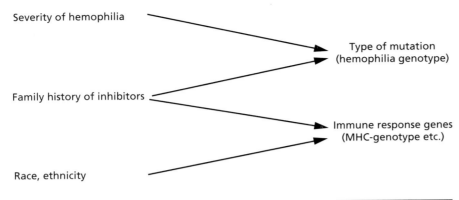

Severity of hemophilia

Family history of inhibitors

Race, ethnicity

Type of mutation
(hemophilia genotype)

Immune response genes
(MHC-genotype etc.)

Figure 10.1 Early indicators of genetic pre-disposition to inhibitor development in hemophilia.

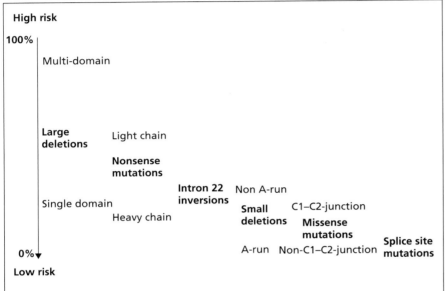

High risk

100%

Multi-domain

Large deletions Light chain

Nonsense mutations

Single domain

Intron 22 inversions Non A-run

Heavy chain **Small deletions** C1–C2-junction

Missense mutations

A-run Non-C1–C2-junction **Splice site mutations**

0%

Low risk

Figure 10.2 Mutation types/subtypes and inhibitor prevalence in hemophilia A according to the data presented in Table 10.1.

Table 10.1 Mutation types and inhibitor prevalence in hemophilia A (Bonn Centre, HAMSTeRS [6]). For each mutation type or subtype the number of individuals is given with the relative inhibitor prevalence (in percent) in brackets.

	Bonn (n=533) (%)	HAMSTeRS (n = 1022) (%)	Total (1555) (%)
Large deletion	15 (33)	86 (42)	101 (41)
Multidomain	3 (100)	23 (87)	26 (88)
Single domain	12 (17)	63 (25)	75 (24)
Nonsense mutations	45 (42)	131 (34)	185 (31)
Heavy chain	21 (13)	61 (18)	81 (17)
Light chain	24 (33)	70 (42)	104 (40)
Intron 22 inversion	179 (21)	no data	179 (21)
Small deletion/insertion	41 (15)	115 (16)	156 (16)
Non A-run	35 (17)	88 (19)	123 (19*)
A-run	6 (0)	27 (4)	33 (3)
Missense mutations	243 (1.5)	669 (6)	912 (5)
Non C1/C2 domain	187 (1)	431 (4)	618 (3)
C1/C2 domain	56 (4)	238 (11)	294 (10)
Splice-site mutations	10 (0)	21 (5)	31 (3)

*Value increases to 21% when in-frame small deletions/insertions are excluded.

domains significantly contribute to the binding of FVIII protein to von Willebrand factor (VWF). During FVIII activation, VWF is cleaved off and the same C1/C2 region binds to the phospholipid membrane to create, with activated factor IX, the X-ase complex. Any changes in the three-dimensional structure of this critical part of the FVIII molecule may affect its immunogenicity.

The HAMSTeRS data show that the inhibitor prevalence in missense mutations is dependent more on the localization of the mutation than on the degree of severity. There is almost no difference in inhibitor prevalence between severe and nonsevere hemophilia A patients with missense mutations, thus indicating that certain regions within the FVIII protein are especially crucial for antigenic integrity.

Besides the small deletions/insertions at series of adenine nucleotides, *splice-site mutations* represent the second mutation type that carries almost no risk for inhibitor formation. The likely explanation is that a very small number of FVIII molecules are still spliced normally and that these few molecules are sufficient to induce immune tolerance.

One of the most important questions for the pathogenesis of inhibitor formation is the following: why is it that not all patients with a single type of null mutation develop an inhibitor? The intron 22 inversion in hemophilia A patients serves as an ideal genetically homogeneous hemophilia cohort to examine possible explanations for this phenomenon. It represents a uniform mutation type and, from the pathogenetic mechanism, the intron 22 inversion appears to be a true null mutation, thus resulting in a complete lack of endogenous FVIII protein in the patient's circulation. Speculated potential reasons for a lack of inhibitor formation include presentation of some maternal FVIII to the fetal immune system *in utero*, thus inducing immune tolerance toward substituted FVIII. In addition, the individual characteristics of a patient's polymorphic immune system may either increase or decrease the risk of inhibitor development. It may also be speculated that an immune response does arise in almost all patients with null mutations but that it is downregulated in two-thirds of the patients by still unknown mechanisms. Solving the question of penetrance of inhibitor formation in hemophilic patients is a key to understanding the pathogenetic mechanism of inhibitor development.

Genetics of the immune system and risk of inhibitor development

Data about the role of immune response genes in inhibitor development are at present available only for hemophilia A. Two studies provide indirect evidence that genes participating in the immune response influence the risk of inhibitor development considerably. Scharrer *et al.* [15] conducted a meta-analysis of three US studies (Kogenate™ [16], Recombinate™ [17], and a US retrospective study [18]) that clearly demonstrated that race influences inhibitor formation. In the ethnic group of American-Africans, the inhibitor incidence among severe hemophilic

patients was twice (51.9%, 14 of 27) that of Caucasians (25.8%, 51 of 191). These findings are supported by the Malmö Inhibitor Brother Pair Study [19]. Cox Gill [20] compared the incidence of inhibitor formation in hemophilic siblings with that among more distant hemophilic relatives and found a much higher incidence in the former (50% vs. 9%). Since the genetic defects of the FVIII gene are expected to be similar in both cohorts, the observed difference in inhibitor incidence must be significantly influenced by the unique genetic profile of the individual's immune system. Candidates for this immunogenetic determinant of inhibitor formation are the MHC classes and other polymorphic genes (e.g., cytokines) that participate in the immune response.

The MHC class II genes DQ, DR and DP are of particular interest because their function is to present extracellular antigens — such as substituted FVIII — to the patient's immune system. However, with respect to the presentation of endogenously truncated and/or immunologically altered FVIII, the MHC class I genes that process intracellular antigens may also play an important role in the genesis of inhibitor formation. In a recent study, the influence of the MHC class I/II genotype on inhibitor formation was exclusively investigated in patients with the homogeneous intron 22 inversion, in order to exclude a bias deriving from different mutation types [2]. A summary of the results is shown in Table 10.2. The MHC class I/II alleles A3, B7, C7, DQA0102, DQB0602, and DR15 could be assigned as risk alleles (relative risk 1.9–4.0), because they occurred more often in inhibitor than in noninhibitor patients. In contrast, the MHC class I/II alleles C2, DQA0103, DQB0603, and DR13 could be assigned as protective alleles (relative risk 0.1–0.2) because

Table 10.2 Common and rare MHC class I and II alleles in severe hemophilia A patients with intron 22 inversion and inhibitor formation according to ref. 2. For the MHC class I loci A, B, and C the number of individuals is given, and for the MHC class II loci DR, DQA, and DQB the number of chromosomes is given.

Allele	Inhibitors No.	%	Noninhibitors No.	%	Relative risk
Common MHC alleles in patients with inhibitor					
A3	11	37.9	9	21.4	2.2
B7	14	48.3	8	19.1	4.0
C7	17	58.6	16	38.1	2.3
DQA0102	20	34.5	16	19.1	2.2
DQB0602	18	31.0	16	19.1	2.7
DR15	19	32.8	17	20.2	1.9
Rare MHC alleles in patients with inhibitor					
C2	1	3.4	6	14.3	0.2
DQA0103	1	1.7	12	14.3	0.1
DQB0603	0	0.0	6	7.1	0.1
DR13	1	1.7	9	10.7	0.1

Table 10.3 MHC class II alleles in severe hemophilia A patients with intron 22 inversion and inhibitor formation according to Hay *et al.* [3].

Allele	Inhibitors		Non-inhibitors		Odds ratio
	n	%	*n*	%	
DQA0102	10	43.5	11	20.0	3.1
DQB0602	7	30.4	9	16.4	ND
DR15	8	34.8	10	18.2	2.4

ND, not determined.

they occurred less often in inhibitor than in noninhibitor patients. These MHC class I/II alleles belonged to extended haplotypes, A3–B7–C7–DQA0102–DQB0602–DR15 and C2–DQA0103–DQB0603–DR13, that were observed more frequently and less frequently, respectively, than in the normal population. However, the number of patients was too small to reach a clear statistical significance.

Inheritance of MHC class I/II alleles as haplotypes might mask those specific MHC alleles that are decisive for the risk for or protection against inhibitor formation. In this context, a finding of Chics *et al.* [21] is of interest. The investigator found a 16 amino acid peptide from the FVIII light chain (amino acids 1706–1721) that could be eluted from a DR15 cell line. Two functional cleavage sites located on the surface of the FVIII molecule bound the peptide. It may be hypothesized that some peptides of the FVIII protein are especially efficient when presented to the patient's immune system, thus leading to the determination of FVIII antibody epitopes. Notably, Hay *et al.* [3] found the same MHC class II alleles to be associated at similar frequencies with inhibitor formation in patients with intron 22 inversions (Table 10.3), thus supporting the concept that the MHC is of some significance for the risk of inhibitor formation. Both studies, however, failed to achieve statistical significance. In addition to the data about possible MHC influences, inhibitor risk may also be determined by non-MHC immunologic genes.

Patients' genetics and characteristics of FVIII antibody epitopes

In hemophilia A, several FVIII antibody epitopes have been characterized. The FVIII A2, A3, and C2 domains are the most immunogenic while the A1 and B domains are, at best, poorly immunogenic. Inhibitory epitopes have been identified in the *a1* region (aa 351–365) [22], the A2 domain (aa 484–508) [23], the *a3* region (aa 1687–1695) [24,25], the A3 domain (aa 1778–1823) [26], and the C2 domains (aa 2181–2243 [27] and aa 2248–2312) [28]. Inhibitors against the C1 domain also have been reported [29]. Interestingly, the antibody epitopes correlate very well with the functional epitopes of ligands that interact with the FVIII protein (reviewed in ref. 30).

In severe hemophilia A, little is known about the relationship between the type and site of the mutation and the localization of the FVIII antibody epitopes. Epitopes have been shown to vary among inhibitor patients with respect to their number and specificity [31,32]. Most hemophilic patients have shown a complex immune response, with two or three epitopes contributing significantly to the inhibitor titer [32]. The mechanism(s) determining the heterogeneous patterns of the various FVIII antibody epitopes are not known. Future studies correlating the type and site of the mutations with epitope characteristics may help define this relationship.

In some mild hemophilia A patients, a direct relationship between the mutation site and the antibody epitope has been clearly established. Fijnvandraat *et al.* [33] described a patient with mild hemophilia A with an Arg593 → Cys mutation in whom the FVIII antibodies were directed against substituted FVIII but not against the mutated endogenous FVIII protein. This led to the interesting phenomenon that D-amino-D-arginine vasopressin (DDAVP) induced a considerable increase in FVIII activity in this individual while infused replacement FVIII did not. Peerlinck *et al.* [32] described two mild hemophilia A patients with a residual FVIII:C of 0.09 IU/mL despite one having an inhibitor titer of 300 Bethesda units (BU) and the other a titer of 6 BU. Both patients had the mutation Arg2150 → His and produced inhibitory antibodies directed against a FVIII domain encompassing the mutation site. By expression studies and functional tests, the mutation at residue 2150 was shown to lead to reduced FVIII binding to VWF, which subsequently decreased FVIII:C [12].

Conclusion

The risk of inhibitor development in hemophilia A is very strongly influenced by specific factor VIII genetic mutation and, to a lesser extent, by the individual's unique immune genotype/phenotype. However, our present knowledge about inhibitor formation is insufficient to delineate the complete pathogenesis. Since individuals' genotypes can now be fairly well determined — allowing for some methodological challenges — and do not change during life, comparison of the genetic profiles of patients with and without inhibitors is fertile ground for future studies. Building large and genetically well-characterized patient cohorts will allow us to form subgroups with more similar genetic backgrounds. This may be necessary to elucidate further factors that influence inhibitor development.

References

1 Schwaab R, Brackmann HH, Meyer C, *et al.* Haemophilia A: mutation type determines risk of inhibitor formation. *Thromb Haemost* 1995; 74: 1402–6.

2 Oldenburg J, Picard J, Schwaab R, *et al.* HLA genotype of patients with severe haemophilia A due to intron 22 inversion with and without inhibitors to factor VIII. *Thromb Haemost* 1997; 77: 238–42.

3 Hay CR, Ollier W, Pepper L, *et al.* HLA class II profile: A weak determinant of factor VIII inhibitor development in severe haemophilia A. UKHCDO Inhibitor Working Party. *Thromb Haemost* 1997; 77: 234–7.

4 Kreuz W, Becker S, Lenz E, *et al.* Factor VIII inhibitors in patients with haemophilia A: epidemiology of inhibitor development and induction of immune tolerance for factor VIII. *Semin Thromb Haemost* 1995; 21: 382–9.

5 Scharrer I, Neutzling O. Incidence of inhibitors in haemophiliacs. review of the literature. *Blood Coagul Fibrinolysis* 1993; 4: 753–8.

6 Resource site: HAMSTeRS version 4. *Nucl Acids Res* 1998; 26: 216–9.

7 Oldenburg J, Brackmann HH, Schwaab R. Risk factors for inhibitor development in haemophilia A. *Haematologica* 2000; 85: 7–13.

8 Young M, Inaba H, Hoyer LW, *et al.* Partial correction of a severe molecular defect in haemophilia A, because of errors during expression of the factor VIII gene. *Am J Hum Genet* 1997; 60: 565–73.

9 Oldenburg J, Schröder J, Schmitt C, *et al.* Small deletion/insertion mutations within poly-A-runs of the factor VIII gene mitigate the severe haemophilia A phenotype. *Thromb Haemost* 1998; 79: 452–3.

10 Becker J, Schwaab R, Moller-Taube A, Characterization of the factor VIII defect in 147 patients with sporadic hemophilia A: family studies indicate a mutation type-dependent sex ratio of mutation frequencies. *Am J Hum Genet* 1996; 58: 657–670.

11 Hay CR, Ludlam CA, Colvin BT, *et al.* Factor VIII inhibitors in mild and moderate-severity haemophilia A. UK Haemophilia Centre Directors Organisation. *Thromb Haemost* 1998; 79: 762–6.

12 Jacquemin M, Lavend'homme R, Benhida A, *et al.* A novel cause of mild/moderate haemophilia A: mutations scattered in the factor VIII C1 domain reduce factor VIII binding to von Willebrand factor. *Blood* 2000; 96: 958–65.

13 Liu ML, Shen BW, Nakaya S, *et al.* Haemophilic factor VIII C1- and C2-domain missense mutations and their modeling to the 1.5-angstrom human C2-domain crystal structure. *Blood* 2000; 96: 979–87.

14 Pratt KP, Shen BW, Takeshima K, *et al.* Structure of the C2 domain of human factor VIII at 1.5 A resolution. *Nature* 1999; 402: 439–42.

15 Scharrer I, Bray GL, Neutzling O. Incidence of inhibitors in haemophilia A patients — a review of recent studies of recombinant and plasma-derived factor VIII concentrates. *Haemophilia* 1999; 5: 145–54.

16 Lusher J, Arkin S, Hurst D. Recombinant FVIII (Kogenate) treatment of previously untreated patients (PUPs) with haemophilia A. Update of safety, efficacy and inhibitor development after seven study years. *Thromb Haemost* 1997; Suppl.: 162.

17 Gruppo R, Chen H, Schroth P, Bray GL. Safety and immunogenicity of recombinant factor VIII (Recombinate) in previously untreated patients (PUPs). A 7.3 year update. *Haemophilia* 1998; 4: 228.

18 Addiego J, Kasper C, Abildgaard C. Increased frequency of inhibitors in African American haemophilia A patients. ASH Nashville. *Blood* 1994 (Suppl.): 239.

19 Astermark J, Berntorp E, White GC, *et al.* The Malmö International Brother Study (MIBS): further support for genetic predisposition to inhibitor development in hemophilia patients. *Haemophilia* 2001; 3: 267–72.

20 Cox Gill J. The role of genetics in inhibitor formation. *Thromb Haemost* 1999; 82: 500–504.

21 Chicz RM, Urban RG, Gorga JC, *et al.* Specifity and promiscuity among naturally processed peptides bound to HLA-DR alleles. *J Exp Med* 1993; 178: 27–47.

22 Foster PA, Fulcher CA, Houghten RA, *et al.* A murine monoclonal anti-factor VIII inhibitory antibody and two human factor VIII inhibitors bind to different areas within a twenty amino acid segment of the acidic region of factor VIII heavy chain. *Blood Coagul Fibrinolysis* 1990; 1: 9–15.

23 Healey JF, Lubin IM, Nakai H, *et al.* Residues 484–508 contain a major determinant of the inhibitory epitope in the A2 domain of human factor VIII. *J Biol Chem* 1995; 270: 14505–9.

24 Tiarks C, Pechet L, Anderson J, *et al.* Characterization of a factor VIII immunogenic site using factor VIII synthetic peptide 1687–1695 and rabbit anti-peptide antibodies. *Thromb Res* 1992; 65: 301–10.

25 Barrow RT, Healey JF, Gailani D, *et al.* Reduction of the antigenicity of factor VIII toward complex inhibitory antibody plasmas using multiply-substituted hybrid human/porcine factor VIII molecules. *Blood* 2000; 95: 564–8.

26 Fijnvandraat K, Celie PH, Turenhout EA, *et al.* A human alloantibody interferes with binding of factor IXa to the factor VIII light chain. *Blood* 1998; 91: 2347–52.

27 Healey JF, Barrow RT, Tamim HM, *et al.* Residues Glu2181–Val2243 contain a major determinant of the inhibitory epitope in the C2 domain of human factor VIII. *Blood* 1998; 92: 3701–9.

28 Scandella D, Gilbert GE, Shima M, *et al.* Some factor VIII inhibitor antibodies recognize a common epitope corresponding to C2 domain amino acids 2248 through 2312, which overlap a phospholipid-binding site. *Blood* 1995; 86: 1811–9.

29 Jacquemin M, Benhida A, Peerlinck K, *et al.* A human antibody directed to the factor VIII C1 domain inhibits factor VIII cofactor activity and binding to von Willebrand factor. *Blood* 2000; 95: 156–63.

30 Lenting PJ, van Mourik JA, Mertens K. The life cycle of coagulation factor VIII in view of its structure and function. *Blood* 1998; 92: 3983–96.

31 Scandella D, Mattingly M, de Graaf S, Fulcher CA. Localization of epitopes for human factor VIII inhibitor antibodies by immunoblotting and antibody neutralization. *Blood* 1989; 74: 1618–26.

32 Peerlinck K, Jacquemin MG, Arnout J, *et al.* Antifactor VIII antibody inhibiting allogeneic but not autologous factor VIII in patients with mild haemophilia A. *Blood* 1999; 93: 2267–73.

33 Fijnvandraat K, Turenhout EA, van den Brink EN, *et al.* The missense mutation Arg593 → Cys is related to antibody formation in a patient with mild haemophilia A. *Blood* 1997; 89: 4371–7.

11 Inhibitors to factor VIII — epidemiology and treatment

Donna DiMichele

Introduction

Given treatment products that are virtually free of transfusion-transmitted disease and the more widespread use of prophylaxis to prevent arthropathy, the development of an inhibitor, a neutralizing antibody to factor VIII (FVIII), in patients with severe hemophilia A (sHA) remains the most significant debilitating therapeutic complication in the developed world. Especially if high titer, an inhibitor precludes access to the safe and effective standard of care and predisposes affected individuals to an unacceptably high level of morbidity and mortality [1].

This chapter will discuss inhibitor epidemiology in sHA relative to the incidence, prevalence, and pathophysiology of this complication. Issues relating to the nature of hemorrhage and its treatment that may potentially affect expression of a genetic or immunologic predisposition to antibody development (Chapters 9 and 10) will be highlighted.

Inhibitor definition and detection

An inhibitor is defined as a polyclonal high-affinity IgG antibody developed and directed against FVIII. It generally refers to that subset of the total antibody pool with the capacity to functionally neutralize FVIII activity. An inhibitor is frequently detected by routine laboratory surveillance using either screening or quantitative inhibitor assays (Chapters 41 and 42). Of these, the most commonly used is the Nijmegen modification of the Bethesda titer [2]. Alternatively, an inhibitor is suspected on the basis of an unexpectedly poor clinical response to standard factor replacement therapy at a time of hemorrhage. The more rigorous the surveillance frequency, the more likely the inhibitor is to be detected before its clinical manifestation [3]. The current recommendation is that inhibitor surveillance be conducted with a minimum frequency of every 3 months during the highest risk period, and every 6 months thereafter.

Inhibitors are classified as high- or low- responding on the basis of (i) the historical preimmune tolerance peak Bethesda titer and (ii) the demonstration of an anamnestic immune response to repeat FVIII exposure subsequent to antibody detection (Table 11.1). Currently, by International Society of Thrombosis and Hemostasis (ISTH) consensus, a high-responding inhibitor is defined by a historical peak titer of at least 5 Bethesda units (BU) and evidence of brisk anamnesis upon FVIII rechallenge [4]. The clinical significance of this

strong and highly reactive immune response is that bleeding can usually no longer be treated with standard FVIII replacement, and products that bypass the hemostatic requirement for FVIII become the necessary therapy of choice (Chapter 14). Conversely, a low-responding inhibitor is defined by a historical peak inhibitor titer of less than 5 BU accompanied by an absent or very attenuated anamnestic response to further FVIII administration [4]. Low-responder patients can frequently continue to use FVIII replacement for hemorrhagic episodes, albeit at a higher dose and/or more frequent dosing schedule than used as standard. The incidence and prevalence of these two distinct immune response patterns are discussed later in this chapter. The conversion of one type of immune response to the other can be observed during the natural history of an inhibitor in a single patient, or, frequently, during immune tolerance therapy (Chapter 13).

Incidence and prevalence of inhibitors

Previously untreated patients (PUPs)

The overall prevalence of inhibitors in hemophilia A (HA) has been reported to be between 3.6% and 21% [5,6]. Retrospective studies of cumulative inhibitor incidence performed at single institutions following nonuniform product exposure have shown that between 20% and 33% of children with severe or moderate HA developed an inhibitor at a median age of 2 years (range 1.7–3.3) after a median of 12 FVIII exposure days (range 11 to 36) (Table 11.2) [1,7–9].

However, it was ultimately the prospective studies of the first- and early second-generation recombinant FVIII (rFVIII) products that first established inhibitor risk, not viral transmission, as the primary safety endpoint in prelicensure clinical trials [10–12]. These three trials, similarly conducted with respect to the trimonthly frequency of inhibitor measurement in PUPs with sHA (defined as "2% FVIII), reported the almost identical cumulative inhibitor risk of about 30%. The median age at inhibitor development was 1.6 years after a median of 10 rFVIII exposure days (Table 11.2) [10–12]. These studies also clearly demonstrated that the first 50 rFVIII exposure days represented the most significant inhibitor risk period. Although more stringently collected, these data did not differ significantly from the previously discussed data from institutional cohorts that were less homogeneous with respect to treatment product exposure.

In the absence of similarly controlled data from PUPs treated with plasma-derived products, the role of product type in inhibitor development continues to be hotly debated and will be discussed later in this chapter.

Historically, high-titer inhibitors (≥5 BU) represented the majority (80–85%) of inhibitors observed in most retrospective cohorts [1,7–9]. In the rFVIII PUP trials, however, these represented only 40–53% of all detected inhibitors [10–12]. Conversely, the phenomenon of transient antibody development was infrequently reported in the historical literature [1,7–9]. However, the transient or disappearing inhibitor (usually defined as a low-titer antibody that resolves over an unspecified time in the absence of intentional immune tolerance therapy) represented 27–55% of all inhibitors observed in the first three rFVIII PUP trials [10–12]. The relative impact of product type and/or frequency of inhibitor measurement on this lower observed frequency of *clinically significant* antibodies remains unclear.

Previously treated patients (PTPs)

The incidence of inhibitor development in sHA patients who have already been treated with over 150–200 infusions with (exposure days to) FVIII is historically considered to be low. For this reason, the FVIII/IX Subcommittee of the ISTH recommended in 1999 that pre-licensure trials of novel FVIII concentrate immunogenicity be conducted in subjects who meet these criteria [13]. Indeed, unusually high FVIII product immunogenicity,

owing to a biochemical alteration during its manufacturing, had previously been detected by an unexpectedly high frequency of inhibitor development in such patients [14,15].

Despite the universal acceptance of this observation, the true incidence of inhibitor development in heavily treated PTPs has never been reliably quantified. Earlier large studies of inhibitor natural history in HA patients receiving largely intermediate-purity plasma-derived FVIII (pdFVIII) suggested that up to 20% of inhibitors may develop after age 30; 10% may still occur after age 40; and almost all will manifest by age 60 [5,16,17]. In one American study, 8 of 1306 (0.6%) prospectively followed hemophilia A patients developed anti-FVIII antibodies (1–13 BU) after 150–250 previous pdFVIII exposure days [5]. In the subsequent experience with monoclonal antibody-purified pdFVIII, several cases of PTP inhibitor development were reported [18]. However, no reliable cohort data exist. A careful review of four published rVIII PTP trials, involving a total of 307 subjects, suggests that five (1.6%) subjects developed a detectable anti-FVIII antibody (3/5 high titer; 2/5 transient, low) [19–21]. However, only one subject (0.3%) met the criteria for a *de novo* nontransient high-titer inhibitor in a previously heavily treated patient [20]. Furthermore, a very low rate of inhibitor development (2–3%) was observed in a Canadian population switched en masse from pdFVIII to rFVIII [22].

In summary, late-onset inhibitor development is a low-frequency event, best estimated at <2%. Only prospective long-term post-licensure pharmacosurveillance studies conducted through all-inclusive national databases can more accurately assess this risk.

Factor VIII epitope specificity of inhibitors

The immunogenicity of FVIII has been well characterized by the initial ground-breaking experiments conducted by Dorothea Scandella [23] and a large body of subsequent work elegantly summarized by Saenko [24]. These definitive studies determined the FVIII epitope specificity of neutralizing antibodies to be localized primarily, but not exclusively, to (i) the A2 domain of the FVIII heavy chain, functionally inhibiting FVIII–factor IX complex formation and (ii) both the C2 domain of the FVIII light chain and the entire light chain itself, functionally inhibiting

Table 11.1 Inhibitors: definition of high- and low-responding pattern of immune response.

High-responding inhibitor
Brisk anamnestic response
"High" antibody titer (≥5 BU)
Not treatable with specific factor replacement

Low-responding inhibitor
Lack of anamnestic response
"Low" antibody titer (<5 BU)
Treatable with higher doses of specific factor replacement

Table 11.2 Hemophilia A inhibitor incidence studies.

Reference	Cumulative inhibitor risk (%)	Hemophilia severity	Median age	Median exposure days	Product
Ehrenforth [3]	33	Severe/moderate	2 years	12	Various
Addiego et al. [8]	28	Severe	1.7 years	11	IP
Ljung et al. [7]	21	Severe	NA	NA	Various
deBiasi et al. [9]	20	Severe/moderate	3.3 years	36	Various
Schwartz [10]	30	Severe	1.6 years	9	Kogenate®
Bray et al. [11]	31	Severe	1.6 years	10	Recombinate®
Lusher et al. [12]	30	Severe	1.3 years	12	ReFacto®

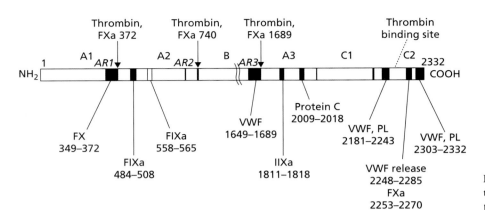

Figure 11.1 Functional inhibitor epitopes on the factor VIII molecules (reproduced with permission from ref. 24).

FVIII–von Willebrand factor and FVIII–phospholipid membrane interactions [24]. The full range of FVIII epitopes known to be the target of neutralizing antibodies is summarized in Figure 11.1.

Several mechanisms by which these antibodies functionally inhibit FVIII have been postulated or characterized. Mechanisms of passive interference include (i) steric hindrance; (ii) immune complex formation and clearance; and (iii) neoepitope recognition [25]. Recent data have also implicated a new class of catalytic antibodies that neutralize FVIII activity through protein hydrolysis [26].

Potential circumstances affecting inhibitor development

Underlying conditions, either host-related or associated with the treatment environment, may impact inhibitor development. Potential host-related risk factors include type and severity of hemophilia, hemophilia genotype, immunogenotype and phenotype, and race. Aspects of the therapeutic environment that have so far been implicated include the following:

- age at first exposure to clotting factor;
- the route, intensity, and method of FVIII administration;
- modification of the immune response to FVIII through breastfeeding or inflammatory/infections costimuli;
- site of hemorrhage;
- perhaps the most controversial of all, type of FVIII product infused (Table 11.3).

Most host- and therapy-related risk factors for inhibitor development have been implicated solely or chiefly on the basis of anecdotal experience and/or preliminary data. Further, many are interrelated. Accordingly, none has been definitively proven to predispose to inhibitor development. It is within this context of the multifactorial nature of inhibitor development and our in-

Table 11.3 Host- and treatment-related factors that may impact on inhibitor development.

Host-related factors
Type and severity of hemophilia
Race
Hemophilia genotype
Immunogenotype/phenotype

Treatment-related factors
Factor VIII product type
Route, intensity, method of factor VIII infusion
Age at first factor VIII exposure
Type/site of hemorrhage
Up-/down-regulation of the immune system at time of factor VIII exposure
Inflammatory costimuli
Breastfeeding

complete knowledge of the roles played by these potential risk factors that each will be discussed.

Host-related risk factors in inhibitor development

Type and severity of hemophilia

Type of hemophilia definitely affects the vulnerability of the affected patient to inhibitor formation. Compared with the incidence of up to 33% in sHA, individuals with hemophilia B are significantly less likely to develop an anti-factor IX antibody (1–7.5%) [27]. The reasons for this discrepancy are speculative and further explored in Chapter 17.

Similarly, the severity of the FVIII deficiency greatly influences inhibitor development in HA. Although severe FVIII deficiency

("0.01 U/mL FVIII) accounts for 50% of all HA, severely affected patients develop 90% of the inhibitors seen in this disease. Inhibitors occurring in patients with mild and moderate hemophilia A are discussed in Chapter 12.

Race

The increased susceptibility of the African-American with sHA to inhibitor development has been documented. In the first North American inhibitor prevalence study, Gill [6] ascertained a prevalence of 21% (23/110) in African-Americans compared with 14% (185/1330) in the Caucasian subcohort. In a subsequent analysis of inhibitor incidence in two rFVIII PUP trials, Addiego [28] reported an incidence of 50% (9/18) in African-American study subjects compared with 29% (35/121) in Caucasians. The underlying etiology of this phenomenon remains unclear.

Genotype and host immune response

The role of the hemophilia A genotype in the host's underlying predisposition to inhibitors has been explored by Schwaab and Oldenburg [29,30]. The predominant role of large and/or multiple deletions and other gene rearrangement mutations in enhancing inhibitor risk and the association of small deletions and missense mutations with reduced risk are discussed in Chapter 10.

The mature host immune response to a foreign antigen is complex and involves mechanisms of antigen processing (MHC class 1 or 2); initial interaction between antigen-presenting cells (APCs) and T cells; T- and B-cell cross-talk; as well as long-term antibody production by plasma cells mediated by memory B cells. The predominance of either coinhibitory or costimulatory signals at the time of these crucial interactions can tilt the immune response toward either immunoreactivity or natural tolerance. Natural tolerance to the FVIII immunogen appears to occur in 65–70% of individuals with sHA. Immune mechanisms postulated to be inducing natural tolerance include FVIII antigen positivity, early fetal exposure to FVIII, T-cell mediated self recognition, as well as non-neutralizing and/or anti-idiotype antibody production [31]. However, the key to effective inhibitor eradication and prevention lies in the collaborative ability of scientists and clinicians to precisely identify and successfully modify the sequence of immunomodulatory events that culminate in the brisk anamnestic production of high-titer neutralizing anti-FVIII antibody. Chapter 9 details this immunology as well as the focus of current investigative efforts in inhibitor pathogenesis.

Host-related factors undoubtedly play a major role in determining inhibitor risk following FVIII exposure. Several studies in sHA brother pairs support this assertion by demonstrating a higher than expected familial inhibitor concordance rate. In the largest of these, the Malmö International Brother Pair Study, concordance for inhibitor development or nondevelopment among 269 brother pairs was 72% [32]. Nonetheless, the intriguing 28% inhibitor discordance rate among siblings (including a set of monozygotic twins) in this cohort points to the potential role of noninherited factors in mediating risk [32].

Treatment-related risk factors in inhibitor development

Type of FVIII concentrate

Among all the treatment-related issues implicated in inhibitor risk, none has been more hotly debated than FVIII product type. The comparative immunogenicity of rFVIII and pdFVIII is central to this debate and the ascertainment of relative risk has been the object of several recent retrospective and prospective studies.

An initial retrospective comparative analysis of inhibitor prevalence among sHA patients in the United States reported no difference between those who received only first-generation rFVIII (24/94, 26%) and those who received only pdFVIII products (13/48, 27%) [33]. Similarly, a retrospective review of inhibitor incidence in Sweden also failed to find a statistically different risk for those who exclusively received rFVIII in the 1990s (10/48; 21%) compared with the population treated with pdFVIII in the 1980s (9/52, 17%) [34].

However, two national prospective studies have since suggested a differential risk between PUPs treated exclusively with one or the other product type. In the French National Cohort Study, the relative risk of inhibitor development on first-generation rFVIII when compared with a locally produced pdFVIII was 2.6 (P = 0.03) [35]. High-titer inhibitors also occurred with a relative risk of 2.9, although incidence was not statistically different between recombinant and plasma-derived cohorts (P = 0.117) [35]. In the ongoing German/Austrian/Swiss study, a trend toward both a higher overall and high-titer inhibitor incidence has been noted in PUPs on rFVIII (39.5% and 18.6% respectively) compared with those receiving plasma-derived products (24.5%, 10.2% respectively) (G. Auerswald, personal communication).

However, since none of these studies has been large enough to accommodate the multifactorial analysis of suspected host- and treatment-related conditions required to assign true relative risk to product type, the role of product type in inhibitor development remains an open question.

Mode of FVIII administration

Preliminary studies of the host immunologic response in mice demonstrate the achievement of a relative tolerance to FVIII following the oral administration of the immunogen prior to intravenous infusion [37]. These studies suggest the immunologic significance of route of FVIII administration in inhibitor development. Moreover, recent anecdotal experience with FVIII infusion in HA patients has implicated a particular mode of intravenous FVIII administration, continuous infusion (CI), as a possible treatment-related risk factor for this complication. The potential significance of CI as a risk factor for inhibitors is amplified by the fact that the proven stability of CI FVIII and its cost-effectiveness [38–40] have led to its becoming an established and widely used therapeutic strategy for the prevention or treatment of life-threatening bleeding during the past decade.

CI was implicated in a cohort of Canadian children with mild hemophilia A who developed inhibitors [41]. In this experience, 4 of 29 (14%) patients developed antibodies during intense factor replacement therapy. Most were high titer and resulted in recurrent or postoperative hemorrhage. All developed in patients treated by CI rather than bolus FVIII infusion. However, median treatment intensity (median total days of factor replacement) differed between the CI group (n = 7; median exposure days = 11) and those treated with bolus therapy (n = 22; median exposure days = 2.5). Retrospective anecdotal experience with CI for major bleeds and surgery in Germany recently revealed the development of inhibitors in 10 patients following CI (five severe, one moderate, and four mild) [42].

Confounding clinical variables frequently mediate the decision to use CI instead of bolus FVIII therapy. They include type of bleed (surgical, intracranial), inflammatory stress, and the need for high therapeutic intensity, all of which are also suspected to contribute to inhibitor development. Therefore, studies that carefully control for these confounders are required to elucidate definitively the role, if any, played by CI FVIII in inhibitor pathogenesis. Until then, the clinician must consider both the proven cost-effectiveness of CI FVIII and the unproven potential for CI-associated neutralizing antibody development in the therapeutic decision-making process.

Neonatal exposure to FVIII

The potential for age at the time of a child's first FVIII exposure to influence inhibitor risk has been suggested by two recent retrospective studies. Lorenzo *et al.* [43] first reported a possible association in a Spanish cohort of 62 sHA patients. In this study, the probability of inhibitor development by age 3 years was 25%. Interestingly, the cumulative inhibitor incidence was inversely proportional to age at first factor exposure; 41% if <6 months; 29% if between 6 and 12 months; and 12% if >12 months (*P* = 0.03) [43].

The Dutch Retrospective Cohort Study corroborated this observation [44]. In a comparable group of 81 sHA children, the same phenomenon relative to cumulative incidence was observed at 100 exposure days: 34% if <6 months; 20% if between 6 and 12 months; and 13% if between 12 and 18 months (*P* = 0.03). No inhibitors were observed in 12 children first treated after age 18 months [44].

Once again, neither cohort was large enough to study the relative importance of this observation in a multivariate inhibitor risk analysis. Consequently, this very interesting initial observation, with the potential to greatly influence treatment practices, awaits confirmation by well-designed prospective studies.

Modification of the immune response: inflammation and breastfeeding

Costimulation of the immune system during antigen presentation is known to boost the immune response to an immunogen. Indeed, anecdotal experience suggests that concomitant infection, immunization, and severe or frequent hemorrhage in a patient receiving FVIII therapy have the potential to stimulate or boost the inhibitor response. Proving the exact role of inflammation in this process is difficult and not yet possible.

Conversely, down-regulation of the immune system prior to or during FVIII administration could theoretically attenuate immunoreactivity. Yee and Lee [45] postulated that, in addition to a potential to tolerize a hemophilic infant to FVIII due to homology between human milk-fat globulin and the FVIII light chain, breast milk cytokines, including transforming growth factor 5 (TGF-5), IL-4 and IL-10, might be immunoprotective. Although this theory has not been specifically studied, a recent retrospective review of the limited Swedish experience failed to demonstrate an inverse correlation between breastfeeding and inhibitor development [34]. Increased understanding of the immune response to FVIII and its regulation will ultimately ascertain if breastfeeding has an additional beneficial role in the hemophilic newborn.

Conclusion

In this chapter, several aspects of inhibitor epidemiology have been reviewed. The role of host- and treatment-related factors in inhibitor pathogenesis has been discussed relative to our current incomplete knowledge of the impact of their combined and temporal interactions on the hemophilic response to FVIII therapy. Questions have been raised. Without doubt, the future study of this immensely important problem will bring answers.

Acknowledgment

This chapter is dedicated to my friend and colleague, Dr Dorothy Scandella.

References

1 Aledort LM, Cohen M, Hilgartner M, Lipton R. Treatment of hemophiliacs with inhibitors: cost and effect on blood resources. *Progr Clin Biol Res* 1984; **150**: 353–65.

2 Verbruggen B, Novakova I, Wessels H, *et al.* The Nijmegen modification of the Bethesda assay for factor VIII:c inhibitors: improved specificity and reliability. *Thromb Haemost* 1995; **73**: 247–51.

3 Ehrenforth S, Kruetz W, Scharrer I, *et al.* Incidence of development of factor VIII and factor IX inhibitors in haemophiliacs. *Lancet* 1992; **339**: 594–8.

4 White GC, Rosendaal F, Aledort LM, *et al.* Definitions in hemophilia. Recommendation of the scientific subcommittee on factor VIII and factor IX of the scientific and standardization committee of

the International Society on Thrombosis and Hemostasis. *Thromb Haemost* 2001; **85**: 560.
5 McMillan C, Shapiro S, Whitehurst D, *et al.* The natural history of factor VIII C inhibitors in patients with hemophilia A. A national co-operative study II. Observations on the initial development of factor VIII C inhibitors. *Blood* 1988; **71**: 344–8.
6 Gill FM. The natural history of factor VIII inhibitors in patients with hemophilia A. In: Hoyer LW, ed. *Factor VIII Inhibitors*. New York: Liss, 1984; 19–28.
7 Ljung R, Petrini P, Lindgren A, *et al.* Factor VIII and factor IX inhibitors in haemophiliacs. *The Lancet* 1992; **339**: 1550–1.
8 Addiego J, Kasper C, Abildgaard C, *et al.* Frequency of inhibitor development in haemophiliacs treated with low-purity factor VIII. *Lancet* 1993; **342**: 462–4.
9 deBiasi R, Rocino A, Papa ML, *et al.* Incidence of factor VIII inhibitor development in hemophilia A patients treated with less pure plasma derived concentrates. *Thromb Haemost* 1994; **71**: 544–7.
10 Schwartz RS, Abildgaard CF, Aledort LM *et al.* Human recombinant DNA-derived antihemophilic factor (factor VIII) in the treatment of haemophilia A. *N Engl J Med* 1990; **323**: 1800–5.
11 Bray GL, Gomperts ED, Courter S *et al.* A multicenter study of recombinant factor VIII (recombinate): safety, efficacy and inhibitor risk in previously untreated individuals with hemophilia A. The Recombinate Study Group. *Blood* 1994; **83**: 2428–35.
12 Lusher JM, Spira J, Rodriguez D. A four-year update of safety and efficacy of an albumin-free formulated B-domain deleted factor VIII (BBD rFVIII, rVIIISQ) in previously untreated severe hemophilia A patients. *Thromb Haemost* 1999; **82**: 1493.
13 White GC, DiMichele D, Mertens K, *et al.* Utilization of previously treated patients (PTPs), noninfected patients (NIPs), and previously untreated patients (PUPs) in the evaluation of new factor VIII and factor IX concentrates. Recommendation of the Scientific Subcommittee on factor VIII and factor IX of the Scientific and Standardization Committee of the International Society on Thrombosis and Hemostasis. *Thromb Haemost* 1999; **81**: 462.
14 Peerlinck K, Armount J, Gilles JG, *et al.* A higher than expected incidence of factor VIII inhibitors in multi-transfused haemophilia A patients treated with an intermediate purity pasteurized factor VIII concentrate. *Thromb Haemost* 1993; **69**: 115–18.
15 Peerlinck K, Arnout J, DiGiambattista M, *et al.* Factor VIII inhibitors in previously treated haemophilia A patients with a double virus-inactivated plasma derived factor VIII concentrate. *Thromb Haemost* 1997; **77**: 80–6.
16 Gill FM. The natural history of factor VIII inhibitors in patients with hemophilia A. *Prog Clin Biol Res* 1984; **150**: 19–29.
17 Sultan Y. Prevalence of inhibitors in a population of 3435 hemophilia patients in France. French Hemophilia Study Group. *Thromb Haemost* 1992; **67**: 600–2.
18 Addiego JE Jr, Gomperts E, Liu SL, *et al.* Treatment of hemophilia A with a highly purified factor VIII concentrate prepared by anti-FVIIIc immunoaffinity chromatography. *Thromb Haemost* 1992; **67**: 19–27.
19 White GC, Courter S, Bray GL, *et al.* A multicenter study of recombinant factor VIII (RecombinateH) in previously treated patient with hemophilia A. *Thromb Haemost* 1997; **77**: 660–7.
20 Seremetis S, Lusher JM, Abildgaard CF *et al.* Human recombinant DNA-derived antihaemophilic factor (factor VIII) in the treatment of haemophilia A: conclusions of a 5-year study of home therapy. *Haemophilia* 1999; **5**: 9–16.
21 Lusher JM, Lee CA, Kessler CM, Bedrosian CL for the ReFacto Phase 3 Study Group. The safety and efficacy of B-domain deleted recombinant factor VIII concentrate in patients with severe haemophilia A. *Haemophilia* 2003; **9**: 38–49.
22 Giles AR, Rivard GE, Teitel J, Walker I. Surveillance for factor VIII inhibitor development in the Canadian hemophilia A population following the widespread introduction of recombinant factor VIII replacement therapy. *Transfus Sci* 1998; **19**: 139–48.
23 Scandella D, DeGraaf Mahoney S, Mattingly M. Epitope mapping of human factor VIII inhibitor antibodies by deletion analysis of factor VIII fragments expressed in Escherichia coli. *Proc Natl Acad Sci USA* 1988; **85**: 6152–6.
24 Saenko EL, Ananyeva NM, Kouiavskaia DV, *et al.* Haemophilia A: effects of inhibitory antibodies on factor VIII functional interactions and approaches to prevent their action. *Haemophilia* 2002; **8**: 1–11.
25 Peerlinck K, Jacquemin M. Characterization of inhibitors in congenital haemophilia. In: Rodriguez-Merchan EC, Lee CA, eds. *Inhibitors in patients with haemophilia*. Oxford: Blackwell Science, 2002; 9–13.
26 Lacroix-Desmazes S, Sooryanarayana, Moreau A, *et al.* Factor VIII inhibitor with catalytic activity towards factor VIII. *Haematologica* 2000; **85** (10 Suppl.): 89–92.
27 Ljung R, Petrini P, Tengborn L, Sjorin E. Haemophilia B mutations in Sweden: a population-based study of mutational heterogenicity. *Br J Haematol* 2001; **113**: 81–6.
28 Addiego JE Jr, Kasper C, Abildgaard *et al.* Increased frequency of inhibitors in African American hemophilia A patients. *Blood* 1994; **1**: 239a.
29 Schwaab R, Brackmann HH, Meyer C *et al.* Haemophilia A. Mutation type determines risk of inhibitor formation. *Thromb Haemost* 1995; **74**: 1402–6.
30 Oldenburg J, Tuddenham E. Genetic basis of inhibitor development in severe haemophilia A and B. In: Rodriguez-Merchan EC, Lee CA, eds. *Inhibitors in Patients with Haemophilia*. Oxford: Blackwell Science, 2002; 21–26.
31 Fijnvandraat K, Bril WS, Voorberg J. Immunobiology of inhibitor development in hemophilia A. *Semin Thromb Haemost* 2003; **29**: 61–8.
32 Astermark J, Berntorp E, White GC, Kroner BL, MIBS Study Group. The Malmö International Brother Study (MIBS): further support for genetic predisposition to inhibitor development in hemophilia patients. *Haemophilia* 2001; **7**: 267–72.
33 DiMichele D, Rothschild C, Sultan Y, Kroner B, Aledort L (members of the ISTH FVIII/IX Subcommittee). Multicenter comparison of inhibitor (INH) development on plasma-derived (pd) vs. recombinant (rec) factor VIII (FVIII) in severe hemophilia A patients (sHA Pts). *Blood* 1999; **1**: 238a.
34 Knobe KE, Sjorin E, Tengborn LI, *et al.* Inhibitors in the Swedish population with severe haemophilia A and B: a 20-year survey. *Acta Paediatr* 2002; **91**: 910–14.
35 Rothschild C, Goudemand J, Demiguel V, *et al.* Effect of type of treatment (recombinant vs. plasmatic) on FVIII inhibitor incidence according to known risk cofactors in previously untreated severe hemophilia A patients (PUPs). *J Thromb Haemost* 2003; July (Suppl.): Abstract OC215.
36 Kreuz W, Ettinghausen CE, Auerswald G, *et al.* Epidemiology of inhibitors and current treatment strategies. *Haematologica* 2003; **88**: EREP04.
37 Rawle F, Labelle AD, Postma L, *et al.* Oral administration of factor VIII contributes to the prevention of anti-factor VIII antibody development after protein infusion, and prolongs factor VIII transgene expression post-adenoviral gene transfer. *Blood* 2003; **102**: Abstract 566.
38 Hathaway WE, Christian MJ, Clarke SL, Hasiba U. Comparison of continuous and intermittent factor VIII concentrate therapy in hemophilia A. *Am J Hematol* 1984; **17**: 85–8.

39 Martinowitz U, Schulman S, Gitel S, *et al.* Adjusted dose continuous infusion of factor VIII in patients with haemophilia A. *Br J Haematol* 1992; **82**: 729–34.

40 DiMichele DM, Lasak M, Miller CH. A study of *in vitro* factor VIII recovery during delivery of four ultra-pure factor VIII concentrates by continuous infusion: A single institution's experience. *Am J Hematol* 1996; **51**: 99–103.

41 Sharathkumar A, Lillicrap D, Blanchette VS, *et al.* Intensive exposure to factor VIII is a risk factor for inhibitor development in mild hemophilia A. *J Thromb Haemost* 2003; **1**: 1228–36.

42 von Auer C, Oldenburg J, Auerswald G, *et al.* The development of inhibitors directed against factor VIII after continuous infusion of factor VIII concentrates in patients with hemophilia A. *J Thromb Haemost* 2003; July (Suppl.): Abstract P1623.

43 Lorenzo JI, Lopez A, Altisent C, Aznar JA. Incidence of factor VIII inhibitors in severe haemophilia: the importance of patient age. *Br J Haematol* 2001; **113**: 600–3.

44 van der Bom JG, Mauser-Bunschoten EP, Fischer K, van den Berg HM. Age at first treatment and immune tolerance to factor VIII in severe hemophilia. *Thromb Haemost* 2003; **89**: 475–9.

45 Yee TT, Lee CA. Oral immune tolerance induction to factor VIII via breast milk, a possibility? *Haemophilia* 2000; **6**: 591.

12 Inhibitors to factor VIII — mild and moderate hemophilia

Kathelijne Peerlinck and Marc G. Jacquemin

Introduction

Until the late 1990s, inhibitors in mild/moderate hemophilia A were considered to be very rare. However, since the publication of Hay *et al.* [1] in 1998 on behalf of the UK Haemophilia Centre Directors' Organisation (now the UK Haemophilia Centre Doctors' Organisation), it has been appreciated that inhibitors in mild/moderate hemophilia are more frequent than previously thought. Clinical problems associated with inhibitors in mild/moderate hemophilia are often considerable, since in the majority of cases adult patients are confronted with a change in phenotype from mild/moderate to severe and they suddenly experience spontaneous severe bleeding. Although some of the risk factors for inhibitor development are similar to those in severe hemophilia, others are specific for mild/moderate hemophilia. The study of the immune response in mild/moderate hemophilia A can help to elucidate some of the mechanisms underlying inhibitor formation and disruption of tolerance. Treatment of bleeding episodes and eradication of inhibitors in mild/moderate hemophilia require specific management, and special attention should be directed to the prevention of this complication.

Incidence and prevalence

Patients with mild/moderate hemophilia are at lower risk of inhibitor development than are severely affected patients. The prevalence of these inhibitors has been estimated to be between 3% and 13% [2–4]. In a prospective study of inhibitor incidence among 1306 hemophilia A patients, only 6% of the inhibitors were found in patients with factor VIII (FVIII) >0.03 IU/mL [5]. Sixteen (28%) of 57 new inhibitors reported between January 1990 and January 1997 in the UK Haemophilia Centre Doctors' Organisation (UKHCDO) inhibitor register arose in patients with mild or moderate hemophilia [1]. The annual incidence of inhibitors in the UK was 3.5 per 1000 registered with severe hemophilia and 0.84 per 1000 patients registered with mild/moderate hemophilia [6].

Clinical presentation

Usually the presence of an inhibitor in patients with mild/moderate hemophilia is suggested by a change in bleeding pattern: patients suddenly start to experience severe spontaneous bleeding whereas they used to bleed only after trauma or surgery. This change in bleeding pattern is explained by cross-reactivity of the inhibitor with the mutated FVIII of the patient, resulting in a residual FVIII:C level of <0.01 IU/mL [7–9]. The bleedings occur often in muscles and joints as in severe congenital hemophilia, but sometimes the bleeding pattern is more reminiscent of acquired hemophilia, with the occurrence of large cutaneous bruising and gastrointestinal and urogenital bleeding [1]. Occasionally there is no change in residual FVIII level but an inhibitor is detected in the Bethesda assay and/or there is lack of efficiency of FVIII transfusions [9–11].

Risk factors

Intensive exposure to factor VIII

Inhibitors in mild/moderate hemophilia occur more commonly later in life and an episode of intensive treatment with factor VIII concentrate (for bleeding, trauma, or surgery) seems to precede detection of the inhibitor in most reported cases. In the series reported by Hay *et al.* [1], 16 out of 26 inhibitors were detected after such intensive replacement therapy, and in this series no particular concentrate was implicated. Intensive exposure to FVIII as a risk factor for inhibitor development in mild hemophilia A was confirmed in a recent publication from Canada [12]. The overall incidence of inhibitors in the study population of boys (aged between 0 and 18 years) with mild hemophilia A (*n* = 54) was 7.4%. When the analysis was restricted to patients exposed to FVIII, the incidence was 14% (4/29), and four out of seven (57%) patients who received FVIII as a continuous infusion developed inhibitors . At this moment, it is not clear whether the risk is confined to high exposure to FVIII alone or whether additional risk is associated with the method of administering the concentrate (bolus injection versus continuous infusion). An answer to this question will probably require a prospective multicenter study.

Genetic background

In severe hemophilia, the risk of inhibitor formation is associated with the type of mutation. More disruptive mutations in the

FVIII gene, such as intron 22 inversions, large-gene deletions and stop codons, are associated with a risk of inhibitor formation of about 35%, compared with only about 5% in those with missense mutations and small deletions [13]. Missense mutations in the light chain are more often (12%) associated with inhibitors than are missense mutations in other parts of the FVIII gene (3.9%) [13]. In patients with mild/moderate hemophilia and inhibitors, certain missense mutations seem to predispose to inhibitor formation. In the series of Hay *et al.* [1], seven out of nine mutations were clustered in a restricted region within 100 bases of the junction between the C1 and C2 domain. The two remaining mutations affected the A2 domain. In most other reported cases of mild/moderate hemophilia, clustering in these regions is confirmed and some particular mutations seem to be over-represented such as Arg2150 → His [1,9,10] and Arg593 → Cys [1,7,14]

Analysis of the immune response to FVIII in mild/moderate hemophilia A

To determine why some mutations located in the A2, C1, or C2 domains of the FVIII molecule are more frequently associated with the presence of inhibitor, the humoral and cellular responses to FVIII were analyzed at the polyclonal and clonal level. Analysis of FVIII produced by patients with mild/moderate hemophilia A demonstrated that mutations at residues Arg2150, Arg2159 or Ala2201 eliminate FVIII epitopes (antigenic determinants) recognized by monoclonal inhibitor antibodies [15–18], which confirmed observations made using patients' polyclonal antibodies [7,10,19].

The T-cell response to FVIII was studied in a mild hemophilia A patient carrying an Arg2150 → His substitution in the C1 domain and who presented with a high-titer inhibitor toward normal but not self FVIII. The FVIII-specific T cells of this patient recognized a peptide encompassing residue Arg2150, the residue mutated in the patient's FVIII gene, and did not recognize recombinant FVIII carrying the substitution Arg2150 → His. Thus, the C1 domain of wild-type FVIII contains T-cell epitopes that are absent in FVIII carrying the mutation Arg2150 → His [20].

These observations demonstrate that Arg2150 → His FVIII and normal FVIII can be distinguished by the immune system not only at the B-cell level but also at the T-cell level. A similar phenomenon may occur in patients carrying some other mutations responsible for mild/moderate hemophilia A and predispose these patients to inhibitor formation.

In most published cases [1,7,9], the inhibitor initially neutralized both mutated self and transfused normal factor VIII, resulting in a basal factor VIII level of <0.01 IU/mL; however, tolerance to self was restored in several of the published patients, resulting in a recovery of the original basal FVIII level and response to desmopressin [1,7,9,10].

Treatment

Bleeding episodes

Bleeding episodes in patients with mild/moderate hemophilia who have developed an inhibitor are often particularly severe and sometimes life-threatening. Bypass therapy with activated prothrombin complex concentrates or recombinant activated factor VII can be used to control bleeding and has the advantage of avoiding anamnesis. Some patients can be treated successfully with D-amino-D-arginine vasopressin (DDAVP), especially those patients whose basal FVIII level did not significantly decrease and whose inhibitor does not seem to cross-react with their endogenous factor VIII [1,9,10] or once adequate circulating FVIII levels have returned. DDAVP does not cause anamnesis in those patients despite the presence of high-responding inhibitors [1].

Inhibitor eradication

Published data on immune tolerance induction in patients with mild/moderate hemophilia and inhibitors are very scarce. In the series reported by Hay *et al.* [1], immune tolerance induction was attempted in eight patients using different regimens. The Malmö regimen (high-dose FVIII combined with cyclophosphamide and intravenous IgG) was used successfully in two patients and with a partial response in a further two patients, the Van Creveld regimen (low-dose FVIII every other day) was used unsuccessfully in one patient and with partial success in a further patient, and the Bonn regimen was used unsuccessfully in one patient and with partial success in another patient. The overall success rate of immune tolerance of two out of eight patients seems lower than the reported success rate in severe hemophilia.

Other reported treatments have included immunosuppressive therapy [8,21,22] and avoidance of re-exposure to factor VIII using desmopressin and bypassing agents to treat bleeding episodes [23]. Currently available data are not sufficient to offer evidence-based advice on the optimal treatment of inhibitors in patients with mild/moderate hemophilia A, and the management of these patients remains controversial at this point.

Prevention

Maximal use of desmopressin for the treatment of patients with mild/moderate hemophilia A is certainly useful to prevent the development of inhibitors in these patients. Avoidance of intensive courses of treatment with FVIII concentrates has to be considered, especially in those patients known to harbor one of the high-risk mutations or having a relative who developed an inhibitor. It is not clear at this moment whether administration of FVIII as bolus injections or as continuous infusion have different risks. Identification of the underlying mutation in patients with mild/moderate hemophilia A is useful to give an indication of their risk of inhibitor formation.

Conclusion

The occurrence of an inhibitor in a patient with mild/moderate hemophilia A is often a dramatic event. Bleeding episodes can be particularly severe, forcing patients to change their lifestyle completely, and may be life-threatening. Avoidance of treatment with FVIII concentrates by using desmopressin where possible is the single most effective way to prevent this complication in mild/moderate hemophilia A patients. It is not clear at this moment whether immune tolerance induction, immunosuppression, or a combination of both should be used to eradicate the inhibitor. Again, avoidance of exposure to FVIII by using bypassing agents [using factor VIII inhibitor bypass activity (FEIBA®; Baxter Healthcare Corporation, Glendale, CA, USA) or rFVIIa] and desmopressin to treat bleeding episodes, might be an interesting option.

References

1 Hay CR, Ludlam CA, Colvin BT, *et al.* Factor VIII inhibitors in mild and moderate-severity haemophilia A. *Thromb Haemost* 1998; **79**: 762–6.

2 Lusher JM, Arkin S, Abildgaard CF, Schwartz RS. Recombinant factor VIII for the treatment of previously untreated patients with haemophilia A. *N Engl J Med* 1993; **328**: 453–9.

3 Sultan Y, and the French Haemophilia Study Group. Prevalence of inhibitors in a population of 3435 haemophilia patients in France. *Thromb Haemost* 1992; **67**: 600–2.

4 Rizza CR, Spooner RGD. Treatment of haemophilia and related disorders in Britain and Northern Ireland during 1976–80: report on behalf of the directors of haemophilia centres in the United Kingdom. *BMJ* 1983; **286**: 929–32.

5 Mc Millan CW, Shapiro SS, Whitehurst D, *et al.* The natural history of factor VIII:c inhibitors in patients with haemophilia A: a national cooperative study. II; observations on the initial development of factor VIII:c inhibitors. *Blood* 1988; **71**: 344–8.

6 Rizza CR, Spooner RJD, Giangrande PLF, on behalf of the UK Haemophilia Centre Doctors' Organisation (UKHCDO). Treatment of Haemophilia In the UK 1981–96. *Haemophilia* 2001; **7**: 349–59.

7 Fijnvandraat K, Turenhout EAM, van den Brink EN *et al.* The missense mutation Arg593 → Cys is related to antibody formation in a patient with mild haemophilia A. *Blood* 1997; **89**: 4371–7.

8 Vlot AJ, Wittebol S, Strengers PFW, *et al.* Factor VIII inhibitor in a patient with mild haemophilia A and an Asn618-Ser mutation responsive to immune tolerance induction and cyclophosphamide. *Br J Haematol* 2002; **117**: 136–40.

9 Santagostino E, Gringeri A, Tagliavacca L, Mannucci P. Inhibitors to factor VIII in a family with mild haemophilia: molecular characterization and response to factor VIII and desmopressin. *Thromb Haemost* 1995; **74**: 619–21.

10 Peerlinck K, Jacquemin M, Arnout J, *et al.* Antifactor VIII antibody inhibiting allogeneic but not autologous factor VIII in patients with mild haemophilia A. *Blood* 1999; **93**: 2267–73.

11 Kesteven PJ, Holland LJ, Lawrie AS, Savidge GF. Inhibitor to Factor VIII in mild haemophilia. *Thromb Haemost* 1984; **52**: 50–2.

12 Sharathkumar A, Lillicrap D, Blanchette VS, *et al.* Intensive exposure to factor VIII is a risk factor for inhibitor formation in mild haemophilia A. *J Thromb Haemost* 2003; **1**: 1228–36.

13 Goodeve AC, Peake IR. The molecular basis of haemophilia A: genotype-phenotype relationships and inhibitor development. *Semin Thromb Haemost* 2003; **29**: 23–30.

14 Thompson AR, Murphy MEP, Liu M, *et al.* Loss of tolerance to exogenous and endogenous factor VIII in a mild haemophilia A patient with an Arg593 to Cys mutation. *Blood* 1997; **90**: 1902–10.

15 Jacquemin M, Benhida A, Peerlinck K *et al.* A human antibody directed to the factor VIII C1 domain inhibits factor VIII cofactor activity and binding to von Willebrand factor. *Blood* 2000; **95**: 156–63.

16 Suzuki H, Shima M, Arai M, *et al.* Factor VIII Ise (R2159C) in a patient with mild haemophilia A, an abnormal Factor VIII with retention of function but modification of C2 epitopes. *Thromb Haemost* 1997; **77**: 862–7.

17 d'Oiron R, Lavergne JM, Lavend'homme R, *et al.* Deletion of Alanine 2201 in the FVIII C2 domain results in mild haemophilia A by impairing FVIII binding to vWF and phospholipids and destroys a major FVIII antigenic determinant involved in inhibitor development. *Blood* 2004; **103**: 155–7.

18 Jacquemin M, Benhida A, Peerlinck K, *et al.* A human antibody directed to the factor VIII C1 domain inhibits factor VIII cofactor activity and binding to von Willebrand factor. *Blood.* 2000; **95**: 156–63.

19 Gilles JG, Lavend'homme R, Peerlinck K, *et al.* Some factor VIII (FVIII) inhibitors recognise a FVIII epitope(s) that is present only on FVIII-vWF complexes. *Thromb Haemost* 1999; **82**: 40–5.

20 Jacquemin M, Vantomme V, Buhot C, *et al.* CD4+ T-cell clones specific for wild-type factor VIII: a molecular mechanism responsible for a higher incidence of inhibitor formation in mild/moderate haemophilia A. *Blood* 2003; **101**: 1351–8.

21 Capel P, Toppet M, Van Remoor E, Fondu P. Factor VIII inhibitor in mild haemophilia. *Br J Haematol* 1986; **62**: 786–7.

22 White B, Cotter M, Byrne M, *et al.* High responding factor VIII inhibitors in mild haemophilia – is there a link with recent changes in clinical practice? *Haemophilia* 2000; **6**: 113–15.

23 Robbins D, Kulkarni R, Gera R, *et al.* Successful treatment of high titer inhibitors in mild haemophilia A with avoidance of factor VIII and immunosuppressive therapy. *Am J Hematol* 2001; **68**: 184–8.

13

Inhibitors to factor VIII/IX: treatment of inhibitors—immune tolerance induction

Charles R.M. Hay

Introduction

Factor VIII/IX inhibitors occur in up to 35% of patients with hemophilia A and 1–2% of patients with hemophilia B [1–4]. Continued treatment with higher than usual doses of FVIII is associated with disappearance of most of these inhibitors, especially those of low titer [5,6]. This leaves about 10% of patients with hemophilia A with troublesome persistent inhibitors, often of high titer. Brackmann and Gormsen's [4] early report that regular administration of high doses of FVIII led to a fall in inhibitor titer inspired more formal attempts to eliminate inhibitors by regular administration of high or very high doses of FVIII, sometimes combined with immunosuppressive therapy [7–9]. Although such techniques have yet to be optimized, they were successful in abolishing approximately 80% of inhibitors in selected patients with severe hemophilia A and a smaller proportion of patients with factor IX (FIX) inhibitors [7–16]. Successful immune tolerance induction (ITI) leads to normalization of the FVIII half-life, a marked improvement in the patient's quality of life, and a considerable reduction in the future cost of treatment. Relapse following successful ITI is uncommon.

Current knowledge of ITI for FVIII and FIX inhibitors is derived from uncontrolled studies of patients treated using various FVIII dosing regimens and the compilations of data from three retrospective surveys of ITI. These surveys include the International Immune Tolerance Registry (IITR), the North American Immune Tolerance Registry (NAITR), and the German Immune Tolerance Registry (GITR) [13–18]. There are no controlled comparisons of the regimens currently used for ITI, and the optimal approach to ITI is disputed. Nevertheless, there is broad agreement on several factors predictive of successful ITI. These will be discussed in the following sections.

Procedure of immune tolerance induction

Tolerance is achieved by the regular administration of FVIII or FIX over a period of between a few months and 2 or more years. Widely differing doses of factor VIII have been used, varying from <50 IU/kg three times a week [9] to 300 IU/kg daily [12]. Intermediate doses of 50 or 100 IU/kg/day are also widely used with success. The regimens in common use are summarized in Table 13.1.

Regimens that combine intensive factor VIII/IX replacement with concomitant immunosuppression have also been described and are outlined in Table 13.1 [9]. The best described of these is the Malmö regimen, in which high-dose FVIII or FIX replacement is combined with cyclophosphamide, high-dose immunoglobulin, and protein A immunoadsorption [9,18]. This regimen is no longer widely used as immunoadsorption may be difficult in small children and clinicians are also reluctant to use cyclophosphamide in this group. Furthermore, the original high success rate has recently not been reproduced as the regimen has increasingly been used in resistant patients with a poor outlook [18].

The classic Bonn regimen described by Brackmann and Gromsen [4] uses factor VIII inhibitor bypass activity (FEIBA®; Baxter Healthcare Corporation, Glendale, CA, USA) prophylaxis twice daily to reduce the frequency of intercurrent bleeding. There is some evidence that FEIBA may reduce, but not prevent, intercurrent bleeding in inhibitor patients undergoing and not undergoing ITI [19,20]. Intercurrent bleeding is thought to be reduced during ITI, even without such use of prophylactic bypass therapy. Recombinant FVIIa (NovoSeven®, Novo Nordisk, Denmark) used as prophylaxis during ITI proved ineffective in one small series [21], possibly because the half-life of thrombin generation of rFVIIa is shorter than that of FEIBA [22].

Intensive FVIII or FIX replacement therapy for ITI may require central venous access and the immediate availability of bypass therapy such as FEIBA or Autoplex® (Baxter) or rVIIa. Further, both interruption of ITI and systemic infection may adversely influence both success and the time taken to achieve tolerance [11,16]. Hence, extraordinary clinical effort to alleviate the likelihood of either should be intrinsic to any ITI regimen.

During immune tolerance therapy, the inhibitor should be quantified using the Bethesda assay at regular intervals until free inhibitor is no longer detectable. Thereafter, FVIII recovery should be measured at frequent intervals until normal (≥66%). When recovery is normal, FVIII half-life should be determined at intervals after a 72-h washout period, until it is also normal (≥8 h). In this way, the restoration of normal FVIII recovery and half-life can be defined as the clinical endpoint of successful ITI.

In North America, ITI is discontinued and FVIII prophylaxis started as soon as tolerance has been demonstrated [15]. In Europe, it is more usual to continue ITI for several months after tolerance is established and then to gradually reduce the FVIII dose to zero over a period of 3 months before starting normal prophylaxis [10–13,16]. This tailing-off procedure is not of proven value in patients shown to be tolerant using hard pharmacoki-

Table 13.1 Commonly used immune tolerance protocols.

Protocol	Therapeutic regimen
Bonn [10]	Phase 1 VIII:C 100 IU/kg twice daily FEIBA 100 U/kg twice daily Phase 2: Tail-off over 3 months when VIII:C half-life normal
Van Creveld [8]	Neutralizing dose: 25–50 IU/kg twice daily for 1–2 weeks Tolerizing dose 25 IU/kg every second day until tolerant
Malmö [9]	Neutralizing continuous infusion of VIII:C to maintain 0.3 IU/mL VIII:C level for 10–14 days Cyclophosphamide 12–15 mg/kg i.v. (days 1 and 2) Cyclophosphamide 2–3 mg/kg orally (days 3–10) Intravenous IgG 2.5–5 g on day 1 and 0.4 g/kg/day on days 4 and 5 + Protein A adsorption if the inhibitor titer is >10 BU/mL before the start of treatment to reduce below 10 BU/mL

netic measures, given that the rate of relapse is very low regardless of whether the patient's FVIII dose is tailed off or stopped abruptly.

The optimum regimen for achieving immune tolerance induction has not as yet been demonstrated. The use of soft nonpharmacokinetic endpoints in the registries and some of the early series, as well as differences in patient selection, make it difficult to compare regimens. High-dose regimens may achieve tolerance more rapidly than low-dose regimens, but it is not clear whether the success rate with frequent high dosing is superior to that obtained using a low-dose regimen, especially in good-risk patients. This is discussed more fully below. Low-dose regimens may be able to be administered more easily than high-dose regimens without the requisite use of central lines. It also may be more acceptable for the patient and parents. Since some parents refuse central lines and since line infection has a major adverse affect on the outcome of ITI, this may sometimes be the decisive factor for choosing a low-dose rather than a high-dose regimen.

Factors influencing the outcome of immune tolerance induction

The various immune tolerance registries were set up to determine predictors of success or failure of ITI and to provide some comparison between regimens. The registries differ in their method of data collection and even their endpoints; accordingly, this limits the extent to which data from different studies may be compared. All registries provide retrospective data that are relatively soft, and reporting bias cannot be excluded. Each registry has used a different standardized questionnaire. The North American Registry (NAITR) [14,15] appears to have

used a less precise definition of success than the other registries but to have collected more detailed data. The German Registry [16] collected no data on the use of low-dose regimens and so provides no insight into their relative efficacy.

Despite these limitations, the registries have established most of the predictors of successful ITI, although a number of questions remain a source of controversy. It is not agreed, for example, how patients should be selected for ITI, which regimen should be used, when to initiate ITI, and when to cease the attempt to tolerize refractory patients.

Inhibitor titer

Both the International Immune Tolerance Registry (IITR) and the NAITR showed that the most important predictor of successful ITI is the inhibitor titer at the start of ITI, which affects both the likelihood of success and the time it takes to achieve tolerance [13–15]. Both the IITR and the NAITR found that an inhibitor titer of <10 BU at the outset of ITI was significantly correlated with successful outcome ($P = 0.001$ and 0.004 respectively) [13–15]. The success rate and time to success for patients starting ITI with an inhibitor titer <10 BU/mL were 85% and 11 months respectively compared with 43% and 15 months in patients with inhibitors >10 BU/mL. Most other studies show a similar relationship between the starting inhibitor titer, outcome, and the time taken to achieve tolerance [8,10,11].

In contrast, the peak historical inhibitor titer appears to be less related to outcome, failing to achieve statistical significance [12,13] even though a low peak historical titer is commonly said to be predictive of successful ITI and a very high peak inhibitor titer (>500 BU/mL) to predict a poor outcome.

The final analysis of the NAITR showed that the peak inhibitor titer after the start of ITI also correlated significantly with outcome. Patients whose peak inhibitor titer was >500 BU/mL prior to attempted ITI usually failed to achieve tolerance [16].

When to start ITI

Although some clinicians believe that ITI should be initiated as soon as possible after the inhibitor is detected, there is no firm scientific basis for this approach. A short interval between inhibitor detection and the initiation of ITI predicted a successful outcome in some studies [11,12] but not others [8,14,15]. If ITI is started at the first opportunity, as is common current practice, ITI will often start during a secondary immune response to FVIII when the inhibitor titer may already be rising rapidly. This may reduce the chance of achieving successful ITI.

Kreuz et al. [11] reported that the greater the number of FVIII exposure days between inhibitor detection and the start of ITI, the longer the treatment to achieve tolerance. This relationship failed to achieve statistical significance in this study and in the NAITR study [12,16], possibly because of low patient numbers in the analysis. It is generally agreed, however, that tolerance may be induced more easily in younger patients whose inhibitors are not long established [8,11–13], although this is disputed by DiMichele and coworkers [14,15].

The likelihood of achieving successful ITI may be enhanced by deliberately deferring the initiation of ITI for a short time until the inhibitor titer has declined below 10 BU/mL and preferably below 5 BU/mL, as ITI is far more successful with a starting titer <10 BU/mL. This usually delays the start of ITI by no more than 3–6 months. During this interval, exposure to FVIII should be avoided or minimized by treating intercurrent bleeding on demand, using bypass therapy, preferably with rVIIa.

Series reporting on regimens in which ITI, either deliberately [23,24] or through circumstance [8], was deferred until the inhibitor titer was <10 BU/mL have all been notably successful. Each of these authors report very similar success rates of 88–100%, despite using widely varying factor VIII dose rates and patient selection criteria.

The dose of factor VIII to be used

The influence of the dose of factor VIII used on the success rate of ITI is disputed. The IITR found that larger doses (≥100 IU/kg/day) were significantly more effective than small doses (≤50 IU/kg/day) [13], particularly in patients with inhibitor titers >10 BU/mL [12]. In contrast, the NAITR found that, although high-dose regimens (≥100 IU/kg/day) achieved tolerance in high responders significantly more rapidly than low-dose regimens (15.9 months vs. 23.6 months), successful outcome was otherwise unrelated to the dose of FVIII employed [14,15]. A meta-analysis of the IITR and NAITR conducted by Kroner [17] showed that the success rate was independent of the dose of FVIII used in patients with a starting inhibitor titer <10 BU/mL and historical peak titer <200 BU/mL (Table 13.2). In this study, higher-dose regimens appeared more effective in those patients with both higher starting titer and historical inhibitor titer. However, the number of patients involved was relatively small, limiting the power of the analysis [17]. These characteristics (starting titer <10 BU/mL and historical peak titer <100–200 BU/mL) may define a good-risk group in whom the dose of FVIII administered is unrelated to the outcome of ITI. This hypothesis is currently the subject of an ongoing multinational randomized clinical trial [25,26].

Further data that support lower starting and historical titers derive from a detailed comparison of the results from the Van Creveld ("50 IU/kg three times per week) and the Bonn (100 IU/kg twice daily) series [8,10,11]. Despite a 15-fold difference in dose rate, both centers reported similar success rates of 88%, suggesting that the two regimens are equally effective [8,10,11]. Kreuz (personal communication) has disputed this, suggesting that the two series are not comparable and that the Van Creveld center used less precise definitions of successful ITI. Further, the Bonn series was not a true cohort study in that only moderate- and high-titer patients were included, low-titer patients being tolerized using a low-dose regimen. The Van Creveld series was a true cohort study, including all patients presenting to the center. Precise entry characteristics were not de-

Table 13.2 Meta-analysis of the IITR and NAITR [17]: the effect of dose, starting inhibitor titer, and historical peak titer ($n = 278$).

Historical titer (BU)	Pre-ITI titer (BU)	Success		
		Dose (IU/kg/day)	n	%
<50	<10	<50	30/36	83
			33/38	87
			18/19	95
		≥200	23/24	96
	10–20	<50	2/3	67
		50–199	11/14	89
		≥200	1/3	33
50–200	<10	<50	8/12	67
		50–199	14/17	82
		≥200	3/4	75
	10–20	50–199	2/6	33
		≥200	3/4	75
	>20	50–199	8/12	67
		≥200	5/7	71
>200	<10	50–199	5/11	45
		≥200	7/7	100
	10–20	50–199	1/3	33
		≥200	3/4	75
	>20	50–199	1/23	4
		≥200	12/18	67

scribed for the Bonn series whereas all patients in the Van Creveld series could be considered good risk using the criteria described above (starting titer <10 BU, peak titer <200 BU/mL). Although the Van Creveld clinic did use clinical criteria when deciding to discontinue ITI, all patients considered tolerant in both series achieved normal recovery and half-life and could therefore be considered tolerant, even when precise and stringent pharmacokinetic criteria are applied. Although a comparison of the two series is possibly limited by differing patient entry characteristics, it appears that high- and low-dose regimens achieve similar results in good-risk patients. High-dose regimens should probably be used for poor-risk patients, since study data evidence suggest superiority in this setting [17].

Factor VIII product type

With the advent of high-purity and recombinant FVIII concentrates, some authors have questioned whether these products are as effective for ITI as older intermediate-purity factor VIII concentrates. This debate originated with the observation of Kreuz *et al.* [27] that six patients in whom ITI was unsuccessful using recombinant factor VIII (rFVIII) responded when plasma-derived factor VIII (pdFVIII) was substituted. However, this is an uncontrolled observation since one cannot be certain that the patients would not have responded had treatment with rFVIII continued. Brackmann [28] has also reported that, between 1990 and 2000, only 50% of patients had been successfully tolerized in his center using the Bonn regimen, a decline in efficacy which he attributed to the change from pdFVIII to rFVIII. However, the individual patient characteristics of this group were not published, and one cannot exclude the possibility that other factors may have influenced the outcome: possible confounders might include a change in referral pattern and/or changing the practice of starting ITI immediately upon recognition in individuals with high-titer inhibitors. These authors have suggested that von Willebrand factor (VWF)-containing concentrate may be more effective for ITI because VWF protects and masks the C2 domain and may thereby prolong the FVIII half-life. Certainly, there is evidence that the patient's endogenous VWF level may influence FVIII half-life in noninhibitor patients [29]. Furthermore, measurement of inhibitor titer seems to vary depending on the concentrate used in the assay, although this is a marked effect only in those uncommon patients who have predominantly anti-C2 inhibitor epitope specificity rather than the more typical mixed anti-A2 and anti-C2 epitope specificity [30–32]. The authors have proposed that this might extend the very short half-life of FVIII during ITI, increasing antigen presentation and ultimately the efficacy of ITI.

There is no other clinical support for this hypothesis, however. Analyses of the NAITR showed similar success rates for patients undergoing ITI using intermediate-purity and high-purity products (67.5% and 71% respectively) [15]. Series in which patients were tolerized exclusively using high-purity products have a similar success rate to those using intermediate-purity products [23,24,33] (Table 13.3).

Infection

It is a common observation that infections of any sort, particularly central venous catheter (CVC) infections, during ITI cause a nonspecific rise in inhibitor titer. This represents a clinical setback in most patients: such a complication may prolong the course of ITI in some patients, and in others may possibly lead to failure of ITI. For this reason, it is important to observe aseptic technique when accessing the CVC. This may be difficult, since ITI is conducted in progressively younger patients, even infants. The median age of the patients in the ongoing international ITI study is only 25 months.

CVC infection is considered such a potentially serious complication of ITI by the Bonn Center that it is currently the practice there to attempt tolerance initially without central venous access. Since their regimen involves the administration of twice-daily FVIII, this is a very demanding regimen. Other centers have reasoned that since the risk of line infection may relate to the frequency with which the port is accessed, an argument can be made for the use of a regimen involving less frequent administration of FVIII (daily or three times weekly). Indeed, it is usual practice outside Germany to administer FVIII either daily or every second day. Such low-dose regimens may be readily accomplished using peripheral veins only, thus avoiding the risk of CVC infection.

ITI in mild hemophilia A

Although the overall risk of developing an inhibitor in mild or moderate hemophilia is low, some kindreds with high-risk mutations have been described [34]. Up to 50% of these kindreds develop inhibitors. These inhibitors frequently cross-react with the patient's endogenous FVIII, resulting in a reduction in their FVIII level to <0.01 IU/dL and resultant risk for severe bleeding. Although these inhibitors may wane naturally, with concomitant restoration of the previous factor VIII level and bleeding pattern, ITI may be considered in those whose inhibitors persist and continue to cause bleeding. There are few data on ITI in this group. All the commonly described regimens have been used [34], although only a 30% success rate was achieved. Inhibitors in this group tend to present later in life (median age of 30 years). This may account for the relatively poor response to ITI observed in this group. Certainly, anecdotal evidence suggests that the response to ITI is much better among those patients with mild/moderate hemophilia whose inhibitors present during childhood.

ITI in hemophilia B

There are few published reports of immune tolerance induction in hemophilia B since factor IX inhibitors are rare. All the regimens previously described for hemophilia B ITI used doses of FIX similar to the doses of FVIII used for ITI of FVIII inhibitors

Table 13.3 Product purity as an outcome predictor of immune tolerance induction (reproduced with permission from ref. 33).

Reference	n	Product	Dose	Success (%)
Brackmann et al. [10]	52	IP (mostly)	High	88
Mauser-Bunschoten et al. [8]	24	IP (mostly)	Low	87
Lusher (pers. comm.)	8	Kogenate	High	63
Gruppo (pers. comm.)	6	Recombinate	High	50
Rothschild (pers. comm.)	8	Recombinate	High	25
Batlle [33]	9	Kogenate	Various	77
Smith et al. [23]	11	Mc/rFVIII	Intermediate	100
Rocino and DiBiasi [24]	12	Mc/rFVIII	High	83
Courter (pers. comm.)	21	Refacto	High	81

IP, intermediate purity; Mc/r FVIII, monoclonal or recombinant FVIII.

[9,18,15]. Considerations unique to ITI in hemophilia B include the risk of treatment-related thrombosis if low-purity pro-thrombin complex concentrates are used to induce tolerance, transfusion reactions, therapy-induced nephrotic syndrome, and a comparatively poor overall response rate to ITI. The risk of treatment-related thrombosis may largely be eliminated by the use of high-purity monospecific FIX concentrates or recombinant FIX. The risk of transfusion reactions cannot be eliminated using this strategy, however, since the reactions are specific for the FIX itself rather than to impurities in the concentrate.

Some patients with a history of allergic reactions have continued ITI with FIX, but most continue to require premedication with antihistamines and steroids [35,36]. These allergic reactions may be very severe and treatment limiting. As they tend to arise early in the treatment course, it is recommended that at least the first 20 treatments should be administered in the hemophilia center. An association between allergic reactions to FIX and nephrotic syndrome has also been reported in patients treated with large doses of FIX for ITI. The nephrotic syndrome has arisen after a median of 9 months of ITI (range 8–36 months) [35–37]. These patients did not respond to steroids but some improved following a dose reduction or discontinuation of ITI [36,37]. The relative risks and benefits of ITI should be carefully considered in patients with FIX inhibitors and the individual's history of reactions in view of the relatively low success rate reported and the high risk of the nephrotic syndrome.

The future

Immune tolerance induction is very costly, often extremely prolonged, and demanding for the family, patient, and managing clinicians. There are no satisfactory treatments for those patients who are resistant to ITI. There is, therefore, a need to develop innovative approaches to eliminate FVIII/IX inhibitors.

Most alternative methods proposed involve either immune suppression or the induction of specific anergy to FVIII/IX by specific targeting of circulating T cells [38,39] or by tolerizing using hybrid FVIII constructs [40] or FVIII peptides [41]. To date, few of these approaches have been tested in humans. Anti-CD40 ligand antibody administered with FVIII appeared to be a promising approach, but its use failed to provide lasting tolerance in mice [38] and was only partially effective in humans [39], with ITI trials being discontinued because thrombosis (possibly caused by monocyte activation) was reported in other studies of anti-CD40 ligand in autoimmune disease. The use of hybrid FVIII molecules, in which the conservative human–porcine substitutions in the A2 and C2 domain yield a low antigenicity recombinant molecule, may provide a valuable approach to both treatment and tolerization of inhibitor patients [40]. These products are still in the earliest stages of development; however, plasma-derived porcine factor VIII has been used successfully to tolerize a low cross-reacting subgroup of patients who, by virtue of their high-level high-responding

inhibitors, would have been difficult to tolerize conventionally [42]. This provides proof of principle that heterologous proteins and peptides may be successfully used for ITI.

References

1 Ehrenforth S, Kreuz W, Scharrer I, et al. Incidence of development of factor VIII and factor IX inhibitors in haemophiliacs. Lancet 1992; 339: 594–8.
2 Addiego J, Kasper C, Abildgaard C, et al. Frequency of inhibitor development in haemophiliacs treated with low-purity factor VIII. Lancet 1993; 342: 462–4.
3 Lusher JM, Arkin S, Abildgaard CF, Schwartz RS. Recombinant factor VIII for the treatment of previously untreated patients with hemophilia A. Safety, efficacy, and development of inhibitors. Kogenate Previously Untreated Patient Study Group. N Engl J Med 1993; 328: 453–9.
4 Brackmann HH, Gormsen J. Massive factor VIII infusion in a haemophilac with factor VIII inhibitor, high responder. Lancet 1977; 2: 933.
5 Rizza CR and Mathews JM. Effect of frequent factor VIII replacement on the level of factor VIII antibodies in haemophiliacs. Br J Haematol 1982; 52: 13–24.
6 Wensley RT, Stevens RF, Burn AI, Delamore IW. Plasma exchange and human factor VIII concentrate in managing haemophilia A with factor VIII inhibitors. BMJ 1980; 281: 1388–9.
7 Brackmann HH. Induced immunotolerance in factor VIII inhibitor patients. Clin Biol Res 1986; 150: 181–95.
8 Mauser-Bunschoten EP, Niewenhuis HK, Roosendaal G, van den Berg HM. Low-dose immune tolerance induction in haemophilia A patients with inhibitors. Blood 1995; 86: 983–8.
9 Nilsson IM, Berntorp E, Zettervall O. Induction of immune tolerance in patients with haemophilia and antibodies to factor VIII by combined treatment with intravenous IgG, cyclophosphamide and factor VIII. N Engl J Med 1988; 318: 947–50.
10 Brackmann HH, Oldenburg J, Schwaab R. Immune tolerance for the treatment of factor VIII inhibitors—twenty years of the Bonn Protocol. Vox Sang 1996; 70: 30–5.
11 Kreuz W, Ehrenforth S, Funk M, et al. Immune-tolerance therapy in paediatric haemophiliacs with factor VIII inhibitors: 14 years follow-up. Haemophilia 1995; 1: 24–32.
12 Mariani G, Ghirardini A, Bellocoo R. Immunotolerance in hemophilia: principal results from the international registry. Thromb Haemost 1994; 72: 1.
13 Mariani G and Kroner BL. International Immune Tolerance Registry, 1997 update. Vox Sang 1999; 77: 25–7.
14 DiMichele DM, Kroner BL, and the ISTH Factor VIII/IX Subcommittee. Analysis of the North American Immune Tolerance Registry (1993–970: current practice implications. Vox Sang 1999; 77: 31–2.
15 DiMichele DM, Kroner B, and the North American Immune Tolerance study Group. The North American Immune Tolerance Registry: practices, outcomes, outcome predictors. Thromb Haemost 2002; 87: 52–7.
16 Lenk H and the Study Group of German Haemophilia Centres. The German National Immune Tolerance Registry, 1997 update. Vox Sang 1999; 77: 28–30.
17 Kroner BL. Comparison of the International Immune Tolerance Registry and the North American Immune Tolerance Registry. Vox Sang 1999; 77: 33–37.

18 Freiberghaus C, Berntorp E, Ekman M, Gunnarsson M, Kjelberg BM, Nilson IM. Tolerance induction using the Malmö treatment model 1982–95. *Haemophilia* 1999; **5**: 32–9.

19 Kreuz W, Escuriola-Ettinghausen C, Martinez I, *et al.* Prophylactic therapy using factor VIII inhibitor bypass activity (FEIBA) in patients with high-titer inhibitors undergoing immune tolerance induction (ITI). *J Thromb Haemost* 2001 (Suppl.): Abstract P2545.

20 Hilgartner M, Makipernaa A, DiMichele DM. Long-term FEIBA prophylaxis does not prevent progression of existing joint disease. *Haemophilia* 2003; **9**: 261–8.

21 Brackmann HH, Effenberger E, Hess R, *et al.* Novoseven in immune tolerance therapy. *Blood Coagul Fibrinol* 2000; **11** (Suppl. 1): S39–S44.

22 Turicek P, Varadi k, Keil B, *et al.* FVIII inhibitor bypassing activity acts by inducing thrombin generation and can be monitored by a thrombin generation assay. *Pathophys Hemostas Thromb* 2003; **33**: 15–22.

23 Smith MP, Spence KJ, Waters EL, *et al.* Immune tolerance therapy for haemophilia A patients with acquired factor VIII alloantibodies: comprehensive analysis of experience in a single institution. *Thromb Haemost* 1999; **81**: 35–8.

24 Rocino A, DiBiasi R. Successful immune tolerance treatment with monoclonal or recombinant factor VIII concentrates in high responding inhibitor patients. *Vox Sang* 1999; **77**: 65–9.

25 Hay CRM. Immunetolerance induction: prospective clinical trials. *Haematologica* 2000; **85** (Suppl. to no. 10): 52–6.

26 DiMichele DM. Immune tolerance therapy dose as an outcome predictor. *Haemophilia* 2003; **9**: 382–6.

27 Kreuz W, Mentzer D, Auerswald G, *et al.* Successful immunetolerance therapy of FVIII inhibitor in children after changing from high to intermediate purity FVIII concentrate. *Haemophilia* 1996; **2** (Suppl. 1): 19.

28 Brackman HH. Factor VIII/von Willebrand complex in haemophilia treatment. *Hematologica* 2003; **88**.

29 Fijnvandraat K, Peters M, Ten Cate JW. Inter-individual variation in half-life of infused recombinant factor VIII is related to pre-infusion von Willebrand factor antigen levels. *Br J Haematol* 1995; **91**: 474–6.

30 Berntorp E, Ekman M, Gunnarsson M, Nilsson IM. Variation in factor VIII inhibitor reactivity with different commercial factor VIII preparations. *Haemophilia* 1996; **2**: 95–9.

31 Suzuki T, Arai M, Amano K, Kagawa K, Fukutake K. Factor VIII inhibitor reactivity with different commercial factor VIII preparations. *Thromb Haemost* 1996; **76**: 749–54.

32 Berntorp E. Immune tolerance induction: recombinant vs. human-derived product. *Haemophilia* 2001; **7**: 109–13.

33 Batlle J, Lopez MF, Brackmann HH, *et al.* Induction of immune tolerance with recombinant factor VIII in haemophilia A patients with inhibitors. *Haemophilia* 1999; **5**: 431–5.

34 Hay CRM, Ludlam CA, Colvin BA, *et al.* Factor VIII inhibitors in mild and moderate-severity haemophilia A. *Thromb Haemost* 1998; **79**: 762–6.

35 Warrier, I. Management of haemophilia B patients with inhibitors and anaphylaxis. *Haemophilia* 1998; **4**: 574–6.

36 Warrier I, Lenk H, Saidi P, *et al.* Nephrotic syndrome in hemophilia B patients with inhibitors. *Haemophilia* 1998; **4**: 248–51.

37 Ewenstein BM, Takemoto C, Warrier I, *et al.* Nephrotic syndrome as a complication of immune tolerance in hemophilia B. *Blood* 1997; **89**: 1115–16.

38 Rossi G, Sarker J, Scandella D. Long-term induction of immune tolerance after blockade of CD40-CD40L interaction in a mouse model of hemophilia A. *Blood* 2001; **97**: 2750–7.

39 Ewenstein BM, Hoots WK, Lusher JM, DiMichele DM. Inhibition of CD40 ligand (CD154) in the treatment of factor VIII inhibitors. *Haematologia* 2000; **10**: 35–9.

40 Barrow RT, Healey JF, Gailani D, *et al.* Reduction in the antigenicity of factor VIII towards complex inhibitory antibody plasmas using multiply-substituted hybrid human/porcine factor VIII molecules. *Blood* 2000; **95**: 564–8.

41 Saint Remy JM. Hemophilia factor VIII therapy. B- and T-cell tolerance: from basic concepts to clinical practice. *Haematologia* 2000; **10**: 89–92.

42 Hay CRM, Laurian Y, Verroust F, *et al.* Induction of immune tolerance in patients with hemophilia A and inhibitors treated with porcine VIIIC by home therapy. *Blood* 1990; **76**: 882–6.

14 Inhibitors to factor VIII: treatment of acute bleeds

Claude Negrier

The treatment of acute bleeds in patients who have developed inhibitors of factor VIII (FVIII) has benefited in the last decades from the development of new drugs, which has dramatically improved the prognosis of patients who experience such events. Several therapeutic agents are available to treat bleeds in hemophiliacs with inhibitors, but no single agent is efficacious in all patients or all circumstances. Although the management of patients with high-responding inhibitors is still complex and remains a medical challenge in some clinical situations, these products may not only ameliorate the pain, but also reduce the risk of muscular and skeletal damage. They also improve the educational and work prospects for these patients as well as enhancing their social participation and quality of life.

Clinical context

Acute bleeds may occur in various clinical contexts, but two characteristics influence product choice to achieve hemostasis. On the one hand, patients with low- or high-titer inhibitors are considered to exhibit the bleeding profile of a severe hemophiliac. This means that they suffer two to four bleeding episodes per month, although some patients demonstrate a decrease in the frequency of bleedings with aging. Most of these bleeds occur spontaneously (in everyday life) and will be successfully treated with home treatment. In contrast, some acute bleeds may be life-threatening or may arise in critical situations such as perioperative periods. Although both types of clinical settings represent acute conditions, the nature of treatment to be administered may be different, depending on the titer of the inhibitor at that moment (Figure 14.1).

Classification between high and low responders

Inhibitors have been classified according to peak historical antibody titer and the presence or absence of immunologic anamnesis. A recent consensus of the FVIII and FIX Standardization Subcommittee of the International Society of Thrombosis and Hemostasis defined high-responding antibodies as those exhibiting a peak historical titer of >5 BU accompanied by brisk anamnesis and the consequent inability to treat hemorrhages routinely with specific factor replacement [1]. Accordingly, a low responder was defined by both a low historical peak titer

(<5 BU) and a lack of anamnesis upon factor re-exposure. As a consequence, these latter patients can usually be treated with higher than usual doses of specific clotting factor concentrate to override the inhibitory effect of the antibody.

Products available

The available therapeutic agents for treatment of acute hemorrhage in hemophiliacs with an inhibitor include high-dose human FVIII concentrate, porcine FVIII concentrate, activated prothrombin complex concentrates (aPCC), and recombinant FVIIa (rFVIIa). In addition, antifibrinolytics and external removal of the inhibitory antibodies may be used as an adjunct therapy.

Human factor VIII concentrates

For nonanamnestic low-titer inhibitors (<5 BU), high doses of FVIII concentrates may be used to achieve hemostasis [2]. Both plasma-derived and rFVIII can be administered with no objective difference in terms of *in vivo* efficacy between these types of products. The dose is targeted to saturate the inhibitor (number of units to be infused = plasma volume in mL × inhibitor titer) and to raise the FVIII plasma concentration to the desired level after inhibitor neutralization [considering a mean recovery of 2 IU/dL/IU infused/kg body weight (b.w.)]. The major advantages of this modality are achievement of a predictable hemostasis according to the plasma level achieved and the ability to undertake biologic monitoring using standard coagulation techniques, if needed. The main disadvantage of this strategy is the subsequent anamnestic response that may occur in some patients, which may decrease the possibility of further use in the next months or years. In general, inhibitors of more than 10 BU cannot be saturated with high-dose FVIII; further, the clinical benefit is not predictable when the titer is between 5 and 10 BU.

Porcine factor VIII

High-purity porcine FVIII (Hyate:C, Ipsen, UK) was developed on the premise that human FVIII inhibitors have a median 15–30% cross-reactivity to porcine FVIII [3]. Porcine FVIII is used for treating serious bleeding in patients with low- or intermediate-level inhibitor titers against the porcine FVIII molecule. Well-selected patients may achieve hemostasis in 80–90% of

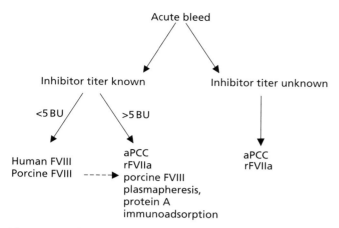

Figure 14.1 Schematic diagram of the therapeutic options for the treatment of acute bleeds according to the inhibitor titer (in Bethesda units/mL).

bleeding episodes, considering a mean recovery of 1.3%/IU injected/kg b.w. [4,5]. The administration of porcine FVIII may be associated with a transient fall in platelet count and allergic reactions in some individuals, partly because of the presence of high-molecular-weight multimers of porcine von Willebrand factor. An anamnestic response commonly occurs in 50–70% of high responders following the infusion of the porcine molecule. This may render the patient completely refractory to further administration for a protracted period of time.

Porcine FVIII is not virally attenuated, although it has not been shown to transmit any viral disease to human recipients. However, the demand for improved side-effect profile and viral safety is driving the development of a porcine product which would be highly purified and would include at least one viral attenuation step. To achieve this end, a recombinant porcine FVIII molecule is under development. At the time of publication, however, porcine FVIII is available only on a named patient basis for life- or limb-threatening bleed (compassionate use protocol).

Activated prothrombin complex concentrates

Activated prothrombin complex concentrates (aPCCs) represented a considerable improvement in inhibitor therapy when they appeared in the 1970s [6]. These products were established as standard first-line treatment for bleeding episodes in high-titer inhibitors. Both of the presently licensed aPCCs are produced by *in vitro* modification of plasma-derived prothrombin complex concentrates (PCCs), resulting in a degree of activation of some of the clotting factors. They contain multiple activated serine protease molecules, of which activated FX and prothrombin represent the main active components in FEIBA® (factor VIII inhibitor bypassing activity; Baxter Healthcare Corporation Glendale, CA, USA), while in Autoplex® T (Nabi Biopharmaceuticals, Boca Raton, FL, USA), FIX and FVII are thought to be the putative active hemostatic proteases [7,8]. However, the

precise mechanism of action of these aPCCs remains poorly understood. This likely explains the difficulty of a standardized therapeutic follow-up *in vivo*.

Kurczynski and Penner [7] reported in 1974 the first significant study on the use of Autoplex T [7]. Single doses of Autoplex T were used to treat 60 bleeds in eight severe hemophilia A inhibitor patients. The largest study assessing the efficacy of Autoplex T was reported by Kantrowitz *et al.* [9]. In this study, 454 infusions of Autoplex T were used to treat 120 bleeding episodes in 60 severe hemophilia A patients with inhibitors. Autoplex T was effective in the treatment of 87% of the reported bleeds.

Sjamsoedin *et al.* [10] studied the effect of FEIBA on joint and muscle bleeding in hemophilia A inhibitor patients (Table 14.1). This randomized double-blind trial compared FEIBA with a nonactivated PCC. Outcome comparison showed that FEIBA produced significantly greater improvements in bleeding control and joint mobility. The largest observational trial on the use of FEIBA was a retrospective multicenter French study [11] Table 14.1. Data were presented on 433 bleeding episodes, including surgical procedures involving 60 patients. Efficacy was good or excellent in 81.3% of treatment episodes, while tolerance (safety) was assessed as good in 98.8% of the cases.

In summary, it can be estimated that both products have been found to achieve effective hemostasis in approximately 80% of bleeds involving joints and soft tissues [9–14].

Both FEIBA and Autoplex T undergo viral inactivation procedures during their manufacturing processes. Minor reactions have been reported in association with both products, mainly consisting of headache, nausea, pruritus, skin rashes, and diarrhea. Anamnestic increases in inhibitor levels have been reported in up to 30% of patients receiving FEIBA, owing to the presence of small amounts of FVIII:C antigen in the material. However, it was shown that in over 50% of the patients who remain on regular FEIBA therapy, the antibody level gradually falls. Autoplex T has also been associated with the development of anamnestic responses in some patients. However, anamnestic responses to aPCCs are not associated with a reduction in their clinical efficacy.

For treatment of acute bleeds, the recommended dose of FEIBA is 50–100 U/kg infused every 8–12 h. Because of the potential for thrombotic complications, a maximum daily dose of 200 U/kg is recommended. Autoplex T is commonly administered at a mean dose of 75 FECU (factor eight correctional units) per kilogram body weight, with the option of repeating doses as required at 8- to 12-h intervals.

Despite many years of experience with these concentrates, there is currently no laboratory test for monitoring the hemostatic efficacy of aPCCs, and dosage must be determined solely by clinical assessment. Future studies will be needed to demonstrate the usefulness of a monitoring system, which would correlate with hemostatic efficacy. However, it was recently proposed that the clinical effect of FEIBA may correlate with circulating thrombin-generating potential, and a fluorogenic substrate assay is being developed to enable monitoring of FEIBA dosage *in vivo* [15].

Table 14.1 Summary of FEIBA efficacy for treatment of various bleeding events (both home and hospital treatments).

Reference	Patients	Bleeding episodes	Dose of Autoplex/FEIBA	Efficacy (%) (time for evaluation)
Kantrowitz et al. [9]	60	120	25–100 FECU/kg 8- to 12-hourly	86 (<36 h)
White [14]	23	54	75 FECU/kg 8- to 12-hourly	85 (72 h)
Sjamsoedin et al. [10]	15	150	88 U/kg	64 (24 h)
Hilgartner and Knatterud [12]	49	165	50–70 U/kg 12-hourly	91 (72 h)
Hilgartner et al. [13]	41	106	50–75 U/kg 12-hourly	79 (36 h)
Negrier et al. [11]	60	433	65–100 U/kg 6- to 12-hourly	81 (up to three doses)

Table 14.2 Summary of home treatment—minor procedures performed with recombinant factor VIIa.

Study	No. of cases	No. of bleeds	Dose (μg/kg)	Achievement of hemostasis	Adverse effects	Mean no. of injections
Key et al. [20]	60	614	90	566 (92%)	32 (3%)	2.2
Laurian et al. [21]	16	147	90–120	90%	1 (0.6%)	3.8
Santagostino et al. [22]	21	53	90	42 (79%)	3 (2.6%)	2

Recombinant factor VIIa

Recombinant factor VIIa (rFVIIa) (NovoSeven, NovoNordisk, Bagsvaerd, Denmark) is produced as a single-chain glycoprotein in genetically modified BHK (baby hamster kidney) cell line. During purification, rFVII is converted to the two-chain activated form. The mode of action of rFVIIa may not be completely understood, but it has been demonstrated that rFVIIa is able to directly activate factor X and increase thrombin production on the surface of activated platelets in the absence of factor VIII or IX. The platelet-specific generation of IIa by rVIIa is thought to localize the hemostatic process to the sites of active bleeding and tissue injury [16,17]. The pharmacokinetic evaluation of rFVIIa demonstrated that the half-life is 2–3 h in adults and 1.30–3 h in children with individual variations [18]. Owing to these pharmacokinetic properties, rFVIIa needs to be administered every 2–6 h. The first description of clinical efficacy occurred in 1988 in a patient with high-titer inhibitor who underwent an open synovectomy [19]. As shown in Table 14.2, initial clinical experience has shown that the treatment of home bleeds usually required a median of more than two rFVIIa injections of 70–90 μg/kg [20–22]. To improve the clinical efficacy of treatment with rFVIIa in high-titer inhibitor patients, attention must be paid to the time of initiating treatment after the onset of bleeding. Early injection of rFVIIa within 1 h following the onset of bleeding has been associated with a better clinical outcome [23].

A few case reports have recently suggested the possibility that higher rFVIIa doses might be more convenient, and perhaps more efficacious, for the treatment of bleeding episodes. It is sug-gested that a full thrombin burst is necessary for the assembly of a tight fibrin structure that efficiently stabilizes the hemostatic plug [24] and induces a complete activation of other clotting factors, including the thrombin-activatable fibrinolytic inhibitor (TAFI) [25]. A prospective and comparative evaluation of bolus megadoses of rFVIIa, i.e., 300 μg/kg, was recently reported by Kenet et al. [26] in three patients with high-titer inhibitors. Pain relief was faster and treatment duration was shorter for the bleeding episodes treated by the megadose protocol. In addition, this increased dose was found to be more convenient and the rFVIIa total consumption per bleeding episode was also significantly lower. No thrombosis was reported in the three patients. The fact that hemostasis was achieved in all patients with a single (83% success rate) or two injections (100% success rate) suggests that this mode of delivering rFVIIa might be more efficacious than with lower doses as previously observed [27].

Since no FVIII is contained in the product, there is no risk of anamnestic response. However, it should be emphasized that, analogous to aPCCs, there is as yet no standardized quantitative laboratory test for measuring the effectiveness of rFVIIa therapy. However, promising results have recently been reported using thromboelastography [28].

All currently used bypassing agents (PCCs, aPCCs, and rFVIIa) for the treatment of patients with high-titer inhibitory antibodies carry the risk of thrombotic complications, including thromboembolism, disseminated intravascular coagulation, and myocardial infarction [29–31]. These complications are rare [32,33] and are considered to be caused by an increase in the concentration of native, or activated, coagulation factors in the recipient. Thrombotic events (e.g., cardiovascular and cerebrovascular) and subclinical disseminated intravascular coagulation (DIC) occur most commonly in patients with underlying atherosclerotic disease and those immobile for long periods. Patients with pre-existing liver disease and premature infants may be particularly susceptible to DIC. In addition, patients undergoing surgery or those who receive repeated high doses of the concentrate should be carefully monitored to minimize the risk of thrombogenicity.

Antifibrinolytics

Tranexamic acid is a structural analog that binds irreversibly to the lysine binding sites on plasminogen, thus inhibiting fibrinolysis. Through the inhibition of the natural degradation of fibrin, it helps to stabilize clots. Although they have a short plasma half-life (~2 h), antifibrinolytic agents may be helpful in the treatment of bleeding from the gastrointestinal tract, menorrhagia, epistaxis, and oral bleeding (including in dental surgery) in inhibitor-developing hemophiliacs [34,35]. It can be administered orally or intravenously, or as a mouth wash. Dosing of tranexamic acid must be reduced in patients with renal dysfunction; further, it is generally advisable not to use tranexamic acid or any other antifibrinolytic drug, including ε-aminocaproic acid (Amicar), for the treatment of hematuria because blood from the upper urinary tract can provoke painful clot retention.

Immunoadsorption

Plasmapheresis or immunoadsorption of plasma with staphylococcal protein A removes immunoglobulins and immune complexes, including inhibitors to FVIII. Although apheresis or immunoadsorption instruments are relatively complex and expensive, the procedure may be cost-effective, given the expense of therapies used to treat patients with inhibitors, particularly in an acute surgical or life-threatening situation. If the inhibitory antibodies are effectively removed, the decrease in the inhibitor titer may render the patient susceptible to be treated by human or porcine FVIII concentrates [36–38].

Management of bleeding situations

The management of bleeding episodes in patients with inhibitors may take advantage of the differential use of the various therapeutic approaches mentioned above. No single product may meet all clinical requirements. The most applicable strategy depends on clinical assessment of severity, knowledge of inhibitor level to human and porcine FVIII and, if the titer is low, whether the patient is a high-or a low responder.

One should therefore consider different clinical scenarios:
• Scenario 1: in low titer and low responders, it seems logical to preferentially use higher than normal doses of human FVIII in all clinical situations. The dose of FVIII is increased proportionate to the inhibitor titer. For major hemorrhages, this strategy can also be used if inhibitor titers are low enough to allow satisfactory plasma levels to be achieved. Porcine FVIII can also be prescribed in limb- or life-threatening bleeds in which there is no significant product cross-reactivity with the patient's inhibitor. Antifibrinolytic agents are useful as local administration such as mouth wash or systemically.
• Scenario 2: in low titer and high responders, one would favor rFVIIa or aPCCs for minor bleeding considering the high efficiency of those products. This strategy allows one to reserve FVIII for further treatment of more critical situations. For major bleeds, high-dose human (or porcine) FVIII concentrate is able to produce effective hemostasis, but it should be recognized that the consequence of such treatment will be a quasisystematic anamnestic response to FVIII molecule after 4–7 days of treatment. This subsequent increase in the inhibitor titer commonly renders the patient refractory to the continuation of factor replacement, although concomitant antibody removal using plasmapheresis or protein A adsorption may be attempted. It is common that the inhibitor titer remains above 5 BU/mL for weeks or months, during which time the patient cannot be treated with FVIII. In this situation, a second-line therapy with aPCC or rFVIIa has to be considered if the bleeding complication needs further treatment.
• Scenario 3: in a patient known to be a high responder with a high-titer inhibitor (>5 BU), minor bleeding may usually be treated with aPCC or rFVIIa (one to four injections as necessary). The treatment of major bleeding in this category of patients represents one of the most challenging situations in the treatment of patients with hemophilia. Considering that an ability to monitor *in vivo* FVIII levels confers predictable correlation with physiologic concentrations, porcine FVIII may be used as first-line therapy if the anti-porcine FVIII inhibitor level is below 5 BU. If anti-porcine inhibitor titers are high or unknown, rFVIIa or an aPCC is preferred. In the case of failure to control the bleeding, immunoadsorption may temporarily reduce the inhibitor, enabling replacement therapy with FVIII for several days. Antifibrinolytic agents can also be used if there are no contraindications (see above).

Conclusion

The management of acute bleeds in patients who have developed inhibitory antibodies remains a medical challenge for those treating hemophilia, particularly in critical medical conditions. Although the administration of human or porcine factor VIII is generally preferred when the inhibitor titer is <5 BU, the anamnestic response may render the patient completely refractory to the clotting factor. Bypassing agents have dramatically improved the home treatment setting, but the impracticality of monitoring for efficacy and the lack of a predictable clinical dose–response represents a major limitation. However, some preliminary positive results using thrombin generating potential or thrombelastographic analysis of whole blood clotting may prove their value in the near future for guiding clinical practice.

References

1 White GC 2nd, Rosendaal F, Aledort LM, *et al.* Factor VIII and factor IX Subcommittee. Definitions in hemophilia. Recommendation of the scientific subcommittee on factor VIII and factor IX of the scientific and standardization committee of the International Society on Thrombosis and Haemostasis. *Thromb Haemost* 2001; **85**: 560.

2 Kasper CK. Human factor VIII for bleeding in patients with inhibitors. *Vox Sang* 1999; **77** (Suppl. 1): 47–8.

3 Kernoff PB. Rationale and evolution of therapy with porcine factor VIII:C. *Am J Med* 1991; **91**: 20–2.

4 Brettler DB, Forsberg AD, Levine PH, *et al.* The use of porcine factor VIII concentrate (Hyate C) in the treatment of patients with inhibitor antibodies to factor FVIII: a multicenter US experience. *Arch Intern Med* 1989; **149**: 1381–5.

5 Hay CR, Lozier JN, Lee CA, *et al.* Safety profile of porcine factor VIII and its use as hospital and home therapy for patients with haemophilia A and inhibitors: the results of an international survey. *Thromb Haemost* 1996; **75**: 25–9.

6 Kurczynski EM, Penner JA: Activated prothrombin concentrate for patients with factor VIII inhibitors. *N Engl J Med* 1974; **291**: 164–7.

7 Turecek PL, Varadi K, Gritsch H, *et al.* Factor Xa and prothrombin: mechanism of action of FEIBA. *Vox Sang* 1999; **77** (Suppl. 1): 72–9.

8 Lundblad RL, Bergstrom J, De Vreker R, *et al.* Measurement of active coagulation factors in Autoplex®-T with colorimetric active site-specific assay technology. *Thromb Haemost* 1998; **80**: 811–15.

9 Kantrowitz JL, Lee ML, McClure DA, *et al.* Early experience with the use of anti-inhibitor coagulant complex to treat bleeding in hemophiliacs with inhibitors to factor VIII. *Clin Ther* 1987; **9**: 405–19.

10 Sjamsoedin LJ, Heijnen L, Mauser-Bunschoten EP, *et al.* The effect of activated prothrombin-complex concentrate (FEIBA) on joint and muscle bleeding in patients with haemophilia A and antibodies to factor VIII. A double-blind clinical trial. *N Engl J Med* 1981; **305**: 717–21.

11 Negrier C, Goudemand J, Sultan Y, *et al.* and the members of the French FEIBA Study Group. Multicenter retrospective study on the utilization of FEIBA in France in patients with factor VIII and factor IX inhibitors. *Thromb Haemost* 1997; **77**: 1113–19.

12 Hilgartner MW, Knatterud GL. The use of factor eight inhibitor by-passing activity (FEIBA immuno) product for treatment of bleeding episodes in haemophiliacs with inhibitors. *Blood* 1983; **61**: 36–40.

13 Hilgartner M, Aledort L, Andes A, Gill J. Efficacy and safety of vapor-heated anti-inhibitor coagulant complex in hemophilia patients. FEIBA Study Group. *Transfusion* 1990; **30**: 626–30.

14 White GC 2nd. Seventeen years' experience with Autoplex/ Autoplex T: evaluation of inpatients with severe haemophilia A and factor VIII inhibitors at a major haemophilia centre. *Haemophilia* 2000; **6**: 508–12.

15 Varadi K, Negrier C, Berntorp E, *et al.* Monitoring the bioavailability of FEIBA with a thrombin generation assay. *J Thromb Haemost* 2003; **11**: 2374–80.

16 Monroe DM, Hoffman M, Oliver JA, Roberts HR. Platelet activity of high dose factor VIIa is independent of tissue factor. *Br J Haematol* 1997; **99**: 542–7.

17 Hoffman M, Monroe DM III, Roberts HR. Activated factor VII activates FIX and FX on the surface of activated platelets: thoughts on the mechanism of action of high dose activated factor VII. *Blood Coagul Fibrinolysis* 1998; **9**: S61–S65.

18 Lindley CM, Sawyer WT, Macik BG, *et al.* Pharmacokinetics and pharmacodynamics of recombinant factor VIIa. *Clin Pharmacol Ther* 1994; **55**: 638–48.

19 Hedner U, Glazer S, Pingel K, *et al.* Successful use of recombinant factor VIIa in patient with severe haemophilia A during synovectomy. *Lancet* 1988; **2**: 1193.

20 Key NS, Aledort LM, Beardsley D, *et al.* Home treatment of mild to moderate bleeding episodes using recombinant factor VIIa (Novoseven) in haemophiliacs with inhibitors. *Thromb Haemost* 1998; **80**: 912–18.

21 Laurian Y, Goudemand J, Negrier C, *et al.* Use of recombinant activated factor VII as first line therapy for bleeding episodes in hemophiliacs with factor VIII or IX inhibitors (NOSEPAC study). *Blood Coagul Fibrinolysis* 1998; **9**: S155–S156.

22 Santagostino E, Gringeri A, Mannucci PM. Home treatment with recombinant activated factor VII in patients with factor VIII inhibitors: the advantages of early intervention. *Br J Haematol* 1999; **104**: 22–6.

23 Lusher JM. Acute hemarthroses: the benefits of early versus late treatment with recombinant activated factor VII. *Blood Coagul Fibrinolysis* 2000; **11**: S45–S49.

24 Blomback B, Carlsson K, Fatah K, *et al.* Fibrin in human plasma gel architectures governed by rate and nature of fibrinogen activation. *Thromb Res* 1994; **75**: 521–38.

25 Lisman T, Mosnier LO, Lambert T, *et al.* Inhibition of fibrinolysis by recombinant factor VIIa in plasma from patients with severe hemophilia A. *Blood* 2002; **99**: 175–9.

26 Kenet G, Lubetsky A, Luboshitz J, Martinowitz U. A new approach to treatment of bleeding episodes in young hemophilia patients: a single bolus megadose of recombinant activated factor VII (Novo-Seven). *J Thromb Haemost* 2003; **1**: 450–55.

27 Lusher J, Ingerslev J, Roberts HR, Hedner U. Clinical experience with recombinant factor VIIa: a review. *Blood Coagul Fibrinolysis* 1998; **9**: 119–28.

28 Sorensen B, Ingerslev J. Whole blood clot formation phenotypes in hemophilia A and rare coagulation disorders. Patterns of response to recombinant factor VIIa. *J Thromb Haemost* 2004; **2**: 102–10.

29 Kohler M. Thrombogenicity of prothrombin complex concentrates. *Thromb Res* 1999; **95**: S13–S17.

30 Peerlinck K, Vermylen J. Acute myocardial infarction following administration of recombinant activated factor VII (Novo seven) in a patient with haemophilia A and inhibitor. *Thromb Haemost* 1999; **82**: 1775–6.

31 Mizon P, Goudemand J, Jude B, Marey A. Myocardial infarction after FEIBA therapy in a hemophilia-B patient with a factor IX inhibitor. *Ann Hematol* 1992; **64**: 309–11.

32 Roberts HR. Clinical experience with activated factor VII: focus on safety aspects. *Blood Coagul Fibrinolysis* 1998; **9**: S115–S118.

33 Ehrlich HJ, Henzl MJ, Gomperts ED. Safety of factor VIII inhibitor bypass activity (FEIBA): 10-year compilation of thrombotic adverse events. *Haemophilia* 2002; **8**: 83–90.

34 Sindet-Pedersen S, Stenbjerg S. Effect of local anti-fibrinolytic treatment with tranexamic acid in hemophiliacs undergoing oral surgery. *J Oral Maxillofac Surg* 1986; **44**: 704–7.

35 Ghosh K, Shetty S, Jijina F, Mohanty D. Role of epsilon amino caproic acid in the management of haemophilic patients with inhibitors. *Haemophilia* 2004; **10**: 58–62.

36 Francesconi M, Korninger C, Thaler E, *et al.* Plasmapheresis: its value in the management of patients with antibodies to factor VIII. *Haemostasis* 1982; **11**: 79–86.

37 Watt RM, Bunitsky K, Faulkner EB, *et al.* Treatment of congenital and acquired hemophilia patients by extracorporeal removal of antibodies to coagulation factors – a review of United States clinical studies. *Transfusion Science* 1992; **13**: 233–53.

38 Freiburghaus C, Berntorp E, Ekman M, *et al.* Immunoadsorption for removal of inhibitors: update on treatments in Malmö-Lund between 1980 and 1995. *Haemophilia* 1998; **4**: 16–20.

Acquired inhibitors to factor VIII

Craig M. Kessler and Ekatherine Asatiani

Acquired inhibitors directed against coagulation factor VIII:C (FVIII:C) interfere and/or neutralize its procoagulant function and result in severe and often life-threatening hemorrhagic complications. These inhibitors are autoantibodies, usually arising in individuals with no prior history of clinical bleeding. Auto-FVIII:C antibodies usually are polyclonal, predominantly immunoglobulin G (IgG) subclasses 1 and 4; they express their neutralizing capacity with type II pharmacokinetics, result in serious clinical bleeding, and require different treatment and immune tolerance strategies. This chapter will review the pathophysiology, clinical picture, and management strategies for this relatively rare acquired condition, which arises in previously noncoagulopathic, nonhemophilic individuals with no previous history of a bleeding diathesis.

Epidemiology

Acquired hemophilia has an estimated prevalence of one per million population per year, with a reported mortality between 6% and 22%. Despite its low prevalence, the condition imposes significant clinical and medical economic challenges because its dramatic complications are frequently life-threatening and its management of bleeding events is always expensive.

The age of onset for acquired hemophilia appears to be distributed in a biphasic pattern, with a small peak in young individuals, primarily postpartum women and those with autoimmune diseases, and the major peak in those aged 60–80 years, mainly males with epithelial and lymphoproliferative malignancies. All of the largest published population series have noted that about 50% of diagnosed individuals were previously healthy with no identified underlying disease state [1–3]. Consistent disease associations have been reported in the other half of the patients and include evolving or pre-existing autoimmune or lymphoproliferative disorders [4].

Pathophysiology and characteristics of autoantibodies to factor VIII

The human factor circulates in the plasma, noncovalently bound to von Willebrand factor (VWF), which chaperones it through the circulation. The sequence of the FVIII:C protein is composed of amino acids grouped into six domains. The most common epitopes for autoantibody (as well as alloantibody) binding appear to lie between amino acids 454–509 and 593 in the A2 domain, between 1804 and 1819 in the A3 domain, and between 2181 and 2243 in the C2 domain [5]. Anti-C2 antibodies inhibit the binding of FVIII to phospholipid and may also interfere with the binding of FVIII to VWF protein, whereas anti-A2 and anti-A3 antibodies impede the binding of factor VIII:C to factor X (FX) and FIXa (FIXa), respectively, in the intrinsic pathway FX activation complex. Autoantibodies binding to sites other than those mentioned above may be clinically silent.

Most antibodies are mixtures of polyclonal IgG1 and IgG4 immunoglobulins, with the IgG4 molecules mainly responsible for inhibiting clotting activity. Kappa light chains predominate. The IgG4 antibodies do not form immunoprecipitates or fix complement; thus, end-organ damage does not occur as it may with alloantibodies against FIX. Cross-reactivity between autoantibodies and heterologous sources of factor VIII:C is limited. This justifies the use of porcine FVIII:C concentrate in the treatment and prevention of bleeding complications in acquired hemophilia.

Interactions between autoantibodies and FVIII:C is characterized by very rapid and nonlinear inactivation of FVIII:C, following type II kinetics [7]. Antibodies are extremely difficult to saturate by addition of FVIII:C; therefore, treatment with human FVIII is usually unsuccessful in the presence of such antibodies. Much less commonly, auto-FVIII:C antibodies may assume a type I pattern of inhibition in which there is linear, second-order kinetics and no residual FVIII:C activity detectable in patient plasma. This type is classically observed with allo-FVIII:C antibodies in congenital hemophilia A [8].

Associated disease states

Auto-FVIII:C antibody inhibitors frequently are associated with disease states thought to arise from a dysregulated immune system. Among such are systemic lupus erythematosus [9,10] and rheumatoid arthritis. Less commonly, acquired hemophilia is associated with organ-specific autoimmune diseases such as myasthenia gravis, multiple sclerosis, Graves' disease and autoimmune hemolytic anemia [11,12]. Asthma, chronic inflammatory bowel disease, pemphigus [13], and graft-vs.-host disease [14] following allogeneic bone marrow transplant have also been reported anecdotally. In contrast to postpartum patients, in whom inhibitors may disappear spontaneously, patients with rheumatoid arthritis usually manifest high-titer inhibitors and require some form of immunosuppressive therapy.

The association between pregnancy and acquired hemophilia has long been recognized. The bleeding disorder usually follows termination of pregnancy, most commonly 1–4 months after delivery, although cases appearing more than 1 year post partum have been described. In addition, the auto-FVIII:C inhibitor may appear during pregnancy in 2–14% of patients. If the inhibitor is low titer ("5 BU), it generally disappears spontaneously over months and does not recur with subsequent pregnancies. High-titer inhibitors (>5 BU) can persist for years despite treatment with corticosteroids, intravenous immunoglobulin, and cytotoxic agents. Mortality rates also tend to be lower in this subgroup of patients, ranging between 0% and 6%. The pathogenesis of these pregnancy-related autoantobody inhibitors directed against FVIII remains unclear.

Approximately 10% of patients with acquired hemophilia have an associated underlying malignancy, most commonly epithelial or lymphoproliferative in nature [3,15]. This association with cancer occurs predominantly in elderly men [16] and, especially when observed in conjunction with lymphoproliferative disorders, is consistent with the broad range of autoimmune phenomena that frequently complicate these conditions. The etiologic role of solid tumor malignancies in acquired hemophilia is not so apparent. In fact, some authors consider that the appearance of FVIII:C autoantibodies in patients with solid tumors may well be an epiphenomenon since these neoplasms occur so commonly in the same elderly cohort as acquired hemophilia. In some cases, the FVIII:C autoantibodies have been observed to arise after treatment for cancer has been initiated. In those cases, it is possible that use of corticosteroids, cytotoxic agents, and biologic response modifiers could have altered host immunity and predisposed the patient to the development of autoimmune phenomena. Alternatively, FVIII:C autoantibody inhibitors could represent a host immune response to the tumor-derived antigens, although no tumor antigen has yet been described to have homology to FVIII:C. The auto-FVIII:C antibody inhibitor may not remit following successful eradication of malignancy process. Conversely, the re-emergence of inhibitors is not a reliable indication of tumor recurrence in patients.

Certain medications, including antibiotics [17] (penicillins, sulfonamides, chloramphenicol), anticonvulsants [18] (diphenylhydantoin), and BCG (bacille Calmette–Guérin) vaccination [19], have well-established associations with development of acquired hemophilia. Frequently, drug-induced anti-FVIII:C antibodies arise after hypersensitivity reactions and remit shortly after withdrawing the offending drug. The pathophysiology of this phenomenon remains unknown in most cases; however, the significant alterations of immune function which are induced by the administration of such medications as interferon (IFN) alpha [20] and fludarabine, may facilitate the appearance of autoantibodies against FVIII:C, as they do for other immune phenomena reported with their use, e.g., autoimmune thrombocytopenic purpura or autoimmune hemolytic anemia.

Clinical manifestation of acquired hemophilia

The clinical picture of acquired hemophilia is characterized by acute onset of severe bleeding in individuals who previously had no history of bleeding diatheses. It is notable that the bleeding pattern is distinctly more severe and anatomically varied than that observed in congenital severe hemophilia A complicated by alloimmune inhibitors directed against FVIII:C. The bleeding is usually spontaneous, although minimal trauma may predispose to disproportionately extensive ecchymoses. Patients may present with overt bleeding or anemia due to occult hemorrhage. The bleeding is accompanied by considerable morbidity and the mortality rate approaches 20%.

Laboratory diagnosis

The activated partial thromboplastin time (aPTT) is prolonged as FVIII, FIX, FXI, and FXII, for which it screens, are decreased in undiluted patient plasma. The prothrombin time (PT) and platelet function are usually normal. To determine if the elevated aPTT is due to a specific clotting factor deficiency or a pathologic circulating anticoagulant, performance of mixing studies is critical. For FVIII:C inhibitory antibodies of the allo- or autovariety, the neutralizing expression of the inhibitor is time and temperature dependent and may require 2 h at 37°C, especially in the case of weak autoantibodies, before an accurate assessment of the inhibitor can be ascertained. A difference of 10 s or greater is indicative of a positive inhibitor screen.

To confirm the neutralization of a specific coagulation factor by auto- or allo-antibody inhibitors, assays for each of the coagulation factors in the involved pathway must be performed. Lupus-like anticoagulants can be distinguished from clotting factor autoantibody inhibitors by the finding of a positive platelet neutralization assay and/or a prolonged dilute Russell's viper venom test (dRVVT), tissue thromboplastin inhibition assay, or kaolin clotting time. The platelet neutralization assay takes advantage of the observation that the phospholipid component of platelet membranes adsorbs out the phospholipophilic lupus-like inhibitor but not an anti-FVIII:C auto- or alloantibody inhibitor. Thus, incubation of patient plasma with washed platelets will result in shortening of an otherwise prolonged aPTT. The dRVVT makes use of an enzyme isolated from the Russell viper that promotes FX activation by direct proteolytic cleavage. This assay monitors the coagulation process from the common pathway distally so that a lupus-like inhibitor, directed against phospholipid in the prothrombinase complex, will prolong the assay. Anti-FVIII:C antibodies do not affect the dRVVT. Similarly, the other two assays for the lupus-like anticoagulant are not prolonged by anti-FVIII:C antibodies.

When the presence of inhibitor is suspected, it is imperative that the specific target is identified and the degree of inhibitory activity quantified. This is accomplished by incubating a source of the specific clotting factor (typically, pooled normal plasma) with increasing dilutions of the patient's plasma at 37°C for 2 h. As the antibody-containing plasma is diluted, the clotting factor concentration will appear to increase although the baseline mixture may yield a normal aPTT or FVIII:C activity level. The inhibitor potency is expressed most commonly worldwide in terms of Bethesda units (BU) [21], where 1.0 BU is the reciprocal dilution of patient test plasma permitting detection of 50% residual FVIII:C activity in a mixture with normal pooled plasma. Less commonly, in Europe, FVIII:C inhibitors are quantitated in new Oxford units, which are derived from neutralizing-mixing studies of patient test plasma with diluted FVIII:C concentrate. One Oxford unit is equivalent to approximately 0.83 BU. The Bethesda assay has been modified by using buffered normal plasma throughout (Nijmegen modification) [22]. This also allows for increased sensitivity of the inhibitor assay to detect low-titer inhibitors, e.g., "0.6 BU.

Other assays for specific clotting factor inhibitors rely on immunologic rather than functional methodologies. These assays are extremely sensitive, but are generally confined to a research setting. Techniques include immunodiffusion and enzyme-linked immunoabsorbent assays (ELISAs) [23], both of which are able to detect antibodies that do not inhibit FVIII:C activity *in vitro* or *in vivo*.

Treatment

There are two major goals for the treatment of acquired hemophilia: the immediate control of acute and chronic bleeding and the long-term suppression/eradication of the autoantibody inhibitor. The first objective is necessary because bleeding episodes are often relentless without reversal of the coagulation deficit, and can be life-threatening. The second objective is required to restore normal hemostasis and can usually be accomplished using some type of immunotherapy. An important caveat is that the level of inhibitor potency is not directly proportional to or predictive of the severity or frequency of bleeding events.

The choice of which of the potential therapeutic agents to administer to reverse bleeding depends on the severity of the bleeding, the clinical setting, the initial and historical peak titers of anti-human FVIII:C and anti-porcine FVIII:C inhibitors, and the degree of cross-reactivity between the anti-FVIII:C autoantibody in patient plasma and exogenous porcine FVIII:C, e.g., does the human inhibitor neutralize porcine FVIII:C? Several strategies, such as administration of desmopressin (intranasal or intravenous) and concentrates of human recombinant FVIII:C (hFVIII:C) or porcine FVIII:C (pFVIII:C), may raise the FVIII:C activity levels adequately in plasmas of individuals with low-titer auto-FVIII:C antibody inhibitors ("5 BU). Individuals with low-titer anti-FVIII:C autoantibody inhibitors are less likely to demonstrate anamnestic rises of their inhibitor titers after exposure to human or porcine FVIII:C replacement products than are allo-FVIII:C antibody inhibitor patients; however, one cannot predict this a priori [24]. If the inhibitor titer is high (>5 BU), or if bleeding persists despite infusions of hFVIII:C or pFVIII:C concentrates, then concentrates of FVIII:C bypassing agents, such as activated prothrombin complex concentrates (aPCCs) or recombinant factor VIIa (rFVIIa), are indicated.

The target level of FVIII:C activity to control most bleeding events should be greater than 50% of normal. It is more feasible with porcine FVIII:C concentrates and more feasible (for hFVIII:C or pFVIII:C) also if the inhibitor titer is <5 BU [25,26]. The recommended dose of hFVIII:C concentrates is 20 IU/kg for each BU of inhibitor plus 40 additional IU/kg intravenously as a bolus. The plasma FVIII:C activity level should be determined 10–15 min after the initial bolus and, if the incremental recovery is not adequate, another bolus dose should be administered [27]. An alternative approach is to administer an initial intravenous bolus of 200–300 IU/kg followed by continuous infusion of about 4–14 IU/kg/h [28]. Human FVIII:C concentrates are not useful if the patient has a high-titer or high-responding inhibitor. The latter may not be known until after the first dose of hFVIII:C concentrate is administered since patients with low-titer inhibitors may be high responders, with the capacity to mount an anamnestic response after exposure to the offending antigen, e.g., FVIII:C.

The factor VIII:C present in intermediate purity concentrates is associated with a large amount of VWF protein, which theoretically protects the FVIII:C from proteolytic inactivation and neutralization by the autoantibodies in the patient's plasma, particularly by antibodies directed against C2 domain. Thus far, this has been more of an *in vitro* consideration than an *in vivo* one, but it is provocative and awaits testing in a clinical setting. A similar argument has been posited for the benefits of D-amino-D-arginine vasopressin (DDAVP) for the treatment of autoantibody FVIII:C inhibitors, albeit low-titer ones. In this situation, DDAVP would be expected to increase both VWF protein and FVIII:C release into the plasma.

Porcine FVIII:C concentrate should be considered as first-line therapy for patients with high titers of acquired anti-FVIII:C autoantibody inhibitors. In contrast to the situation in allo-FVIII:C antibody inhibitors, the cross-reactivity between anti-human FVIII:C autoantibodies and pFVIII:C is usually minimal and rarely neutralizing enough to obviate the use of pFVIII:C concentrate. While the package insert for pFVIII:C concentrate (Hyate-C) states that the best results in FVIII:C inhibitor patients occur with inhibitor titers less than 50 BU against hFVIII, this does not appear operative for auto-FVIII:C antibody inhibitors [26]. A study of 64 patients with acquired hemophilia from 47 centers in Europe and North America reported that the overall control of bleeding was considered excellent in 41%, good in 38%, and fair or poor in 21% [26]. The simplified approach to dosing consists of infusing 50–100 IU/kg pFVIII:C concentrate as an intravenous bolus when the anti-human FVIII:C antibody titer is less that 50 BU/mL and 100–200 IU/kg for inhibitors between 50 and 100 BU/mL. After the initial bolus is deemed effective, pFVIII:C also can be administered as a continuous infusion. If the recoveries (incremental rise in FVIII:C activity levels after administering pFVIII:C) are substantially less than expected and/or the circulating half-life of pFVIII:C activity shortens after multiple doses of pFVIII:C concentrate, a search for anamnestic rises in anti-FVIII:C antibody titers should be initiated.

Other less common but potential adverse effects of pFVIII:C include thrombocytopenia (<10% incidence) and allergic reactions. The thrombocytopenia is rarely severe, is usually dose related, and may be associated with *in vivo* platelet clumping/agglutination (pseudothrombocytopenia). The occurrence of typical allergic transfusion reactions also appears to be dose dependent (particularly at doses >100 IU/kg), and anaphylaxis fortunately is a rare occurrence [2]. In the relatively uncommon situation in which the auto-human FVIII:C autoantibody cross-reacts significantly with pFVIII:C and neutralizes pFVIII:C activity, or if a patient receiving pFVIII:C concentrate has developed refractoriness, severe thrombocytopenia, or allergic transfusion reactions, it is necessary to select another hemostatic agent to control bleeding. These alternative replacement therapies are "bypassing" agents and include recombinant human factor VIIa (rFVIIa) and two activated prothrombin complex concentrates (aPCCs).

The successful use of rFVIIa in acquired hemophilia is essentially anecdotal [29], in the absence of any prospective, randomized, controlled trials. The recommended regimen for acquired hemophilia-related bleeding is rapid intravenous bolus administration of 90–120 μg/kg rFVIIa, repeated every 2–3 h depending on clinical response. Continuous infusion of rFVIIa is being explored as a means of simplifying the demands of frequent dosing and of reducing cost of product. Overall, rFVIIa concentrate is well tolerated despite the small number of venous and arterial thrombotic complications (myocardial infarction, deep venous thrombosis and pulmonary emboli, and disseminated intravascular coagulation).

Activated prothrombin complex concentrates have been used extensively in the treatment of bleeding episodes in patients with both allo- and auto-FVIII:C antibody inhibitors. The most commonly prescribed and most readily available commercially aPCCs are FEIBA and Autoplex. The exact mechanism(s) by which the aPCCs circumvent the anti-FVIII:C antibody and affect coagulation is not completely clear. Most experience with aPCCs has been reported in patients with allo-FVIII:C antibody inhibitors [30]. The recommended dose for both products is 50–200 IU/kg/day administered in divided intravenous bolus doses. The most frequent adverse reactions to the activated prothrombin complex concentrates include thrombogenic events and infrequent allergic reactions. The severe headaches associated with Autoplex administration appear to be related to the rate of infusion.

The primary aim in long-term management of acquired hemophilia is to eradicate the FVIII:C autoantibodies so that further bleeding can be averted. Although in some clinical situations (postpartum women and individuals developing acquired hemophilia as a reaction to certain medications) FVIII:C autoantibodies may remit spontaneously, most published guidelines and algorithms recommend early initiation of eradication therapy. This can be achieved through immunomodulation, employing immunosuppressive medications or administration of intravenous gammaglobulin, and by physically removing antibodies.

Administration of intravenous immunoglobulin (IVIG) in large doses often mediates a rapid decline in autoantibody titers, which is probably mediated by the presence of anti-idiotypic antibodies in the i.v. immunoglobulin, derived from the pooled plasmas of thousands of normal donors. The usual administered dose is 2 g/kg divided in either two or five daily intravenous transfusions [31]. At this time, i.v. immunoglobulin is not considered front-line single-agent therapy for eradication of FVIII:C autoantibody inhibitors, but it may be useful adjunctive therapy along with immunosuppressants, as part of an immune tolerance induction regimen (ITI), or with extracorporeal plasmapheresis.

The most frequently successful immunosuppression of auto-FVIII:C antibodies has been accomplished using corticosteroids as the cornerstone, either as a single agent or in combination with either azathioprine or cyclophosphomide. Steroids usually have been dosed at prednisone 1 mg/kg/day, administered over 3–6 weeks, with less than a 50% success rate of complete remission [32]. Patients who respond to steroids fall into a good prognostic category. Interestingly, the acquired hemophilia of pregnancy is often resistant to steroids and yet remits spontaneously.

Other immunosuppressive medications have been employed for particularly refractory autoantibody inhibitor eradication. These have included cyclosporin [35], FK506 (tacrolimus), azathioprine, mycophenolate mofetil (CellCept) and sirolimus (rapamycin). Controlled studies have not been performed to confirm their safety and efficacy in sufficiently large populations.

The successes of autoantibody eradication with plasmapheresis/exchange protocols and the use of cytotoxic regimens stimulated interest in employing a combined approach to facilitate the long-term resolution of this difficult bleeding disorder. One such protocol included combination of hFVIII:C concentrate, cyclophosphamide, and methylprednisolone with 95% success rate of inhibitor eradication over a mean of 4.7 weeks, with a low recurrence rate [36]. These excellent results remain to be tested in a randomized manner but are extremely promising and should be considered in most acquired patients.

Introduction of Rituximab, a chimeric monoclonal antibody that targets the CD20 antigen, has opened new horizons in the treatment of benign hematologic diseases, such as immune thrombocytopenic purpura, cold agglutinin disease [37], and acquired hemophilia [38]. Anecdotal case reports justify a randomized prospective trial that would define the exact role of this costly modality of treatment in management of acquired hemophilia.

Additional new treatment modalities for acquired hemophilia await development. Theoretically, they could include the manufacture via recombinant technology of a preparation of combined rFII–rFX, which could provide an alternative to rFVIIa concentrate for refractory auto-FVIII:C inhibitors, the development of recombinant pFVIII:C concentrate (currently in phase I clinical trials), and, eventually, the development of a human–porcine FVIII:C hybrid molecule, with porcine-derived amino acid substitutions in the A2, A3, and C2 domains of the human FVIII:C molecule, areas which serve as the epitopes for auto-human FVIII:C antibody inhibitors. Finally, modification of the immune system may be possible to eradicate the autoantibody. Anti-CD40 ligand monoclonal antibodies were used with some success with allo-FVIII:C antibodies before being withdrawn from the clinical arena because of hypercoagulability adverse events in a rheumatoid arthritis population. This approach remains to be tested for auto-FVIII:C antibodies. All of these strategies are provocative and suggest that the future for treatment of the auto-FVIII:C antibody inhibitors in acquired hemophilia is promising.

References

1 Green D, Lechner K. A survey of 215 non-hemophilic patients with inhibitors to factor VIII. *Thromb Haemost* 1981; **45**: 200–3.
2 Kessler CM, Ludlam CA. The treatment of acquired factor VIII inhibitors: worldwide experience with porcine factor VIII concentrate. International Acquired Hemophilia Study Group. *Semin Hematol* 1993; **30**: 22–7.
3 Rizza CR, Spooner RJ, Giangrande PL. Treatment of haemophilia in the United Kingdom 1981–1996. *Haemophilia* 2001; **7**: 349–59.
4 Hay CR. Acquired haemophilia. *Baillière's Clin Haematol* 1998; **11**: 287–303.
5 Barrow RT, Healey JF, Jacquemin MG, *et al.* Antigenicity of putative phospholipid membrane-binding residues in factor VIII. *Blood* 2001; **97**: 169–74.
6 Carmona E, Aznar JA, Jorquera JI, *et al.* Detection of two different anti-factor VIII/von Willebrand factor antibodies of the IgA class in a hemophilic patient with a polyclonal factor VIII inhibitor of the IgG class. *Thromb Res* 1991; **63**: 73–84.
7 Green D, Blanc J, Foiles N. Spontaneous inhibitors of factor VIII: kinetics of inactivation of human and porcine factor VIII. *J Lab Clin Med* 1999; **133**: 260–4.
8 Jacquemin MG, Desqueper BG, Benhida A, *et al.* Mechanism and kinetics of factor VIII inactivation: study with an IgG4 monoclonal antibody derived from a hemophilia A patient with inhibitor. *Blood* 1998; **92**: 496–506.
9 Schulman S, Langevitz P, Livneh A, *et al.* Cyclosporine therapy for acquired factor VIII inhibitor in a patient with systemic lupus erythematosus. *Thromb Haemost* 1996; **76**: 344–6.
10 Soriano RM, Matthews JM, Guerado-Parra E. Acquired haemophilia and rheumatoid arthritis. *Br J Rheumatol* 1987; **26**: 381–3.
11 Hoyle C, Ludlam CA. Acquired factor VIII inhibitor associated with multiple sclerosis, successfully treated with porcine factor VIII. *Thromb Haemost* 1987; **57**: 233.
12 Sievert R, Goldstein ML, Surks MI. Graves' disease and autoimmune factor VIII deficiency. *Thyroid* 1996; **6**: 245–7.
13 Sohngen D, Specker C, Bach D, *et al.* Acquired factor VIII inhibitors in nonhemophilic patients. *Ann Hematol* 1997; **74**: 89–93.
14 Seidler CW, Mills LE, Flowers ME, Sullivan KM. Spontaneous factor VIII inhibitor occurring in association with chronic graft-versus-host disease. *Am J Hematol* 1994; **45**: 240–3.
15 Sallah S, Wan JY. Inhibitors against factor VIII in patients with cancer. Analysis of 41 patients. *Cancer* 2001; **91**: 1067–74.
16 Hauser I, Lechner K. Solid tumors and factor VIII antibodies. *Thromb Haemost* 1999; **82**: 1005–7.
17 Klein KG, Parkin JD, Madaras F. Studies on an acquired inhibition of factor VIII induced by penicillin allergy. *Clin Exp Immunol* 1976; **26**: 155–61.
18 O'Reilly RA, Hamilton RD. Acquired hemophilia, meningioma, and diphenylhydantoin therapy. *J Neurosurg* 1980; **53**: 600–5.
19 Ferri GM, Vaccaro F, Caccavo D, *et al.* Development of factor VIII: C inhibitors following vaccination. *Acta Haematol* 1996; **96**: 110–11.
20 Mauser-Bunschoten EP, Damen M, Reesink HW, *et al.* Formation of antibodies to factor VIII in patients with hemophilia A who are treated with interferon for chronic hepatitis C. *Ann Intern Med* 1996; **125**: 297–9.
21 Kasper CK, Aledort L, Aronson D, *et al.* Proceedings: a more uniform measurement of factor VIII inhibitors. *Thromb Diath Haemorrh* 1975; **34**: 612.
22 Verbruggen B, Novakova I, Wessels H, *et al.* The Nijmegen modification of the Bethesda assay for factor VIII: C inhibitors: improved specificity and reliability. *Thromb Haemost* 1995; **73**: 247–51.
23 Sanchez-Cuenca JM, Carmona E, Villanueva MJ, Aznar JA. Immunological characterization of factor VIII inhibitors by a sensitive micro-ELISA method. *Thromb Res* 1990; **57**: 897–908.
24 Kessler CM. An introduction to factor VIII inhibitors: the detection and quantitation. *Am J Med* 1991; **91**: 1S–5S.
25 Cohen AJ, Kessler CM. Acquired inhibitors. *Baillière's Clin Haematol* 1996; **9**: 331–4.
26 Morrison AE, Ludlam CA, Kessler C. Use of porcine factor VIII in the treatment of patients with acquired hemophilia. *Blood* 1993; **81**: 1513–20.
27 Kasper CK. Human factor VIII for bleeding in patients with inhibitors. *Vox Sang* 1999; **77** (Suppl. 1): 47–8.
28 Blatt PM, White GC, McMillan CW, Roberts HR. Treatment of anti-factor VIII antibodies. *Thromb Haemost* 1977; **38**: 514–23.
29 Hay CR, Ludlam CA, Colvin BT, *et al.* Factor VIII inhibitors in mild and moderate-severity haemophilia A. UK Haemophilia Centre Directors Organisation. *Thromb Haemost* 1998; **79**: 762–6.
30 Negrier C, Goudemand J, Sultan Y, *et al.* Multicenter retrospective study on the utilization of FEIBA in France in patients with factor VIII and factor IX inhibitors. French FEIBA Study Group. Factor Eight Bypassing Activity. *Thromb Haemost* 1997; **77**: 1113–19.
31 Sultan Y, Kazatchkine MD, Maisonneuve P, Nydegger UE. Anti-idiotypic suppression of autoantibodies to factor VIII anti-haemophilic factor by high-dose intravenous gammaglobulin. *Lancet* 1984; **2**: 765–8.
32 Green D, Rademaker AW, Briet E. A prospective, randomized trial of prednisone and cyclophosphamide in the treatment of patients with factor VIII autoantibodies. *Thromb Haemost* 1993; **70**: 753–7.
33 Shaffer LG, Phillips MD. Successful treatment of acquired hemophilia with oral immunosuppressive therapy. *Ann Intern Med* 1997; **127**: 206–9.
34 Lian EC, Larcada AF, Chiu AY. Combination immunosuppressive therapy after factor VIII infusion for acquired factor VIII inhibitor. *Ann Intern Med* 1989; **110**: 774–8.
35 Schulman S, Langevitz P, Livneh A, *et al.* Cyclosporine therapy for acquired factor VIII inhibitor in a patient with systemic lupus erythematosus. *Thromb Haemost* 1996; **76**: 344–6.
36 Nemes L, Pitlik E. New protocol for immune tolerance induction in acquired hemophilia. *Haematologica* 2000; **85**: 64–8.
37 Engelhardt M, Jakob A, Ruter B, *et al.* Severe cold hemagglutinin disease CHD successfully treated with rituximab. *Blood* 2002; **100**: 1922–3.
38 Wiestner A, Cho HJ, Asch AS, *et al.* Rituximab in the treatment of acquired factor VIII inhibitors. *Blood* 2002; **100**: 3426–8.

16 Hemophilia B—molecular basis

Peter M. Green

Introduction

Hemophilia B is caused by defects in, or an absence of, coagulation factor IX (FIX). The fact that there are two types of hemophilia that can be caused by a lack of either factor VIII (FVIII) or FIX was first recognized in 1952 by Biggs *et al.* [1], who also gave FIX the alternative name of Christmas factor (hence Christmas disease), after the eponymous patient in whom the disease was first identified. Hematologic tests were developed that enabled accurate classification of these patients, and to some extent enabled carrier testing of female relatives. However, because of the X-linked genes involved and the characteristic variable X inactivation, hematologic assays in females often gave rise to equivocal results: a low FIX coagulant level may indicate a carrier, but a "normal" level would not necessarily indicate a noncarrier.

Early on in the burst of human gene cloning activity in the 1980s came the isolation and characterization of the FIX gene [2]. The gene is described as "average" size, spanning 34 kb and comprising eight exons [3]—based on parameters set by the Human Genome Project, which now calculates an average gene size of 27 kb and nine exons [4]. In 1985, the entire FIX genomic sequence was established [5], one of the longest contiguous human sequences to have been so elucidated at that time.

After the genomic structure was determined, it was recognized that the exon structure of FIX was closely related to the protein domain structure. This supports the theory of Walter Gilbert that the introns evolved as a means of facilitating domain shuffling [6]. The FIX protein is a member of the chymotrypsin-like superfamily of serine proteases. It has other domains in common with various coagulation proteins, but in particular its domain structure matches that of FVII, FX, and protein C, and it is thought that they all share a common ancestor [7]. The first exon encodes the prepeptide (also called the signal or leader sequence). This is a region of hydrophobic amino acids that is required by all secreted proteins to allow passage through the endoplasmic reticulum and into the extracellular medium. The prepeptide is cleaved off, following secretion, by a prepeptidase between residues Cys–19 and Thr–18.

The prepeptide is followed by another signaling peptide: the propeptide encoded in exon b. This 18-residue sequence is the signal for modification, post-translationally, at 12 glutamic acid residues by a vitamin K-dependent gamma-carboxylase to produce γ-carboxyglutamic acid [8]. This so-called "Gla" domain region is a high-affinity calcium-binding region and is the first

domain of the mature protein after the propeptide is cleaved by a specific propeptidase. Residues 3–11 are important for binding to phospholipid membranes on the endothelial cell surface [9,10]. There is also contact between FVIII and a region of the Gla domain including Phe25 [11].

The third and shortest exon encodes a hydrophobic region that forms an α-helix, the function of which is still unclear. Exons d and e both encode domains homologous to epidermal growth factor. The former has been shown to be an important high-affinity calcium-binding region, particularly aspartate residues 47, 49, and 64 (beta hydroxylated) and glutamine 50 [12,13], while the latter epidermal growth factor (EGF) domain is involved in interacting with the cofactor, FVIII [14]. A salt bridge between residues Glu78 and Arg94 in the two EGF domains has also been shown to be essential for FVIII binding [15].

Exon f encodes the activation peptide, which, upon activation, is cleaved by FXI or FVII in the presence of tissue factor after Arg145 and Arg180. The two remaining peptides (145-residue light chain and 234-residue heavy chain) of FIX are then held together by a single disulfide bridge (Cys132–Cys289). Exons g and h encode the catalytic domain of the protein including the catalytic triad of His221, Asp269, and Ser365, as well as Asp359 at the bottom of the substrate-binding pocket, which binds basic residues in the substrate (FX). Additionally, Lys316 is essential for specific binding of FX [16], while there appears to be a binding site for low-density lipoprotein receptor-related protein at residues Phe342–Asn346 [17].

Mutation detection in the factor IX gene

The first detection of a mutation in the FIX gene was actually achieved prior to gene cloning: the Chapel Hill mutation [18] was first identified in 1983 by protein sequencing as an Arg145 to histidine amino acid change. However, following the characterization of the gene, several mutations were identified via a pre-screening using Southern blotting [19,20]. Inevitably, this technique resulted in a swathe of deletions being reported, as they were the easiest to detect using these methods. It was only when polymerase chain reaction (PCR) testing became routine with the commercial availability of *Taq* polymerase in the late 1980s that full mutation screening became really feasible. This resulted in an explosion in reporting in the literature of new mutations. Different groups have preferred different mutation scanning technologies, which have evolved over the years. These include denaturing gradient gel electrophoresis (DGGE) [21], single-strand conformational polymorphism (SSCP) [22] (and its variant, dideoxy fingerprinting, ddF [23]), heteroduplex analysis [24], chemical cleavage of mismatch (CCM) [25], and genome amplification with transcript sequencing (GAWTS) [26]. Today, however, it is fair to say that DNA sequencing has become so simple, rapid, and inexpensive that it is probably the most widely used method to identify novel mutations in the FIX gene.

Hemophilia B is a mutationally heterogeneous disorder: essentially every family harbors a different mutation. Consequently, each individual must have his gene sequenced in order to elucidate the pathogenic mutation. This mutational heterogeneity is both useful and awkward: useful because there is an enormous number of naturally occurring mutations that can cause hemophilia B, giving the scientist plenty of data to work with; and awkward because complete gene screening is required for every individual family before rapid, accurate carrier (and prenatal) diagnoses can be performed. However, this problem has largely been circumvented in the UK by the introduction of a national hemophilia B mutation database in the early 1990s [27,28]. This research-led effort to identify mutations in all hemophilia families in the UK involved the collaboration of many hemophilia centers and resulted in a database containing hematologic, pedigree, and mutation details of about 80% of the UK hemophilia B patients. This resource has proven invaluable for carrier and prenatal screening of affected relatives. This, in turn, verifies the accuracy of the data, improving its usefulness and reliability over time. This database model has also been adopted by several other countries.

In addition to confidential patient databases like that described for the UK, there is also an anonymous worldwide mutation database for hemophilia B (http://www.kcl.ac.uk/ip/petergreen/hemBdatabase.html). It was initiated in 1990 by Brownlee [29] and is updated annually by country coordinators. The latest edition of the database contains over 2500 patient entries, of which 896 are unique. A summary of the different types of mutation that cause hemophilia B is shown in the pie chart in Figure 16.1. About two-thirds of the alterations are missense mutations (amino acid changing).

Mutation hotspots

Figure 16.2 shows mutations that occur in more than five individuals from the world database. There may be several reasons for these "hotspots."

First, it has been shown in some cases that patients with the same mutation have the same haplotype (genetic background across the gene or further). This was first clearly shown with the Ile397 → Thr mutation, which occurs in 41 individuals [30]. Many of these patients have been shown to have the same polymorphic markers across the gene, which make up a rare haplotype. Indeed, it was shown that although today the majority of people with this mutation live in the USA, a few individuals in France share the same mutation and haplotype, implying that the mutation originated in northern Europe a few hundred years ago and was carried to the USA by early settlers [31]. A more detailed examination of the haplotype background of another mutation (17810, A → G) has been carried out in UK patients [32]. This study identifies a "founder" for this English mutation, who probably lived about 450 years ago, while relatives who emigrated to Canada, New Zealand, and the USA more recently may explain the wide geographic distribution of this genotype. Further, two additional occurrences of this same mutation have been shown to be independent based on the intragenic haplotype. This phenomenon confirms the pathogenic nature of this intronic mutation. Further instances of "mini-founder" effects have been identified at the Gly60 → Ser and Thr296 → Met sites, although these represent only a proportion, not all, of the changes found at these sites [31]. As might be expected, all of these "mini-founder" mutations cause a mild to moderate disease, since a severe mutation would be unlikely to have survived over many generations.

Another cause of clustering is the well-known effect of CpG sites: thus Arg29 → Stop, Arg333 → Stop, etc. (shaded in Figure 16.2) are all mutations of the type CpG → TpG (on one strand or the other). CpG sites are targets for methylation, and methylcytosine can deaminate to produce thymine. This initially creates a T.G mismatch, which is usually repaired correctly to C.G, but in a minority of cases the G will be repaired to an A, thus establishing a mutation [33,34]. Consequently, CpGs are underrepresented in the FIX gene, as they have been selected against: those that remain are largely at critical sites such as proteolytic cleavage sites [35]. What is perhaps surprising is that several CpG sites in which the mutation would create a stop codon are under-represented (notably Arg116 → Stop, of which there are only 13 cases). Other potential CpG → TpG changes in the gene may not lead to a clinically significant lower FIX:C level since they have not been observed at all; further, the two changes at Arg403 to Trp and Gln have only been recorded in 10 and six patients respectively, perhaps because they lead to very mild phenotypes and are thus under-reported.

"Coldspots" also exist in the gene, in which missense muta-

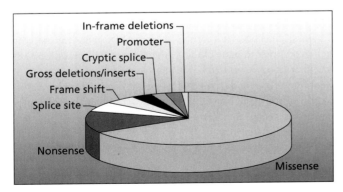

Figure 16.1 Pie chart of types of factor IX mutations. The different types of factor IX mutation reported in the 12th edition of the hemophilia B mutation database are shown in pie chart format, including gross deletions/rearrangements.

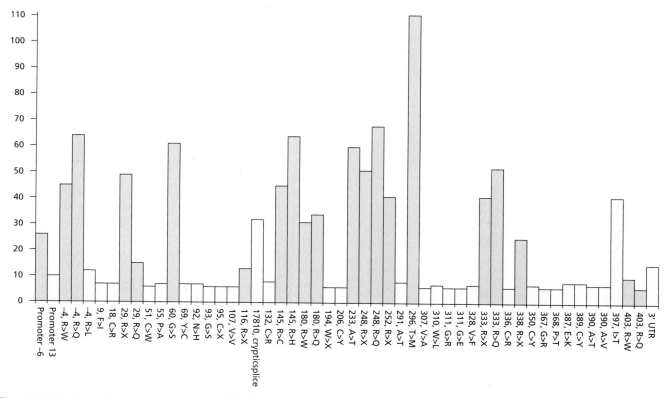

Figure 16.2 Bar chart of repeat mutations in factor IX. All mutations reported more than five times in the 12th edition of the hemophilia B mutation database are shown along the X-axis against the number of cases reported on the Y-axis. The bars shaded represent mutations at CpG sites.

tions are rare or absent. These correlate with parts of the protein that are not required for catalytic activity and which are cleaved off during processing or activation. Examples include the activation peptide, which contains only the well-known amino acid dimorphism at Ala/Thr148, and several missense mutations adjacent to the cleavage sites (Ala146) as well as the prepeptide (Cys−19). However, there are a few missense mutations in the latter domain, which may affect the hydrophobicity of the prepeptide, thus inhibiting its migration through the endoplasmic reticulum and causing the protein to remain intracellular (e.g., Ile−30 → Asn) [36]. In the case of Gly-26 → Val, however, the effect may well be on the efficiency of the donor splice site as a new GT donor site is created. It is also apparent that some regions are under-represented by missense mutations. These regions have been described as "spacer" regions, a term coined to indicate the loose conservation status of these amino acids and the fact that they are merely required to position other more critical regions of the protein [37].

Protein-truncating mutations and the inhibitor complication

Deletions and nonsense and frameshift mutations are often described as truncating mutations, and many splice-site mutations also fit in this category. As long ago as 1983 [19,38] it was pro-

posed that deletions would be likely to predispose patients to develop inhibitors; this became the rationale for screening such patients for deletions (four out of five were indeed found to have large deletions; the fifth was later shown to have a frameshift mutation) [39]. Subsequent studies have reinforced this hypothesis, so that it is now widely accepted in both hemophilias to screen for deletions to ascertain high risk for inhibitor development [40].

Promoter mutations

Leyden-type hemophilia B is characterized by low levels of FIX in infancy and early childhood, which gradually rise to normal or near-normal levels by adulthood. The rise is correlated with the rise in testosterone through puberty. Mutations in these patients have been characterized; without exception they occur in the promoter region of FIX (specifically from −21 to +13 with respect to the transcription start; Table 16.1). Base changes at −26 result in "standard" hemophilia B with no postpubertal improvement [41,42]. This phenomenon has been explained at least partly by the fact that the Leyden mutations disrupt transcription factor binding sites, reducing transcription, which is then compensated for by an androgen response element [43,44]. Mutations at −26, however, disrupt both the androgen response element and an overlapping

Table 16.1 Promoter mutations in the factor IX gene. All of the mutations reported to date in the 12th edition of the hemophilia B mutation database that lie in the promoter region of the factor IX gene are shown. The right-hand column lists known binding sites that are disrupted by the mutation.

Mutation	Binding site
−26, G → C	HNF4/ARE
−26, G → A	HNF4/ARE
−23, C → T	HNF4/ARE
−21, T → G	HNF4
−20, T → A	HNF4
−20, T → C	HNF4
−19, G → C	HNF4
−6, G → C	Unknown
−6, G → A	Unknown
−5, A → T	Unknown
−5, A → G	Unknown
6, T → A	C/EBP
7, T → C	C/EBP
8, −T	C/EBP
8, T → C	C/EBP
9, C → G	C/EBP
12, A → G	C/EBP
13, −A	C/EBP
13, A → C	C/EBP
13, A → G	C/EBP

ARE, androgen response element; HNF4, hepatic nuclear factor 4; C/EBP, CCAAT enhancer-binding protein.

transcription factor binding site, thereby blocking any testosterone-mediated amelioration.

Mosaicism

It is possible that a woman with a normal FIX phenotype who is the mother of an isolated case will have a higher than average risk of passing on the disease to further children. This will occur if she has gonadal mosaicism, i.e., a proportion of her germline contains the pathogenic mutation and the remainder does not; she may also have the mutation in a proportion of all cells in her body, in which case she would also have somatic mosaicism. This creates a problem for accurate genetic counseling, particularly if it is unknown how often germline mosaicism occurs. Work on Duchenne muscular dystrophy (DMD) has highlighted the problem, since "noncarrier" mothers were found to have a 20% risk of having a second affected child whenever they transmitted the affected haplotype [45]. Although DMD is also an X-linked disorder, it is caused, largely, by gross deletions, and this may influence the frequency of mosaicism, thus making it impossible to draw conclusions in relation to other disorders. For hemophilia B, one study has attempted to address this question by searching for mosaicism in mothers of one or two affected individuals but no other family history [46]. Out of 47 potential opportunities to detect gonadal mosaicism, none was detected. Of course, this does not mean it cannot happen in hemophilia B, but the odds of it occurring were calculated at <0.062. The fact that it can and does happen is evidenced by two anecdotal reports in the literature [47,48].

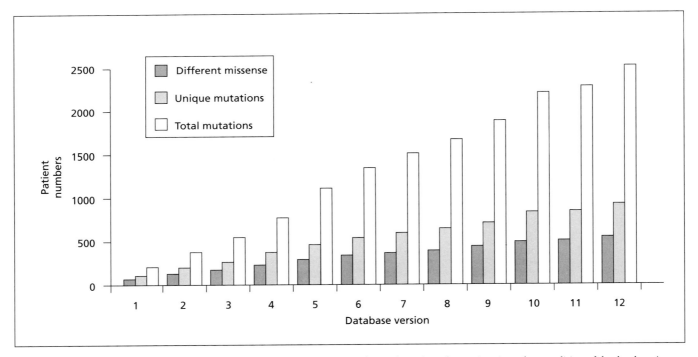

Figure 16.3 Bar chart showing number of new mutations reported each year. The total number of mutations in each new edition of the database is shown as white blocks; in front of these are the total number of different mutations in the database for each edition; and, finally, in the foreground are the number of different missense mutations in each edition of the database.

Summary

The FIX mutation database, now in its 12th edition, continues to attract new entries every year: the chart (Figure 16.3) shows the number of mutations submitted each year along with the number of different mutations and different missense mutations. It can be seen that, although novel missense mutations are still appearing each year, and "saturation" has not yet been achieved, the numbers of new ones appearing each year does appear to be leveling off. This is perhaps not that surprising when one considers that 523 amino acid subsitutions affecting 224 residues have already been identified among the 380 amino acids of the activated FIX in hemophilia B patients.

The database is not only useful as a research aid but can give an indication of the severity of disease that a particular mutation can confer, particularly when many patients have already been identified with a given mutation. This is especially useful when, for example, a Leyden-type mutation is found in a child that is an isolated case. However, it is also useful to know the mutation prior to replacement therapy, e.g., to know the likelihood of developing inhibitors, which will take on a new significance with the dawn of gene therapy.

References

1 Biggs R, Douglas AS, Macfarlane RG, *et al*. Christmas disease: a condition previously mistaken for haemophilia. *Br Med J* 1952; **2**: 1378–82.

2 Choo KH, Gould KG, Rees DJG, Brownlee GG. Molecular cloning of the gene for human anti-haemophilic factor IX. *Nature* 1982; **299**: 178–80.

3 Anson DS, Choo KH, Rees DJG, *et al*. The gene structure of human anti-haemophilic factor IX. *EMBO J* 1984; **3**: 1053–60.

4 Lander ES, Linton LM, Birren B, *et al*. Initial sequencing and analysis of the human genome. *Nature* 2001; **409**: 860–921.

5 Yoshitake S, Schach BG, Foster DC, *et al*. Nucleotide sequence of the gene for human factor IX (antihemophilic factor B). *Biochemistry* 1985; **24**: 3736–50.

6 Gilbert W. Why genes in pieces? *Nature* 1978; **271**: 501.

7 Leytus SP, Foster DC, Kurachi K, Davie EW. Gene for human factor X: a blood coagulation factor whose gene organisation is essentially identical with that of factor IX and protein C. *Biochemistry* 1986; **25**: 5098–102.

8 Handford PA, Winship PR, Brownlee GG. Protein engineering of the propeptide of human factor IX. *Protein Eng* 1991; **4**: 319–23.

9 Cheung WF, Hamaguchi N, Smith KJ, Stafford DW. The binding of human factor IX to endothelial cells is mediated by residues 3–11. *J Biol Chem* 1992; **267**: 20529–31.

10 Freedman SJ, Blostein MD, Baleja JD, *et al*. Identification of the phospholipid binding site in the vitamin K-dependent blood coagulation protein factor IX. *J Biol Chem* 1996; **271**: 16227–36.

11 Blostein MD, Furie BC, Rajotte I, Furie B. The Gla domain of factor IXa binds to factor VIIIa in the tenase complex. *J Biol Chem* 2003; **278**: 31297–302,

12 Handford PA, Baron M, Mayhew M, *et al*. The first EGF-like domain from human factor IX contains a high-affinity calcium binding site. *EMBO J* 1990; **9**: 475–80.

13 Handford PA, Mayhew M, Baron M, *et al*. Key residues involved in calcium-binding motifs in EGF-like domains. *Nature* 1991; **351**: 164–7.

14 Nishimura H, Takeya H, Miyata T, *et al*. Factor IX Fukuoka. Substitution of ASN92 by His in the second epidermal growth factor-like domain results in defective interaction with factors VIIa/X. *J Biol Chem* 1993; **268**: 24041–6.

15 Christophe OD, Lenting PJ, Kolkman JA, *et al*. Blood coagulation factor IX residues Glu78 and Arg94 provide a link between both epidermal growth factor-like domains that is crucial in the interaction with factor VIII light chain. *J Biol Chem* 1998; **273**: 222–7.

16 Kolkman JA, Mertens K. Surface-loop residue Lys316 in blood coagulation Factor IX is a major determinant for Factor X but not antithrombin recognition. *Biochem J* 2000; **350**: 701–7.

17 Rohlena J, Kolkman JA, Boertjes RC, *et al*. Residues Phe342-Asn346 of activated coagulation factor IX contribute to the interaction with low density lipoprotein receptor-related protein. *J Biol Chem* 2003; **278**: 9394–401.

18 Noyes CM, Griffith MJ, Roberts HR, Lundblad RL. Identification of the molecular defect in factor IX Chapel Hill: substitution of histidine for arginine at position 145. *Proc Natl Acad Sci USA* 1983; **80**: 4200–2.

19 Giannelli F, Choo KH, Rees DJ, *et al*. Gene deletions in patients with haemophilia B and anti-factor IX antibodies. *Nature* 1983; **303**: 181–2.

20 Matthews RJ, Anson DS, Peake IR, Bloom AL. Heterogeneity of the factor IX locus in nine hemophilia B inhibitor patients. *J Clin Invest* 1987; **79**: 746–53.

21 Attree O, Vidaud D, Vidaud M, *et al*. Mutations in the catalytic domain of human coagulation factor IX: rapid characterization by direct genomic sequencing of DNA fragments displaying an altered melting behavior. *Genomics* 1989; **4**: 266–72.

22 Demers DB, Odelberg SJ, Fisher LM. Identification of a factor IX point mutation using SSCP analysis and direct sequencing. *Nucl Acids Res* 1990; **18**: 5575.

23 Sarkar G, Yoon HS, Sommer SS. Dideoxy fingerprinting (ddE): a rapid and efficient screen for the presence of mutations. *Genomics* 1992; **13**: 441–3.

24 Chen SH, Schoof JM, Weinmann AF, Thompson AR. Heteroduplex screening for molecular defects in factor IX genes from haemophilia B families. *Br J Haematol* 1995; **89**: 409–12.

25 Montandon AJ, Green PM, Giannelli F, Bentley DR. Direct detection of point mutations by mismatch analysis: application to haemophilia B. *Nucl Acids Res* 1989; **17**: 3347–58.

26 Stoflet ES, Koeberl DD, Sarkar G, Sommer SS. Genomic amplification with transcript sequencing. *Science* 1988; **239**: 491–4.

27 Montandon AJ, Green PM, Bentley DR, *et al*. A new strategy for carrier prenatal diagnosis and molecular studies in haemophilia B. In: Albertini A, Lenfant CL, Mannucci PM, Sixma JJ, eds. *Biotechnology of Plasma Proteins. Current Studies in Hematology and Blood Transfusion* No. 58. Basel: Karger, 1991; 88–93.

28 Saad S, Rowley G, Tagliavacca L, *et al*. First report on UK database of haemophilia B mutations and pedigrees. UK Haemophilia Centres. *Thromb Haemost* 1994; **71**: 563–70.

29 Giannelli F, Green PM, High KA, *et al*. Haemophilia B: database of point mutations and short additions and deletions. *Nucl Acids Res* 1990; **18**: 4053–9.

30 Thompson AR, Bajaj SP, Chen SH, MacGillivray RT. "Founder" effect in different families with haemophilia B mutation. *Lancet* 1990; **335**: 418.

31 Ketterling RP, Bottema CD, Phillips JA, Sommer SS. Evidence that descendants of three founders constitute about 25% of hemophilia B in the United States. *Genomics* 1991; **10**: 1093–6.

32 Anagnostopoulos T, Morris AP, Ayres KL, *et al.* DNA variation in a 13-Mb region including the F9 gene: inferring the genealogical history and causal role of a hemophilia B mutation (IVS 5+13 A→G). *J Thromb Haemost* 2003; **1**: 2609–14.

33 Zell R, Fritz HJ. DNA mismatch-repair in Escherichia coli counteracting the hydrolytic deamination of 5-methyl-cytosine residues. *EMBO J* 1987; **6**: 1809–15.

34 Brown TC, Jiricny J. Different base/base mispairs are corrected with different efficiencies and specificities in monkey kidney cells. *Cell* 1988; **54**: 705–11.

35 Green PM, Montandon AJ, Bentley DR, *et al.* The incidence and distribution of CpG–TpG transitions in the factor IX gene. A fresh look at CpG mutational hotspots. *Nucl Acids Res* 1990; **18**: 3227–31.

36 Green PM, Mitchell VE, McGraw A, *et al.* Haemophilia B caused by a missense mutation in the prepeptide sequence of factor IX. *Hum Mutat* 1993; **2**: 103–7.

37 Bottema CD, Ketterling RP, Ii S, *et al.* Missense mutations and evolutionary conservation of amino acids: evidence that many of the amino acids in factor IX function as "spacer" elements. *Am J Hum Genet* 1991; **49**: 820–38.

38 Giannelli F, Brownlee GG. Cause of the "inhibitor" phenotype in the haemophilias. *Nature* 1986; **320**: 196.

39 Green PM, Bentley DR, Mibashan RS, *et al.* Molecular pathology of haemophilia B. *EMBO J* 1989; **8**: 1067–72.

40 Giannelli F, Green PM, Naylor JA. A genetic view on the etiology of the inhibitor complication. *Blood* 1996; **87**: 2612.

41 Crossley M, Ludwig M, Stowell KM, *et al.* Recovery from hemophilia B Leyden: an androgen-responsive element in the factor IX promoter. *Science* 1992; **257**: 377–9.

42 Morgan GE, Rowley G, Green PM, *et al.* Further evidence for the importance of an androgen response element in the factor IX promoter. *Br J Haematol* 1997; **98**: 79–85.

43 Reitsma PH, Bertina RM, Ploos van Amstel JK, *et al.* The putative factor IX gene promoter in hemophilia B Leyden. *Blood* 1988; **72**: 1074–6.

44 Crossley M, Brownlee GG. Disruption of a C/EBP binding site in the factor IX promoter is associated with haemophilia B. *Nature* 1990; **345**: 444–6.

45 van Essen AJ, Abbs S, Baiget M, *et al.* Parental origin and germline mosaicism of deletions and duplications of the dystrophin gene: a European study. *Hum Genet* 1992; **88**: 249–57.

46 Green PM, Saad, S, Lewis, CM, Giannelli F. Mutation rates in humans I: overall and sex-specific rates obtained from a population study of haemophilia B. *Am J Hum Genet* 1999; **65**: 1572–9.

47 Taylor SA, Deugau KV, Lillicrap DP. Free in PMC Somatic mosaicism and female-to-female transmission in a kindred with hemophilia B (factor IX deficiency). *Proc Natl Acad Sci USA* 1991; **88**: 39–42.

48 Sommer SS, Knoll A, Greenberg CR, Ketterling RP. Germline mosaicism in a female who seemed to be a carrier by sequence analysis. *Hum Mol Genet* 1995; **4**: 2181–2.

17 Inhibitors in hemophilia B

Indira Warrier

Introduction

Inhibitor (antibody) development against coagulation factor VIII (FVIII) or IX is a devastating complication of hemophilia treatment in very young children. Inhibitors are not known to increase bleeding symptoms in hemophilia, but management of bleeding episodes becomes a lot more challenging and therapeutic results are unpredictable in inhibitor patients. The incidence of inhibitors varies with the type and severity of hemophilia. Inhibitors are much more common in hemophilia A than in hemophilia B. This is in a way fortunate, because inhibitor development in hemophilia B is complicated by yet another problem: anaphylaxis occurring simultaneously with inhibitor. This unique problem has further complicated management of inhibitors in hemophilia B.

Prevalence of FIX inhibitors

The prevalence of factor IX (FIX) inhibitors in hemophilia B patients (1.5–3%) is 5–10 times lower than the prevalence of FVIII inhibitors in hemophilia A (15–52%) [1–4]. The reason for this difference is not clearly understood. One of the reasons cited is the higher percentage (60%) of severe phenotypes in hemophilia A (FVIII <1%) than in hemophilia B (30%). Two recent surveys conducted in the USA in 1995 and 1997 have shown a prevalence of FIX inhibitors in the range of 1.5–2.7% [5,6] among cohorts in which the prevalence of severe phenotype was 30–37% of all hemophilia B. If only severe patients are included to calculate the prevalence, the percentage of inhibitors increases to 9% (52/573). Investigators from Sweden have reported the highest prevalence of FIX inhibitors (23%) [7].

A second possible reason for lower inhibitor prevalence in hemophilia B may be related to the molecular size of FIX protein, which is one-fifth the size of FVIII. It is postulated that, because of its smaller size, there are fewer epitopes against which antibodies can form. However, no information is reported in the current literature regarding target epitopes in FIX inhibitor patients.

A third possible reason for the lower prevalence is the much higher protein concentration of FIX in the circulation compared with FVIII (5 µg/mL vs. 100 ng/mL for FVIII) [8]. Patients with even the severest phenotype may have minute amounts that are adequate for induction of immunologic tolerance. A fourth possible explanation may be related to the structure of FIX and its similarity to other vitamin K-dependent factors. Because of considerable conservation of amino acid sequence among the vitamin K-dependent factors, the presence of other prothrombin complex components (FII, FVII, and FX) may confer some tolerance to FIX. These possible factors are summarized in Table 17.1.

Large deletions and mutations leading to the loss of coding information are much more frequently associated with inhibitors. In hemophilia B, large deletions account for only 1–3% of all hemophilia B patients, but constitute 50% in inhibitor patients [8].

In 1995, two of our patients with severe hemophilia B developed anaphylaxis while receiving high-purity FIX product. FIX assays obtained at the time of anaphylactic episodes showed no increase in FIX level. A Bethesda inhibitor assay showed the presence of FIX inhibitor in both individuals, which peaked at 6.4 Bethesda units (BU) in one patient and 30 BU in the second patient [9]. Similar case histories were reported contemporaneously by several centers in the USA and abroad [10,11]. An international registry for FIX inhibitors under the auspices of the International Society of Thrombosis And Hemostasis (ISTH) was established in 1998 in response to these reports of anaphylactic reactions occurring at the time of FIX inhibitor development in patients with hemophilia B.

Although accrual in the registry has been limited, combining data collected from published reports and the registry yields 52 FIX inhibitor patients in the USA. Twenty-four of these patients (46%) had experienced anaphylaxis at the time of inhibitor development. Seventy-five percent of 36 (27/36) non-US patients have reported anaphylaxis with inhibitors. However, the total number of non-US FIX inhibitors may be erroneously low owing to under-reporting of uncomplicated FIX inhibitor patients to the registry (Table 17.2).

General characteristics of factor IX inhibitors

Unlike FVIII inhibitors, FIX inhibitors are not well characterized. From what is known about the inhibitors, they are predominantly of the IgG4 subclass. They do not fix complement and have equal affinity to both heavy and light chains of FIX. A Japanese study showed an IgG1 antibody in addition to an IgG4 antibody in a patient with FIX inhibitor at the time of anaphylaxis [10,12,13].

Table 17.1 Lower incidence of factor IX (FIX) inhibitors.

1 Fewer severely affected persons
2 FIX is one-fifth the size of FVIII
3 Higher FIX protein (5 µg/mL vs. 100 ng/mL)
4 Structural analogy to other vitamin K-dependent factors
5 Nature of FIX mutation

Table 17.2 Demographic data of factor IX inhibitor patients.

Median age 19.5 months (9–16 months)
Median exposure 11 days (2–180 days)
Median inhibitor titer 30 BU (1–1156 BU)
Various ethnic and racial groups are affected
Various FIX products (including ultrapure products have been used)

Hypothesis related to anaphylaxis with factor IX inhibitor development

Although the reasons for anaphylaxis at the time of inhibitor development in hemophilia B are not entirely clear, several hypotheses can be considered. One hypothesis is related to the smaller molecular size of FIX. FIX, with a molecular mass of 55 000, distributes to extravascular spaces, and this feature of FIX may in some way be contributing to anaphylaxis, perhaps by influencing antigen presentation.

A second hypothesis is based on the higher exogenous protein load with FIX infusions (5 µg/mL). Whether the quantity or tissue distribution of immune complexes formed with the development of FIX inhibitor is contributing to anaphylaxis is not known at present.

A third hypothesis relates to possible IgE-mediated hypersensitivity. Skin and radioallergosorbent (RAST) testing in a few patients have suggested IgE-mediated reactions, and further study is warranted [14].

A fourth possible explanation postulates that the IgG1 antibody formed at the time of inhibitor development may activate complement and thereby play an active role in the immunologic mechanisms leading to anaphylaxis. Against this argument is the observation that two subjects studied at our center did not show complement activation.

Finally, the nature of the FIX mutation itself may play a role in determining relative immunogenicity: large deletions represent 50% of the FIX genotypes among hemophilia B inhibitor patients. Whether lack of any FIX gene product leads to absence of tolerance is not known at present. It has been suggested that complete gene deletions confer the greatest risk for anaphylaxis, with a minimum risk of 26% [15]. It has been postulated that the complete absence of FIX protein results in inhibitor formation while a codeletion of a neighboring immune modulatory gene results in anaphylaxis. This is an attractive hypothesis since FIX gene deletions are often very large—sometimes greater than a megabase in length [14].

If deletion of immune modulatory genes is the explanation, it still does not explain why all such individuals with similar mutations do not develop inhibitors. At present, no answer is forthcoming. It is possible that a combination of factors in addition to genetic factors may be contributing to this unique complication of anaphylaxis in hemophilia B patients.

Management

Management of hemophilia B inhibitor patients itself is challenging and it is even more difficult if inhibitor development is associated with anaphylaxis. Hence, treatment should be attempted only at a hemophilia treatment center that is well equipped and has experienced staff to handle such an emergency. There are two goals for the treatment of these patients: treatment of acute bleeding episodes and eradication of the inhibitor by immune tolerance induction (ITI).

First goal—treatment of acute bleeding episodes

Treatment of acute bleeding episodes in patients with inhibitors and anaphylaxis should be attempted at a hemophilia treatment center with experienced staff. Unless fully desensitized, the hemophilia patient with inhibitor and anaphylaxis will be unable to receive the commonly used bypassing agents prothrombin complex concentrates (PCCs) or activated PCCs, because these products contain FIX. Several of the subjects in the registry have received alternate FIX products and have had anaphylaxis with the second FIX product as well. Thus, for those hemophilia B inhibitor patients who have demonstrated anaphylaxis, infusion with PCCs or aPCCs does not appear to be the treatment of choice. Another bypassing agent, recombinant factor VIIa (rFVIIa), has been used successfully for treatment of acute bleeding episodes and surgery and *is* the treatment of choice for those with inhibitors and anaphylaxis. However, the relatively short half-life of rFVIIa does not lend itself to use as a prophylactic agent. The recommended dose of rFVIIa is 90–120 µg/kg every 2 h until bleeding stops. Once the bleeding stops, the interval between doses can be increased. Treatment of a bleeding episode will likely require several doses of rFVIIa.

Studies are ongoing to determine the most appropriate dosing regimen for rFVIIa in inhibitor patients (three doses of 90 µg/kg compared with one dose of 270 µg/kg). Several of the patients in the registry have received rFVIIa with excellent results [9]. No serious adverse effects with rFVIIa have been reported in hemophilia B patients with inhibitors [10]. The disadvantages of rFVIIa include the following:
1 the need for multiple doses, hence;
2 the requirement for easy venous access in children (necessitating surgical placements of a port or externalized catheter);
3 the lack of a suitable and easy laboratory test to monitor response to treatment;
4 the high cost of multiple doses.

If the current dose finding study determines that one large dose (270 µg/kg) is as effective as three 90 µg/kg doses, many of the above mentioned disadvantages will be mitigated.

Second goal—eradication of the inhibitors by immune tolerance induction

Experience with immune tolerance induction (ITI) in hemophilia B inhibitor patients is limited for several reasons. These include the low prevalence of FIX inhibitors, the thrombogenicity of PCCs, the lack of availability of high-purity FIX products until recently, and the lack of a well-defined standardized method for ITI. In addition, FIX inhibitor patients with anaphylaxis require desensitization to FIX first (similar to other allergens). In addition, ITI attempted in individuals with prior anaphylaxis/or allergy to FIX has been associated with a renal complication of membranous nephropathy.

Of the 88 FIX inhibitor patients in the International Registry, ITI has been attempted in 34 patients and was successful in only five individuals (14%). Those who achieved tolerance either had low titers or had no allergy to FIX concentrates. The only reported success with ITI in hemophilia B subjects prior to the description of anaphylaxis is from the late Professor Nilsson's group [16]. The Malmö treatment protocol for ITI pioneered by this group, consists of the following interventions:
• removal of the patient's anti-FIX antibody by extracorporeal adsorption to staphylococcal protein A followed by treatment with cyclophosphamide intravenously or orally;
• daily administration of FIX concentrate in an attempt to achieve a factor concentration level of 40–100 IU/dL for 2–3 weeks;
• intravenous gammaglobulin administration on days 4–9;
• institution of a prophylactic regimen once inhibitor is undetectable.

Of seven patients treated with this regimen, four had complete responses after one course. Two patients required two courses, one of whom failed to respond; the other experienced recurrence of the inhibitor after 6 months. No allergic reactions to the infused FIX products were reported.

Disadvantages of immune tolerance induction

Failure of ITI is reported in hemophilia B inhibitor patients with and without anaphylaxis [6]. In addition, a unique problem of membranous nephropathy/nephrotic syndrome has been reported in hemophilia B inhibitor patients with anaphylaxis [17–21].

Nephrotic syndrome

The International Registry lists 13 cases of nephrotic syndrome in hemophilia B inhibitor patients on ITI. Anaphylaxis to FIX products was reported in 11 of these 13 individuals (85%): four are from the USA, three each from Germany and Sweden, and one from each of the Netherlands, Spain, and Japan. Nephrotic syndrome has *not* been reported in hemophilia B inhibitor patients who are not on ITI. In each case, nephrotic syndrome symptoms typically developed after 8–9 months of ITI. Renal biopsy was performed in 2 of the 13 subjects, and revealed membranous glomerulonephritis. Immunohistochemical staining for FIX, which was carried out on the biopsy specimen in one case, failed to show FIX-containing deposits.

Clinical features common to nephrotic syndrome included young age (<12 years), anaphylaxis at the time of inhibitor development, exposure to high and repeated doses of FIX (100–325 U/kg) daily, FIX deficiency because of either deletion or stop codon abnormality, poor response to immune suppression with steroids and cyclophosphamide, and resolution of proteinuria with decrease or cessation of FIX infusions.

Despite the vastly greater and longer clinical experience with ITI in hemophilia A patients with inhibitors, nephrotic syndrome has never been reported in hemophilia A patients on ITI. There are no clear-cut explanations for this difference. However, several hypotheses are offered. These include:
• The smaller molecular size of FIX. Unlike the higher-molecular-weight FVIII molecule, which complexes with von Willebrand factor and remains intravascular, FIX is more readily distributed to extravascular spaces. This unique feature of FIX, i.e., extravascular dissemination, may contribute to membranous nephropathy.
• Exposure to exogenous protein. Hemophilia B inhibitor patients on ITI are exposed to much larger amounts of exogenous protein when treated with even standard doses of FIX (5 µg/mL vs. 100 ng/mL). The protein load exposure becomes even higher in patients on ITI. This protein load may in some way influence the subepithelial deposition in the kidney as has been seen in other drug-induced membranous nephropathies.
• Genetic predisposition. A third hypothesis links the development of nephrotic syndrome with the patient's genetic predisposition for inhibitor development and concurrent anaphylaxis. A lack of primary immunologic tolerance because of the absence of any FIX gene product has been commonly cited as one of the reasons for development of inhibitors and perhaps also for anaphylaxis. Whether there is also a codeletion of an immune regulatory gene adjacent to FIX gene contributing to immune-mediated nephropathy is unknown at present.

The occurrence of nephrotic syndrome in the context of ITI among 13 hemophilia B subjects with FIX inhibitors, anaphylaxis, and biopsy-proven membranous nephropathy (in two patients) suggests a direct causal relationship between ITI and nephrotic syndrome. The cogency of the argument is further strengthened by the observation that cessation of the offending agent alone resulted in resolution of the nephropathy.

Long-term sequelae of this unique complication are unknown at present. Nephrocalcinosis and urinary calculus has been observed in one patient. This suggests that these patients need long-term follow-up even after complete resolution of nephropathy.

Practical suggestions/guidelines

Although there are more questions than answers for the recently described problems of anaphylaxis and nephrotic syndrome in hemophilia B inhibitor patients, hematologists can use certain guidelines when treating young patients with severe hemophilia B. Specifically, these include:
• Identifying the patient at risk by genotyping at the time of diagnosis and counseling the family accordingly. Those with large deletions or stop codon abnormalities can then be monitored during the early period of treatment at a medical facility equipped to handle life-threatening emergencies.
• Discussing these unique problems with the family at the time of initial diagnosis and counsel as needed.
• Considering ITI only when there are no other treatment options available and shortening the ITI intervention as much as possible.
• During ITI, monitoring closely for nephrotic syndrome by routine urinalysis and serum albumin level determination.
• Treating bleeding episodes in hemophilia B inhibitor patients with rFVIIa early and without delay in order to avoid repeated dosing and to prevent target joint development.

Conclusions

Anaphylaxis concurrent with inhibitor development is a unique problem in hemophilia B. Similar to FVIII inhibitors in hemophilia A, FIX inhibitors occur early in life. Inhibitor development and anaphylaxis are commonly seen in hemophilia B patients with either FIX gene deletions or stop codon abnormalities. The success rate with ITI is poor in this group and nephrotic syndrome is seen as a complication of ITI. Currently, rFVIIa is the most likely treatment of choice in these patients with acute bleeding. Studies to determine the most appropriate dosing or rFVIIa need to be performed.

Other innovative treatment options, including the use of monoclonal antibody (anti-CD20) and immune suppression/modulation (as used by our bone marrow transplant colleagues), need to be investigated in these challenging hemophilia B inhibitor patients with anaphylaxis. Further studies are also required to determine the characteristics of FIX inhibitors and mechanism of anaphylaxis at inhibitor development.

References

1 Briët E. Factor IX inhibitor in hemophilia B patients: Their incidence and prospects for development with high purity factor IX products. *Blood Coagul Fibrinol* 1991; **2**: 47–50.

2 Ljung RC. Gene mutations and inhibitor formation in patients with hemophilia B. *Acta Hematol* 1995; **94**: 49–52.

3 Schwarzinger I, Pabinger I, Korninger C, et al. Incidence of inhibitors in patients with severe and moderate hemophilia A treated with FVIII concentrates. *Am J Hematol* 1987; **24**: 241–5.

4 Ehrenforth S, Kreuz W, Shcarrer I, et al. Incidence of development of factor VIII and factor IX inhibitors in hemophiliacs. *Lancet* 1992; **339**: 594–8.

5 Katz J. Prevalence of FIX inhibitors among patients with hemophilia B: results of large scale North American survey. *Haemophilia* 1996; **2**: 38–31.

6 Warrier I. ITI in hemophilia B: Possibilities and problems. International Monitor of *Haemophilia* 2000; **8**(2): 3–6.

7 Ljung R, Petrini P, Tengborn L, Sjorin E. Haemophilia B mutations in Sweden: A population based study of mutational heterogeneity. *Br J Haematol* 2001, **113**: 81–86.

8 High KA. Factor IX: molecular structure, epitopes, and mutations associated with inhibitor formation. In: Aledort LM, Hoyer LW, Lusher JM, et al., eds. *Inhibitors to Coagulation Factors*. New York: Plenum Press, 1995: 79–86.

9 Warrier I, Ewenstein BM, Koerper MA, et al. FIX inhibitors and anaphylaxis in hemophilia B. *J Pediatr Haematol Oncol* 1997, **19**: 23–7.

10 Sawamoto Y, Shima M, Yamamoto M, et al. Measurement of anti-factor IX IgG subclass in haemophilia B patients who developed inhibitors with episodes of allergic reactions to FIX concentrates. *Thromb Res* 1996; **83**: 279–86.

11 Bergmann F, Vester U, Rose M, et al. Behandlungs-saltervativen Bei Hemmokörperhäemophilie B: Erfahrungen mit dem Einsatz von reckombinatem Factor VII a (rFVIIa). In: Scharrer I, Schramm W, eds. *Haemophilie-Symposium, Hamburg Berlin*. Heidelberg: Springer-Verlag; 1994: 126–9.

12 Pike IM, Yount WJ, Purtz EM, et al. Immunochemical characterization of a monoclonal G₄ human antibody to factor IX. *Blood* 1972; **40**: 1–10.

13 Örstavik KH, Miller CH. IgG subclass identification of inhibitors to FIX in haemophilia B patients. *Br J Haematol* 1988; **68**: 451–4.

14 Kettering RP, Vielhaber EL, Lind TJ, et al. The rates and patterns of deletions in the human factor IX gene. *Am J Hum Genet* 1994; **54**: 201–13.

15 Thorland EC, Drost JB, Lusher JM, et al. Anaphylactic response to FIX replacement therapy in hemophilia B patients: complete gene deletions confer the highest risk. *Haemophilia* 1999; **5**: 101–5.

16 Nilsson IM, Berntorp E, Freiburghaus C. Treatment of patients with factor VIII and FIX inhibitors. *Thromb Haemost* 1993; **70**: 56–9.

17 Ewenstein MB, Takemoto C, Warrier I, et al. Nephrotic syndrome as a complication of immune tolerance in hemophilia B. *Blood* 1997; **89**: 115–16.

18 Lenk H, Bierback U, Schille R. Inhibitor to FIX in hemophilia B and nephrotic syndrome in the course of immune tolerance treatment. *Haemophilia* 1996; **2**(1): 164 (Abstract # 397).

19 Pollman H. A hemophilia B patient with complete FIX gene deletion and a high titer antibody against FIX. *Haemophilia* 1996; **2**(1): 72 (Abstract # 274).

20 Tengborn L, Hansson S, Fasth A, et al. Anaphylactoid reaction and nephrotic syndrome—a considerable risk during FIX treatment in patients with hemophilia B and inhibitors—a report on the outcome of two brothers. *Haemophilia* 1998; **4**: 854–9.

21 Perez R, Martinez ML, Sosa R. Nephrotic syndrome in a 12 year old hemophilia B patient in the course of immune tolerance. *Haemophlia* 2000; **6**: 311 (Abstract).

18 Treatment of inhibitors in hemophilia B

Simon A. Brown

Introduction

Although the management of inhibitors in hemophilia B follows the same general principles as the management of inhibitors in hemophilia A, namely the control of bleeding and eradication of the inhibitor, there are significant differences that make this rare complication of hemophilia B a major therapeutic challenge. The low prevalence of inhibitor development after factor IX (FIX) replacement therapy, at less than 4% [1], means that experience in managing individuals with this complication is limited. In addition, the clinician is faced with the apparently unique features of anaphylactoid reactions following FIX concentrate administration in individuals who develop FIX inhibitors, and the potential development of nephrotic syndrome during immune tolerance induction (ITI).

Historical perspective

Factor IX inhibitor development in hemophilia B was described shortly after the differentiation of Christmas disease (hemophilia B) from classical hemophilia (hemophilia A) [2]. Early experience with FIX inhibitors demonstrated the possibility of swamping the inhibitor with excess FIX replacement therapy to achieve hemostasis during surgical procedures and acute bleeds. Such replacement therapy was usually complicated by an anamnestic antibody response, after which hemostatic levels of FIX were difficult to maintain. In an attempt to prevent or delay the onset of the anamnestic response, immunosuppressive therapy was given concomitantly with FIX replacement therapy: this potentially allows the administration of FIX replacement therapy and attainment of therapeutic FIX levels over longer periods, but this approach is not universally successful [3]. In 1981, Inga Marie Nilsson and her colleagues in Malmö, Sweden, described a successful surgical procedure in a patient with a FIX inhibitor, utilizing immunoadsorption of the FIX inhibitor with a protein A–Sepharose column, cyclophosphamide, and FIX replacement therapy. Subsequently, the addition of intravenous (i.v.) immunoglobulin to this protocol effected immune tolerance in an individual with hemophilia B complicated by a FIX inhibitor; this was the birth of the Malmö protocol for ITI [4]. Despite this encouraging start to ITI for inhibitors in hemophilia B, it is now recognized that the outcome of ITI is poor when compared with patients with a FVIII inhibitor complicating their hemophilia A. Major contributing factors to the poor results of ITI in hemophilia B inhibitor patients are the occurrence of allergic reactions to infused FIX concentrates and the associated complication of nephrotic syndrome during ITI.

Control of bleeding

The management of acute bleeds and hemostatic prophylaxis for surgery in individuals with FIX inhibitors is dependent on the inhibitor titer, type of anamnestic response (high- or low-responding), and history of allergic reactions. For individuals with a low titer (<5 BU/mL) and low-responding inhibitor, high-dose infusions or continuous infusion of FIX concentrate can swamp the FIX alloantibody and maintain hemostatic plasma levels of FIX. However, if a low-titer FIX inhibitor has been associated with allergic reactions following FIX infusions and the patient has not been adequately desensitized, the logical therapeutic agent is recombinant activated factor VII (rFVIIa). Individuals with a high-titer or high-responding inhibitor without a history of allergic reactions after FIX infusions can be managed with either activated prothrombin complex concentrates (aPCCs) or rFVIIa in order to secure hemostasis. aPCCs may result in an anamnestic response, are contraindicated in individuals with a history of allergy to FIX, and are plasma-derived concentrates: these factors should be considered when therapeutic decisions are being made, and are why rFVIIa is considered first-line therapy in this patient group.

Studies evaluating the safety and effectiveness of APCCs and rFVIIa in patients with inhibitors include only small numbers of patients with FIX inhibitors [5–7]. This makes it difficult to assess differences between these hemostatic agents in patients with FIX inhibitors, or to assess whether there is any significant difference in response between individuals with FIX or FVIII inhibitors. Therefore, the rationale for therapy with APCCs and rFVIIa is predominantly based on data from patients with FVIII inhibitors. Bolus infusions of rFVIIa, as frequently as 2-hourly, remain the standard mode of administration and have been used for surgical prophylaxis and the treatment of acute bleeds, both under medical supervision and at home [6,8,9]. The recommended dose of rFVIIa is 90–120 μg/kg given every 2 h initially, but higher doses have been used, especially in children, in whom the half-life of rFVIIa is shorter than in adults [10]. Delivery of rFVIIa by continuous infusion remains controversial. Comparison of

101

two rates of rFVIIa continuous infusion, 16.5 mg/kg/h and 50 mg/kg/h, has shown the higher dose rate to be effective for surgical prophylaxis whereas the lower rate of infusion failed to provide adequate hemostasis [11,12]. Further variability in the efficacy of rFVIIa administered by continuous infusion has been reported, with a reduced efficacy for bleeds or surgery involving the oral cavity [13]. The use of rFVIIa and aPCCs for prophylaxis in individuals with inhibitors has been studied but remains controversial. There has been one case report of the use of daily rFVIIa infusions for prophylaxis [14], but this is insufficient data to recommend it as standard therapy—especially when one considers that the half-life of rFVIIa is approximately 2–3 h. Similarly, the aPCC product FEIBA has been used for prophylaxis in inhibitor patients, but the results reported to date are inconsistent [15]. Published data on the use of aPCCs in individuals with FIX inhibitors are limited [5,16]. In these two reports, a total of three patients with FIX inhibitors were treated with FEIBA, and one patient suffered a myocardial infarction after the second dose of FEIBA [5].

Immunosuppression has been used in conjunction with FIX concentrate infusions to blunt the anamnestic response, but this form of adjunctive therapy does not predictably reduce the immune response and may result in significant immunosuppression [3]. Alternatively, immunoadsorption of the FIX inhibitor is another therapeutic option and has been used to decrease FIX inhibitor levels prior to surgery, during acute bleeds, and before ITI. In a series from Malmö, five patients with FIX inhibitors were treated nine times with immunoadsorption with a protein A column [17]. The range of FIX inhibitor titer before immunoadsorption was 13.5–159 BU/mL, and after immunoadsorption was 0–7.2 BU/mL. Two surgical procedures were completed without excess bleeding and three acute bleeds were effectively stopped. However, there were two complications: one thrombotic cardiac event related to FIX infusion and a case of compartment syndrome secondary to intravenous cannula placement. Protein A immunoadsorption is practical because the majority of FIX alloantibodies are IgG (mostly IgG4 and IgG1), and protein A binds all IgG except for IgG3 [18]. Accordingly, immunoadsorption with protein A columns may not be successful in all cases, for example in cases of non-IgG FIX alloantibodies [19]. Potentially this problem could be resolved by specific FIX alloantibody adsorption using a FIX–Sepharose column [20].

Individuals in whom on-demand therapy with rFVIIa remains the only therapeutic option, owing to failure of ITI and/or a history of severe allergic reactions, will benefit from other forms of therapy. Physiotherapy can aid recovery from acute bleeds and help in the prevention of further musculoskeletal bleeds. In addition, appropriate use of immobilization of joints during acute bleeds and the use of braces can be helpful in the management and recovery of acute bleeds. The development of chronic synovitis in these individuals remains a real problem, and chemical or radioactive synoviorthesis should be considered for this complication. Despite the challenges faced by these few individuals, a multidisciplinary team approach to this complex therapeutic challenge can help to optimize both medical and social outcomes.

Immune tolerance induction

The eradication of inhibitors that have developed in individuals with hemophilia remains the optimum therapy for this complication of factor concentrate replacement therapy. Patients have been described in whom either high-responding FIX inhibitors have been converted to low-responding inhibitors [4] or the inhibitor has become undetectable after several years of on-demand therapy with FIX concentrates [19,21]. However, the first successful ITI protocol for FIX inhibitors in hemophilia B, the Malmö protocol, resulted from the addition of i.v. immunoglobulin to the combination of FIX concentrate infusions and cyclophosphamide, with or without immunoadsorption [22]. The Malmö protocol consists of cyclophosphamide [12–15 mg/kg body weight (b.w.)] intravenously on days 1 and 2, then 2–3 mg/kg b.w. orally for a further 8 to 10 days), i.v. immunoglobulin (0.4 g/kg b.w. intravenously, daily for 5 days), and FIX concentrate given to initially increase the FIX level to 40–100 IU/dL, and then to maintain a FIX level of 30–80 IU/dL. Disappearance of the inhibitor is followed by twice-weekly prophylaxis with FIX concentrate. Immunoadsorption using a protein A column is used prior to the commencement of this combination therapy if the initial FIX inhibitor level is >10 BU/mL. Inhibitors in both hemophilia B and hemophilia A (administering FVIII concentrate rather than FIX concentrate for the latter) have been successfully eradicated with this form of ITI [23]. A series of nine patients with FIX inhibitors (eight with high-titer inhibitors) who have been treated with this protocol have been reported. The initial response rate was six complete responses, but one patient relapsed after 6 months, giving a final response rate of 56% (five out of nine). Seven of these individuals received a median of one course of ITI (range one to three courses), with a mean of 23 days of FIX concentrate per course of ITI (range 8–53 days) [24]. In two patients with a FIX inhibitor managed using the Malmö protocol, delivery of the FIX concentrate by continuous infusion resulted in failure of ITI [25].

The Malmö protocol is the most studied regimen of ITI in FIX inhibitor patients. However, other ITI regimens, based on the low- and high-dose ITI protocols used in patients with hemophilia A complicated by a FVIII inhibitor, have been tried in patients with FIX alloantibodies (Table 18.1). Doses of FIX concentrate in these reports range from 25 IU/kg b.w. given three times a week to 200 IU/kg b.w./day, with additional plasmapheresis and/or immune modulators in some cases [26–31]. The success rate for ITI with these regimens is <30% (Table 18.1). Unfortunately, owing to the small number of hemophilia B patients with FIX inhibitors who have undergone ITI, no meaningful analysis of prognostic factors has been possible. However, two factors stand out from the North American data: first, all five patients with a family history of FIX inhibitor failed ITI, and, second, central venous access complications and adverse

Table 18.1 Experience with immune tolerance induction (ITI) in hemophilia B complicated by a FIX inhibitor. Data from Malmö not included (see text). Inhibitor titer defined as low if <5 Bethesda units (BU)/mL.

Titer of inhibitor (high or low)	Completed ITI	Success	Failure	ITI regimen (including dose of FIX concentrate U/kg)	Notes	Source (reference)
High (n=13) and low	16	5	11	FIX 25–200 U/kg/day. Plasmapheresis (n = 2) Immune modulators (n = 8)		N. America [29]
Low	2	0	2	FIX 130 U/kg/day initially. Plasmapheresis + steroids FIX 50 U/kg for 6 days/week	Subsequent relapse after 40 months	Australia [27,28]
High	2	1	1	FIX 25 U/kg three times/week FIX 220 U/kg/alternate day	Relapse 2 months after low-dose ITI	Japan [30]
Unknown	2	0	2	Unknown		Germany [26]
High and low	2	1	1	Unknown	Failure due to nephrotic syndrome Success in patient with low-titer inhibitor	Japan [31]

events were more common among individuals failing ITI, with 79% of the adverse reactions being severe allergic reactions [29]. The poor success rate of ITI and high incidence of allergic reactions — the latter being associated with the development of the nephrotic syndrome during ITI — mean that ITI for FIX inhibitors remains a major clinical challenge.

Anaphylaxis and the nephrotic syndrome

The association between FIX inhibitor development and severe anaphylactic reactions is a significant problem [32,33]. The management of the initial anaphylactic reaction depends on its severity, but, as the reactions can be life-threatening, management includes fluid replacement, antihistamines, steroids, oxygen, and epinephrine. Desensitization with increasing doses of FIX concentrate has been performed and, if successful, allows the continued administration of FIX concentrates [31,32,34]. However, although desensitization has been associated with disappearance of the FIX inhibitor without formal ITI, in the majority of cases the inhibitor persists [31,32]. The treatment of bleeding episodes in individuals who have experienced anaphylactic reactions will depend on the associated FIX inhibitor titer and whether there has been a response to desensitization. Individuals have been treated for bleeding episodes with FIX concentrates and PCCs, with or without desensitization [32]. However, rFVIIa is the logical treatment for bleeding episodes in those individuals who have not been adequately desensitized and/or who still have a high-titer or high-responding FIX inhibitor.

A history of anaphylactic reaction is important with respect to ITI. As mentioned previously, a history of allergic reactions in FIX inhibitor patients appears to be associated with a poor outcome of ITI [29]. One reason for this poor response to ITI in this group of patients is the development of nephrotic syndrome [35]. The development of nephrotic syndrome during ITI for FIX inhibitors has been reported to occur between 7 and 13 months after the start of ITI [31,35–38]. Attempts to treat the nephrotic syndrome have included reducing the dose of FIX, interrupting ITI, stopping FIX infusions, and the administration of corticosteroids and cyclophosphamide; the response has been quite variable, ranging from complete recovery to continued proteinuria and hypoalbuminemia. The pathogenesis of nephrotic syndrome remains unknown. There has been only one report of a renal biopsy in an individual with nephrotic syndrome secondary to ITI in hemophilia B [39], and this demonstrated a membranous glomerulonephritis. It has been postulated that the nephrotic syndrome is secondary to immune complex deposition, but an attempt to demonstrate FIX deposition in the renal biopsy failed, although only one anti-FIX antibody was utilized in this analysis. In addition to the unresolved pathogenesis of nephrotic syndrome in these patients, the etiological factors also remain unclear. In two brothers with severe hemophilia B, both of whom developed FIX inhibitors and who were treated with ITI, only the younger brother developed nephrotic syndrome [36]. This was despite the fact that both brothers suffered allergic reactions to FIX infusions and that the FIX concentrate and ITI regimen used for attempted ITI were identical. Despite these unresolved questions, regular urinalysis should form part of the standard care of individuals undergoing ITI for FIX inhibitors.

Acquired factor IX deficiency

Acquired FIX deficiency can be immune or nonimmune mediated. The nonimmune form has been well characterized in individuals with nephrotic syndrome [40]. By contrast, acquired autoimmune hemophilia B is rare, although the true incidence is unknown. Cases of acquired autoimmune hemophilia B are associated with a similar spectrum of medical conditions as seen in acquired hemophilia A, with cases associated with other autoimmune disorders, gastrointestinal disease, postoperative situations, postpartum status, and with no underlying disorder [41–43]. Three cases of acquired FIX inhibitors were seen in individuals with hemophilia A and a FVIII inhibitor who were treated with FEIBA [44]. Acquired FIX inhibitors have been described in adults and children [42,43,45]. Treatment of acquired FIX inhibitors follows the same principles as for acquired hemophilia A, with both spontaneous remission and responses to immunosuppression described [42,43,45].

Future developments

Inhibitors in individuals with hemophilia B continue to pose significant clinical problems. These issues may have an impact on the development of gene transfer and warrant attempts at improving the outcome of ITI in this group of patients who remain severely affected by their inhibitors. Concern about inhibitor development as a result of FIX gene transfer protocols may have a major impact on those individuals who have high-risk FIX gene mutations and previously untreated individuals with hemophilia B. Early gene therapy protocols excluded individuals with gross FIX gene deletions. However, despite these concerns, there is a growing body of work that suggests that tolerance to FIX can occur with gene transfer and that this is dependent on the vector type and route employed, for example hepatic or *in utero* [46,47]. With respect to ITI, a better understanding of the immunologic processes involved in the development of anaphylaxis and the nephrotic syndrome may allow the refinement of desensitization and ITI protocols to minimize or prevent the occurrence of the latter. Potentially murine models utilizing FcR receptor knock-out mice may provide some answers. Studies with this type of knock-out model have demonstrated that IgG can mediate anaphylaxis, and FcRgII –/– knock-out mice develop glomerulonephritis associated with proteinuria [48]. Potentially, interbreeding between FIX knock-out mice and the FcR receptor knock-out mice may allow a model for these complications to be developed. In addition, new immunomodulatory therapies may have a role in preventing inhibitor development or as new agents to be used in ITI. Such agents include the chimeric molecule mCTLA4Ig [49] and anti-CD40 antibody (which interfere with antigen presenting cell–T-cell costimulatory interactions), and a monoclonal antibody against CD20-positive B cells.

References

1 Sultan Y. Prevalence of inhibitors in a population of 3435 hemophilia patients in France. French Hemophilia Study Group. *Thromb Haemost* 1992; **67**: 600–2.

2 Soulier JP, Larrieu MJ. Differentiation of hemophilia into two groups. *N Engl J Med* 1953; **249**: 547.

3 Allain J-P, Frommel D. Failure of immunosuppression in a severe haemophilia B patient with specific antibody. *Thromb Haemost* 1976; **36**: 86–9.

4 Hedner U, Nilsson IM. Induced tolerance in hemophilia patients with antibodies against IX:C. *Acta Med Scand* 1983; **214**: 191–7.

5 Negrier C, Goudemand J, Sultan Y, et al. Multicenter retrospective study on the utilization of FEIBA in France in patients with factor VIII and factor IX inhibitors. French FEIBA Study Group. Factor Eight Bypassing Activity. *Thromb Haemost* 1997; **77**: 1113–19.

6 Lusher JM, Roberts HR, Davignon G, et al. A randomized, double-blind comparison of two dosage levels of recombinant factor VIIa in the treatment of joint, muscle and mucocutaneous haemorrhages in persons with haemophilia A and B, with and without inhibitors. rFVIIa Study Group. *Haemophilia* 1998; **4**: 790–8.

7 Hilgartner MW, Knatterud GL. The use of factor eight inhibitor bypassing activity (FEIBA immuno) product for treatment of bleeding episodes in hemophiliacs with inhibitors. *Blood* 1983; **61**: 36–40.

8 Key NS, Aledort LM, Beardsley D, et al. Home treatment of mild to moderate bleeding episodes using recombinant factor VIIa (Novoseven) in haemophiliacs with inhibitors. *Thromb Haemost* 1998; **80**: 912–18.

9 Shapiro AD, Gilchrist GS, Hoots WK, et al. Prospective, randomised trial of two doses of rFVIIa (NovoSeven) in haemophilia patients with inhibitors undergoing surgery. *Thromb Haemost* 1998; **80**: 773–8.

10 Cooper HA, Jones CP, Campion E, et al. Rationale for the use of high dose rFVIIa in a high-titer inhibitor patient with haemophilia B during major orthopaedic procedures. *Haemophilia* 2001; **7**: 517–22.

11 Smith MP, Ludlam CA, Collins PW, et al. Elective surgery on factor VIII inhibitor patients using continuous infusion of recombinant activated factor VII: plasma factor VII activity of 10 IU/mL is associated with an increased incidence of bleeding. *Thromb Haemost* 2001; **86**: 949–53.

12 Ludlam CA, Smith MP, Morfini M, et al. A prospective study of recombinant activated factor VII administered by continuous infusion to inhibitor patients undergoing elective major orthopaedic surgery: a pharmacokinetic and efficacy evaluation. *Br J Haematol* 2003; **120**: 808–13.

13 Mauser-Bunschoten EP, Koopman MM, Goede-Bolder AD, et al. Efficacy of recombinant factor VIIa administered by continuous infusion to haemophilia patients with inhibitors. *Haemophilia* 2002; **8**: 649–56.

14 Saxon BR, Shanks D, Jory CB, Williams V. Effective prophylaxis with daily recombinant factor VIIa (rFVIIa-Novoseven) in a child with high titre inhibitors and a target joint. *Thromb Haemost* 2001; **86**: 1126–7.

15 Brown SA, Aledort LM, Astermark J, et al. Unresolved issues in prophylaxis. *Haemophilia* 2002; **8**: 817–21.

16 Giddings JC, Bloom AL, Kelly MA, Spratt HC. Human factor IX inhibitors: immunochemical characteristics and treatment with activated concentrate. *Clin Lab Haematol* 1983; **5**: 165–75.

17 Freiburghaus C, Berntorp E, Ekman M, et al. Immunoadsorption for removal of inhibitors: update on treatments in Malmö-Lund between 1980 and 1995. *Haemophilia* 1998; **4**: 16–20.

18 Kronwall G, Williams RD. Difference in antiprotein A activity among IgG subgroups. *J Immunol* 1969; **103**: 828.

19 Carroll RR, Panush RS, Kitchens CS. Spontaneous disappearance of an IgA anti-factor IX inhibitor in a child with Christmas disease. *Am J Hematol* 1984; **17**: 321–5.

20 Theodorsson B, Hedner U, Nilsson IM, Kisiel W. A technique for specific removal of factor IX alloantibodies from human plasma: partial characterization of the alloantibodies. *Blood* 1983; **61**: 973–81.

21 Ohkubo Y, Takahashi Y, Sugimoto M, Nishino M, Nishimura T, Yoshioka A, *et al.* Disappearance of inhibitor to factor IX in a patient with severe haemophilia B and immunological characterization of the inhibitor. *Clin Lab Haematol* 1988; **10**: 177–85.

22 Nilsson IM, Sundqvist SB. Suppression of secondary antibody response by intravenous immunoglobulin and development of tolerance in a patient with haemophilia B and antibodies. *Scand J Haematol* 1984; **40** (Suppl.): 203–6.

23 Berntorp E, Astermark J, Carlborg E. Immune tolerance induction and the treatment of hemophilia. Malmö protocol update. *Haematologica* 2000; **85**: 48–50; discussion p. 1.

24 Freiburghaus C, Berntorp E, Ekman M, *et al.* Tolerance induction using the Malmö treatment model 1982–1995. *Haemophilia* 1999; **5**: 32–9.

25 Tengborn L, Berntorp E. Continuous infusion of factor IX concentrate to induce immune tolerance in two patients with haemophilia B. *Haemophilia* 1998; **4**: 56–9.

26 Lenk H. The German National Immune Tolerance Registry, 1997 update. Study Group of German Haemophilia Centres. *Vox Sang* 1999; **77** (Suppl. 1): 28–30.

27 Barnes C, Rudzki Z, Ekert H. Induction of immune tolerance and suppression of anaphylaxis in a child with haemophilia B by simple plasmapheresis and antigen exposure. *Haemophilia* 2000; **6**: 693–5.

28 Barnes C, Brewin T, Ekert H. Induction of immune tolerance and suppression of anaphylaxis in a child with haemophilia B by simple plasmapheresis and antigen exposure: progress report. *Haemophilia* 2001; **7**: 439–40.

29 DiMichele DM, Kroner BL. The North American Immune Tolerance Registry: practices, outcomes, outcome predictors. *Thromb Haemost* 2002; **87**: 52–7.

30 Suzuki N, Watanabe J, Kudoh T, *et al.* Successful induction of immune tolerance in a patient with haemophilia B with inhibitor. *Haemophilia* 2003; **9**: 340–2.

31 Shibata M, Shima M, Misu H, *et al.* Management of haemophilia B inhibitor patients with anaphylactic reactions to FIX concentrates. *Haemophilia* 2003; **9**: 269–71.

32 Warrier I, Ewenstein BM, Koerper MA, *et al.* Factor IX inhibitors and anaphylaxis in hemophilia B. *J Pediatr Hematol Oncol* 1997; **19**: 23–7.

33 Warrier I, Ewenstein BM, Koerper MA, *et al.* Factor IX inhibitors and anaphylaxis in haemophilia B. *Haemophilia* 1996; **2**: 259–61.

34 Dioun AF, Ewenstein BM, Geha RS, Schneider LC. IgE-mediated allergy and desensitization to factor IX in hemophilia B. *J Allergy Clin Immunol* 1998; **102**: 113–17.

35 Ewenstein BM, Takemoto C, Warrier I, *et al.* Nephrotic syndrome as a complication of immune tolerance in hemophilia B. *Blood* 1997; **89**: 1115–16.

36 Tengborn L, Hansson S, Fasth A, *et al.* Anaphylactoid reactions and nephrotic syndrome—a considerable risk during factor IX treatment in patients with haemophilia B and inhibitors: a report on the outcome in two brothers. *Haemophilia* 1998; **4**: 854–9.

37 Lenk H, Bierbach U, Schille R. Inhibitor to factor IX and nephrotic syndrome in the course of immune tolerance treatment. *Haemophilia* 1996; **2** (Suppl. 1): 104.

38 Pollmann H. A haemophilia B patient with complete factor IX gene deletion and a high titre antibody against FIX. *Haemophilia* 1996; **2** (Suppl. 1): 72.

39 Dharnidharka VR, Takemoto C, Ewenstein BM, Rosen S, Harris HW. Membranous glomerulonephritis and nephrosis post factor IX infusions in hemophilia B. *Pediatr Nephrol* 1998; **12**: 654–7.

40 Natelson EA, Lynch EC, Hettig RA, Alfrey CP, Jr. Acquired factor IX deficiency in the nephrotic syndrome. *Ann Intern Med* 1970; **73**: 373–8.

41 Kyriakou DS, Alexandrakis MG, Passam FH, *et al.* Acquired inhibitors to coagulation factors in patients with gastrointestinal diseases. *Eur J Gastroenterol Hepatol* 2002; **14**: 1383–7.

42 Miller K, Neely JE, Krivit W, Edson JR. Spontaneously acquired factor IX inhibitor in a nonhemophiliac child. *J Pediatr* 1978; **93**: 232–4.

43 Ozsoylu S, Ozer FL. Acquired factor IX deficiency. A report of two cases. *Acta Haematol* 1973; **50**: 305–14.

44 Panicucci F, Sagripanti A, Conte B, *et al.* Inhibitor to factor IX following activated prothrombin–complex concentrate treatment. *Thromb Haemost* 1981; **45**: 96.

45 Berman BW, McIntosh S, Clyne LP, *et al.* Spontaneously acquired Factor IX inhibitors in childhood. *Am J Pediatr Hematol Oncol* 1981; **3**: 77–81.

46 Waddington SN, Buckley SM, Nivsarkar M, *et al.* In utero gene transfer of human factor IX to fetal mice can induce postnatal tolerance of the exogenous clotting factor. *Blood* 2003; **101**: 1359–66.

47 Mingozzi F, Liu YL, Dobrzynski E, *et al.* Induction of immune tolerance to coagulation factor IX antigen by in vivo hepatic gene transfer. *J Clin Invest* 2003; **111**: 1347–56.

48 Bolland S, Ravetch JV. Spontaneous autoimmune disease in Fc(gamma)RIIB-deficient mice results from strain-specific epistasis. *Immunity* 2000; **13**: 277–85.

49 Qian J, Collins M, Sharpe AH, Hoyer LW. Prevention and treatment of factor VIII inhibitors in murine hemophilia A. *Blood* 2000; **95**: 1324–9.

19 Pharmacokinetics

Sven Björkman and Erik E. Berntorp

Why pharmacokinetics?

Treatment with a drug aims to produce a certain pharmacologic effect for a certain time. This requires that the drug attains an appropriate concentration at its site of action and is then eliminated from this site when the effect is no longer desired. The processes governing drug concentrations are summarized as the *pharmacokinetics* of the drug. The relationship between drug concentration at the site of action and an observable effect is then the *pharmacodynamics* of the drug. The pharmacokinetics and pharmacodynamics together determine the necessary dose, dosing intervals, and mode of administration of the drug. If a drug is prescribed according to general guidelines with or without empirical adjustment of the dosing, then the "black box" of pharmacokinetics and pharmacodynamics remains unopened. In many instances this can be entirely justified. However, treatment of hemophilia is eminently suited to optimization by pharmacokinetic methods. The therapeutic plasma levels of factor VIII (FVIII) or factor IX (FIX) in various clinical situations are reasonably known and the methods to achieve, maintain, and monitor these levels are well established. The aim of this chapter is to review the pharmacokinetics of FVIII and FIX and to give an outline of clinical applications to optimize the treatment of hemophilia. Several published review articles by our group have recently examined this subject extensively and will frame this discussion [1–4].

Assays and plasma levels

Coagulation factors are precursors of enzymes or cofactors in the coagulation cascade. Plasma concentrations of these proteins are difficult to measure and sometimes irrelevant since molar concentrations may not directly translate into biologic activity. Consequently, their "concentrations" in plasma are normally determined by bioassays and expressed as coagulant activities in international units (U) per milliliter or deciliter. For FVIII and FIX the coagulant activities will be denoted FVIII:C and FIX:C respectively. Since the word "concentration" is obviously inappropriate to refer to coagulant activity, the word "level" will be used throughout the subsequent discussion. By definition, 1 U/mL, 1 kU/L, or 100 U/dL is the average coagulation factor level in healthy individuals.

The methods currently used to measure FVIII:C and FIX:C are the one-stage assay and the chromogenic substrate assay.

The one-stage assay is performed by mixing the sample plasma with plasma deficient in the assayed factor and measuring the resultant coagulation time after addition of calcium and a coagulation-activating agent [5]. In the chromogenic substrate assay, FVIII or FIX activates factor X and the formed factor Xa acts on a synthetic substrate to release *p*-nitroaniline, which, in turn, is measured by spectrophotometry [6].

Discrepancies between different bioassays may complicate the interpretation of pharmacokinetic data since they affect the determination of both administered dose and the corresponding plasma levels. The problems are most pronounced for the measurement of the *in vitro* potency of a factor concentrate. The greatest difference between traditional one-stage assays and the chromogenic assay has been observed for B-domain-deleted (BDD) recombinant FVIII [7], in that FVIII:C measured by the one-stage assay may be only half of that determined by the chromogenic assay. Therefore, these difficulties must be overcome. Guidelines on how to minimize the assay problems for FVIII have been published [8].

The advantage of defining plasma levels using bioassays is that these levels as functions of time represent the kinetics of the desired coagulant effect. Pharmacokinetics properly deals with drug concentrations. Applying pharmacokinetic calculations to coagulant activity values, while questionable in principle, is, nonetheless, very convenient in practice.

Methods, definitions and applications of pharmacokinetics

The following parameters are normally used to characterize the disposition or "pharmacokinetics" of the coagulation factors [1,2]:
- *Clearance (CL)*. CL is the capacity of the body to eliminate a substance, usually expressed as the volume of plasma that is cleared of substance in 1 min or 1 h. The best-known CL in the medical literature is creatinine clearance. However, the concept can be applied to any substance, either endogenous or exogenous. The CL of a drug is normally calculated as dose divided by the area under the plasma concentration curve (AUC). During a constant rate infusion this corresponds to rate of infusion divided by plasma concentration at steady state.
- *Volume of distribution (V)*. This is defined as the amount of drug in the body divided by the plasma concentration. Thus, it represents the apparent volume of plasma in which a drug is dis-

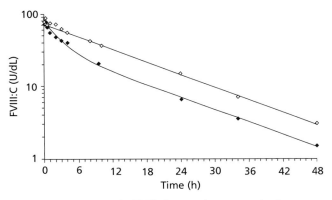

Figure 19.1 Representative FVIII:C versus time curves after intravenous administration of FVIII to adult patients with severe haemophilia A [12]. The upper curve (open symbols) is practically monophasic. After some slight early irregularities, it declines with a single half-life of 10 h. The exponential equation describing the curve is $C(t) = 72 \times e^{-0.067 \times t}$, where $C(t)$ is the "concentration" of FVIII:C as a function of time and t is time. The lower curve (closed symbols) is obviously biphasic. The two half-lives are 1.9 and 10 h and the exponential equation is $C(t) = 45 \times e^{-0.36 \times t} + 34 \times e^{-0.066 \times t}$. The early phase contributes 20% of the area under the curve.

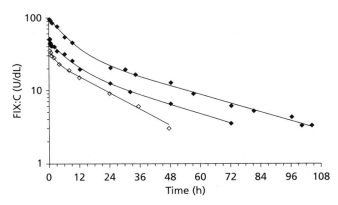

Figure 19.2 Representative FIX:C versus time curves after intravenous administration of FIX to adult patients with severe haemophilia B. They are taken from three different studies. Uppermost curve: plasma-derived FIX was given in a dose of 80 U/kg [9]. The curve is described by the function $C(t) = 63 \times e^{-0.15 \times t} + 35 \times e^{-0.023 \times t}$. The half-lives of the phases are 4.7 and 30 h. Middle curve: plasma-derived FIX was given in a dose of 50 U/kg [32]. The curve is described by the function $C(t) = 26 \times e^{-0.13 \times t} + 20 \times e^{-0.024 \times t}$. The half-lives of the phases are 5.2 and 28 h. Lower curve (open symbols): recombinant FIX was given in a dose of 50 U/kg [33,34]. The curve is described by the function $C(t) = 10 \times e^{-0.51 \times t} + 26 \times e^{-0.043 \times t}$. The half-lives of the phases are 1.4 and 16 h. Lower levels of FIX:C were obtained after administration of recombinant as compared with plasma-derived FIX in spite of the dose being the same. This is reflected by the clearance values calculated from the three curves: plasma-derived FIX 4.0 and 4.9 mL/h/kg, respectively, and recombinant FIX 8.0 mL/h/kg.

tributed (or diluted) in the body. If, for example, 1500 U of injected FVIII increases the plasma level immediately afterwards by 0.5 U/mL, then the FVIII appears to have been distributed into 3000 mL of plasma. Since drugs in general diffuse gradually from the circulation into various organs and tissues, V normally increases over time after the injection. At distribution equilibrium, V is the volume of distribution at steady state (V_{dss}). The higher the V_{dss}, the more extensive is the distribution of the drug away from the plasma space.

• *Mean residence time (MRT)*: This represents the average lifetime of the drug molecules in the body. The MRT depends on both distribution and elimination and can be calculated very simply as V_{dss} divided by CL.

• *Half-life ($t_{1/2}$)*: The processes of distribution and elimination also govern the half-life of a drug. However, the plasma concentration curve of a drug normally shows several half-lives (or phases), at least one early phase owing to distribution and the "terminal" phase representing elimination. Half-lives are determined by fitting an exponential equation to the plasma concentration versus time values (or in simple cases a linear function to log plasma concentration versus time values, which is equivalent). This curve-fitting is illustrated in Figures 19.1 and 19.2.

• *In vivo recovery (IVR)*: This parameter has been used only for coagulation factors. IVR is calculated as observed peak FVIII:C or FIX:C divided by the expected peak activity. The expected activity is the dose divided by the plasma volume of the patient. As will be described below, the assumption that the initial V equals the plasma volume may be approximately valid for FVIII:C but not for FIX:C [1,2,9]. A second problem is that the plasma volume of a subject is seldom accurately known. It is, for instance, not linearly related to total body weight [10]. A third problem is that of a "postinfusion activation" (see below for FVIII) that

makes the IVR dependent on the early blood sampling schedule in the pharmacokinetic study [1,2,11,12].

CL and V (V_{dss}) are often normalized to the body weight of the patient and expressed as, for example, mL/h/kg and L/kg. However, CL and V are seldom directly proportional to body weight, thus this normalization may not always diminish interindividual variance.

The pharmacokinetic parameters as such are useful to describe the *in vivo* behavior of FVIII and FIX and to compare preparations of coagulation factors. [1,2,11,12]. Of greater clinical interest, however, is that they can be used to calculate plasma levels of FVIII:C or FIX:C at any time during a treatment [13–15]. This will be illustrated below. Most commonly trough (minimum) and peak levels, i.e., levels found immediately before and after administration of a dose, during ongoing treatment, are discussed.

Pharmacokinetics of FVIII

In healthy persons, FVIII is presumably produced mainly in the liver and circulates in the plasma bound to the von Willebrand factor (VWF) [16]. In patients with hemophilia A, this complex is rapidly formed between infused FVIII and endogenous VWF. The binding of FVIII to VWF protects FVIII from degradation [17,18]. Thus, FVIII infused as a highly purified or recombinant concentrate is cleared much faster in patients with severe von Willebrand's disease, who lack functional VWF, than in patients with hemophilia A [19,20]. The very high molecular weight of the FVIII–VWF complex practically confines it to the plasma space. It can be calculated [2] that only about 14% of the body load of FVIII is extravascular at steady state.

When FVIII is given to adult patients as short-term infusions (typically 5–15 min duration), plasma FVIII:C levels, on average, rise by 0.020–0.025 U/mL for every U/kg administered. Thus, an infusion of 50 U/kg will normally give a peak plasma level of 1.0–1.3 U/mL. This corresponds to an initial volume of distribution (V) of 0.04–0.05 L/kg. The plasma disposition curve of FVIII:C is often approximately monophasic (Figure 19.1). Even if an irregular early phase can be discerned, it seldom contributes much to the total area under the curve. This early phase may result from more than one process: some (very limited) distribution of FVIII to intra- or extravascular sites and/or rapid clearance of high-molecular weight forms and aggregates of FVIII by the reticuloendothelial system. In addition, the peak plasma FVIII:C is often found 10–15 min after the end of the FVIII infusion, or sometimes even 1–2 h later [1,2,4,11,12]. The reason for this postinfusion rise in activity is not known.

The pharmacokinetics of FVIII:C in patients with hemophilia is summarized in Table 19.1. The parameter values apply under normal physiologic conditions and in the absence of inhibitors (antibodies) to FVIII. The presence of inhibitors may give a low IVR and/or a rapid clearance of FVIII:C [2,11,21]. The differences between plasma-derived and the presently available types of recombinant FVIII are marginal, even though some of them were statistically significant in comparative cross-over studies.

There is wide inter-individual variation in the pharmacokinetics of FVIII:C. In adult patients, the CL of plasma-derived FVIII:C typically varies between 1.8 and 6 mL/h/kg and $t_{1/2}$ between 8 and 23 h [1,2,12,22]. Some of the variance can be explained by physiologic factors. Since binding of FVIII to VWF protects the former molecule from degradation, variability in the plasma concentration of endogenous VWF likely explains one source of variability in CL and $t_{1/2}$. Accordingly, it has been demonstrated that the CL of B-domain deleted recombinant FVIII correlates negatively, and the $t_{1/2}$ positively, with VWF levels in patients with hemophilia A [23]. Blood group may also play a role, independently of associated VWF level; in one study

FVIII:C showed a significantly shorter mean elimination $t_{1/2}$ in patients with group O than in patients with group A [24].

Factor VIII pharmacokinetic data are available for children of school age and upwards but not for small children or infants. Chronological age is a substitute parameter for the changes in body weight and composition that take place during growth and that actually affect the pharmacokinetics of FVIII. Growing into adulthood may increase the body proportion of fat, which plays no part in the distribution and elimination of a coagulation factor. Thus it has been observed that the weight-adjusted CL of FVIII:C (i.e., in mL/h/kg) decreases with the age of the patients [25]. In a later study [14], it was found that a doubling of body weight (from 40 to 80 kg) was associated with only a 42% increase in CL and a 60% increase in V_{dss}. A positive correlation also exists between age and terminal $t_{1/2}$ of FVIII:C. IVR, when calculated assuming that plasma volume is a constant proportion of total body weight, tends to increase with the weight of the patient [12,26,27]. This is likely explained by the fact that plasma volume as a fraction of total body weight decreases with weight [10].

Crossover studies on different FVIII concentrates indicate that the pharmacokinetics of FVIII:C remains fairly constant within an individual, i.e., intra-individual variation in pharmacokinetics is lower than the inter-individual variation [12,28].

Pharmacokinetics of factor IX

Factor IX is produced by the liver and circulates in the plasma as a free molecule. Owing to its low molecular weight (55 kDa) it also readily diffuses into the interstitial fluid [29]. FIX also binds rapidly and reversibly to the vascular endothelium, with a half-maximal binding concentration similar to its normal concentration in plasma [30,31]. There are conflicting data in the literature on the pharmacokinetics of FIX:C. One reason for this is that many studies have been performed with inadequate blood sampling protocols, yielding biased or imprecise results [1,9]. A second reason is the difference in pharmacokinetics between plasma-derived and recombinant FIX (see below).

When plasma-derived FIX is given to adult patients as short-term infusions (typically 5–15 min duration), plasma FIX:C levels on average rise by 0.010–0.014 U/mL for every U/kg administered. Thus, an infusion of 50 U/kg will normally give a peak plasma level of 0.5–0.7 U/mL. This corresponds to an initial volume of distribution of 0.07–0.10 L/kg, which exceeds the plasma volume. Binding to the endothelium causes immediate disappearance of some of the infused FIX from the plasma. FIX:C then declines in a clearly biexponential fashion (Figure 19.2), in which the distribution phase of the curve represents diffusion of FIX into interstitial fluid. Thus, the V_{dss} of FIX is three- to fourfold greater than the plasma volume.

Table 19.2 summarizes methodologically adequate single-dose pharmacokinetic studies on FIX:C in patients with hemophilia. It can be seen that the terminal $t_{1/2}$ of FIX:C is longer than that of FVIII:C. The presently available recombinant FIX differs in both biochemistry and pharmacokinetics from plasma-

Table 19.1 Reported mean pharmacokinetic parameter values of factor VIII (FVIII), compiled from studies on plasma-derived FVIII concentrates (pdFVIII, range of mean values from six studies), full-length recombinant FVIII (rFVIII, one study) and B-domain deleted FVIII (rFVIII SQ, one study). Data are taken from ref. 2.

	CL (mL/h/kg)	V_{dss} (L/kg)	MRT (h)	Terminal $t_{1/2}$ (h)
pdFVIII	2.4–3.4	0.04–0.06	14–21	11–15
rFVIII	2.5	0.05	21	16
rFVIII SQ	3.2	0.05	16	11

Table 19.2 Reported mean pharmacokinetic parameter values of factor IX (FIX), compiled from studies with plasma-derived FIX concentrates (pdFIX, range of mean values from five studies) or recombinant FIX (rFIX, two studies; CL and V_{dss} are given in only one of them). Data are taken from ref. 2.

	CL (mL/h/kg)	V_{dss} (L/kg)	MRT (h)	Terminal $t_{1/2}$ (h)
pdFIX	3.8–4.3	0.11–0.15	34–45	29–34
rFIX	8.4	0.22	25–26	18–20

derived FIX, with a higher CL. Its IVR is approximately two-thirds that of plasma-derived FIX [33].

Inter-individual variance in the pharmacokinetics of plasma-derived FIX:C is difficult to estimate since the applicable studies include only very few patients. No correlates or causes of inter-individual variation in the standard pharmacokinetic parameters have as yet been identified. In a large study on recombinant FIX administered to 55 patients aged 4–56 years [33,34], both CL (in mL/h) and V_{dss} (in L) were linearly correlated (but not directly proportional) to body weight, consequently increasing during childhood and adolescence but remaining fairly constant during adulthood. Owing to the similar rises in CL and V_{dss}, neither MRT (= V_{dss}/CL) nor $t_{1/2}$ showed any significant regression with either body weight or age.

Application of pharmacokinetics to treatment of hemophilia

Clinical pharmacokinetics is the application of pharmacokinetic principles to the therapeutic management of patients [35]. Adjusting the dosage of a drug according to the requirement of the individual patient, which in turn is based on a knowledge of the pharmacokinetics of the drug in that particular patient, is often referred to as "tailoring" the dose. Target plasma levels of FVIII:C or FIX:C, as well as the need for dose tailoring, are very different for different clinical situations. These will therefore be dealt with separately. Common to all situations, however, is the fact that coagulation factor concentrates are a precious resource, expensive and/or of limited availability, which should not be wasted by inappropriate dosing.

Treatment of bleedings and prophylaxis and treatment during and after surgery

Guidelines for therapy and optimal dosing for bleeding in hemophilia have been developed on behalf of the World Health Organization (WHO) and the World Federation of Hemophilia (WFH) [36]. The therapeutic FVIII:C or FIX:C level (in this case the peak level after the first dose) recommended for most bleedings, such as joint, muscle, and retroperitoneal bleedings or hematuria, is 0.3–0.5 U/mL. The treatment should be continued

for 1–4 days, depending on the severity of the bleeding. For intracranial bleeding the initial peak level should minimally be 0.6–0.8 U/mL and the treatment period at least 7–10 days.

The doses of FVIII and FIX can be calculated from the IVR data given above. Thus, for FVIII, the dose (in U/kg) = 50 × (required rise in U/mL FVIII:C), and for FIX the dose (in U/kg) = 100 × (required rise in U/mL FIX:C). A fairly standardized recommended dosage for an adult patient with an ordinary bleeding is 15–25 U/kg for FVIII and 30–50 U/kg for FIX, with repeat dosing as required every 12–24 h (however, a single dose of at least 30 U/kg FVIII is often sufficient for joint bleedings).

Guidelines for dosing in surgery have also been developed and endorsed by the WHO and WFH [36]. For major surgery, the preoperative peak factor level should be 0.8–1.0 U/mL for FVIII:C and 0.5–0.8 U/mL for FIX:C. This peak level applies during days 1–3 and is then tapered off until day 12. The dosing interval for the first 4–6 days is 8–12 h for FVIII and 12–18 h for FIX. For minor surgery, peak levels can be lower by 40–50% and the total treatment duration shortened. In certain cases, higher levels and increased frequency of administration may be required.

Administration of FVIII or FIX as a continuous infusion is becoming popular since maintaining a steady therapeutic plasma level of coagulation factor in this way requires less factor concentrate than maintaining a therapeutic trough level by intermittent injections [2,37]. With a given dosing interval the saving is greater the shorter the $t_{1/2}$ of the factor activity (since the shorter the $t_{1/2}$, the higher the peak levels must be in order to maintain the desired trough level) [38]. There are as yet no universally accepted dosage recommendations for coagulation factor infusions.

The dosage recommendations above include a certain margin of safety and the patient is monitored clinically in most situations. Dose tailoring can be performed by assays of plasma coagulation factor and suitable dose adjustments without elaborate pharmacokinetic calculations.

Prophylactic treatment

Long-term clinical experience indicates that prophylactic treatment which aims to produce trough levels of FVIII:C or FIX:C of 0.01 U/mL is often adequate to prevent bleedings in patients with severe hemophilia [39,40]. The recommended standard doses to achieve this are 25–40 U/kg FVIII three times weekly in hemophilia A and 25–40 U/kg FIX twice weekly in hemophilia B. It is, however, clear that the dosage requirement of FVIII or FIX for prophylactic treatment varies considerably between individuals. There are some patients with biochemically severe disease (i.e., a factor level of <0.01 U/mL) who suffer few bleedings, maintain normal joint function, and sometimes do not require prophylactic treatment. On the other hand, patients with severely damaged joints may require higher trough levels of FVIII:C or FIX:C [3,14,15,39,40]. Dosing during prophylactic treatment must therefore be adjusted according to clinical outcome in terms of bleeding frequency or change in joint status. In

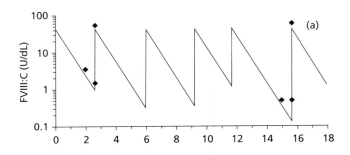

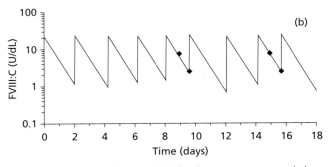

Figure 19.3 Predicted plasma FVIII:C levels in a patient on prophylactic therapy with FVIII [13]. The single-dose curve $C(t) = 56 \times e^{-1.48 \times t}$ (where time, t, is in days) was obtained after a dose of 2300 U [12]. Multiple-dose curves were consequently plotted from the equations $C(t) = (\text{given dose}/2300) \times 56 \times e^{-1.48 \times t}$, which were added over time, each new curve starting when a new dose was given. (a) Originally prescribed dosing of 2000 U twice weekly. (b) Dose tailored to give a trough level of 1 U/dL (0.01 U/mL); 1000 U every 2 days. Diamonds are measured control values. The two values at 0.5 U/dL are essentially "blank," or baseline, readings in the assay.

Table 19.3 Calculated dose requirements of FVIII, plasma-derived FIX, and recombinant FIX in 70-kg patients to maintain trough plasma levels of 0.01 U/mL during regular prophylactic treatment. Calculations were performed for average values of pharmacokinetic parameters (FVIII: CL 3.0 mL/h/kg, terminal $t_{1/2}$ 12 h; plasma-derived FIX: CL 4.0 mL/h/kg, terminal $t_{1/2}$ 31 h; recombinant FIX: CL 8.4 mL/h/kg, terminal $t_{1/2}$ 19 h) and also for 1.5-fold lower and higher clearances (values in parentheses). Some doses are obviously unrealistic, in particular administration of coagulation factor every third day to patients in which the CL is higher than average.

Schedule	Dose needed (U)	Annual consumption (kU/year)*
Factor VIII		
Daily	113 (56; 268)	41 (21; 98)
Every other day	588 (204; 2590)	107 (37; 473)
Every third day	2600 (588; 22 800)	316 (72; 2770)
By continuous infusion	50† (34; 76)	18 (12; 28)
Plasma-derived FIX		
Daily	105 (60; 206)	38 (22; 75)
Every other day	297 (148; 790)	54 (27; 144)
Every third day	626 (270; 2260)	76 (33; 274)
By continuous infusion	67† (45; 101)	25 (16; 37)
Recombinant FIX		
Daily	234 (131; 469)	85 (48; 171)
Every other day	794 (365; 2260)	145 (67; 413)
Every third day	2140 (781; 9090)	261 (95; 1110)
By continuous infusion	141† (94; 212)	52 (34; 77)

*kU = 1000 U.
†U/day.

spite of this, pharmacokinetics can be regarded as a valuable tool to optimize dosing of FVIII and FIX.

An example of dose tailoring in a patient with hemophilia A is shown in Figure 19.3. A 0.01 U/mL trough level was aimed for and attained. Concomitantly, the consumption of FVIII was lowered from 4000 to 3500 U per week. Several studies [13–15,34] have shown that the cost-effectiveness of prophylactic treatment can be improved considerably in this way. The raised trough levels in conjunction with (normally) decreased consumption of factor concentrate during optimized dosing are chiefly due to shorter injection intervals and lower doses at each injection, which result in lower peak levels. There is no indication that lower peak levels would result in less effective prophylactic treatment. After all, the original idea of prophylactic treatment [39,40] was to mimic the situation in moderate hemophilia, i.e., a constant coagulation factor level of 0.01–0.05 U/mL with no peaks at all.

Table 19.3 shows calculated annual consumption, with various dose intervals, of FVIII, plasma-derived FIX or recombinant FIX in hypothetical "average" adult patients (70 kg, pharmacokinetic parameters as in Tables 19.1 and 19.2) as well as in patients with extreme values of CL and $t_{1/2}$. In practice, the dosing would have to be adjusted to available vial sizes. The sharp in-

crease in dose requirement with prolongation of the dose interval should be noted. For example, if the $t_{1/2}$ of the coagulation factor is 12 h then the level will decrease by three-quarters during 24 h. Shifting the single-dose curve upwards from 0.01 U/mL at 24 h to 0.01 U/mL at 48 h thus requires a quadrupling of the dose (and to 0.01 U/mL at 72 h another quadrupling). During repeated dosing, the degree of accumulation (i.e., how much the previously given doses will contribute to the total FVIII:C or FIX:C level) will also influence these dose ratios. Long-term prophylaxis by continuous infusion would be very economical as regards factor consumption but is not technically feasible at the time of writing. The choice between injection schedules must balance practical and ethical issues against cost and availability of factor concentrates.

Conclusion

The pharmacokinetics of FVIII and FIX have been extensively investigated and their therapeutic plasma levels are well defined in most situations. Applied pharmacokinetics has therefore become an established tool for dosing in the treatment of hemophilia.

References

1 Björkman S, Carlsson M. The pharmacokinetics of factor VIII and factor IX: methodology, pitfalls and applications. *Haemophilia* 1997; **3**: 1–8.

2 Björkman S, Berntorp E. Pharmacokinetics of coagulation factors. Clinical relevance for patients with haemophilia. *Clin Pharmacokin* 2001; **40**: 815–32.

3 Björkman S. Prophylactic dosing of factor VIII and factor IX from a clinical pharmacokinetic perspective. *Haemophilia* 2003; **9** (Suppl. 1): 101–10.

4 Berntorp E, Björkman S. The pharmacokinetics of clotting factor therapy. *Haemophilia* 2003; **9**: 353–59.

5 Hedner U, Nilsson IM. Methods. In: Nilsson IM. *Haemorrhagic and Thrombotic Diseases*: London: John Wiley & Sons, 1974: 209–35.

6 Rosén S. Assay of factor VIII:C with a chromogenic substrate. *Scand J Haematol* 1984; **33** (Suppl. 40): 139–45.

7 Mikaelsson M, Oswaldsson U, Sandberg H. Influence of phospholipids on the assessment of factor VIII activity. *Haemophilia* 1998; **4**: 646–50.

8 Barrowcliffe TW. Recommendations for the assay of high-purity factor VIII concentrates. *Thromb Haemost* 1993; **70**: 876–7.

9 Björkman S, Carlsson M, Berntorp E. Pharmacokinetics of factor IX in patients with haemophilia B: methodological aspects and physiological interpretation. *Eur J Clin Pharmacol* 1994; **46**: 325–32.

10 Feldschuh J, Enson Y. Prediction of the normal blood volume. Relation of blood volume to body habitus. *Circulation* 1977; **56**: 605–12.

11 Allain JP. Principles of in vivo recovery and survival studies. *Scand J Haematol* 1984; **33** (Suppl. 41): 123–30.

12 Björkman S, Carlsson M, Berntorp E, Stenberg P. Pharmacokinetics of factor VIII in humans: obtaining clinically relevant data from comparative studies. *Clin Pharmacokin* 1992; **22**: 385–95.

13 Carlsson M, Berntorp E, Björkman S, Lindvall K. Pharmacokinetic dosing in prophylactic treatment of hemophilia A. *Eur J Haematol* 1993; **51**: 247–52.

14 Carlsson M, Berntorp E, Björkman S, Lethagen S, Ljung R. Improved cost-effectiveness by pharmacokinetic dosing of factor VIII in prophylactic treatment of haemophilia A. *Haemophilia* 1997; **3**: 96–101.

15 Carlsson M, Björkman S, Berntorp E. Multidose pharmacokinetics of factor IX: implications for dosing in prophylaxis. *Haemophilia* 1998; **4**: 83–8.

16 Lenting P, van Mourik JA, Mertens K. The life cycle of coagulation factor VIII in view of its structure and function. *J Am Soc Hematol* 1998; **92**: 3983–96.

17 Weiss HJ, Sussman II, Hoyer LW. Stabilization of factor VIII in plasma by the von Willebrand factor. *J Clin Invest* 1977; **60**: 390–404.

18 Noe DA. A mathematical model of coagulation factor VIII kinetics. *Hemostasis* 1996; **26**: 289–303.

19 Tuddenham EGD, Lane RS, Rotblat F, *et al.* Response to infusions of polyelectrolyte fractionated human factor VIII concentrate in human haemophilia A and von Willebrand´s disease. *Br J Haematol* 1982; **52**: 259–67.

20 Lethagen S, Berntorp E, Nilsson IM. Pharmacokinetics and hemostatic effect of different factor VIII/von Willebrand factor concentrates in von Willebrand´s disease type III. *Ann Hematol* 1992; **65**: 253–9.

21 Allain JP, Frommel D. Antibodies to factor VIII. V. Patterns of immune response to factor VIII in hemophilia A. *Blood* 1976; **47**: 973–82.

22 Smith KJ, Lusher JM, Cohen AR, Salzman P. Initial clinical experience with a new pasteurized monoclonal antibody purified factor VIIIC. *Semin Hematol* 1990; **27** (Suppl. 2): 25–9.

23 Fijnvandraat K, Peters M, Ten Cate JW. Inter-individual variation in half-life of infused recombinant factor VIII is related to pre-infusion von Willebrand factor antigen levels. *Br J Haematol* 1995; **91**: 474–6.

24 Vlot AJ, Mauser-Bunschoten EP, Zarkova AG, *et al.* The half-life of infused factor VIII is shorter in hemophiliac patients with blood group O than in those with blood group A. *Thromb Haemost* 2000; **83**: 65–9.

25 Matucci M, Messori A, Donati-Cori G, *et al.* Kinetic evaluation of four factor VIII concentrates by model-independent methods. *Scand J Haematol* 1985; **34**: 22–8.

26 Aronstam A, McLellan DS, Wassef M, Mbatha PS. Effect of height and weight on the in vivo recovery of transfused factor VIII C. *J Clin Pathol* 1982; **35**: 289–91.

27 Rousell RH, Kasper CK, Schwartz RS. The pharmacology of a new pasteurized antihemophilic factor concentrate derived from human blood plasma. *Transfusion* 1989; **29**: 208–12.

28 Nilsson IM, Berntorp E. Clinical efficacy of clotting factor concentrates: survival, recovery and haemostatic capacity. In: Smit Sibinga C Th, Das PC, Mannucci PM, eds. *Coagulation and Blood Transfusion* (Proceedings of the Fifteenth Annual Symposium for Blood Transfusion, Groningen 1990). Dordrecht: Kluwer Academic Publishers, 1991: 193–206.

29 Thompson AR. Factor IX concentrates for clinical use. *Semin Thromb Haemost* 1993; **19**: 25–36.

30 Heimark RL, Schwartz SM. Binding of coagulation factors IX and X to the endothelial cell surface. *Biochem Biophys Res Commun* 1983; **111**: 723–31.

31 Stern DM, Drillings M, Nossel HL, *et al.* Binding of factors IX and IX$_a$ to cultured vascular endothelial cells. *Proc Nat Acad Sci USA* 1983; **80**: 4119–23.

32 Berntorp E, Björkman S, Carlsson M, *et al.* Biochemical and in vivo properties of high purity factor IX concentrates. *Thromb Haemost* 1993; **70**: 768–73.

33 White G, Shapiro A, Ragni M, *et al.* Clinical evaluation of recombinant factor IX. *Semin Hematol* 1998; **35** (Suppl. 2): 33–8.

34 Björkman S, Shapiro AD, Berntorp E. Pharmacokinetics of recombinant factor IX in relation to age of the patient: Implications for dosing in prophylaxis. *Haemophilia* 2001; **7**: 133–9.

35 Rowland M, Tozer TN. *Clinical Pharmacokinetics: Concepts and Applications*, 3rd edn. Baltimore: Williams & Wilkins 1995.

36 Rickard KA. Guidelines for therapy and optimal dosages of coagulation factors for treatment of bleeding and surgery in haemophilia. *Haemophilia* 1995; **1** (Suppl. 1): 8–13.

37 Schulman S. Continuous infusion. *Haemophilia* 2003; **9**: 368–75.

38 Hay CRM, Doughty HI, Savidge GF. Continuous infusion of factor VIII for surgery and major bleeding. *Blood Coagul Fibrinolysis* 1996; **7** (Suppl. 1): S15–9.

39 Nilsson IM, Berntorp E, Löfqvist T, Pettersson H. Twenty-five years' experience of prophylactic treatment in severe haemophilia A and B. *J Intern Med* 1992; **232**: 25–32.

40 Löfqvist T, Nilsson IM, Berntorp E, Pettersson H. Haemophilia prophylaxis in young patients—a long-term follow-up. *J Intern Med* 1997; **241**: 395–400.

20 Work-up of a bleeding child

Victor S. Blanchette and Walter H.A. Kahr

Introduction

Cessation of bleeding is dependent on the formation of a stable hemostatic plug at sites of vessel injury. The hemostatic plug is composed primarily of platelets and fibrin. Excessive bleeding may reflect quantitative and/or qualitative abnormalities of platelets, and/or the coagulation proteins, and/or components of the vessel wall. These abnormalities may be inherited (congenital) or acquired.

The work-up of a child referred because of unusual or excessive bleeding should always include: (i) a comprehensive medical history including a specific bleeding history; (ii) a family history; (iii) a detailed physical examination; and (iv) selected laboratory tests. The results of these investigations usually allow an accurate diagnosis to be made in children referred for evaluation of abnormal bleeding. Of note, the interpretation of hemostatic test results in children requires that attention be paid to the effect of age on a number of coagulation parameters, an effect that is most pronounced during the first 6 months of life [1–3].

This review begins with a brief description of platelet plug formation in normal hemostasis and some common laboratory tests, fibrin formation being discussed in detail in Chapter 1. Subsequently, a practical approach to the evaluation of a child referred because of abnormal bleeding, including a commentary on specific hemostatic laboratory tests, is presented. Some selected common, as well as rare, inherited bleeding disorders are also discussed.

The hemostatic system

The hemostatic system is a delicate balance between procoagulant forces (forces that promote hemostatic plug formation at sites of vessel injury) and anticoagulant forces (coagulant protein inhibitors and the fibrinolytic system). Disturbances of this balance may result in abnormal bleeding. Current opinion regarding hemostatic plug formation at sites of vessel injury is summarized below.

Platelet plug formation

The initiating event in hemostatic plug formation is the adhesion of circulating platelets to exposed subendothelium. The high-molecular-weight hemostatic multimeric forms of the glycoprotein von Willebrand factor (VWF) play a critical role in this first event by linking platelets through the glycoprotein GPIb component of the GPIb/IX/V receptor to collagen in the subendothelium (Figure 20.1). Adhesion is further augmented by additional interactions involving the GPIa/IIa (integrin $\alpha_2\beta_1$) and GPVI receptors on platelets and collagen in the exposed subendothelium. As a result of this initial adhesive process, platelets become activated resulting in the release of multiple proteins, ADP and thromboxane A_2, causing local aggregation and recruitment of additional platelets to the site of vessel injury, and forming the hemostatic plug (primary hemostasis). Key mediators in platelet aggregation include platelet GPIIb/IIIa receptors (integrin $\alpha_{IIb}\beta_3$) with the ligands fibrinogen and VWF (Figure 20.1), the latter being of greater importance under conditions of higher shear. Activated platelets provide the anionic phospholipid surface necessary for the tenase and prothrombinase complexes to accelerate coagulation (described in Chapter 1). The platelet plug is then stabilized by the formation of cross-linked fibrin strands (secondary hemostasis).

Tests assessing the contribution of platelets toward hemostatic plug formation include enumeration of the circulating platelet count in blood samples, visualization of platelets in a blood smear, the skin bleeding time, platelet aggregation tests, platelet flow cytometry, and platelet electron microscopy. The Platelet Function Analyzer, PFA-100®, merits discussion as it may substitute for the skin bleeding time, which is an invasive and poorly reproducible test.

Fibrin formation

The end product of the soluble coagulation reaction is the formation of insoluble fibrin. The integrity of the soluble coagulation factors can be measured using patient's plasma in screening coagulation tests that may be affected by quantitative and/or qualitative abnormalities of coagulation proteins. Although these tests have their limitations owing to the absence of platelets and cells, in addition to the artificial testing conditions, they are readily available in a routine clinical laboratory and can provide useful information in the assessment of coagulopathies. These screening tests include the activated partial thromboplastin time (aPTT), prothrombin time or PT [reflected by the international normalized ratio (INR)], and the thrombin time (TT). Since reptilase clots fibrinogen in the presence of heparin, the reptilase time is useful to distinguish heparin contamination from afibrinogenemia and dysfibrinogenemia.

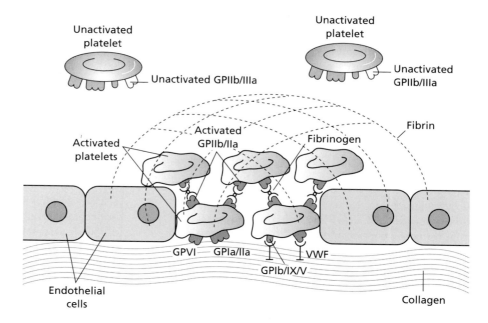

Figure 20.1 Schematic representation of a hemostatic plug. See text for details.

Evaluation of the child with abnormal bleeding or a suspected bleeding disorder

Medical history, including bleeding history

The initial evaluation of a child referred with abnormal bleeding, or because of a suspected bleeding disorder, should include a detailed history including a specific bleeding history. The medical history should include a list of all medications, including herbal supplements, that the child may be taking. The age of the child is important since bleeding disorders presenting in newborn infants (defined for the purpose of this review as infants less than or equal to 4 months of age) are significantly distinct from those encountered in older infants and children [4]. It is useful to separate patients into those who are ill at the time of initial presentation and those who are well; the former group often includes children in hospital who have acquired bleeding disorders secondary to a variety of conditions, e.g., bacterial or viral sepsis, renal and/or liver disease. In such patients, several components of the hemostatic system may be perturbed (platelets, coagulation factors, and inhibitors), which may together contribute to abnormal bleeding [5–8]. By contrast, abnormal bleeding in otherwise well infants and children is more likely to reflect underlying single defects (inherited or acquired) of platelets or coagulation proteins.

The bleeding history is of great value in the assessment of children with abnormal bleeding or a suspected bleeding disorder. Mucocutaneous bleeding is the hallmark of the inherited or acquired platelet disorders and includes symptoms such as easy bruising, recurrent and/or prolonged epistaxis, menorrhagia and prolonged bleeding following cuts, dental extractions, or other surgical procedures (e.g., circumcision).

Table 20.1 Hospital for Sick Children criteria for significant mucocutaneous bleeding symptoms (reproduced from ref. 27 with permission).

A significant mucocutaneous bleeding history requires any one of the following:
- recurrent nose bleeds requiring medical treatment (packing, cautery, DDAVP, etc.) or leading to anemia
- oral cavity bleeding lasting for at least 30 min, or restarting over the next 7 days or requiring medical treatment
- skin laceration bleeding lasting for at least 30 min, restarting over the next 7 days or requiring medical treatment
- menorrhagia requiring medical attention or leading to anemia
- prolonged bleeding associated with, or following, dental extraction or other oral surgery
- spontaneous gastrointestinal hemorrhage requiring medical attention or leading to anemia, unexplained by local causes (e.g., ulceration or portal hypertension)
- prolonged bleeding from other skin or mucous membrane surfaces requiring medical treatment (e.g., eye, ear, respiratory tract, genitourinary tract)

We have noted that bleeding histories are often poorly taken, leading in some cases to excessive and unnecessary investigations. In our pediatric center, we use a defined pediatric bleeding questionnaire based on criteria for significant mucocutaneous bleeding (Table 20.1) adapted from International Society on Thrombosis and Hemostasis (ISTH) significant mucocutaneous bleeding criteria for use in individuals with suspected von Willebrand disease (VWD). This bleeding questionnaire is comprehensive, easy to administer, and reproducible [9]. When using the questionnaire to classify children as "bleeders" or "normal," it should be recognized that young children may simply not have had sufficient opportunity, i.e., time, to declare symptoms that would classify them as "bleeders"; repeat assessments over time may therefore be both appropriate and necessary, particularly if there is a history of unusual or prolonged bleeding, or if the family history is positive for abnormal bleeding. The site and pattern of bleeding may yield important clues regarding an underlying etiology. For example, bleeding from multiple sites in an ill child should raise the suspicion of disseminated intravascular coagulation (DIC) secondary to an underlying disorder such as sepsis or anoxia, whereas a history suggestive of delayed bleeding, particularly into a joint such as an ankle, knee, or elbow, in a boy would be very suggestive of hemophilia A [factor VIII (FVIII) deficiency] or B (FIX deficiency). Mucocutaneous purpura in an otherwise well child after a viral infection may indicate idiopathic thrombocytopenic purpura (ITP). A history of prolonged bleeding from the umbilical cord with delayed wound healing in a newborn infant is suggestive of FXIII deficiency. Excessive menstrual bleeding in an adolescent girl may be the first sign of von Willebrand disease (VWD). Intracranial hemorrhage, if occurring in the newborn period, may be the first clue to an underlying severe coagulation bleeding disorder such as FXIII, FX, FIX, FV, FVIII, FVII, or fibrinogen deficiency. Other causes of intracranial hemorrhage in a newborn include birth trauma, DIC, connective tissue disorders (Ehlers–Danlos syndrome), congenital thrombocytopenia, and neonatal alloimmune thrombocytopenia, which is observed in 1–2 per 1000 newborns [10].

Family history

A detailed family history should be taken for all children referred for evaluation of a possible bleeding disorder. Specific questions regarding sites and patterns of bleeding should be asked of the child's parents, siblings and any other affected relatives. A positive family history for bleeding should be taken into consideration when deciding about repeat or additional testing in children referred because of abnormal bleeding. The family history may provide important clues regarding potential inheritance of an underlying bleeding disorder, e.g., a sex-linked inheritance pattern in a boy with hemophilia or an autosomal dominant inheritance pattern in a family with type 1 VWD. One example in which the family history can be very informative is the rare type 2N VWD variant [11,12]. In this condition, circulating FVIII coagulant levels (FVIII:C) are disproportionately low in comparison with circulating VWF antigen (VWF:Ag) and ristocetin cofactor (VWF:RCo) levels, because of an abnormality in VWF that results in a markedly decreased affinity for FVIII [13]. Patients may be labeled incorrectly as having mild/moderate hemophilia A [14] with potentially significant adverse effects if bleeding episodes are treated with a recombinant FVIII concentrate (devoid of functional VWF) rather than a VWF-containing concentrate such as Humate P. The inheritance pattern for type 2N VWD is autosomal recessive, and the presence of a typical laboratory profile plus a family history consistent with a recessive mode of inheritance should

prompt consideration of this relatively rare coagulation disorder.

Physical examination

The physical examination is often of limited use in the diagnosis of children with suspected bleeding orders. If present, the finding of purpura and/or petechiae in areas other than the lower limbs should raise the suspicion of a platelet disorder. In a boy, evidence of current or past bleeding into joints is suggestive of a diagnosis of hemophilia. Certain physical findings may point to specific, albeit relatively rare, bleeding disorders, e.g., telangiectasias in patients with hereditary hemorrhagic telangiectasia, oculocutaneous albinism in cases with Hermansky–Pudlak syndrome, skeletal abnormalities in patients with thrombocytopenia absent radius (TAR) syndrome, joint laxity and scarring in patients with Ehlers–Danlos syndrome, and cataracts in some patients with inherited macrothrombocytopenia (Fechtner and Alport syndromes) [15,16].

Laboratory evaluation

Laboratory evaluation should begin with screening laboratory tests unless the history and available laboratory results already performed are strongly suggestive of a specific bleeding disorder. For example, in a young boy with a positive family history for hemophilia A, the initial laboratory evaluation should include measurement of FVIII:C in addition to screening coagulation tests.

Screening coagulation tests should include measurement of a complete blood count (including a platelet count), examination of a blood smear, an aPTT, and an INR. If the child has a history of mucocutaneous bleeding, a screen to confirm or refute a diagnosis of VWD should be initiated. Such a screen should include measurements of FVIII:C, VWF:Ag, and VWF:RCo, VWF multimer analysis, and, if available, measurement of the closure time using the PFA-100 (see below). A skin bleeding time is not recommended as an initial screen in all patients referred for evaluation of abnormal bleeding. The result of screening laboratory tests taken together with the child's medical and family history should be used to decide about repeat testing or further specialized tests. Three laboratory tests/scenarios deserve special commentary because of their importance in the context of evaluation of the child with abnormal bleeding.

Enumeration of the circulating platelet count

The platelet count is typically measured in a sample of venous blood collected into ethylenediaminetetraacetic acid (EDTA) anticoagulant. Automated blood cell counters are usually more accurate than manual platelet counting (coefficient of variation 10–25%). However, at low platelet counts (less than 20×10^9 platelets/L), a manual platelet count is more accurate and is recommended [17,18]. A newborn infant's blood is often collected by heel puncture, and a low platelet count may sometimes be caused by clot formation at the time of sample collection and thus be an artifact. For this reason, it is recommended that the unexpected finding of thrombocytopenia (platelet count 100×10^9/L or less) in a newborn infant based on a heelstick sample be confirmed on a venous blood sample.

It is important that newly diagnosed thrombocytopenia be confirmed by careful examination of a blood smear. This will allow determination of pseudothrombocytopenia in samples collected into EDTA anticoagulant due to EDTA-induced *in vitro* agglutination of platelets by antibodies [19]. Pseudothrombocytopenia can be prevented by using a different anticoagulant (e.g., citrate or heparin) or by preparing a blood film directly from a heel puncture. Automated counters may also exclude megathrombocytes resulting in spurious thrombocytopenia, as automated counters often exclude platelets if they are larger than 30–35 fL [20]. Although rare, a gray platelet syndrome (α-granule deficiency) could be identified with a blood film showing pale gray-appearing platelets, whereas leukocyte inclusions could indicate a May Hegglin anomaly, or Sebastian or Fechtner syndrome [16]. The blood smear is very important in the diagnosis of hemolytic uremic syndrome (HUS) and thrombotic thrombocytopenic purpura (TTP), where the presence of red blood cell schistocytes may be the only clue to the etiology of the thrombocytopenia. Schistocytes may also be observed in a sick child with DIC and are usually accompanied by worsening thrombocytopenia and a coagulopathy (prolonged aPTT and INR).

Bleeding time and PFA-100

The skin bleeding time is one of oldest tests of global platelet function used to investigate bleeding disorders, and template devices are available for use in children and newborn infants as well as adults [3,21]. It has become recognized, however, that the use of the bleeding time as a routine screening test is not warranted. The test is highly operator dependent, poorly reproducible, and a poor predictor of bleeding risk [22–24]. The bleeding time is usually not prolonged in hemophiliacs, may be prolonged in patients with type 1 VWD, and is prolonged in patients with certain platelet function disorders.

A recently developed *in vitro* measure of primary, platelet-related hemostasis, that of the determination of the closure time using the platelet function analyzer PFA-100, may be more useful as a screening test for bleeding disorders than the bleeding time. The test is quantitative, simple, rapid, and reproducible, and measures, under high-shear conditions, the time taken for a platelet plug to occlude a microscopic aperture in a membrane coated with platelet agonists [25]. Like the bleeding time, the closure time is not prolonged in hemophiliacs [26]. However, the PFA-100 is particularly useful for screening for VWD in children and adults, and is just as sensitive as the bleeding time in detecting platelet function disorders [27,28]. The test is well suited for use in pediatric subjects, being less invasive than the bleeding time and requiring only 0.8 mL of citrated whole blood for each measurement.

Assessment of heparin contamination

Contamination of blood samples by heparin, especially in children such as ill, very low-birthweight infants and children in intensive care units, is a clinically significant problem. It is usually the most frequent cause of a prolonged aPTT. Heparin binds to antithrombin present in plasma samples, thereby enhancing inactivation of thrombin and FXa and, to a lesser extent FIXa, FXIa, and FXIIa. At very high plasma heparin concentrations, the PT is also prolonged. A prolonged aPTT due to heparin contamination will also result in a prolonged thrombin clotting time (TT) in which thrombin is added to citrated plasma. Heparin contamination in a plasma sample can be confirmed by normalization of the TT in the presence of protamine sulfate, which acts to neutralize any heparin present in the sample [29]. Alternatively, the snake venom reptilase (from *Bothrops atrox*), which is not inhibited by heparin, can be used instead of thrombin when measuring the TT. An abnormal TT but normal reptilase clotting time indicates heparin contamination [30]. A heparin-degrading enzyme (from *Flavobacterium heparinum*), heparinase (Hepzyme, Dade Behring), has recently been utilized to remove heparin from plasma samples prior to measuring aPTT [31,32]. Heparin-binding cellulose can also be added to remove heparin from specimens whereby the heparin–cellulose is removed from plasma by centrifugation (ECTEOLA-cellulose, Inotech Biosystems International, Inc.) [33]. Finally, if individual clotting factor levels need to be measured in heparin-containing specimens, removal or neutralization of heparin can be accomplished prior to measuring the factor activity.

Other assessments

Once the results of screening coagulation tests are available, they can be used to recommend repeat testing and/or additional, more specialized tests. In our experience of 388 children followed in a large pediatric bleeding disorders clinic, the three commonest groups of children with inherited bleeding disorders are boys with hemophilia A or B (47%), children with VWD (35%), and those with inherited platelet function defects (13%). Less common are the rare congenital coagulation factor disorders, e.g., FXIII, FXI, FX, FVII, FV, prothrombin, or fibrinogen deficiencies (5%). Selected inherited bleeding disorders are discussed below.

Hemophilia

The diagnosis of hemophilia requires the documentation of circulating FVIII (hemophilia A) or FIX (hemophilia B) levels below the normal for the age of the subject. Traditionally, individuals with hemophilia are classified as having severe, moderate, or mild disease, based on circulating factor levels of less than 1% (less than 0.01 IU/mL), 1–5% (0.01–0.05 IU/mL) and 5–50% (0.05–0.5 IU/mL) respectively. In some countries, the value of less than 2% (less than 0.02 IU/mL) is used to define the severe form of the disorder. The majority of per-

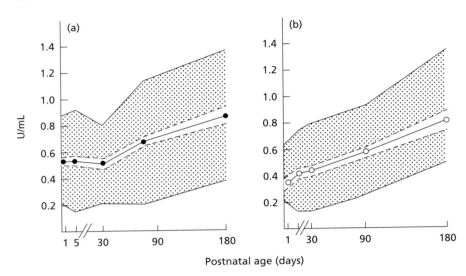

Figure 20.2 Factor IX levels in healthy full-term infants (a) and healthy premature infants (b) during the first 6 months of life. (a) Factor IX levels in 118 full-term infants. (b) Factor IX levels in 137 healthy premature infants (30–36 weeks' gestation). The inner line represents the mean values, the inner clear area the 95% confidence interval, and the shaded area 95% of all values. The mean adult factor IX levels are 1.09 ± 0.27 U/mL. Figure adapted from refs 1 and 2.

sons with hemophilia have circulating factor levels below 30% (0.3 IU/mL).

In our experience, the diagnosis of severe hemophilia is made within the first year of life because of testing at or around the time of birth in boys with a positive family history of the disorder, or because of abnormal bruising/bleeding that prompts laboratory investigation of the hemostatic system. Typical bleeding symptoms in the first month of life include prolonged bleeding from heelpricks performed for blood sampling, hematomas at the site of intramuscular injections of vitamin K, or postcircumcision bleeding [34]. Beyond the first month of life, there is a quiescent period of about 6 months, after which excessive bruising and prolonged bleeding from cuts in the oral cavity are relatively uncommon [34]. Hemarthroses in the first year of life are relatively uncommon and are usually trauma related. Male infants with these symptoms in the first year of life should be investigated for a possible underlying bleeding disorder including hemophilia A or B. Although, in our experience, the aPTT is always prolonged in boys with severe hemophilia, this screening laboratory test can be normal in boys with mild or even moderate hemophilia and it is therefore strongly recommended that, if a diagnosis of hemophilia is suspected, FVIII and FIX levels be specifically measured together with VWF.

The diagnosis of mild/moderate hemophilia is often delayed and may occur only after investigation for unusual bleeding in the setting of invasive procedures such as tonsillectomy. It is also important to remember that the diagnosis of mild hemophilia B in the first 6 months of life is compromised by the fact that levels of FIX, like other vitamin K-dependent factors, are reduced in early life and only reach adult levels at the age of 6 months [2,21] (Figure 20.2). Repeat testing after an interval of 6–12 months may therefore be appropriate in selected cases of suspected mild FIX deficiency. In contrast, patients with mild hemophilia A can reliably be diagnosed at any time since plasma FVIII levels are the same in newborns and adults.

Table 20.2 Classification of von Willebrand disease.

Type	Frequency	Comment
1	~80%	Partial quantitative deficiency of VWF
2	15–20%	Qualitative defects of VWF
2A		Variants with decreased platelet-dependent function associated with the selective absence of high-molecular-weight VWF multimers
2B		Variants with increased affinity for binding platelet GPIb leading to a reduction of high-molecular-weight VWF multimers
2M		Variants with decreased platelet-dependent function associated with a normal distribution of VWF multimers
2N		Variants with markedly decreased affinity for factor VIII
3	Rare	Virtually complete absence of VWF

von Willebrand disease

von Willebrand disease (VWD) is caused by qualitative and/or quantitative defects of the multimeric glycoprotein, von Willebrand factor (VWF) [35]. A current classification of VWD is presented in Table 20.2 [36]. Accurate diagnosis of the type 2 (qualitative) and type 3 (severe quantitative) variants is generally possible following measurement of the following variables: VWF:Ag, VWF:RCo, F VIII:C, and VWF multimer analysis. By contrast, diagnosis of the more common type 1 VWD is much more difficult, and in many cases the distinction between type 1 VWD and patients with normal VWF is unclear. Repeat testing is often required to determine whether an individual has type 1 VWD. Part of the problem is that the 95% confidence interval of the normal laboratory range for VWF can vary between 50% and 200% of the mean level, and clinical bleeding is variable even at low VWF levels [37]. In addition, the mean VWF:Ag and VWF:RCo levels are 20–25% lower in group O than in nongroup O subjects [27,38], and this difference should be taken into consideration when evaluating subjects for possible type 1 VWD. In our clinic, the diagnostic laboratory criteria for type 1 VWD are as follows: (i) levels of VWF:Ag below the 95% lower confidence limit for appropriate ABO type on at least two determinations, or levels of VWF:RCo below the 95% lower confidence limit for appropriate ABO type on at least two determinations, with a VWF:Ag level below the ABO-adjusted 95% lower confidence limit on at least one determination; and (ii) normal pattern of VWF multimer distribution. Because of the large variability of VWF levels and bleeding symptoms, Sadler [37] has suggested restricting the labeling of a person as having type 1 VWD to those individuals with very low VWF levels (less than 15%), frequent bleeding symptoms, and a dominant mode of inheritance. VWD can be further classified according to the type of qualitative defect in VWF:

• decreased platelet-dependent function with an absence of high-molecular-weight VWF multimers in type 2A VWD;
• mutations in VWF causing increased affinity of VWF for platelet GPIb, resulting in depletion of platelets and VWF in type 2B VWD;
• decreased platelet-dependent functions with normal VWF multimers in type 2M VWD;
• decreased affinity of VWF for FVIII in type 2N VWD, a condition that resembles mild hemophilia due to the decreased plasma FVIII levels.

A rare condition that resembles type 2B VWD is the platelet-type or pseudo-VWD caused by mutations in the platelet GPIbα gene causing enhanced binding of GPIbα to VWF [39–41]. Enhanced ristocetin-induced platelet aggregation (RIPA) is observed in both type 2B VWD and platelet-type VWD. Platelet aggregation studies at low concentrations of ristocetin (0.5 mg/mL) using normal platelets and patient's plasma, or patient's platelets and normal plasma, allow one to differentiate between the two conditions [42].

Platelet disorders

Platelet disorders encompass a wide spectrum of bleeding disorders, which may be inherited or acquired and include quantitative and/or qualitative defects [15,43]. Although the most common causes of thrombocytopenia and/or platelet dysfunction in children are due to acquired causes such as DIC, immune thrombocytopenia purpura (ITP), HUS, TTP, uremia, and liver disease [44,45], these will not be discussed here. Like VWD, platelet disorders present as primary hemostatic defects characterized by easy bruising, epistaxis, menorrhagia, and excessive bleeding from trauma and dental or surgical interventions. Physical findings include increased bruising, especially in areas other than the lower limbs in young children, and petechiae in

patients with severe quantitative and/or qualitative platelet disorders.

In the view of some experts, inherited disorders of platelet function manifested as mild mucocutaneous bleeding may be more common in the general population than has previously been appreciated. Such patients may remain undiagnosed throughout life and are simply considered to be "easy bruisers" or "bleeders." Congenital platelet disorders can be classified according to the type of qualitative defect present. For example, platelet adhesion and aggregation defects include the Bernard–Soulier syndrome (GPIb/IX/V deficiency), and Glanzmann thrombasthenia (GPIIb/IIIa deficiency) respectively. Abnormalities of platelet receptors for agonists include collagen receptors (GPVI, GPIa/IIa), ADP receptors (P2Y$_{12}$) or the thromboxane A$_2$ receptor. Platelet granule deficiencies involving dense granules (δ-granules) include isolated δ-granule deficiency, Hermansky–Pudlak syndrome, Chediak–Higashi syndrome, and Wiskott–Aldrich syndrome, whereas α-granule defects are seen in gray platelet syndrome, Quebec platelet disorder, and Paris–Trousseau syndrome [15]. Various abnormalities in platelet signal transduction pathways have also been identified. Defective platelet phospholipid translocation resulting in decreased platelet procoagulant activity has been described in Scott syndrome [46]. Congenital platelet disorders may be associated with normal platelet counts (e.g., Hermansky–Pudlak syndrome) or thrombocytopenia (e.g., platelet-type VWD). A useful working classification of inherited thrombocytopenias that is based on platelet size has been proposed by the Italian Gruppo di Studio delle Piastrine [47]. Examples of conditions with small, normal and large-sized platelets are Wiskott–Aldrich syndrome (small platelets), congenital amegakaryocytic thrombocytopenia (normal sized platelets), and the nonmuscle myosin heavy chain IIA (MYH9 gene) group of platelet disorders such as the May–Hegglin anomaly and the Sebastian, Fechtner, and Epstein syndromes (large platelets). On occasion, accompanying physical findings such as oculocutaneous albinism (e.g., Hermansky–Pudlak and Chediak–Higashi syndromes) or limb abnormalities in infants with the thrombocytopenic absence radius (TAR) syndrome allow the identification of these inherited platelet disorders.

Screening laboratory tests for inherited platelet disorders should include a complete blood count with accurate enumeration of the platelet count and a careful examination of the peripheral blood smear. In selected patients in whom the medical and/or family history is suggestive of a platelet disorder, and in whom an alternate explanation for bleeding symptoms such as VWD has been excluded, evaluation of the bleeding time and/or a closure time using the PFA-100 combined with platelet aggregation studies (platelet-rich plasma with agonists ADP, collagen, arachidonic acid, ristocetin, and epinephrine) [48] should be performed. In our experience, the bleeding time or PFA-100 closure time is always prolonged in patients with the severe forms of platelet function defects such as Glanzmann thrombasthenia or Bernard–Soulier syndrome and should be followed by platelet aggregation studies. In Glanzmann thrombasthenia, platelets aggregate only with ristocetin, whereas in Bernard–Soulier syndrome platelets aggregate with all agonists except ristocetin. Confirmatory testing using flow cytometry for the quantitation of GPIIb/IIIa and GPIb/IX/V receptors on platelets is useful since, for both of these conditions, quantitative receptor defects are usually more common than qualitative defects (not detected by flow cytometry). Dense (δ) granule platelet storage pool disorders can be identified using whole-mount electron microscopy whereas transmission electron microscopy is useful to exclude α-granule disorders such as gray platelet syndrome [49,50]. Finally, molecular and cytogenetic testing can be performed for some of the congenital platelet disorders where gene defects have been identified (e.g., Glanzmann thrombasthenia, Bernard–Soulier syndrome, Wiskott–Aldrich syndrome, X-linked macrothrombocytopenia with dyserythropoietic anemia, MYH9 gene mutations, Hermansky–Pudlak syndrome, Paris–Trousseau syndrome, and others) [51]. Such DNA analyses of congenital platelet defects are limited to specialized laboratories.

Summary

The correct and timely diagnosis of an inherited bleeding disorder in a child is important. This goal can best be achieved by combining a careful history, a detailed physical examination, and selected laboratory tests. Once a diagnosis is made, the child (if of an appropriate age) and/or parents or guardians can be counseled about the severity and anticipated natural history of the disorder plus available management options, both specific (e.g., factor concentrate therapy in boys with hemophilia) and nonspecific (e.g., DDAVP, antifibrinolytic therapy in children with type 1 VWD or congenital platelet disorders). It is important that the advice given be accurate in order to not create unnecessary anxiety in the child and/or parents, or lead to inappropriate restriction of physical activities (e.g., sporting activities in children with mild type 1 VWD). In many cases, this information is best provided by healthcare personnel with expertise in the field of pediatric hemostasis, and children suspected to have inherited disorders should be referred to specialized groups for evaluation and counseling.

Acknowledgment

We would like to thank Dr Margaret L. Rand for significant contributions to this chapter including the tables and Figure 20.1.

References

1 Andrew M, Paes B, Milner R, *et al.* Development of the human coagulation system in the full-term infant. *Blood* 1987; **70**: 165–72.

2 Andrew M, Paes B, Milner R, *et al.* Development of the human coagulation system in the healthy premature infant. *Blood* 1988; **72**: 1651–7.

3 Andrew M, Vegh P, Johnston M, *et al.* Maturation of the hemostatic system during childhood. *Blood* 1992; **80**: 1998–2005.

4 Zipursky A, deSa D, Hsu E, *et al.* Clinical and laboratory diagnosis of hemostatic disorders in newborn infants. *Am J Pediatr Hematol Oncol* 1979; **1**: 217–26.

5 Eberst ME, Berkowitz LR. Hemostasis in renal disease: pathophysiology and management. *Am J Med* 1994; **96**: 168–79.

6 Levi M, Ten Cate H. Disseminated intravascular coagulation. *N Engl J Med* 1999; **341**: 586–92.

7 Lisman T, Leebeek FW, de Groot PG. Haemostatic abnormalities in patients with liver disease. *J Hepatol* 2002; **37**: 280–7.

8 Monagle P, Andrew M. Acquired disorders of hemostasis. In: Nathan DG, Orkin SH, Ginsburg D, Look AT, eds. *Nathan and Oski's Hematology of Infancy and Childhood*, Vol. 2 (6th edn). Philadelphia: WB Saunders; 2003: 1631–67.

9 Hedlund-Treutiger I, Dean JA, Lillicrap D, *et al.* Evaluation of a bleeding history questionnaire in patients with von Willebrand disease. *Haemophilia* 2000; **6**: 218–19.

10 Dreyfus M, Kaplan C, Verdy E, *et al.* Frequency of immune thrombocytopenia in newborns: a prospective study. Immune Thrombocytopenia Working Group. *Blood* 1997; **89**: 4402–6.

11 Nishino M, Girma JP, Rothschild C, *et al.* New variant of von Willebrand disease with defective binding to factor VIII. *Blood* 1989; **74**: 1591–9.

12 Mazurier C, Dieval J, Jorieux S, *et al.* A new von Willebrand factor (vWF) defect in a patient with factor VIII (FVIII) deficiency but with normal levels and multimeric patterns of both plasma and platelet vWF. Characterization of abnormal vWF/FVIII interaction. *Blood* 1990; **75**: 20–6.

13 Mazurier C, Meyer D. Factor VIII binding assay of von Willebrand factor and the diagnosis of type 2N von Willebrand disease—results of an international survey. On behalf of the Subcommittee on von Willebrand Factor of the Scientific and Standardization Committee of the ISTH. *Thromb Haemost* 1996; **76**: 270–4.

14 Schneppenheim R, Budde U, Krey S, *et al.* Results of a screening for von Willebrand disease type 2N in patients with suspected haemophilia A or von Willebrand disease type 1. *Thromb Haemost* 1996; **76**: 598–602.

15 Cattaneo M. Inherited platelet-based bleeding disorders. *J Thromb Haemost* 2003; **1**: 1628–36.

16 Heath KE, Campos-Barros A, Toren A, *et al.* Nonmuscle myosin heavy chain IIA mutations define a spectrum of autosomal dominant macrothrombocytopenias: May–Hegglin anomaly and Fechtner, Sebastian, Epstein, and Alport-like syndromes. *Am J Hum Genet* 2001; **69**: 1033–45.

17 Hanseler E, Fehr J, Keller H. Estimation of the lower limits of manual and automated platelet counting. *Am J Clin Pathol* 1996; **105**: 782–7.

18 Haung ML, Ho CH. Diagnostic value of an automatic hematology analyzer in patients with hematologic disorders. *Adv Ther* 1998; **15**: 137–41.

19 Bizzaro N. EDTA-dependent pseudothrombocytopenia: a clinical and epidemiological study of 112 cases, with 10-year follow-up. *Am J Hematol* 1995; **50**: 103–9.

20 Racchi O, Rapezzi D. Megathrombocytes and spurious thrombocytopenia. *Eur J Haematol* 2001; **66**: 140–1.

21 Andrew M, Castle V, Mitchell L, Paes B. Modified bleeding time in the infant. *Am J Hematol* 1989; **30**: 190–1.

22 Rodgers RP, Levin J. A critical reappraisal of the bleeding time. *Semin Thromb Haemost* 1990; **16**: 1–20.

23 Lind SE. The bleeding time does not predict surgical bleeding. *Blood* 1991; **77**: 2547–52.

24 De Caterina R, Lanza M, Manca G, *et al.* Bleeding time and

bleeding: an analysis of the relationship of the bleeding time test with parameters of surgical bleeding. *Blood* 1994; **84**: 3363–70.

25 Jilma B. Platelet function analyzer (PFA-100): a tool to quantify congenital or acquired platelet dysfunction. *J Lab Clin Med* 2001; **138**: 152–63.

26 Carcao MD, Blanchette VS, Dean JA, *et al.* The Platelet Function Analyzer (PFA-100): a novel in-vitro system for evaluation of primary hemostasis in children. *Br J Haematol* 1998; **101**: 70–3.

27 Dean JA, Blanchette VS, Carcao MD, *et al.* von Willebrand disease in a pediatric-based population—comparison of type 1 diagnostic criteria and use of the PFA-100 and a von Willebrand factor/collagen-binding assay. *Thromb Haemost* 2000; **84**: 401–9.

28 Favaloro EJ. Clinical application of the PFA-100. *Curr Opin Hematol* 2002; **9**: 407–15.

29 Cumming AM, Jones GR, Wensley RT, Cundall RB. *In vitro* neutralization of heparin in plasma prior to the activated partial thromboplastin time test: an assessment of four heparin antagonists and two anion exchange resins. *Thromb Res* 1986; **41**: 43–56.

30 Funk C, Gmur J, Herold R, Straub PW. Reptilase-R—a new reagent in blood coagulation. *Br J Haematol* 1971; **21**: 43–52.

31 van den Besselaar AM, Meeuwisse-Braun J. Enzymatic elimination of heparin from plasma for activated partial thromboplastin time and prothrombin time testing. *Blood Coagul Fibrinolysis* 1993; **4**: 635–8.

32 Harenberg J, Reichel T, Malsch R, *et al.* Multicentric evaluation of heparinase on aPTT, thrombin clotting time and a new PT reagent based on recombinant human tissue factor. *Blood Coagul Fibrinolysis* 1996; **7**: 453–8.

33 Thompson AR, Counts RB. Removal of heparin and protamine from plasma. *J Lab Clin Med* 1976; **88**: 922–9.

34 Baehner RL, Strauss HS. Hemophilia in the first year of life. *N Engl J Med* 1966; **275**: 524–8.

35 Lillicrap D, Dean JA, Blanchette VS. von Willebrand disease. In: Lilleyman JS, Hann IM, Blanchette VS, eds. *Pediatric Hematology*, 2nd edn. London: Churchill Livingstone; 1999: 601–9.

36 Sadler JE, Mannucci PM, Berntorp E, *et al.* Impact, diagnosis and treatment of von Willebrand disease. *Thromb Haemost* 2000; **84**: 160–74.

37 Sadler JE. Von Willebrand disease type 1: a diagnosis in search of a disease. *Blood* 2003; **101**: 2089–93.

38 Gill JC, Endres-Brooks J, Bauer PJ, *et al.* The effect of ABO blood group on the diagnosis of von Willebrand disease. *Blood* 1987; **69**: 1691–5.

39 Miller JL, Castella A. Platelet-type von Willebrand's disease: characterization of a new bleeding disorder. *Blood* 1982; **60**: 790–4.

40 Weiss HJ, Meyer D, Rabinowitz R, *et al.* Pseudo-von Willebrand's disease. An intrinsic platelet defect with aggregation by unmodified human factor VIII/von Willebrand factor and enhanced adsorption of its high-molecular-weight multimers. *N Engl J Med* 1982; **306**: 326–33.

41 Miller JL, Cunningham D, Lyle VA, Finch CN. Mutation in the gene encoding the alpha chain of platelet glycoprotein Ib in platelet-type von Willebrand disease. *Proc Natl Acad Sci USA* 1991; **88**: 4761–5.

42 Favaloro EJ. Laboratory assessment as a critical component of the appropriate diagnosis and sub-classification of von Willebrand's disease. *Blood Rev* 1999; **13**: 185–204.

43 Michelson AD. The clinical approach to disorders of platelet number and function. In: Michelson AD, ed. *Platelets*. Amsterdam: Academic Press; 2002: 541–5.

44 Wilson DB. Acquired platelet defects. In: Nathan DG, Orkin SH, Ginsburg D, Look AT, eds. *Nathan and Oski's Hematology of Infancy and Childhood*, Vol. 2, 6th edn. Philadelphia: WB Saunders; 2003: 1597–630.

45 Cines DB, Blanchette VS. Immune thrombocytopenic purpura. *N Engl J Med* 2002; **346**: 995–1008.

46 Weiss HJ, Lages B. Family studies in Scott syndrome. *Blood* 1997; **90**: 475–6.

47 Balduini CL, Cattaneo M, Fabris F, *et al.* Inherited thrombocytopenias: a proposed diagnostic algorithm from the Italian Gruppo di Studio delle Piastrine. *Haematologica* 2003; **88**: 582–92.

48 Yardumian DA, Mackie IJ, Machin SJ. Laboratory investigation of platelet function: a review of methodology. *J Clin Pathol* 1986; **39**: 701–12.

49 Witkop CJ, Krumwiede M, Sedano H, White JG. Reliability of absent platelet dense bodies as a diagnostic criterion for Hermansky–Pudlak syndrome. *Am J Hematol* 1987; **26**: 305–11.

50 Israels SJ, McNicol A, Robertson C, Gerrard JM. Platelet storage pool deficiency: diagnosis in patients with prolonged bleeding times and normal platelet aggregation. *Br J Haematol* 1990; **75**: 118–21.

51 Balduini CL, Iolascon A, Savoia A. Inherited thrombocytopenias: from genes to therapy. *Haematologica* 2002; **87**: 860–80.

Care of the child with hemophilia

Rolf Ljung

The goal of treatment of a child with hemophilia should be to ensure that both the family and the affected child perceive themselves as healthy, despite the diagnosis of hemophilia. The World Health Organization (WHO) defines health as a state of complete physical, psychological, and social well-being. The aim of this chapter is to consider various aspects of the medical and psychosocial care of children with hemophilia.

Medical care

Diagnosis

Healthcare professionals are highly aware that hemophilia is a hereditary disorder. However, in many countries today, what is less well recognized is that the majority of babies born with hemophilia actually represent sporadic cases, i.e., the families in question have no known history of hemophilia. This lack of knowledge is a major cause of delay in diagnosis of the disorder, since physicians simply overlook the risk of hemophilia in previously unaffected families.

Once a definite diagnosis has been made based on the results of clotting assays, it is recommended that the mutation in the family be characterized. The information that is now available regarding different types of mutations can help us identify subgroups of hemophilia A and hemophilia B patients that are at high or low risk of developing inhibitors directed against factor VIII (FVIII) or FIX [1–3]. Studies have not yet shown that special treatment regimens should be used for the individuals in these subgroups. However, in as much as there is a risk of inhibitor formation, caution should be observed when considering therapeutic options for patients who are also exposed to other established or suspected risk factors for inhibitor development. Such factors may include frequent and extensive administration of high doses of factor concentrate, or treatment during concomitant inflammatory states. Nevertheless, administration of FVIII/FIX concentrates as treatment for a bleed should not be avoided, even if a patient is at risk of developing inhibitors. A child with hemophilia B due to a complete gene deletion runs a substantial risk of an anaphylactoid reaction to FIX infusions [4]. Such a response usually occurs after one of the first 10–20 infusions, therefore it is suggested that healthcare professionals who administer this type of treatment are also prepared to deal with an allergic reaction.

Treatment

The most important aspect of the care of children with hemophilia is the treatment regimen that is used, which varies considerably between countries owing to differences in the level of healthcare that is generally available [5]. The quality of FVIII or FIX replacement therapy in a country usually evolves from sporadic or on-demand treatment of bleeding episodes, to secondary prophylaxis for those with frequent bleeds, and finally to individually tailored primary prophylaxis for all children with severe or moderate hemophilia [6–8]. According to a joint statement made by the WHO and the World Federation of Hemophilia (WFH), initiating prophylactic treatment at an early age is considered to be the optimal form of therapy for a child with hemophilia [9]. Today, the most refined regimens involve primary prophylaxis, in which treatment is begun at 12–18 months of age, before the onset of bleeding into joints or other serious bleeds. The rationale behind such an early start is that even a small number of joint bleeds can result in irreversible damage, as well as damage that progresses despite prophylactic therapy [10]. It has also been shown that the time point at which prophylaxis is begun is an independent factor in the evaluation of joint outcome [11]. In most cases, an early therapeutic approach is initiated by giving a dose of approximately 50 IU/kg once or twice a week via a peripheral vein, with the aim of increasing the frequency of administration as soon as possible. The ultimate goal is to reach full-scale primary prophylaxis, which usually involves the following: in hemophilia A, FVIII is administered at a dose of 20–40 IU/kg/day every second day or three times weekly; in hemophilia B, FIX is given at a dose of 20–40 IU/kg/day every third day or twice weekly [7,12]. However, both the dose and the dose interval have to be individually tailored for each child owing to pharmacokinetic differences between patients. The level of the lowest concentrations is more important than the peak level after injection [13]. However, it is the clinical outcome, not the achieved trough level, that determines whether the given dose is adequate [14]. In practical use, the sizes of the vials available can also influence the size of the dose administered, especially in young children. From both a medical and a social perspective, it is best if children with hemophilia can be treated at home by their parents, and that particular objective has already been accomplished for most of those patients in countries that have a well-developed system of care for people with hemophilia [15].

Table 21.1 Some items that are recommended to be considered at biannual/annual check-ups of children with hemophilia.

Physical examination, including orthopedic joint score

Feedback on "daily log book" or similar registration of bleeds and treatments

Education of the child and/or parents in venous access

Surveillance of central venous lines (position of catheter, rtPA/urokinase installation in catheter, blood culture, education of the child and/or parents in aseptic techniques)

Laboratory surveillance including blood counts, FVIII/IX levels 24 or 48 h after treatment (when on prophylaxis), FVIII/IX peak values after infusion of prescribed dose, inhibitor analysis

Sociomedical aspects (quality of life, leisure activities, absence from school)

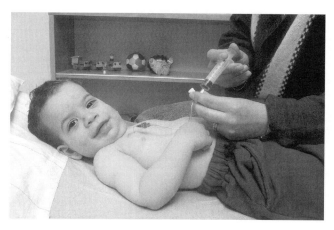

Figure 21.1 An implantable central venous line facilitates injections in children with difficult venous access in peripheral veins.

Monitoring treatment

To ensure a high quality of care, children with severe hemophilia should be examined once or twice a year by a pediatrician at a comprehensive hemophilia care center. The same applies to children with mild hemophilia, although the check-ups can be done less frequently in such cases. The basic items that are recommended to be included in a biannual or annual check-up are listed in Table 21.1. Several different joint evaluation tools are available, for instance orthopedic score, plain X-ray, and MRI (magnetic resonance imaging) scores [16–18].

Venous access

Easy venous access is a prerequisite of administering blood factor concentrates to young children with hemophilia A (FVIII) or hemophilia B (FIX), regardless of whether this is done at the time of a bleed or as a prophylactic measure. For a child receiving on-demand treatment at home, it is preferable that the FVIII/FIX concentrate be given by the parents as soon as a bleed occurs. In such a situation, safe and easy access to a vein is essential, and the same is true for children on a prophylactic regimen. The first choice of access should be a peripheral vein. However, that can be very difficult or even impossible to accomplish in very young children, thus it may be necessary to consider a central venous line (Figure 21.1). Introduction of a central venous catheter entails risks that must be weighed against the potential benefits for individual patients. Medical indications may include poor access to a peripheral vein for a planned therapy, especially the daily injections that are required for immune tolerance induction (ITI) in patients with inhibitors. An example of a combined medical and social indication is when a central venous line would enable parents to treat a young child at home. Implantation of a central venous catheter solely on psychological grounds should be discouraged—a child who is merely afraid of venipuncture needs to be helped in some other way.

Several reports have described various adverse effects associated with the use of central venous catheters in patients with he-

mophilia [19,20], and infections were the most frequently mentioned complications in those subjects. Table 21.2 shows the rates of infections that have been observed in some of the larger studies conducted in recent years. It appears that noninhibitor patients fall into two major categories: those with approximately 0.2 infections per 1000 days, and those with roughly 1.0 (range 0.7–1.7) infections per 1000 days [19–22]. In the best of hands, a patient without inhibitors who has a Port-A-Cath and is on regular prophylaxis will probably have at most one catheter-related infection every 10 years, although this rate varies greatly between different centers. In an equivalent patient who has developed inhibitors, it can be expected that there will be about one infection per 12–24 months of use [19]. Notwithstanding this, easy venous access is imperative for these patients, both for the treatment of acute bleeds and for immune tolerance induction (ITI).

The rates of clinically manifest thrombosis have been low in the large series of patients who have been documented, but it should be noted that routine venography was not performed in most of those series. A few recent reports in the literature have indicated that thrombosis may be a more serious problem than previously assumed [23–26]. Alarmingly, in one of the cited studies [24], venography provided evidence of thrombosis in 8 out of 15 children who had a central venous line (tunneled subclavian catheter). However, none of these eight patients had abnormal venograms or clinical signs of thrombosis until their catheters had been in place for at least 48 months, which suggests that the risk of catheter-related thrombosis increases after many years of use. Development of thrombosis may be related to the site of the catheter (jugular or subclavian vein), the type of concentrate used, or some genetic thrombophilic factors [27].

The final decision to use a central venous catheter must be a compromise between the following: the medical goal, the bleeding tendency and the social situation of the patient, and familiarity with the devices at the particular hemophilia center. The number of complications can be reduced by taking adequate

Table 21.2 The rates of infections in recently studied series of hemophilia patients using central venous lines.

Reference	Number of patients (*n*)	Rate of infections per 1000 patient days	Comments
Blanchette *et al.* [32]	19	0.7	Three patients with inhibitors, three HIV-positive
Perkins *et al.* [33]	35	1.2 (central access) 0.7 (peripheral device)	7/32 patients with inhibitors, 2/32 with VWD
Ljung *et al.* [34]	53	0.19	Eleven patients with inhibitors
Sanagostino *et al.* [35]	15	0.3	Two patients with inhibitors, 13 on prophylaxis
Miller *et al.* [36]	41	0.14	Includes external catheters
McMahon *et al.* [20]	58	1.6 (without inhibitors) 4.3 (with inhibitors)	77/86 had Port-A-Caths; 37/58 patients with hemophilia
Tusell (personal communication, 2002)	20 35	0.28 (prophylaxis) 0.68 (ITI)	Port-A-Caths used for prophylaxis, on-demand treatment, or ITI

measures to maintain asepsis, both at the time of implantation and during subsequent use, and also by adopting explicit basic routines for surveillance of the systems and repeatedly educating the users [28]. In many cases, a central venous line is indispensable for appropriate treatment, and several series on record have clearly demonstrated the benefits of these devices for hemophilic children and their families. Early in treatment, it may be advisable to use a peripheral vein once a week and successively increase the frequency of infusions [29]. If this approach is not successful, and the child has frequent bleeds, it is usually easier for both the parents and the doctor to make the decision to choose a central venous catheter, and also to accept the potential future complications of the device.

Medication

In developed countries, most children with hemophilia are treated with recombinant FVIII/IX concentrates [30,31]. Drugs containing acetylsalicylic acid should not be used to relieve pain, because they inhibit platelet function and therefore have an adverse effect on coagulation. Consequently, preparations containing acetaminophen (paracetamol), alone or in combination with codeine, are recommended as analgesics. Anti-inflammatory drugs such as celecoxib and rofecoxib can in certain cases be useful to reduce joint pain and synovial inflammation. Plasma volume expanders such as dextran should be avoided, and similar preparations also have a negative impact on platelet function and the coagulation proteins von Willebrand factor (VWF) and fibrinogen.

Psychological care

In countries with limited resources for medical care, it is natural to focus on hemophilia itself and literally on how to help patients survive from day to day. In most countries with well-developed healthcare, the ability to treat this disease has improved dramatically during the last decades owing to the in-

troduction of FVIII and FIX concentrates. Therefore, in those nations, the focus should be switched from the disorder per se to the healthy aspects of the child with hemophilia. The connotation of the word 'hemophilia' and the description of the condition have a markedly negative influence on how it is perceived by the parents and later on by the child. This disease has a dramatic history, and the attitudes of healthcare professionals and older people with hemophilia are still affected by the way the disorder used to be managed, even in industrialized countries.

The initial information given to a family with a child who has been diagnosed with hemophilia will have a pronounced impact on how this family, and in time the child himself, will cope with the disease and how it will influence daily life. Ideally, this information should be given to both parents, if possible together with older siblings. If advanced hemophilia care is available, the most important message to convey in the first discussion is that a person with hemophilia can lead a practically normal life and have a normal life expectancy. It is of the essence that children who are old enough to understand the situation do not feel that, by not being healthy, they have caused problems for their parents and made them unhappy. A young child lives in the here and now, whereas the parents have a totally different time perspective and are more extensively influenced by existential thoughts. Parents usually assume that they are to blame for the condition of their child, and it is easier for them to cope if there is a logical explanation for the disease. The mother might be a genetic carrier; thus, it is obvious that she may feel responsible for her child's hemophilia, even though totally irrelevant events in the past are mentioned as potential causes of the disorder.

Consequently, to achieve an optimal outcome of the crisis reaction, it is important to try to discover whether the parents think that they have done something wrong in the past that might have given rise to the disease.

The initial counseling should be repeated at subsequent meetings with the parents to ensure that they have received all relevant information. Positive facts about prophylactic treatment strategies and the prospect of being able to use gene therapy to cure hemophilia should be given together with straightforward information about possible complications, such as the development of inhibitors. Furthermore, it is important that the same doctor and nurse communicate with the family during this sensitive period in order to avoid the uncertainty and frustration that can result from slight differences in the way that individual care providers present the same information.

The child suffering from hemophilia is not the only person who is influenced by the disease; there is also a profound psychosocial effect on all members of the family. Overprotection may become a serious problem, and the strong natural urge to safeguard the child can instead cause difficulties for the entire family. Indeed, in extreme cases, the misguided love of the parents may be more harmful to a son with hemophilia than the disorder itself. Therefore, it is essential that the pediatric hemophilia team work together with the families to support and promote normal behavior.

Social care

Hemophilia identification cards

In conjunction with the diagnosis, a patient with hemophilia should be issued a card that states the type of the disease that the bearer has, and that also provides information about how to contact the hemophilia treatment center. It is important that the patient always carries the card and shows it when consulting a physician or undergoing dental work.

Vaccinations

Children with hemophilia can be vaccinated like any other children, but the vaccines must be given subcutaneously, not intramuscularly. Moreover, in countries where low-purity concentrates or cryoprecipitates are used for treatment, vaccination against hepatitis A and B is recommended.

Daycare center attendance

Attending a daycare center is no problem for a hemophilic child, although it is recommended that the staff of the facility have access to some extra resources. The family has to avoid overprotection, and daycare or other activity groups can provide just the social training and stimulation that the child needs.

School

Other students and the school staff should be informed that a child has hemophilia, preferably by the parents and the child, if necessary together with the staff of the hemophilia center. If adequate prophylaxis is given, no other resources are required for medical reasons, although it is important to coordinate prophylactic treatment with the scheduling of physical education. Also, the study and vocational counselor should be told about any limitations that the disease imposes on the choice of profession for the child.

Leisure activities

A child with hemophilia who is on adequate prophylaxis can enjoy virtually normal free-time activities, but it is best to steer clear of contact sports that involve a high risk of traumatic events. Regardless of the mode of therapy, parents should be encouraged to stimulate the interest of the child in certain suitable sports (such as swimming) at an early age. A hemophilic baby can wear a protective cap or helmet from the time he begins to stand up, until he has learned to walk steadily. However, as the child grows older, a helmet may be a social stigma that should be avoided. Parents and other people who take care of a young hemophilic child should be continually encouraged to observe and reminded to focus on the healthy side of the child.

References

1 Schwaab R, Brackmann HH, Meyer C, et al. Hemophilia A: mutation type determines risk of inhibitor formation. *Thromb Haemost* 1995; **74**: 1402–6.
2 Giannelli F, Choo KH, Rees DJ, et al. Gene deletions in patients with haemophilia B and anti-factor IX antibodies. *Nature* 1983; **303**: 181–2.
3 Ljung RC. Gene mutations and inhibitor formation in patients with hemophilia B. *Acta Haematol* 1995; **94**: 49–52.
4 Warrier I, Ewenstein BM, Koerper MA, et al. Factor IX inhibitors and anaphylaxis in hemophilia B. *J Pediatr Hematol Oncol* 1997; **19**: 23–7.
5 Aledort L. Unsolved problems in haemophilia. *Haemophilia* 1998; **4**: 341–5.
6 Van Den Berg HM, Fischer K. Prophylaxis for severe hemophilia: experience from Europe and the United States. *Semin Thromb Haemost* 2003; **29**: 49–54.
7 Nilsson IM, Berntorp E, Lofqvist T, Pettersson H. Twenty-five years' experience of prophylactic treatment in severe haemophilia A and B [see comments]. *J Intern Med* 1992; **232**: 25–32.
8 Aledort LM, Haschmeyer RH, Pettersson H. A longitudinal study of orthopaedic outcomes for severe factor-VIII-deficient haemophiliacs. The Orthopaedic Outcome Study Group. *J Intern Med* 1994; **236**: 391–9.
9 Berntorp E, Boulyjenkov V, Brettler D, et al. Modern treatment of haemophilia. *Bull World Health Org* 1995; **73**: 691–701.
10 Kreuz W, Escuriola Ettingshausen C, Funk M, Schmidt H, Kornhuber B. When should prophylactic treatment in patients with haemophilia A and B start? The German experience. *Haemophilia* 1998; **4**: 413–17.
11 Astermark J, Petrini P, Tengborn L, et al. Primary prophylaxis in severe hemophilia should be started early but can be individualized. *Br J Haematol* 1999; **105**: 1109–13.
12 Ljung RC. Can haemophilic arthropathy be prevented? *Br J Haematol* 1998; **101**: 215–19.
13 Carlsson M, Berntorp E, Bjorkman S, Lindvall K. Pharmacokinetic dosing in prophylactic treatment of hemophilia A. *Eur J Haematol* 1993; **51**: 247–52.
14 Björkman S. Prophylactic dosing of factor VIII and IX from a clinical pharmacokinetic perspective. *Haemophilia* 2003; **9**: 101–10.
15 Ljung R. Second workshop of the European Paediatric Network for Haemophilia Management, 17–19 September 1998, Vitznau, Switzerland. *Haemophilia* 1999; **5**: 286–91.

16 Pettersson H, Ahlberg A, Nilsson IM. A radiologic classification of hemophilic arthropathy. *Clin Orthop* 1980; **149**: 153–9.

17 Manco-Johnson M, Nuss R, Funk S, Murphy J. Joint evaluation instruments for children and adults. *Haemophilia* 2000; **6**: 649–57.

18 Kilcoyne R, Nuss R. Radiological assessment of haemophilic arthropathy with emphasis on MRI findings. *Haemophilia* 2003; **9**: 57–64.

19 Ljung R, van den Berg M, Petrini P, *et al.* Port-A-Cath usage in children with haemophilia: experience of 53 cases. *Acta Paediatr* 1998; **87**: 1051–4.

20 McMahon C, Smith J, Khair K, *et al.* Central venous access devices in children with congenital coagulation disorders; complications and long-term outcome. *Br J Haematol* 2000; **110**: 461–8.

21 Blanchette VS, Al Musa A, Stain AM, *et al.* Central venous access devices in children with hemophilia: an update. *Blood Coagul Fibrinolysis* 1997; **8** (Suppl. 1): S11–14.

22 Yee T, Beeton K, Griffioen A, *et al.* Experiences of prophylaxis treatment in children with severe haemophilia. *Haemophilia* 2002; **8**: 76–82.

23 Blanchette VS, Al Trabolsi H, Stain AM, *et al.* High risk of central venous line-associated thrombosis in boys with haemophilia (abstract). *Blood* 1999; **94**: 234a.

24 Journeycahe JM, Quinn CT, Miller KL, *et al.* Catheter related deep venous thrombosis in children with haemophilia. *Blood* 2001; **98**: 1717–31.

25 Vidler V, Richards M, Vora A. Central venous catheter-associated thrombosis in severe haemophilia. *Br J Haematol* 1999; **104**: 461–4.

26 Koerper MA, Esker S, Cobb L. Asymptomatic thrombosis of innominate vein in haemophilic children with subcutaneous venous access devices (ports) (Abstract). *National Haemophilia Foundation 48th Annual Meeting.* San Diego, CA, 1996.

27 Ettingshausen C, Kurnik K, Schobess R, *et al.* Catheter related thrombosis in children with haemophilia A. Evidence of a multifactorial disease. *Blood* 2002; **99**: 449–500.

28 Ljung R. Central venous lines in haemophilia. *Haemophilia* 2003; **9** (Suppl. 1): 88–93.

29 Petrini P. How to start prophylaxis. *Haemophilia* 2003; **9** (Suppl. 1): 83–7.

30 Ljung R, Aronis-Vournas S, Kurnik-Auberger K, *et al.* Treatment of children with haemophilia in Europe: a survey of 20 centres in 16 countries. *Haemophilia* 2000; **6**: 619–24.

31 Lusher JM, Arkin S, Abildgaard CF, Schwartz RS. Recombinant factor VIII for the treatment of previously untreated patients with hemophilia A. Safety, efficacy, and development of inhibitors. Kogenate Previously Untreated Patient Study Group. *N Engl J Med* 1993; **328**: 453–9.

32 Blanchette VS, al Musa A, Stain AM, *et al.* Central venous access catheters in children with haemophilia. *Blood Coagul Fibrinolysis* 1996; **7** (Suppl. 1): S39–44.

33 Perkins JL, Johnson VA, Osip JM, *et al.* The use of implantable venous access devices (IVADs) in children with hemophilia. *J Pediatr Hematol Oncol* 1997; **194**: 339–44.

34 Ljung R, Petrini P, Lindgren AK, Berntorp E. Implantable central venous catheter facilitates prophylactic treatment in children with haemophilia. *Acta Paediatr* 1992; **81**: 918–20.

35 Santagostino E, Gringeri A, Muca Perja M, Mannucci PM. A prospective clinical trial of implantable central venous access in children with haemophilia. *Br J Haematol* 1998; **102**: 1224–8.

36 Miller K, Buchanan GR, Zappa S, *et al.* Implantable venous access devices in children with hemophilia: a report of low infection rates [see comments]. *J Pediatr* 1998; **132**: 934–8.

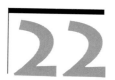

22 The neonate with hemophilia

Angela Thomas and Elizabeth Chalmers

Introduction

The neonatal period spans the first 28 days of life of a liveborn infant of any gestation. Although acquired disorders of coagulation are more frequent during this period, severe forms of congenital factor deficiencies, such as hemophilia A and B, often present in the early neonatal period and are a particular challenge from both the diagnostic and management point of view. There should be a high index of suspicion of such disorders in an otherwise healthy infant who presents with unusual bleeding. The proportion of children with hemophilia who are diagnosed in the neonatal period has improved significantly over the past 40 years. Baehner and Strauss [1] reported in 1966 that fewer than 10% of severe hemophiliacs were identified in the newborn period despite unusual bleeding in 22%. Subsequent studies have shown that between 52% and 68% of babies with severe hemophilia are diagnosed as neonates [2–4]. However, even among those with a positive family history, up to 59% are diagnosed only at the time of the first bleed [4], and the diagnosis is delayed despite unusual bleeding in up to 87.5% [1,4,5]. The normal baby is adapted for the trauma of birth. Levels of coagulation proteins, their inhibitors, and fibrinolytic proteins are age specific and at birth are physiologically balanced to help protect against the risk of bleeding with such trauma. However, in a baby with hemophilia, the balance is altered and the risk of bleeding during birth is significantly increased. Birth is one of the most critical times for intracerebral bleeding in patients with hemophilia [6] and can be the first presenting sign of the disease. In around 50% of individuals with hemophilia, there is no family history at birth and therefore preventive measures cannot be instituted. However, if the fetus is known to have or be at risk of having hemophilia, it is important to take proactive steps to reduce birth trauma. This is usually advised for male infants, but care should also be taken with female infants of known carriers as their factor levels may be significantly reduced and predispose to bleeding in certain circumstances.

Family history and genetics of hemophilia

Hemophilia A and B are inherited as X-linked recessive bleeding disorders. A number of cohort studies have examined the initial presentation of these conditions and have found that in 42–57% of cases there is no apparent prior family history of hemophilia [1–4,7]. It is estimated from molecular studies that at least 30% of newly diagnosed cases of hemophilia occur as a consequence of a new mutation, affecting either the male propositus or a female carrier in whom there may be no personal history of bleeding problems [8]. It is also evident from published studies that even where there is a positive family history of hemophilia, the history is not always recognized and a proportion of such cases are diagnosed only after they present with clinically overt bleeding symptoms [3].

Hemostatic challenges in the neonatal period

Precipitating factors for bleeding specific to the neonatal period are mostly associated with birth trauma [6,9]. One study showed that in nearly 600 000 unselected infants of nulliparous mothers, the rate of intracranial hemorrhage (ICH) was higher among infants delivered by vacuum extraction, forceps, or cesarean section during labor than infants delivered spontaneously or by elective cesarean section [10]. This suggests that the common risk factor for hemorrhage is abnormal labor. Although no information was given regarding outcome or coagulation status of these infants, it would seem reasonable to extrapolate these results and assume that these types of birth are more risky for babies with hemophilia. This has been supported by several studies [6,9] in which instrumentation, particularly vacuum extraction, has been associated with an increase in both ICH and extracranial hemorrhage (ECH) (Figures 22.1 and 22.2).

The majority of bleeds occur within the first week of birth [6] and include excessive oozing from puncture sites, including heelpricks, extracranial hemorrhage such as subgaleal bleeds and cephalhematomas, and intracranial bleeding. Bleeding from the umbilical stump is rare but unusual bruising can be seen with minimal trauma (see Plate 2, facing p. 212) and large hematomas secondary to intramuscular vitamin K can occur.

A recent review of neonatal bleeding in babies with hemophilia noted that the commonest site of bleeding is the cranium, with ICH accounting for 27% of all bleeds and ECH 13% [11]. However, in one Swedish series, 75% of all cranial hemorrhages were extracranial, and it is possible that ECH is under-reported [4]. Iatrogenic bleeding included bleeding from puncture sites (vascular, capillary, and intramuscular) in 16% of infants and from circumcision in 30% [11]. This latter figure will be considerably lower in countries where early circumcision is not cus-

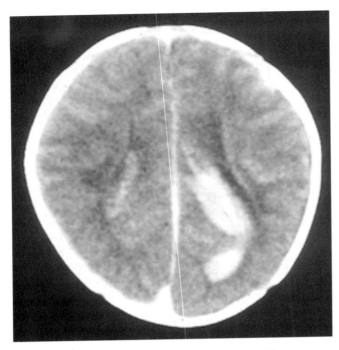

Figure 22.1 Intraventricular hemorrhage in a neonate with hemophilia.

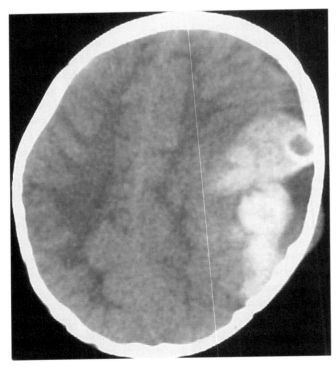

Figure 22.2 Subdural hemorrhage in a neonate with hemophilia.

tomary. Umbilical stump bleeding was rare (6%), as were gastrointestinal/mouth bleeds, parenchymal bleeds, joint bleeds, or ecchymoses (<5%).

The incidence of ICH in neonates with hemophilia is reported as being 1–4% [11] and is usually related to birth trauma, regardless of the mode of delivery. The consequences can be devastating, with death or subsequent neurologic deficit as the outcome [5,6,12,13]. ECH also occurs either alone or in conjunction with an ICH and can be life-threatening owing to hypovolemic shock. A 22.8% mortality rate with subgaleal hemorrhages in all newborns has been reported [14]. Although the majority of bleeds occur and are identified before 1 week of age, many infants are now discharged from hospital early, some even within 24 h. Signs and symptoms of ICH can be nonspecific and include symptoms such as lethargy, poor feeding, and irritability. In those in whom the diagnosis of hemophilia is unsuspected, general advice only will have been given and the diagnosis of ICH may be delayed.

Raising the awareness of the need for full investigation of neonates with unexpected or unusual bleeding, including liaison with a hematologist experienced in this area, is the key to early identification of unsuspected hemophilia. Life-threatening bleeds can be treated appropriately and early diagnosis will help to prevent further bleeding or delay in treatment in the future. Neonatologists rarely come across babies with hemophilia and therefore are unfamiliar with their presentation in this period. Bleeding in the neonatal period, even in hemophilia, is rare and therefore most undiagnosed babies with hemophilia do not present at this time. Many hematologists who predominantly care for adults are also unaware of problems in the neonate or have not been involved in their care.

Investigation and management of a neonate with a positive family history of hemophilia

Perinatal management

The safe outcome for the neonate at risk of hemophilia is highly dependent on appropriate management during the perinatal period. Good communication between the involved obstetrician, hematologist, and pediatrician is crucial, particularly if the delivery is to take place at a site distant from a hemophilia center. Although the uptake of prenatal diagnosis in hemophilia is low, fetal sexing by ultrasound scanning will usually have been undertaken during the second trimester of pregnancy to determine if the fetus is male.

Delivery

The optimal mode of delivery for an at-risk male fetus has been the subject of significant controversy but current practice in most centers is to consider vaginal delivery as the initial approach, unless there are specific obstetric contraindications. In order to avoid additional head trauma, it is recommended that instrumental interventions, including forceps, vacuum extraction, and the use of scalp electrodes, are avoided and early recourse to cesarean delivery is advised where labor fails to progress. Although vacuum extraction should be avoided, where the head is deeply engaged in the pelvis, 'lift-out' forceps may be less traumatic than cesarean section, provided the operator is experienced in the procedure [15]. These recommendations are based on findings from a small number of individual studies in which cranial bleeding in the early neonatal period appeared to be strongly associated with trauma at the time of delivery, particularly the use of vacuum extraction [6,9]. Nevertheless, it should be noted that in a review of 102 published cases of neonatal cranial bleeding, 19/47 (40%) followed apparently spontaneous vaginal delivery and such bleeds have also been recorded following cesarean section for obstetric reasons [11,16].

Diagnostic investigations

Following delivery, cord blood should be obtained for coagulation screening and factor VIII (FVIII) or factor IX (FIX) assays. Testing cord blood avoids potential trauma to the neonate, but care is required to avoid contamination with maternal blood or activation of the sample prior to testing. In the event that cord blood is not obtained, a venous sample should be obtained from the neonate.

The hemostatic system in the neonate differs significantly from that observed in older children and adults and is often described as being physiologically immature at birth. This affects the levels of many procoagulant proteins and results in prolongation of baseline coagulation parameters, including the activated partial thromboplastin time (aPTT) [17]. It is therefore important that all coagulation investigations are interpreted using reference ranges that take into account both the gestational and postnatal age of the infant. Such reference ranges are also machine and reagent specific and, while larger laboratories may derive their own local reference ranges, smaller centers may be dependent on previously published ranges which may not reflect current technology and must therefore be interpreted with care.

Hemophilia A and B classically result in an isolated prolongation of the aPTT and the diagnosis is confirmed by measurement of FVIII and FIX levels respectively. In the neonate, FVIII levels are within the normal adult range in both term and preterm infants, whereas FIX levels are reduced to around 50% of adult values at term and are further reduced in preterm neonates [17,18]. It is therefore possible to confirm a diagnosis of hemophilia A in a neonate regardless of the gestational age or the severity of the condition. If the levels of FVIII are borderline, measurement should be repeated at 6 months or older as mild hemophilia A may initially give normal values. It is also usually possible to diagnose severe and moderate hemophilia B, but confirmation of mild hemophilia B is complicated by overlap with normal values, necessitating repeat testing at around 6 months of age, or molecular analysis if the genetic defect is known.

Vitamin K

Intramuscular vitamin K remains the preferred regimen for the prevention of vitamin K deficiency bleeding in many countries. The administration of vitamin K by this route should be delayed until diagnostic tests for hemophilia are completed. If hemophilia is confirmed or there is likely to be a delay in obtaining results, vitamin K should be administered according to an oral regimen. Heel-stab sampling for other neonatal screening procedures carries the risk of iatrogenic bleeding and should be performed with care.

Routine cranial scanning

One of the most devastating bleeds in the neonate with hemophilia is ICH. Early diagnosis will allow prompt treatment with the aim of stopping the bleed and therefore limiting the damage and long-term sequelae. Such bleeds can be diagnosed by cranial ultrasound, which is a noninvasive procedure that can be done at the cot-side. Although the majority of bleeds can be diagnosed by this method, subdural hematomas can be missed, as can posterior fossa hemorrhages. A normal scan therefore will not exclude all bleeds. It has been shown that in up to 10% of neonates without hemophilia, ICH can occur during birth and that, of those, only 0.4% develop symptoms in the first year of life [19]. It is not known, however, whether these children had an underlying coagulation or anatomical defect. Routine scanning may therefore pick up bleeds of uncertain significance and may miss some significant bleeds. It would seem appropriate to treat an ICH identified on routine scanning in a hemophilic neonate since the consequences can be serious or fatal, but whether all hemophilic neonates should have routine cranial ultrasound is not known. A survey of hemophilia centers in the UK regarding management of neonatal hemophilia showed that only 41% of those responding would routinely perform cranial ultrasonography on babies with severe hemophilia; 21% would perform a cranial ultrasound only in the presence of clinical signs suggestive of bleeding [20]. If symptoms compatible with a bleed develop after a negative ultrasound scan, a follow-up CT (computed tomography) or MRI (magnetic resonance imaging) scan should be performed.

Counseling

Once a diagnosis of hemophilia has been made, it is important that the families of affected infants are referred promptly to their local hemophilia treatment center. Neonatal bleeding problems not infrequently present following discharge from hospital, and it is therefore important that prior to discharge parents are adequately counseled regarding the diagnosis and are informed about potential problems, including those which could relate to major bleeding, particularly ICH.

Female carriers

Female infants who are potential carriers of hemophilia appear to be at low risk of bleeding during the neonatal period. Occasional patients will, however, have particularly low factor levels due to extreme lyonization, and any abnormal bleeding should be appropriately investigated.

Investigation of abnormal bleeding in the absence of a positive family history

The hemorrhagic neonate

The majority of hemorrhagic problems observed during the neonatal period are due to acquired hemostatic disorders. Thrombocytopenia and acquired coagulopathies due to disseminated intravascular coagulation (DIC), liver disease, and vitamin K deficiency are commonly observed in the context of underlying illness and in sick preterm neonates. This is in contrast to the typical presentation of an inherited coagulation disorder, which is more likely to be seen in a term infant with isolated bleeding problems.

Recognition of abnormal bleeding is crucial, particularly as signs are often subtle or nonspecific, and it is vital that in the presence of unexplained bleeding appropriate investigations are initiated to exclude hemophilia and other inherited bleeding disorders. It is also important that coagulation investigations include specific factor assays and not just baseline coagulation screening tests, which can be misleading owing to the physiologic prolongation of these parameters during the neonatal period. In the presence of major hemorrhage, DIC may coexist with an underlying inherited defect, which may further complicate the results obtained.

Problems with diagnosis

Unfortunately, the published literature highlights ongoing problems with delayed recognition and inadequate investigation of abnormal bleeding in this age group. In 1988, Yoffe reported that a diagnosis of hemophilia was delayed, in some cases for several months, in six of eight infants presenting with intracranial hemorrhage [5]. More recently in 2001, Myles reported two infants presenting with intracranial hemorrhage in whom neurosurgery was undertaken before a definitive diagnosis was reached [21].

Failure to initiate appropriate investigations has also been highlighted in a survey from the USA published in 1999, in which neonatologists and hematologists were questioned regarding how they would investigate neonates presenting with ICH. Among neonatologists, only 23% reported that they would specifically request FVIII and FIX assays in a term neonate presenting with ICH, and the figure dropped to 3% in preterm infants. The figures were higher when the same questions were asked of hematologists—64% and 39% respectively—but in many centers hematologists may not be actively involved in initiating these investigations. In the light of this it is now advised by the Medical and Scientific Advisory Council (MASAC) of the National Hemophilia Foundation in the USA that all neonates with intracranial hemorrhage should be specifically investigated for the presence of an underlying bleeding disorder.

Treatment of hemophilia during the neonatal period

Choice of product

In the presence of acute bleeding or where prophylactic management is deemed necessary, treatment should be initiated with an appropriate factor concentrate. This applies regardless of severity, as desmopressin (DDAVP) is contraindicated during the neonatal period due to the risk of hyponatremia [22]. The choice of product should be governed by issues of safety and availability. In the developed world, recombinant FVIII and FIX concentrates are now widely available and neonates should have the highest priority to receive these products. This is based on the likelihood that recombinant technology will be associated with the lowest risk of transmitting viral infections [23]. In those parts of the world where recombinant products are not available, high-purity, virucidally inactivated, plasma-derived products remain the preferred treatment. Where prothrombin complex concentrates (PCCs) are used for the treatment of hemophilia B, it should be noted that an increased risk of DIC has been reported in neonates treated with these products.

As FVIII and FIX concentrates, particularly recombinant products, are not widely available outside hemophilia treatment centers, it is important that arrangements are made to secure a supply of an appropriate product prior to the delivery of a potentially affected neonate. Although fresh-frozen plasma (FFP) is not recommended for the treatment of neonatal hemophilia, it may have a role in the presence of major hemorrhage where hemophilia is suspected but confirmatory investigations are not yet available or where other products are unavailable.

Dosing regimens

Dosing regimens for neonates are largely based on those used for older children and adults, as there is little published information available regarding the pharmacokinetics of replacement therapy in this age group [24]. In view of this, careful monitoring of factor levels is likely to be particularly important. In a single case report describing replacement therapy in a preterm neonate with hemophilia A, FVIII recovery was similar to that seen in older children whereas the half-life was at the lower end of the expected range [25].

Prophylactic treatment

Given that the incidence of ICH in neonates with severe or moderate hemophilia is 1–4% and the outcome of such bleeds can be fatal or severely disabling, some have advocated prophylactic factor replacement for all known hemophilic neonates and for those in whom the diagnosis is highly likely [26,27]. Prophylactic use of factor concentrate is well established in the older hemophiliac both for preventing spontaneous bleeds, particularly joint bleeds, and after injury before bleeding has taken place, especially when that injury could result in ICH. In the neonate, the head and brain have been subjected to significant stress but unlike traumatic head injuries the stress is physiologic. Nevertheless, ICH occurs and the risk is increased in deliveries requiring instrumentation or cesarean section during labor [6,9]. However, there is some evidence that early treatment increases the likelihood of inhibitor formation, with 34–41% developing inhibitors when treated at <6 months of age, compared with 0% when treated at >18 months of age [28,29]. Until the reasons for inhibitor development have been further elucidated, universal prophylactic treatment of neonates with hemophilia cannot be recommended. However, in those with a traumatic delivery, immediate treatment should be considered, and in addition a high index of suspicion of ICH should be maintained. In a UK survey of hemophilia centers, only 19% of responders said they would consider prophylaxis in all severe cases but up to 62% following instrumental delivery [20]. In a survey in the USA, 89% of pediatric hematologists favored early prophylaxis with factor concentrates [30].

Hepatitis B vaccination

Even where infants are receiving recombinant products, routine vaccination against hepatitis B continues to be recommended at the present time [23].

Conclusion

Hemophilia A and B are rare disorders but can present in the neonatal period with catastrophic bleeding. If the diagnosis is missed, not only is appropriate treatment not instituted at the time, but further bleeds may occur, with attendant morbidity or even mortality, before the diagnosis is eventually made. Although there has been a significant improvement in making an early diagnosis, cases are still missed despite a positive family history or unusual bleeding in a well neonate. It is important to encourage liaison between obstetricians, neonatologists, and hematologists in the management of the known hemophilia carrier and between hematologists and neonatologists when abnormal bleeding in a neonate occurs. The importance of family history can be emphasized during genetic counseling of the mother so that appropriate information is given and help sought. Medical staff in attendance also need to be aware of the importance of a family history of bleeding. Written protocols for the management of the hemophilia carrier should be available in institutions where such mothers are delivered, and protocols for the investigation of a bleeding neonate available in all neonatal units. Prospective studies collecting data on neonatal bleeding episodes, the contribution of routine cranial imaging, and analysis of early exposure to FVIII concentrate and inhibitor development may help determine best management in the future.

References

1 Baehner RL, Strauss H. Hemophilia in the first year of life. *N Engl J Med* 1966; **275**: 524–8.
2 Chambost H, Gaboulaud V, Coatmelec B, et al. What factors influence the age at diagnosis of hemophilia? Results of a French cohort study. *J Paediatr* 2002; **141**: 548–52.
3 Conway JH, Hilgartner MW. Initial presentation of paediatric hemophiliacs. *Arch Pediatr Adolesc Med* 1994; **148**: 589–94.
4 Ljung R, Petrini P, Nilsson IM. Diagnostic symptoms of severe and moderate haemophilia A and B. *Acta Paediatr Scand* 1990; **79**: 196–200.
5 Yoffe G, Buchanan GR. Intracranial hemorrhage in newborn and young infants with hemophilia. *J Paediatr* 1988; **113**: 333–6.
6 Klinge J, Auberger K, Auerswald G, et al. Prevalence and outcome of intracranial haemorrhage in haemophiliacs—a survey of the paediatric group of the German Society of Thrombosis and Haemostasis (GTH). *Eur J Pediatr* 1999; **158**: S162–5
7 Pollmann H, Richter H, Ringkamp H, Jurgens H. When are children diagnosed as having severe haemaphilia and when do they start to bleed? A 10-year single centre PUP study. *Eur J Pediatr* 1999; **158**: S166–70.
8 Giannelli F, Green PM. The molecular basis of haemophilia A and B. *Baillière's Haematol* 1996; **9**: 211–28.
9 Ljung R, Lindgren A-C, Petrini P, Tengborn L. Normal vaginal delivery is to be recommended for haemophilia carrier gravidae. *Acta Paediatr* 1994; **83**: 609–11.
10 Towner D, Castro MA, Eby-Wilkens E, Gilbert WM. Effect of mode of delivery in nulliparous women on neonatal intracranial injury. *New Engl J Med* 1999; **341**: 1709–14.
11 Kulkarni R, Lusher JM. Intracranial and extracranial hemorrhages in newborns with hemophilia. *J Pediatr Hematol Oncol*; 1999; **21**: 289–95.
12 Khair K, Baxter B, Fields P, et al. Intracranial haemorrhage in a tertiary pediatric centre: a survey of 100 children with severe haemophilia. *Haemophilia* 2002; **8**: 522–6.
13 Kletzel M, Miller CH, Becton D, et al. Postdelivery head bleeding in hemophilic neonates. *Arch J Dis Child* 1989; **143**: 1107–10.
14 Plauche WC. Subgaleal haematoma. A complication of instrumental delivery. *JAMA* 1980; **244**: 597–8.
15 Kadir RA, Economides DL. Obstetric management of carriers of haemophilia. *Haemophilia* 1997; **3**: 81–6.
16 Michaud JL, Rivard GE, Chessex P. Intracranial hemorrhage in a newborn with hemophilia following elective caesarean section. *Am J Pediat Hematol Oncol* 1991; **13**: 473–5.
17 Andrew M, Paes B, Milner R, et al. Development of the coagulation system in the full-term infant. *Blood* 1987; **70**: 165–72.
18 Andrew M, Paes B, Milner R, et al. Development of the human coagulation system in the healthy premature infant. *Blood* 1988; **80**: 1998–2005.
19 Heibel M, Heber R, Bechinger D, Kornhuber HH. The early diagnosis of perinatal cerebral lesions in apparently normal full term newborns by ultrasound of the brain. *Neuroradiology* 1993; **35**: 85–91.
20 Chalmers EA. On behalf of the UKHCDO Paediatric Working Party.

Management of neonates with inherited coagulation disorders. A survey of current practice. *Haemophilia* 2002; **8**: 488.

21 Myles LM, Massicotte P, Drake J. Intracranial hemorrhage in neonates with unrecognized hemophilia A: A persisting problem. *Pediatr Neurosurg* 2001; **34**: 94–7.

22 Williams MD, Chalmers EA, Gibson BES. Guideline: The Investigation and Management of Neonatal Haemostasis and Thrombosis. *Br J Haematol* 2002; **119**: 295–309.

23 UKHCDO. Guideline for the selection and use of therapeutic products to treat haemophilia and other hereditary bleeding disorders. *Haemophilia* 2003; **9**: 1–23.

24 Rickard KA. Guidelines for therapy and optimal doses of coagulation factors for treatment of bleeding and surgery in haemophilia. *Haemophilia* 1995; **1** (Suppl. 1): 8–13.

25 Gale RF, Hird MF, Colvin BT. Management of a premature infant with moderate haemophilia A using recombinant factor VIII. *Haemophilia* 1998; **4**: 850–3.

26 Berry E. Intracranial haemorrhage in the haemophiliac neonate —

the case for prophylaxis. URL http://www.haemophilia-forum.org/lock/Discussion/990426.htm.

27 Buchanan GR. Factor concentrate prophylaxis for neonates with haemophilia. *J Pediatr Hematol Oncol* 1999; **21**: 254–9.

28 Lorenzo JI, López A, Altisent C, Aznar JA. Incidence of factor VIII inhibitors in severe haemophilia: the importance of patient age. *Br J Haematol* 2001; **113**: 600–3.

29 Van der Bom JG, Mauser-Bunschoten EP, Fischer K, van den Berg HM. Age at first treatment and immune tolerance to factor VIII in severe haemophilia. *Thromb Haemost* 2003; **89**: 475–9

30 Kulkarni R, Lusher JM, Henry RC, Kallens DJ. Current practices regarding new-born intracranial haemorrhage and obstetrical care and mode of delivery of pregnant haemophilia carriers: a survey of obstetricians, neonatologists and haematologists in the United States, on behalf of the National Hemophilia Foundation's Medical and Scientific Advisory Council. *Haemophilia* 1999; **5**: 410–15.

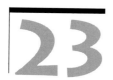

Products used to treat hemophilia: evolution of treatment for hemophilia A and B

Inge Scharrer and Thomas Becker

Blood transfusions were first used in 1840 for successful management of postoperative bleeding complications. Transfusion did not subsequently achieve widespread acceptance as a therapeutic modality because of a high rate of fatal reactions caused by blood group incompatibility following transfusion of donor blood. Approximately 50% of blood transfusions performed between 1850 and 1900 were reportedly fatal to the recipient.

In 1900, Karl Landsteiner discovered the first three human blood groups, A, B, and C (later called O), allowing physicians to rule out incompatibility reactions by first conducting compatibility tests [1].

In 1908, Ottenberg used for the first time a blood test for compatibility before performing a human blood transfusion. He is the first to note that human blood groups are inherited according to Mendel's law. He also showed that group O blood can be given to group A and B patients, establishing the concept of the "universal donor."

Handling blood and plasma was made much easier in 1914 by the discovery that sodium citrate inhibits coagulation. In 1915, Richard Lewisohn described the minimum amount of citrate required to prevent blood from clotting, making indirect transfusion possible and practical and allowing blood to be stored for later transfusion [2]. This discovery subsequently made it possible to set up blood bank systems.

In 1923 and 1929 Feissly showed that plasma is superior to whole blood for treating hemophilia, but plasma and blood remained in short supply until the blood bank system was set up during World War II [3].

Bernard Fantus, director of therapeutics at the Cook County Hospital in Chicago, set up the first hospital blood bank in the USA in 1937. His pioneering act was followed by the establishment of hospital and community blood banks across the USA over the next few years. The main driving force for this was the "Plasma for Britain" program launched by the US government in 1940, a nationwide program for the collection of blood. The program also resulted in enough plasma to conduct major surgery in hemophilia patients for the first time [4]. The widespread use of blood and plasma transfusions also resulted in the transmission of hepatitis viruses. Beeson's classic description of transfusion-transmitted hepatitis was published in 1943.

The main drawback of plasma substitution therapy for hemophilia A was the low quantity of factor VIII (FVIII) that was capable of being administered by this route. Precipitation of a globulin from platelet-free plasma with water at a low pH was the first major step toward developing substitution therapy. The globulin combated the bleeding tendency in hemophilic subjects more effectively than plasma (globulin was the term used at the time to describe a water-insoluble protein). This globulin was called antihemophilic globulin. Two years later, Brinkhous [5] demonstrated that hemophilia patients were deficient in this globulin, which he dubbed antihemophilic factor.

Much higher concentrations of this protein were found in fraction I of the alcohol-mediated plasma fractionation done by Cohn *et al.* [6] in 1940, with the primary aim of obtaining albumin as a plasma expander.

The efficacy of this fraction (which mainly contained fibrinogen in addition to FVIII) in hemophiliacs was limited owing to the instability of its antihemophilic activity. This prompted Blombäck *et al.* [7] to extract subfraction I-0 with stable FVIII for the treatment of hemophilia. Nilsson [8] was the first to administer this subfraction to children for preventive management of severe hemophilia, in 1958.

Until 1947, hemophilia was believed to be a single entity. Pavlowsky's [9] successful treatment of one hemophiliac subject with the blood of another hemophiliac was the first indication that hemophilia embraced two different clinical entities. This was confirmed in 1952 on the basis of further clinical studies by Biggs [10], who introduced the term Christmas disease. Development of the thromboplastin generation test and the partial thromboplastin time test also provided the diagnostic means of differentiating between the two types of hemophilia. Cramer *et al.* [11] coined the terms hemophilia A and B. Prothrombin complex products to treat hemophilia B became available in 1958. Prothrombin complex factors (II, VII, IX, X) were either precipitated together by Cohn fractionation using a specific alcohol concentration or isolated by calcium phosphate adsorption of plasma and remained the gold standard for treating hemophilia B until the early 1990s as factor IX (FIX) complex concentrate [12]

Despite continuing progress in purifying Cohn fraction I, the FVIII concentrate thus produced remained in short supply during the 1950s and early 1960s owing to a lack of plasma [7]. A solution was attempted by extracting FVIII from bovine and porcine plasma and using it for therapeutic purposes. Scientists nevertheless succeeded in the biochemical characterization of FVIII and determined its basic kinetic properties. It was also determined that plasma FVIII activity correlated with clinical response. Treatment protocols were developed on the basis of these insights.

However, the side-effects of treatment with blood and plasma products also became evident. The risk of transmitting hepatitis became apparent as early as the 1940s [13]. Anticoagulant (inhibitor) formation in a hemophilic subject was first reported in 1941 [14]. In 1947 Craddock and Lawrence [15] hypothesized that this anticoagulant was an antibody produced by the hemophilic subject against the exogenous antihemophilic factor. The anticoagulant was assayed semiquantitatively by mixing different proportions of hemophilic plasma and healthy plasma and identified by electrophoresis as belonging to the gammaglobulin fraction of plasma. The Oxford method for quantitative assay was introduced in 1959 [16], and it was shown that the FVIII antibody is primarily composed of immunoglobulin 4 (IgG4). Until the end of the 1960s, it was difficult if not impossible to treat bleeds in hemophilia patients with inhibitors. The two main treatment options were to override the inhibitor by administering elevated FVIII doses or to give the patient porcine FVIII [16]. Most inhibitor patients (approximately 85%) were not cross-reactive to porcine FVIII, but many were allergic or developed thrombocytopenia [17]. These serious side-effects were attributable to the insufficient purity of the porcine FVIII products available at the time. This problem was solved in 1981 with the launch of the first high-purity porcine FVIII concentrate (Hyate C, Speywood Laboratories, Wrexham, UK [18]).

Another side-effect of treatment with blood and plasma products was declining hematocrit, attributable to hemolysis caused by the antierythrocyte antibody present in the products. Furthermore, allergic reactions occurred in up to 80% of those patients treated.

Until the early 1960s, scientists believed in the impossibility of commercial availability of FVIII concentrates. Two events in 1964 helped to achieve the breakthrough making modern substitution therapy feasible. Plasmapheresis became established in the USA to harvest plasma for fractionation. Pool *et al.* [19] discovered that slowly thawed frozen plasma contained a precipitate rich in FVIII. This cryoprecipitate, as it was called, was easily produced by any blood bank or plasmapheresis workstation and could be carried out before Cohn plasma fractionation without any loss of other plasma components. In the years to come, all plasma fraction suppliers launched commercial FVIII concentrates with a specific activity of approximately 1 U FVIII per mg of protein (Table 23.1). By 1972, the USA had enough FVIII to treat all cases of acute bleeding in hemophilia patients.

Sufficient availability and the possibility of storing freeze-dried concentrates in a refrigerator for long periods facilitated the introduction of home treatment in the early 1970s and widespread prophylaxis [20]. The first measure to reduce the risk of hepatitis B infection dates back to 1971 and was the introduction of hepatitis B surface antigen (HBsAg) testing of donated blood and plasma [21].

New products for treating hemophilia were launched in the early 1970s. An activated prothrombin concentrate (APCC, Hyland, Travenol Laboratories) for treating bleeds in inhibitor patients was developed. An aPCC is a multicomponent system composed of nonactivated and activated prothrombin complex factors. aPCCs have now been an integral part of inhibitor ther-

Table 23.1 Specific FVIII activity of plasma fractions and concentrates.

Product	Year	Specific activity (U/mg)
Plasma	1940	0.001
pH precipitation	1962	0.05
Cryoprecipitate	1965	0.1
Factor VIII concentrate	1965	0.2
Intermediate-purity factor VIII concentrate (cryoprecipitate + further purification)	1970–80	1.5–50
High-purity FVIII concentrate (cryoprecipitate + chromatographic separation)	1980–2000	50–200
Monoclonal	1987	2500
Recombinant	1992	4000

apy for more than 30 years. The main representative of this class, FEIBA (factor eight inhibitor bypassing activity, Baxter), has reported response rates of 88–96% [22]. In 1999, factors II and Xa were identified as the key compounds responsible for FEIBA's effects.

In 1974, Cash *et al.* [23] showed that the synthetic vasopressin analog desmopressin acetate (DDAVP) raises plasma FVIII and von Willebrand factor (VWF) activity three- to sixfold and is therefore a suitable alternative to FVIII concentrates for treating mild hemophilia and mild von Willebrand syndrome.

Modern plasma-derived factor VIII and IX concentrates

To eliminate viruses present in products despite hepatitis B screening, attempts to develop suitable virus inactivation methods were initiated in the late 1970s. One reason for these efforts was that the hepatitis B screening had pointed to the existence of unknown hepatitis-causing organisms, which were dubbed non-A/non-B hepatitis viruses (NANB).

Applied to clotting factor concentrates, the pasteurization process developed for albumin in 1948 (heating for 10 h at 60°C in an aqueous solution) resulted in heavy losses as the method significantly reduced the FVIII content.

Nevertheless, a pasteurized FVIII product entered clinical tests in 1979 and was launched in 1981 in which FVIII was heated for 10 h at 60°C in an aqueous solution containing glucose as stabilizer, a process that destroyed hepatitis B virus (HBV) [24].

The development of alternative virus inactivation methods was enormously accelerated by the advent of HIV (human immunodeficiency virus) and the HIV catastrophe among hemophilia patients in the period from 1980 to 1984. By 1987, all registered FVIII and FIX complex concentrates were subjected to at least one virus inactivation or virus reduction method during manufacture, for safe elimination of HIV, hepatitis C virus (HCV), and HBV. These methods include thermal inactivation

Table 23.2 Virus transmission via blood products since 1985 [26].

Product	Inactivation	Transmission of	Number of transmissions	Year
PPSB	β-Propiolactone + UV	HIV	>10	1989/90
Factor VIII	Solvent/detergent	HAV	>80	1991 onwards
Intravenous Ig	Cohn fractionation	HCV	>250	1993/94
PPSB	Pasteurization	HBV	>30	1994
Factor VIII	Solvent/detergent	HAV	>3	1995/96

(pasteurization, dry heating, steam treatment) and the solvent/detergent (S/D) method using an organic solvent (tri(*n*-butyl)phosphate) and a detergent (Tween 80). The S/D method is easy to use and generates high yields of FVIII and FIX. Although it is effective against enveloped viruses only, it is highly effective and is now the most commonly used method. Hepatitis A virus transmission occurred in the 1990s in association with FVIII concentrates treated with the S/D method only (Table 23.2).

Modern plasma concentrates are considered safe in terms of transmission of HIV, HBV, and HCV. The measures conducted during the manufacturing process have contributed to this situation, as have the various individual donor plasma and production pool test methods launched in the course of the past two decades. Thanks to effective donor screening and the testing of each individual plasma donation for anti-HIV1/2 antibodies, there has not been a single report of HIV transmission via FVIII concentrates since 1986. A setback occurred in 1990 when a method previously considered effective (β-propiolactone plus UV light) was associated with HIV transmission in hemophilia B patients receiving a FIX complex product [25].

Compulsory testing of all plasma donations for the presence of virus markers (ALT, HBsAg, anti-HIV-1) was introduced in 1984. ELISA for detection of anti-HCV antibodies was introduced into the blood and plasma screening program in 1991. Official recommendations for polymerase chain reaction (PCR) testing of plasma for HCV-RNA were issued in 1999. Most manufacturers also test their products for HIV, HBV, HAV, and parvovirus B19 genome as well. To ensure that the manufacturing process eliminates both enveloped and nonenveloped viruses, the authorities recommend the performance of two independently active virus reduction measures [26]. Most manufacturers have now complied with this recommendation.

Following the development of effective virus inactivation measures for the manufacture of FIX complex concentrates, more effective purification steps were implemented, resulting in the launch of the first pure FIX concentrates in the early 1990s (Immunine, Baxter Healthcare Corporation; AlphaNine, Alpha Therapeutic Corporation).

The purity of FVIII concentrates was further enhanced by the integration of immunoaffinity chromatography into the manufacturing process. The use of monoclonal antibodies against FVIII or against VWF increased the specific activity (ratio of factor VIII activity to protein quantity) to more than 2500 IU/mg (Table 23.1).

Two monoclonally purified FVIII concentrates were available in 1990 (Monoclate, Armour; Hemofil M, Baxter Healthcare Corporation), followed in 1992 by the first monoclonally purified FIX concentrate (Mononine, Armour Pharmaceutical).

A number of immunohemolytic reactions were seen in hemophilia A patients given plasma-derived FVIII concentrates in the 1970s and 1980s [27]. Cryoprecipitate and intermediate-purity factor VIII concentrates in particular contained anti-A and anti-B antibodies that reacted with red blood cells of blood groups A, B, and AB. Most of these cases occurred associated with the high dose levels required for treating inhibitors by immune tolerance induction or prior to major surgery [28].

The European Pharmacopoeia specifies indirect Coombs testing for anti-A and anti-B hemagglutinins for the FVIII concentrates sold today. Levels must be below 1:64 in concentrates prediluted to 3 IU/mL. While genetically engineered concentrates are hemagglutinin-free by definition, FVIII concentrates containing VWF display levels of up to 1:32. This is unsurprising given that VWF adsorbs hemagglutinins and hence prevents their complete elimination in the FVIII purification process. The risk of immunohemolysis in subjects given these concentrates for immune tolerance induction or in preparation for surgery is particularly high for small children owing to the high dose levels involved.

The life expectancy of hemophiliacs now approximates that of the normal population thanks to the availability of sufficient quantities of pure, safe factor concentrates, established prophylaxis regimens, home treatment, and access to effective therapeutic options for patients who develop inhibitors, inhibitor formation being the most serious side-effect that exists today.

Recombinant factor concentrates

The cloning of the FVIII gene (cDNA) and the subsequent derivation of the full amino acid sequence by two study groups [29,30] represented a milestone in hemophilia therapy. For subsequent synthesis by gene technology, the FVIII gene was transfected in a vector to mammalian cells that express and secrete the FVIII protein in a special culture medium in bioreactors. Mammalian cells are essential for protein expression because only they have the capacity to perform the necessary posttranslational glycosylation of the FVIII molecule. Chinese hamster ovary cells (CHO cells) and baby hamster kidney cells (BHK cells) have proven to be highly suitable for the synthesis of FVIII, which, with a molecular weight of 320 000, is the largest molecule ever produced by genetic engineering. The FVIII produced using these cell lines was not biochemically different from plasma-derived FVIII.

Recombinant FVIII concentrate was given to the first patient in 1987. The subsequent clinical trials led to product approval in the USA in 1992 (Recombinate, Baxter Healthcare Corporation) [31]. The second concentrate came to market a year later after completion of the clinical trial program (Kogenate, Bayer). Both these concentrates used albumin during manufacture (cell culture) and in the final product as a stabilizer. This is because high-purity FVIII is unstable and albumin has shown to be the ideal stabilizer for FVIII but also for other biotechnologically engineered products. Albumin allows FVIII concentrates to be stored for several months at room temperature. Albumin is obtained from human or bovine plasma. The use of plasma-derived albumin does little to compromise the safety benefits gained through the production of FVIII by gene technology, as there have been no reports of virus transmission since albumin was first used in the 1940s. This is due to virus reduction in Cohn fractionation—albumin is not produced until the end of the procedure—and to effective pasteurization. Nevertheless, efforts were initiated to replace albumin by other stabilizers. The first second-generation FVIII concentrate received European marketing authorization in 1999. This second-generation product contained histidine and polysorbate 80 in the final product instead of albumin, but continued to use serum albumin in the cell culture (ReFacto, Wyeth, Genetics Institute). This concentrate contains not the full-length FVIII molecule but a molecule shortened through the absence of the B domain, called B domain-deleted FVIII (BDDFVIII, molecular weight 170 000). The B domain seems to be unnecessary for the physiologic effects of FVIII, whereas deletion significantly reduces the complexity of the procedure required to synthesize the relevant cell line. Kogenate was likewise upgraded to a second-generation concentrate, which was approved in 2000. This full-length FVIII concentrate contains sucrose instead of albumin as the stabilizer in the final formulation (Kogenate SF/Kogenate Bayer, Bayer) [32].

The now inevitably overdue improvement in the recombinant concentrates was the elimination of albumin and any other foreign proteins in the manufacturing process. This was made possible by adjusting the cell culture to a serum albumin-free medium. The first third-generation concentrate manufactured entirely without added foreign animal or human protein during synthesis or in the final formulation was approved in the USA in 2003 (Advate, Baxter Healthcare Corporation) [33]. The same applies to the manufacture of the FVIII-specific antibodies used in immunoaffinity chromatography for the purification process. This represents the utmost of what can be achieved in terms of the virus safety of FVIII concentrates with the technical means available today.

The cloning of the FIX gene in 1982 and elucidation of its nucleotide and protein sequence in 1984 made it possible to produce FIX by genetic engineering. However, the development of a suitable cell line transfected with the FIX gene was highly complex as the FIX molecule requires extensive post-translational modification. Years of intensive research activity culminated in 1995 with the production of a biologically active FIX with CHO cells, which came to market in 1999 following successful completion of the requisite clinical trials (BeneFIX, Genetics Institute) [34]. This concentrate is manufactured and formulated without added animal or human proteins. A mixture of polysorbate 80 and sucrose is used for stabilization of the FIX in the final product. Hence, the only recombinant FIX concentrate available to date already matches the safety attributes of the third-generation FVIII concentrate.

Alternatives to aPCCs were also sought for the treatment of bleeds in patients with inhibitors. These had to be agents resulting in effective hemostasis, or fibrin formation, without relying on FVIII or FIX (bypassing agents).

Factor VIIa was identified as meeting these requirements after Hedner and Kiesel [35] successfully treated two patients with inhibitors with plasma-derived FVIIa in 1983. The extremely low FVII plasma concentration of 500 ng/mL was an obstacle in the way of manufacturing a commercial therapeutic agent. This factor and the risk of virus transmission in plasma-derived products prompted efforts to manufacture the activated factor VII by genetic engineering, especially since the relevant cDNA had been isolated.

1988 saw the first successful treatment of a patient with recombinant FVIIa (NovoSeven, Novo Nordisk) [36]. The product was granted European marketing authorization in 1996 after years of studies [37]. The main mechanism of action of rFVIIa was elucidated in 1997; it converts FX straight to FXa on the surface of activated platelets without the intervention of tissue factor or FVIII and FIX [38]. This concentrate now made it possible to systematically treat hemophilia A and B patients with recombinant products, both for treating the actual disease and for the management of bleeds occurring as a result of the formation of inhibitors on therapy with a recombinant FVIII or FIX concentrate.

Conventional aPCCs still have plenty of potential for development. FII and FXa are mainly responsible for the effects of an aPCC in the treatment of patients with inhibitors. Therefore, a recombinant partial prothrombin complex was developed, consisting of these factors at a molar ratio of 37 500:1. A CHO cell line was used for manufacturing the recombinant FXa (rFXa) and a BHK cell line was used for the recombinant FII (rFII). The recombinant complex demonstrated bypassing activity both *in vitro* and in a rabbit model [39]. It is unfortunately not possible at this time to produce sufficient quantities of rFII for a clinical concentrate with the established engineered tissue culture cells. It may be possible to overcome this problem using transgenic animals, which have already been used with success to obtain vitamin K-dependent proteins (FIX, protein C). This prospect belongs to the distant future, however.

References

1 Landsteiner K. On agglutination of normal human blood. *Transfusion* 1961; **1**: 5–8.

2 Van Creveld S. Transfusion in hemophilia. In: *The Hemophiliac and his World*, Proceedings of the Fifth Congressional World Federation of Hemophilia, Montreal 1968. *Bibl Haemat* 1968; **34**: 1–8.

3 Feissly R. Études sur l'hemophilie. *Bull Mem Soc Med Hop Paris* 1923; **47**: 1778–83.

4 Craddock CG, Fenninger LD, Simmons B. Hemophilia. Problem of surgical intervention for accompanying diseases: Review of the literature and report of a case. *Ann Surg* 1948; **128**: 888–903.

5 Brinkhous KM. A study of the clotting defect in hemophilia: the delayed formation of thrombin. *Am J Med Sci* 1939; **198**: 509–16.

6 Cohn EJ, Strong LE, Hughes WL, *et al.* Preparation and properties of serum and plasma proteins. IV. A system for the separation into fractions of the protein and lipoprotein components of biological tissues and fluids. *J Am Chem Soc* 1946; **68**: 459–75.

7 Blombäck B, Blombäck M, Nilsson IM. Role on the purification of human antihemophilic globulin. *Acta Chem Scand* 1958; **12**: 1878.

8 Nilsson IM. Treatment of haemophilia A and v. Willebrand's disease. *Bibl Haematol* (Switzerland) 1965; **23**: 1307–12.

9 Pavlovsky A. Contribution to the pathogenesis of hemophilia. *Blood* 1947; **2**: 185–91.

10 Biggs R, Douglas AS, Macfarlane RG, *et al.* Christmas disease: a condition previously mistaken for hemophilia. *Br Med J* 1952; **2**: 1378–82.

11 Cramer R, Flückiger P, Gasser C, *et al.* Hemophilia B. Two cases of hereditary hemophilia due to a deficiency of a new clotting factor (Christmas factor). *Acta Haematol* 1953; **10**: 65–76.

12 Soulier JP. The history of PPSB. *Vox Sang* (Switzerland) 1984; **461**: 58–61.

13 Beeson PB. Jaundice occurring one to four months after transfusion of blood or plasma. *JAMA* 1943; **121**: 1332–4.

14 Lawrence JS, Johnson JB. The presence of a circulating anticoagulant in a male member of a hemophiliac family. *Trans Am Clin Climatol Assoc* 1941; **57**: 223.

15 Craddock CG, Lawrence JS. A report of the mechanism of the development and action of an anticoagulant in two cases. *Blood* 1947; **6**: 505.

16 Biggs R, Bidwell E. Method for the study of antihaemophilic globulin inhibitors with reference to six cases. *Br J Haematol* 1959; **5**: 379–395.

17 Kernoff PBA, Thomas ND, Lilley PA. Clinical experience with polyelectrolyte-fractionated porcine factor VIII concentrate in the treatment of haemophiliacs with antibodies to factor VIII. *Blood* 1984; **63**: 31–41.

18 Eyster ME, Bowman HS, Haverstick JN. Adverse reactions to factor VIII infusions. *Ann Intern Med* 1977; **872**: 248.

19 Pool JG, Hershgold EJ, Pappenhagen AR. High-potency antihaemophilic factor concentrate prepared from cryoglobulin precipitate. *Nature* 1964; **203**: 312.

20 Rabiner SF, Telfer MC. Home transfusion for patients with hemophilia A. *N Engl J Med* 1970; **283**: 1011–15.

21 Wallace J, Barr A, Milne GR. Which techniques should be used to screen blood donations for hepatitis B surface antigen? *Br Med J* 1975; **2** (5968): 412–14.

22 Hilgartner MW, Knatterud GL. The use of factor eight inhibitor by-passing activity (FEIBA immuno) product for treatment of bleeding episodes in hemophiliacs with inhibitors. *Blood* 1983; **611**: 36–40.

23 Cash JD, Gader AM, da Costa J. Proceedings: The release of plasminogen activator and factor VIII to lysine vasopressin, arginine vasopressin, I-desamino-8-d-arginine vasopressin, angiotensin and oxytocin in man. *Br J Haematol* 1974; **272**: 363–4.

24 Heimburger N, Schwinn H, Gratz P, *et al.* Faktor VIII-Konzentrat, hochgereinigt und in Lösung erhitzt. *Arzneim Forsch* 1981; **31**: 619–22.

25 Nübling CM, Chudy M, Löwer J. Virus testing of plasma pools and blood products by nucleic acid amplification. *Hämostaseologie* 1996; **16**: 274–6.

26 Committee for Proprietary Medicinal Products (CPMP). Note for guidance for viral validation studies. CPMP/268/96, 1996.

27 Hach-Wunderle V, Teixidor D, Zumpe P, *et al.* Anti-A in factor VIII concentrate: a cause of severe hemolysis in a patient with acquired factor VIII:C antibodies. *Infusionstherapie* 1989; **16**: 100–1.

28 Brackmann HH, Oldenburg J, Schwaab R. Immune tolerance for the treatment of factor VIII inhibitors—twenty years' "Bonn protocol". *Vox Sang* 1996; **70** (Suppl. 1): 30–5.

29 Wood WI, Capon DJ, Simonsen CC, *et al.* Expression of active human factor VIII from recombinant DNA clones. *Nature* 1984; **312**: 330–7.

30 Toole JJ, Knopf JL, Wozney JM, *et al.* Molecular cloning of a cDNA encoding human antihaemophilic factor. *Nature* 1984; **312**: 342–7.

31 White GC, McMillan CW, Kingdon HS, *et al.* Use of recombinant antihemophilic factor in the treatment of two patients with classic hemophilia. *N Engl J Med* 1989; **3203**: 166–70.

32 Boedeker BG. Production processes of licensed recombinant factor VIII preparations. *Semin Thromb Haemost* 2001; **274**: 385–94.

33 Mitterer A, Kaliwoda M, Kumar HPM, Kashi RS. Recombinant FVIII manufactured without the use of animal/human derived substances (rAHF-PFM). *Blood* 2002; **100**: 92b [Abstract].

34 Haase M. Human recombinant factor IX: safety and efficacy studies in hemophilia B patients previously treated with plasma-derived factor IX concentrates. *Blood* 2002; **100**: 4242; author reply 4242–3.

35 Hedner U, Kiesel W. Use of human factor VIIa in the treatment of two hemophilia A patients with high-titer inhibitors. *J Clin Invest* 1983; **716**: 1836–41.

36 Negrier C, Lienhart A. Overall experience with NovoSeven. *Blood Coagul Fibrinolysis* 2000; **11** (Suppl. 1): S19–24.

37 Scharrer I. Recombinant factor VIIa for patients with inhibitors to factor VIII or IX or factor VII deficiency. *Haemophilia* 1999; **54**: 253–9.

38 Monroe DM, Hoffman M, Oliver JA, *et al.* Platelet activity of high-dose factor VIIa is independent of tissue factor. *Br J Haematol* 1997; **993**: 542–7.

39 Himmelspach M, Richter G, Muhr E, *et al.* A fully recombinant partial prothrombin complex effectively bypasses FVIII *in vitro* and *in vivo*. *Thromb Haemost* (Germany) 2002; **88**: 1003–11.

24 Products used to treat hemophilia: recombinant products

Akira Yoshioka

After the human factor VIII (FVIII) gene was cloned and expressed in cell culture by two independent biotechnology groups in 1984 [1–4], two pharmaceutical companies developed large-scale production methods for full-length, recombinant FVIII (rFVIII) preparations (Kogenate by Miles-Cutter/Bayer Corporation, and Recombinate by Baxter Healthcare). These were licensed in the early 1990s [5,6].

Interest in developing genetically engineered recombinant clotting factors was driven by the desire for "safer" therapeutic products following the tragic epidemics of blood-borne transmitted diseases in the 1970s and 1980s. The main advantages of these recombinant products are viral safety, independence from plasma supply, and very small volume.

Following intensive preclinical evaluation, clinical trials were undertaken worldwide, which demonstrated that rFVIII is comparable to plasma-derived (pd) FVIII not only in the characteristics of FVIII itself but also in the safety and efficacy of treatment for hemorrhagic episodes. Subsequently, no significant adverse events have been reported.

The first-generation rFVIII proteins were stabilized with bovine or human serum albumin (HSA) either in preparation or in final formulation. Although no viral transmissions have been documented and confirmed with albumin after more than 50 years of clinical use, manufacturers nevertheless worked toward developing products containing minimum amounts of human- or animal-derived components.

Thus, second-generation therapies have been produced in which the HSA in the final vial is replaced by nonprotein stabilizers. Third-generation products lack added bovine and/or human protein in either the cell culture procedure or the final vial. The second-generation types were ReFacto, produced by Genetics Institute/Wyeth and Kogenate FS/Kogenate Bayer, produced by Bayer Corporation. The third-generation types are BeneFIX (rFIX, produced by Genetics Institute/Wyeth), and Advate (rFVIII) recently licensed for use by Baxter Bioscience (Table 24.1).

Recombinant factor VIII

The FVIII gene is one of the largest to be cloned, including 186 kilobase pairs. FVIII messenger RNA (mRNA) encodes a precursor protein of 2351 amino acids. The mature FVIII protein contains 2332 amino acids with a molecular weight of about 300 kDa and with six domains, designated as A1–A2–B–A3–C1–C2 from the amino to carboxy terminus [3]. The B domain between A2 and A3 contains 19 of the 25 potential glycosylation sites on the molecule and has no known functional role in hemostatic activity (FVIII clotting activity, FVIII:C) [7].

rFVIII: Kogenate (Helixate) and Kogenate FS (Kogenate Bayer, Helixate NexGen)

An established baby hamster kidney (BHK) cell line was transfected with human FVIII cDNA and secreted full-length rFVIII into the culture medium without the addition of von Willebrand factor (VWF) [2]. The secreted rFVIII was then subjected to multiple purification steps, including ion-exchange, size exclusion, and immunoaffinity chromatography using a murine monoclonal anti-FVIII antibody. Thus, Kogenate contained trace amounts of hamster protein (51 ng/1000 IU of FVIII:C) and murine IgG (1–27 ng/1000 IU of FVIII:C) from the manufacturing process, as well as HSA (100 mg/1000 IU of FVIII:C) as stabilizer [8]. The purification steps for Kogenate had the capacity to remove and inactivate viruses even though the cultures were believed to be virus-free. The whole process, which included chromatography steps and heat treatment, was validated for a 12-log reduction of relevant model viruses. The first generation of Kogenate is no longer manufactured.

Kogenate FS/Kogenate Bayer (Helixate NexGen distributed by Aventis Behring through a license agreement) are produced as second-generation concentrates using the same production cell line and cell culture process as the first-generation Kogenate. A solvent/detergent stage (S/D) using tri-*n*-butyl phosphate and Triton X-100 has been included early in the preparation. Unlike the original Kogenate, the second-generation products are stabilized in the final formulation with sucrose prior to lyophilization [9].

In validated viral spiking studies, the manufacturing process has been shown to have the potential to reduce model enveloped viruses by >16.4 logs. In addition, the spiking studies have demonstrated that the Kogenate FS processing steps may have potential to remove the prions responsible for the transmissible spongiform encephalopathies (TSEs) [10].

Clinical trials in previously treated patients

Pre-license clinical trials of Kogenate in 56 previously treated patients (PTPs) with hemophilia A began in 1988. Stage I safety

Table 24.1 Summary of recombinant FVIII and FIX products commercially available (2003).

Products (manufacturer/distributor)	Cell line	Gene	Protein in culture medium	Murine MAbs	Stabilizer in final vial	Viral inactivation/removal	Generation
Kogenate FS Kogenate Bayer (Bayer Corp.) Helixate FS Helixate NexGen (Aventis Behring)	BHK	FVIII	HSA	Yes	Sucrose	SD	2
Recombinate (Baxter) Bioclate (Aventis Behring)	CHO	FVIII, VWF	BSA Insulin Aprotinin	Yes	HSA	No	1
Advate (Baxter)	CHO	FVIII, VWF	No	Yes	Sugar etc.	SD	3
ReFacto (Wyeth)	CHO	BDD FVIII	HSA	Yes	No	SD	2
BeneFIX (Wyeth)	CHO	FIX	No	No	Sucrose Amino acids rh-Insulin Vitamin K	NF	3

BDD, B domain deleted; BHK, baby hamster kidney; BSA, bovine serum albumin; CHO, Chinese hamster ovary; HSA, human serum albumin; MAbs, monoclonal antibodies; NF, nanofiltration; SD, solvent/detergent.

and pharmacokinetic studies and stage II safety and efficacy studies showed that Kogenate was safe and clinically effective for the treatment and prevention of hemorrhage in hemophilia A patients and that its behavior *in vitro* was similar to that of pd-FVIII concentrates [6].

The first clinical trials of a sucrose-formulated full-length rFVIII-FS (Kogenate FS) were conducted in 35 PTPs with severe hemophilia A (FVIII:C <2 IU/dL) in North America and Europe. RFVIII-FS displayed a pharmacokinetic profile similar to that of Kogenate. Safety and efficacy during home treatment were evaluated in 71 patients [11]. Of 2585 bleeding episodes, 93.5% were treated with one or two infusions and 80.5% of responses were rated as excellent or good. No *de novo* inhibitor development was observed. Overall, rFVIII-FS provided excellent hemostatic effect, was well tolerated, and caused no significant adverse reactions. Hemostasis was excellent to good in the 30 surgical procedures ranging from minor (port placement/tooth extraction) to major (orthopedic endoprosthesis/brain tumor excision) surgery [12].

Clinical trials in previously untreated patients

In January 1989, a study of Kogenate in previously untreated patients (PUPs) was initiated. A total of 101 PUPs were enrolled, treated and followed; 64 were severe (FVIII clotting activity, FVIII:C <2 U/dL), 16 moderate (2–5 U/dL), and 21 mild (>5 U/dL) [13]. Follow-up was evaluated every 3 months. At the end of December 1996, the cohort had been monitored for up to 8 years (median 4.8 years) since first exposure to rFVIII and had

received 13 029 infusions, or a total of 10.8 million units of Kogenate. Although the response to treatment was judged excellent and the product was well tolerated, the development of FVIII inhibitors in 21 (21/101 = 20.8%, 19 severe and two moderate cases) of PUPs caused concern. Lusher *et al.* [13] reported that the cumulative probability of inhibitor development was 24.8% by day 451 after first infusion with Kogenate and 36.1% after 18 exposure clays (Figure 24.1).

Twelve of the 21 children developing inhibitors had high titers (>10 BU/mL) and nine had low titers. The median exposure was 9 days (range 3–41 days). Inhibitors in seven of the children with low-titer and one with high-titer antibodies were transient, disappearing despite continued episodic treatment with Kogenate. Five of eight with high-titer inhibitors were placed on immune tolerance induction (ITI) protocols with Kogenate and had excellent response [14]. Kogenate was licensed for use in the USA in early 1993.

A prospective, international clinical trial of rFVIII-FS was conducted in 31 PUPs and minimally treated patients (MTPs) with severe hemophilia A in home therapy and surgery [15]. The patients received a total of 2729 infusions (mean 88; range 6–274) for bleeding episodes, surgery, or prophylaxis. No unexpected drug-related adverse events were observed. Four patients (12.9%) developed an inhibitor after a median of 8 exposure days (range 3–12 days). One patient successfully underwent ITI. The inhibitors in two patients disappeared spontaneously with on-demand treatment, while the inhibitor titer remained low in one patient. Twenty-nine patients (93%) with more than 20 exposure days were regarded as low risk for inhibitor

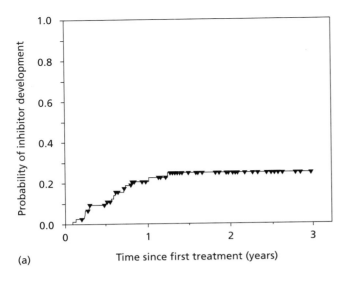

(a)

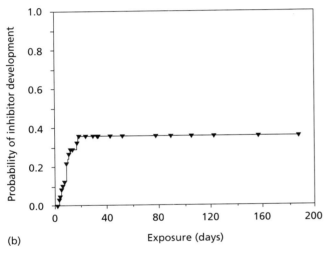

(b)

Figure 24.1 Cumulative probability of development of FVIII inhibitor in 77 PUPs with severe or moderate hemophilia A from the time of initial treatment with Kogenate (a) and according to the number of days of exposure to FVIII treatment (b). Each triangle denotes a patient without inhibitor formation. Used with permission from Lusher *et al.* [13].

development. The incidence of inhibitor formation was consistent with previous experience with other rFVIII or pd-FVIII preparations.

rFVIII: Recombinate (Bioclate) and Advate

The synthesis of Recombinate differs from that of Kogenate in several respects.

Recombinate is manufactured by Genetics Institute/Baxter Healthcare in Chinese hamster ovary (CHO) cells that are co-transfected with cDNAs for both human FVIII and VWF. Co-transfection is found necessary to enhance the yield and to stabilize rFVIII [16]. The rFVIII in the conditioned medium contains added bovine proteins and is then purified by a combina-

tion of immunoaffinity and ion-exchange chromatography. VWF is removed by the same method as that used with Hemofil M (Baxter) [17]. HSA is added to the final product as stabilizer. Recombinate is heat-treated to 40°C for 8 h in the presence of polysorbate 80 and imidazole. The production process has been validated to inactivate or exclude 7 logs of relevant model viruses.

An advanced category, full-length rFVIII, plasma/albumin-free (rFVIII-PFM) preparation (named Advate) has been developed by Baxter Bioscience, without the need for additional animal- or human-derived materials in cell culture, purification, or final formulation. The production of this third-generation concentrate is based largely on the original Recombinate purification process.

Clinical trials in previously treated patients

Recombinate was first infused into two PTPs with severe hemophilia A in 1987. Both patients tolerated the product well and both received the rFVIII at home for a year with clinical success and no adverse reactions [5].

Subsequently, a prospective, open-label clinical study was conducted. Pharmacokinetic studies demonstrated consistent *in vivo* recovery and biological half-life over time (14.7 h), similar to those of pd-FVIII (Hemofil M).

In phase II studies in 55 PTPs, excellent clinical responses were noted, and no FVIII inhibitors developed during >18 months' observation. The response to home treatment was judged as excellent or good in 3195 (91.2%) of 3481 bleeding episodes evaluated. Hemostasis was excellent in all 24 cases with surgical procedures [18].

Pivotal phase II/III studies in PTPs in adults, adolescents, and pediatric patients with hemophilia A have suggested that rFVIII-PFM is bioequivalent to Recombinate based on pharmacokinetic parameters, immunogenicity, efficacy, and safety [19]. In addition, interim data from PTP continuation studies after completion of the phase II/III studies also showed excellent to good hemostatic efficacy in the majority of cases of bleeding episodes [20] as well as in 42 surgical procedures [21].

Clinical trials in previously untreated patients

A Recombinate PUPs study commenced in 1990. Seventy-nine patients with severe hemophilia A (FVIII:C ″2 U/dL) were enrolled. Hemostatic response was excellent with 92% of bleeding episodes responding to one or two infusions [22].

Inhibitor antibodies occurred in 22 (30.6%) out of these 72 PUPs, nine with peak titer ≥5 BU/mL and 13 with titer <5 BU/mL. Survival analysis showed that the probability of remaining inhibitor free in this group of patients was 88.4% after 8 exposure days, 73.6% after 10 exposure days, and 61.6% after 25 exposure days (Figure 24.2). The inhibitor disappeared in 12 patients (11 with low titers) and postinfusion recovery values were normalized.

Recombinate was licensed for use in the USA in December

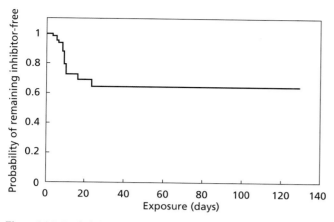

Figure 24.2 Probability of remaining inhibitor-free as a function of Recombinate exposure days for 72 assessable study subjects. Used with permission from Bray *et al.* [22].

1992. Bioclate was distributed by Aventis Behring through a license agreement. The third generation rFVIII-PFM preparation, Advate, was licensed for use in the USA in 2003. A study assessing rFVIII-PFM in PUPs began in April 2004.

rFVIII: ReFacto

The heavily glycosylated B-domain of FVIII seems to be unnecessary for hemostatic activity of the FVIII molecule [7]. B domain-deleted rFVIII (BDDrFVIII, rFVIIISQ) is more readily secreted by CHO cells and is much more stable because of reduced susceptibility to proteolysis. Thus, HSA is not needed as stabilizer in the final product, although it is utilized in the cell culture medium.

rFVIIISQ, trade name ReFacto (Wyeth), is essentially identical to pd FVIII in terms of functional properties and VWF binding kinetics [23]. The production process includes virus inactivation using solvent/detergent (S/D) and immunoaffinity chromatography [24].

Clinical trials in previously treated patients

Phase I (four patients) and phase II (12 patients) prelicense clinical studies were conducted in 1993 and 1994 in patients with severe hemophilia A. These demonstrated that rFVIIISQ had a pharmacokinetic profile equivalent to full-length, monoclonal antibody-purified pd-FVIII (Octonativ-M, Pharmacia) and was similar in hemostatic efficacy and safety [25].

By January 1998, 113 PTPs (median age 26 years, range 8–73) had been followed in Europe and the USA [26]. Overall, a median dose of 29.5 IU/kg had been given for bleeding episodes. In this study, 71% of episodes were resolved with one infusion, and 93% were resolved with 1–3 infusions. Thus, it was concluded that rFVIIISQ was safe and efficacious for PTPs with hemophilia A, for on-demand and/or prophylactic treatment. One PTP developed an inhibitor with a peak titer of 12.6 BU/mL after

93 exposure days and 3 years into the study. The patient is still being treated successfully with increased doses of rFVIIISQ.

Hemostatic efficacy in 22 surgical procedures was rated excellent in all cases and blood loss during surgery was similar to that observed in nonhemophiliacs undergoing the same types of procedures [25].

Clinical trials in previously untreated patients

By September 1999, 101 severe PUPs were enrolled in a safety and efficacy study. Of 1362 bleeding episodes treated in this study, 65% were resolved with a single infusion and 92% were resolved with 1–3 infusions. Forty surgical procedures in 30 patients were performed, with excellent hemostasis.

Overall, 30 (29.7%) PUPs developed FVIII inhibitor antibodies after a median of 12 exposure days (range 3–49). Sixteen of these 30 patients had high-titer antibodies (here defined as ≥ 5 BU/mL) and 14 had low (<5 BU/mL) and/or transient titers [14]. The high-titer inhibitor rate was 16%, which is similar to the rate of the other two full-length rFVIII concentrates.

rFVIIISQ was licensed in European countries in 1998 and in the USA in 2000.

Advantages and disadvantages of rFVIIISQ

As noted above, HSA is not added to the final product as a stabilizer. In addition, rFVIIISQ employs a novel delivery system, in which various potencies are prepackaged in self-contained syringes.

A disadvantage of rFVIIISQ appears to be that the usual one-stage clotting assays for FVIII:C based on the aPTT give much lower than expected recovery values in recipients (on average, 50% less). In contrast, chromogenic substrate assays, which are used in very few clinical laboratories for FVIII:C assays, give expected recovery values. It has therefore been recommended that one-stage assays should be performed in recipients of rFVIIISQ using a vial of the therapeutic material as reference standard, thus essentially adopting a "like versus like" assay principle [26].

Comments on inhibitor development with rFVIII concentrates

The results of several prospective trials of rFVIII in PUPs that were carefully monitored with laboratory inhibitor assays at regular 3-monthly intervals suggested that the incidence of inhibitor development in infants and children with severe hemophilia A may be much higher than previously thought. The cumulative incidence in patients receiving rFVIII concentrates appeared to be in the order of 25%. A much lower incidence has been reported in patients receiving various types of pd-FVIII concentrates [27], although figures vary from 10% to 52%.

Vermylen [28] elegantly reviewed the development of hemophilic inhibitors and indicated that there is probably enough evidence to suggest that repeated switching from one type of FVIII product to another facilitates a multifactorial immune response. In a more recent review, however, there was no evidence for increased inhibitor incidence in patients changing from pd-FVIII to rFVIII [29]. It therefore remains unclear whether pd-FVIII offers a protective effect against inhibitor development, perhaps by influencing immunomodulatory mechanisms of the immune system or by the blockade of epitopes by VWF. Furthermore, rFVIII may appear to potentiate the risk of developing inhibitors because this product is increasingly being used for continuous infusion, particularly in patients with moderate to mild disease who have previously had limited exposure to replacement therapy. It may also be pertinent in this context that intensive FVIII gene analysis in three rFVIII PUPs studies demonstrated that inhibitors were present more commonly in patients with large gene deletions, nonsense mutations, or the intron 22 inversion [30].

Recombinant factor IX

The FIX gene and cDNA were cloned in 1982 [31,32] and expression of rFIX in CHO cells was reported in 1986 [33].

The unique challenge in the development of rFIX protein for clinical use was the need for post-translational modifications, such as α-carboxylation, sulfation, and propeptide cleavage. For its manufacturing process, the Genetics Institute uses a CHO cell line that has been cotransfected with a rFIX cDNA expression plasmid and a cDNA expression plasmid encoding an engineered form of the protease PACE (paired basic amino acid cleaving enzyme). PACE is necessary for the proper cleavage of the signal peptide and secretion of FIX [34].

Another challenge has been to develop methods to eliminate foreign proteins from the production process. Now all CHO cells used in the synthesis of rFIX are grown in serum-free medium containing only amino acids, salts, rh-insulin and vitamin K. Thus, a major advantage of the product, trade-named BeneFIX, is that it is virtually risk free in terms of transmission of bloodborne viruses and spongiform agents [34].

Pharmacokinetic studies

A double-blind, randomized, crossover study was conducted in 11 patients with hemophilia B. The elimination half-lives of the rFIX and monoclonal antibody-purified pd-FIX were 17.7 h and 18.1 h respectively. *In vivo* recovery of rFIX, however, was 28% lower than that of pd-FIX ($P < 0.05$). This difference was probably due to the difference in sulfation of Tyr155 and phosphorylation of Ser158, suggesting that these residues are important in the clearance of FIX. There was no evidence of increased thrombogenicity with rFIX in this study [34].

Clinical trials in previously treated patients

An open-label, multicenter study to evaluate the long-term safety, efficacy and pharmacokinetics of rFIX concentrate has been performed. In 56 patients (46 with severe hemophilia B), hemostatic efficacy was rated as excellent or good in the majority of bleeding episodes and surgical procedures. Eighty percent (854 of 1070) of new bleeding episodes were treated with a single infusion of rFIX [34].

One patient developed a low-titer FIX inhibitor after 39 exposure days to rFIX. The peak titer was 1 BU/mL and the inhibitor disappeared after 11 months [34]. Clinical responses during 13 different surgical procedures ($n = 24$), including orthotopic liver transplantation, were rated as excellent or good in 97% of cases [35].

Clinical trials in previously untreated patients

By June 1999, 60 PUPs were enrolled in an open-label, multinational, multicenter study to evaluate safety and efficacy. In 50 PUPs with follow-up inhibitor assays, two developed inhibitors with anaphylactoid reactions, which is well known to be a unique feature of the FIX inhibitor response in 50% of patients on exposure to any FIX-containing product [36]. In view of the lower recovery values following rFIX infusion, dosage recommendations for BeneFIX are as follows:

Number of FIX units required = body weight (kg) × desired FIX increase (%) × 1.2

It should be noted that even lower recoveries may be seen in infants and young children [14].

Conclusion

rFVIII and rFIX preparations are now increasingly in clinical use in Europe, the USA, Japan, and elsewhere for patients with hemophilia. Clinical experience indicates that the incidence of inhibitors is probably not increased in PTPs or in PUPs. New, second- and third-generation rFVIII or rFIX preparations, without HSA as a stabilizer and with no animal or human proteins used in manufacture, are currently available commercially.

The greatest difficulty that has emerged with the increasing use of recombinant factor preparations for the treatment of hemophilia has been cost. This has led to a debate that has only been possible in the developed world [17,37].

The choice of product for replacement therapy must take into account three facts: (i) plasma-derived factors are becoming ever safer; (ii) recombinant factors cost two to three times as much as plasma-derived factors; and (iii) the limited capacity to produce recombinant factors often causes periods of shortage [38]. In the UK and Italy, priority is given for the use of recombinant factors to PUPs and to patients without blood-borne infections despite previous exposure to plasma-derived factors [39].

Finally, as with any new technology, well-designed protocols and continued surveillance for any unexpected long-term complications are necessary.

References

1 Gitschier J, Wood WI, Goralka TM, et al. Characterization of the human factor VIII gene. *Nature* 1984; **312**: 326–30.

2 Wood WI, Capon DJ, Simons CC, et al. Expression of active human factor VIII from recombinant DNA clones. *Nature* 1984; **312**: 330–7.

3 Vehar GA, Keyt B, Eaton D, et al. Structure of human factor VIII. *Nature* 1984; **312**: 337–42.

4 Toole JT, Knopf JL, Wozney JM, et al. Molecular cloning of a cDNA encoding human antihaemophilic factor. *Nature* 1984; **312**: 342–7.

5 White GC, McMillan CW, Kingdon HS, Shoemaker CB. Use of recombinant antihemophilic factor in the treatment of two patients with classic hemophilia. *N Engl J Med* 1989; **320**: 166–70.

6 Schwartz RS, Abildgaard CF, Aledort LM, et al. Human recombinant DNA-derived antihemophilic factor (factor VIII) in the treatment of hemophilia A. *N Engl J Med* 1990; **323**: 1800–5.

7 Toole JT, Pittman DD, Orr EC, et al. A large region (= 95kDa) of human factor VIII is dispensable for in vitro procoagulant activity. *Proc Natl Acad Sci USA* 1986; **83**: 5939–42.

8 Yoshioka A. Advances in hemophilia and other coagulation disorders: Recombinant factor VIII preparations. *Int J Pediatr Hematol Oncol* 1994; **1**: 491–7.

9 Jiang R, Monroe T, McRogers R, Larson PJ. Manufacturing challenges in the commercial production of recombinant coagulation factor VIII. *Haemophilia* 2002; **8** (Suppl. 2): 1–5.

10 Lee DC, Millar JLA, Petteway SR Jr. Pathogen safety of manufacturing process for biological products: special emphasis on Kogenate Bayer. *Haemophilia* 2002; **8** (Suppl. 2): 6–9.

11 Abshire TC, Brackmann H-H, Scharrer I, et al. Sucrose formulated recombinant human antihemophilic factor FVIII is safe and efficacious for treatment of hemophilia A in home therapy. *Thromb Haemost* 2000; **83**: 811–16.

12 Scharrer I, the Kogenate Bayer Study Group. Experience with Kogenate Bayer in surgical procedures. *Haemophilia* 2002; **8** (Suppl. 2): 15–18.

13 Lusher JM, Arkin S, Abildgaard CF, Schwartz RS. Recombinant factor VIII for the treatment of previously untreated patients with hemophilia A. *N Engl J Med* 1993; **328**: 453–9.

14 Lusher JM. Recombinant clotting factors. A review of current clinical status. *Bio-Drugs* 2000; **13**: 289–98.

15 Giangrande PLF, for the Kogenate Bayer Study Group. Safety and efficacy of Kogenate Bayer in previously untreated patients (PUPs) and minimally treated patients (MTPs). *Haemophilia* 2002; **8** (Suppl. 2): 19–22.

16 Kaufman RJ, Wasley LC, Dorner AJ. Synthesis, processing and secretion of recombinant human factor VIII expressed in mammalian cells. *J Biol Chem* 1988; **263**: 6352–62.

17 Gomperts ED, Lundblad R, Adamson R. The manufacturing process of recombinant factor VIII, Recombinate. *Transf Med Rev* 1992; **6**: 247–51.

18 White GC, Courter S, Bray GL, et al. A multicenter study of recombinant factor VIII (Recombinate) in previously treated patients with hemophilia A. *Thromb Haemost* 1997; **77**: 660–7.

19 Hoots K, Blanchette V, Shapiro A, et al. for the rAHF-PFM Clinical Study Group. Clinical evaluation of an advanced category recombinant FVIII, antihemophilic factor (recombinant) plasma/albumin-free method (rAHF-PFM) in pediatric previously treated patients. Poster presented at XIX Congress of ISTH, 2003, Birmingham, UK.

20 Shapiro A, Collins P, Tarantino M, et al. Continuing clinical evaluation of an advanced category recombinant FVIII, antihemophilic factor (recombinant) plasma/albumin-free method (rAHF-PFM) in previously treated patients. Poster presented at XIX Congress of ISTH, 2003, Birmingham, UK.

21 Astermark J, Négrier C, Schroth P, et al. for the rAHF-PFM Clinical Study Group. Clinical evaluation of an advanced recombinant FVIII, antihemophilic factor (recombinant) plasma/albumin-free method (rAHF-PFM) in surgical settings. Poster presented at XIX Congress of ISTH, 2003, Birmingham, UK.

22 Bray GL, Gomperts ED, Courter S, et al. A multicenter study of recombinant factor VIII (Recombinate): safety, efficacy, and inhibitor risk in previously untreated patients with hemophilia A. *Blood* 1994; **83**: 2428–35.

23 Sandberg H, Almstedt A, Brandt J. Structural and functional characteristics of a B-domain deleted recombinant factor VIII molecule, r-VIII SQ. *Thromb Haemost* 2001; **85**: 93–100.

24 Charlebois TS, O'Connell BD, Adamson SR, et al. Viral safety of B-domain deleted recombinant factor VIII. *Semin Hematol* 2001; **38** (Suppl. 4): 32–9.

25 Lusher JM, Lee CA, Kessler CM, Bedrosian CL – for the Refacto 3 Study Group. The safety and efficacy of B domain deleted recombinant factor VIII concentrate in patients with severe haemophilia A. *Haemophilia* 2003; **9**: 38–49.

26 Mikaelsson M, Oswaldsson U, Jankowski MA. Measurement of factor VIII activity of B-domain deleted recombinant factor VIII. *Semin Hematol* 2001; **38** (Suppl. 4): 13–23.

27 Scharrer I, Bray GL, Neutzling O. Incidence of inhibitors in haemophilia A patients – a review of recent studies of recombinant and plasma-derived factor VIII concentrates. *Haemophilia* 1999; **5**: 145–54.

28 Vermylen J. How do some haemophiliacs develop inhibitors? *Haemophilia* 1998; **4**: 538–42.

29 Scharrer I, Ehrlich HJ. Lack of evidence for increased inhibitor incidence in patients switched from plasma-derived to recombinant factor VIII. *Haemophilia* 2001; **7**: 346–8.

30 Williams IJ, Peake IR, Goodeve AV. Recombinant PUP mutation study: relationship between factor VIII mutation and inhibitor development. *Haemophilia* 1998; **4**: 228.

31 Kurachi K, Davie EW. Isolation and characterization of a cDNA coding for human factor IX. *Proc Natl Acad Sci USA*: 1982; **79**: 6461–4.

32 Choo GH, Gould KG, Rees DJ, Brownlee GG. Molecular cloning of the gene for human anti-haemophilic factor IX. *Nature* 1982; **299**: 178–80.

33 Kaufman RJ, Wasley IC, Furie BC, et al. Expression, purification, and characterization of recombinant gamma-carboxylated factor IX synthesized in Chinese hamster ovary cells. *J Biol Chem* 1986; **261**: 9622–8.

34 White GC, Beebe A, Nielsen B. Recombinant factor IX. *Thromb Haemost* 1997; **78**: 261–5.

35 White G, Shapiro A, Ragni M, et al. Clinical evaluation of recombinant factor IX. *Semin Hematol* 1998; **35** (Suppl. 2): 33–8.

36 Warrier I. Factor IX inhibitor and anaphylaxis In: Rodriguez-Merchan EC, Lee CA, eds. *Inhibitors in Patients with Haemophilia.* Oxford: Blackwell Science, 2002: 87–91.

37 Lee C. Recombinant clotting factors in the treatment of hemophilia. *Thromb Haemost* 1999; **82**: 516–24.

38 Mannucci PM, Tuddenham EGD. The hemophiliacs—from royal genes to gene therapy. *N Engl J Med* 2001; **344**: 1773–9.

39 United Kingdom Haemophilia Centre Doctors' Organisation (UKHCDO). Guidelines on the selection and use of therapeutic products to treat haemophilia and other hereditary bleeding disorders. *Haemophilia* 2003; **9**: 1–23.

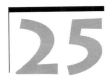

Products used to treat hemophilia: plasma-derived coagulation factor concentrates

Paul L.F. Giangrande

Introduction

The development of blood products for the treatment of hemophilia has dramatically altered the prognosis for those patients who live in affluent countries and have regular access to safe products. The median life expectancy for people with severe hemophilia increased fivefold from only 11 years during the period 1831–1920 to 56.8 years during the period 1961–1980 [1]. In more recent years, infection with HIV and hepatitis C (HCV) has had a significant negative impact [2,3]. Access to treatment also improves the quality of life of patients, at least in part by facilitating access to normal education and employment [4]. In recent years, the relative merits of plasma versus recombinant products have been a major topic of debate. [5,6]. The arguments focus primarily on safety with regard to transmission of pathogens, which must be of prime concern in the selection of products for the treatment of hemophilia. The recent experience of an acute and worldwide shortage of recombinant factor VIII has certainly served to focus minds on the fact that the number of manufacturing plants is very limited, particularly so in the cases of recombinant factor IX and recombinant factor VIIa. However, one important positive consequence of the progressive switch to recombinant products in developed countries is that this will help to secure effective and safe treatment for people in developing countries. As patients in more affluent parts of the world such as North America, Europe, Australia, and Japan convert inexorably to recombinant products, manufacturers of plasmaderived products will be forced to seek new markets in the developing world and these will also have to be competitively priced. It is clear that there will continue to be a global requirement for plasma-derived as well as recombinant coagulation factor concentrates for many years to come.

Cryoprecipitate

Although coagulation factor concentrates are now regarded as the treatment of choice for hemophilia in developed countries, it must be recognized that cryoprecipitate stills forms the mainstay of treatment for patients in many less affluent countries around the world. The discovery by Judith Pool in 1964 that a fraction of thawed plasma contained factor VIII was a major landmark in the development of products for the treatment of hemophilia. Cryoprecipitate is prepared by slow thawing of fresh-frozen plasma (FFP) at 4°C for 24 h, when cryoprecipitate appears as an insoluble precipitate and is separated by centrifugation. It contains significant quantities of factor VIII, von Willebrand factor (VWF), fibrinogen, and factor XIII (FXIII) (but not factors IX or XI). Current AABB (American Association of Blood Banks) standards call for a minimum standard of 80 IU FVIII per pack (and 150 mg fibrinogen). However, in practice the coagulation factor content of individual packs in developing countries is variable and is usually not controlled. The yield of FVIII from plasma can be enhanced by controlling several variables, and in one study packs with a FVIII content of 150 IU or more were produced using an automated device with computer-controlled temperature cycling [7]. However, the most significant problem with cryoprecipitate is that it cannot be easily subjected to viral inactivation procedures (such as heat or solvent/detergent treatment) and this inevitably translates into a risk of transmission of viral pathogens that is not insignificant with repeated exposure. For example, a study based on data from Venezuela estimated a cumulative risk of 40% for HIV and almost 100% for HCV over a lifetime (60 years) of treatment with cryoprecipitate [8]. The use of this product in the treatment of congenital bleeding disorders cannot therefore be recommended in countries that can afford coagulation factor concentrates. Certain steps can at least be taken to minimize the risk of transmission of viral pathogens. These include careful selection of donors and producing packs from single donors. Once collected, the plasma should be quarantined until the donor has been recalled and retested for markers of infection: if the donor does not return, the plasma should not be used. Polymerase chain reaction (PCR) testing is a technology that has a potentially much greater relevance for the production of cryoprecipitate than of concentrates, as the latter are subjected to viral inactivation steps. Quality control, involving the monitoring of FVIII content, is also very important.

Much of what has been written about cryoprecipitate applies to the use of FFP, which is a source of all coagulation factors. As it contains factor IX (FIX), it is still used for the treatment of hemophilia B in countries unable to afford the use of plasmaderived FIX concentrate. Packs of FFP subjected to some form of virucidal treatment (including solvent/detergent treatment) are already available. The possibility of severe allergic reactions to infused plasma, including transfusion-related acute lung injury (TRALI) attributed to cytotoxic antibodies of donor origin in the infused plasma, has been recognized for some time [9]. An additional benefit of solvent/detergent-treated FFP is a significant decrease in the incidence of such allergic reactions [10].

Principles of manufacture

There are some common steps involved in the manufacture of coagulation factor concentrates. Plasma proteins such as albumin, coagulation factor concentrates, and immune globulin preparations are manufactured from large pools of human plasma, primarily by the Cohn cold ethanol fractionation method. This method, developed by Edwin Cohn in Boston in the 1940s, involves the sequential precipitation of specific proteins under varying conditions of ethanol and pH conditions.

In the case of FVIII, cryoprecipitate is produced using a standard ethanol/dry ice process for snap freezing and the cryoprecipitate is extracted by thawing at 4°C. Antihemophilic factor (AHF) is extracted from the cryoprecipitate by dissolving in a buffer. Fibrinogen is removed from the resulting supernatant by precipitation, followed by precipitation of FVIII from supernatant. FVIII is then purified by chromatographic techniques, using either ion-exchange chromatography or immunoaffinity chromatography.

Factor IX is prepared by anion-exchange chromatography in the presence of heparin, applied to cryoprecipitate-depleted plasma, or the use of immunoaffinity chromatography.

The coagulation protein (FVIII or FIX) is then freeze-dried and lyophilized concentrate is bottled under sterile conditions. At some stage, either as a final step or during the manufacturing process, a specific virucidal step such as heat treatment and/or solvent/detergent treatment is applied (see below).

Quality control is an essential element in the manufacturing process, and each batch of product is randomly sampled and analyzed for FVIII (or FIX) clotting activity, electrolyte concentration, pyrogenicity, sterility, and toxicity. If found to comply with all release parameters, the bottles are labeled with a batch number and bottle number before being issued for use. Regulatory agencies such as the FDA and EMEA generally conduct some form of independent oversight of this process by routine monitoring of the manufacturers' test results or by conducting their own tests.

The plasma used for fractionation may be recovered plasma, typically derived from whole blood procured from volunteer donors, or source plasma, usually collected from paid donors who undergo periodic plasmapheresis. In the past, plasma for fractionation from paid donors was considered to be at higher risk of viral infection than plasma from voluntary donors drawn from the same population. However, this can no longer be considered to be the case. Donor selection procedures are designed to identify and exclude donors at risk of being infected with pathogenic viruses. Exclusion criteria include a history of blood-borne infection, intravenous drug use, and high-risk sexual behavior. The quarantining of plasma until a donor appears for retesting (inventory hold) is an additional precaution that may be taken. Nucleic acid testing (NAT) is now mandatory for hepatitis C, but is employed for detection of other viruses such as HIV, parvovirus B19, and both hepatitis A and B by an increasing number of manufacturers.

The establishment of a "plasma master file" for plasma-derived products is a relatively new concept that has been pioneered by the European regulatory authorities (EMEA). This contains details of all donations in a batch of products. This permits tracing of blood donations through the screening procedure right up to intravenous administration. Within Europe, the plasma master file will replace that part of the marketing authorization application (MAA) describing the raw material plasma (annexe IIC) and will make the arrangements for movement of plasma, intermediates, and products across member states both easier and more transparent. Two particular issues deserve further consideration: purity of product and the number of virucidal steps.

Product purity

Product purity should not be confused with concentrate safety or efficacy. Purity simply refers to the percentage of the desired ingredient (e.g., FVIII) in concentrates relative to other ingredients present. Concentrates on the market vary widely in their purity from around 5.0 IU FVIII mg/protein in intermediate-purity concentrates to 2000 in the case of high-purity concentrates. Generally, products that are produced at higher purity tend to be associated with low manufacturing yields and therefore cost more. High-purity products are more readily soluble, which makes them more convenient for home treatment and also facilitates administration by continuous infusion if desired in the setting of surgery. The incidence of allergic reactions is also probably lower with high-purity products. However, there is no clear evidence that modern high-purity concentrates offer a higher margin of safety with regard to transmission of pathogens. Several studies have suggested that the use of high-purity concentrates retards the decline in CD4+ lymphocyte counts in HIV-positive individuals, but this has not been a consistent finding [11–14]. However, it has not been clearly demonstrated that any resulting change in CD4+ lymphocyte is associated with a slowing in the rate of progression to AIDS or death and any such positive effect of high-purity products is insignificant when compared with the immune reconstitution associated with highly active antiretroviral therapy (HAART). One advantage of less pure FVIII concentrates products is that they usually contain significant quantities of von Willebrand factor (VWF) so that they may be useful in the treatment of that condition. Examples of concentrates suitable for the treatment of von Willebrand disease include 8Y (BPL), Alphanate (Alpha), Fanhdi (Grifols), Hemate P (Aventis Behring), and VWF concentrate (LFB) [15]. None of the brands of plasma-derived high-purity FVIII or recombinant concentrates contains VWF.

Although it would be fair to say that the current general consensus is that the incidence of inhibitor development is very similar among patients treated with recombinant and plasma-derived products [16–18], there is some evidence that the use of a concentrate containing VWF results in a lower incidence of inhibitor development and a better response in patients with inhibitors undergoing immune tolerance [19,20].

In the case of FIX concentrates, high-purity concentrates have been shown to induce less activation of coagulation than prothrombin complex concentrates [21]. The latter should no longer be employed in the routine management of hemophilia B in view of case reports of thrombosis (including venous thromboembolism, disseminated intravascular coagulation, and myocardial infarction) associated with their use [22–24].

Methods of viral inactivation and elimination

The introduction of heat treatment and solvent/detergent treatment in the mid-1980s effectively eliminated the risk of transmission of HIV and HCV (hepatitis C) through the use of plasma-derived products [25–27]. Although highly effective against a wide range of viruses with a lipid envelope (including West Nile virus), solvent/detergent treatment with such agents as TNBP and Triton X-100 does not inactivate nonenveloped viruses such as hepatitis A [28,29]. Furthermore, some viruses (such as human parvovirus B19 virus) are relatively resistant to both types of physical process [30,31]. While infection with parvovirus is rarely of clinical significance, it is naturally of concern that this hardy DNA virus is resistant to physical virucidal treatments.

There are no screening tests available for the detection of prions, including the presumed causative agent of variant Creutzfeldt–Jakob disease (vCJD), and precautions are largeliform based on donor exclusion. All regulatory authorities have regulations in place to exclude donors who have spent defined periods in countries considered to be at high risk of bovine spongiform encephalitis (BSE) or vCJD, such as the UK. Furthermore, these pathogenic protein particles are completely resistant to conventional heat and solvent/detergent treatment. It is therefore reassuring that plasma fractionation techniques appear quite fortuitously to eliminate substantial amounts of prions [32]. No cases of either the classical or variant form of Creutzfeldt–Jakob disease have ever been reported in a subject with hemophilia. By contrast, nanofiltration is also highly effective in eliminating prions in experimental conditions. Nanofiltration was originally developed as an alternative method of removing a wide range of viruses, including parvovirus B19. It is a relatively simple manufacturing step that consists of filtering protein solution through membranes of a very small pore size, typically 15–40 nm, under conditions that retain viruses by a mechanism largely based on size exclusion [33]. Nanofiltration has also been demonstrated not to induce protein alteration (e.g., neoantigenicity) and the yield of filtered protein is not adversely affected. Nanofiltration of FVIII products is also possible nowadays, despite a relatively large molecular weight of 330 kDa compared with 60-kDa FIX. The Planova filtration device is particularly suitable for FVIII preparations and is composed of hollow-fiber microporous membranes made of naturally hydrophilic cuprammonium-regenerated cellulose, housed in a polycarbonate body. It is an efficient method of removing more than four to six logs of a wide range of viruses, and has the added advantage of having no adverse, denaturing effect on plasma proteins.

All virus inactivation and removal steps have their limitations. It is recommended that two distinct and effective steps that are complementary be incorporated into the plasma product manufacturing process [15]. European guidelines recommend that at least one step effectively inactivates or removes nonenveloped viruses. A 2001 recommendation from the Committee for Proprietary Medicinal Products (CPMP) states that [15]:

. . . for all plasma-derived medicinal products, it is an objective to incorporate effective steps for inactivation/removal of a wide range of viruses of diverse physicochemical characteristics. In order to achieve this, it will be desirable in many cases to incorporate two distinct effective steps which complement each other in their mode of action such that any virus surviving the first step would be effectively inactivated/removed by the second. At least one of the steps should be effective against nonenveloped viruses. Where a process step is shown to be reliably effective in inactivating or removing a wide range of viruses including enveloped and non-enveloped viruses of diverse physicochemical characteristics and the process contains additional stages reliably contributing to the inactivation/ removal of viruses, a second effective step would not be required.

It is recommended that all patients receiving plasma-derived concentrates be vaccinated against hepatitis A and B as an additional precaution [34]. It is noteworthy that an outbreak of hepatitis B occurred as recently as 1994 in a group of anticoagulated patients given a pasteurized prothrombin complex concentrate to reverse the effects of warfarin [35].

Potency and labeling issues

Assays of coagulation factors have been standardized by the establishment of international standards by the World Health Organization (WHO). These standards define the international unit (IU) and are available in limited quantities for calibration of local, commercial, national, and supranational standards— these in turn are used to assay therapeutic concentrates and plasma samples from patients and hence all such measurements can be recorded in IU. When the first international standards for each coagulation factor were established, they were calibrated against fresh normal plasma from a large number of donors, and so 1 IU is approximately equivalent to the amount of each factor in 1 mL of average normal plasma. An important principle in biologic standardization is that of "like versus like." For many biologic substances, not just coagulation factors, reproducibility between laboratories, and between assay methods, is greatest when test and standard are of similar composition. It has been found in several collaborative studies that plasma standards are unsuitable for assay of coagulation factor concentrates and vice versa. There are therefore two WHO standards for all the principal coagulation factors, one for the assay of therapeutic concentrates and the other for assay of plasma samples.

The current (sixth) WHO FVIII standard was prepared from a full-length recombinant product, containing albumin, but is used to calibrate both plasma-derived and recombinant products. Other standards are the US Mega and European Pharmacopoeia (EP) standards, which are working standards calibrated against the WHO standard in multicenter studies. The current US Mega (2) and EP (3) standards are identical, shared from the same large batch of a plasma-derived concentrate. In the USA, most manufacturers use the Mega standard to assay their product, whereas most manufacturers in Europe use an internal house standard calibrated against the WHO standard. All three assay methods are still in use, although the two-stage method is used by only a few manufacturers. Most US manufacturers use the one-stage method, although most European manufacturers of plasma-derived concentrates now use the chromogenic method, which is the recommended method of the EP and of the ISTH. In the case of plasma-derived products, significant discrepancies are typically observed between the results of one-stage and chromogenic assays found with the "Method M" products; the former giving potencies around 25–30% higher than those obtained with the chromogenic method [36]. Assays of plasma samples following infusions of concentrates are carried out for pharmacokinetic studies or to check the hemostatic level of the patient, especially before and after surgery. As these samples consist of plasma, they are normally assayed against plasma standards, which may be local pools, commercial standards which are calibrated against the appropriate WHO plasma standards. Postinfusion plasmas can, however, also be considered as concentrates "diluted" in the patient's deficient plasma, and as such a concentrate standard, diluted in deficient plasma, may be more appropriate [37].

Selection of products

The World Federation of Hemophilia (WFH) has published a guide [38] for the assessment of clotting factor concentrates that deals with all types of available products but focuses primarily on plasma-derived products. The UK Hemophilia Centre Doctors' Organisation (UKHCDO) has also published relevant guidelines [15]. It is beyond the scope of this chapter to include details of all the available coagulation factor concentrates, but the WFH guide also includes a registry of all coagulation factor concentrates. This is updated on an annual basis and is also available through the WFH website (wwfh.org). The registry includes information on: donors (nationality, whether paid or voluntary); method of obtaining plasma; serologic tests on donors; testing of mini-pools for viruses using PCR amplification; location of fractionation facilities; methods of fractionation; methods of viral inactivation/elimination; levels of purification; identity of distributor and manufacturer; and intended area of distribution (domestic or export).

Consideration needs to be given to both the plasma source and the manufacturing process. Cost alone should certainly not be the deciding factor when choosing products. As regards the plasma source, the plasma supplier should be licensed by the relevant national health authority and the donor epidemiology

scrutinized. At the very least, blood testing should include screening of individual donations (not just mini-pools of plasma) for HIV, HBV, and HCV, preferably using NAT technology. Evidence of a robust quality assurance system for the performance of viral screening tests is vital. Products should be subjected to well-validated viral inactivation/removal steps. Data relating to stability data and shelf-life may also be important. Clinical reports of previous use are also important, including details of where the product is currently available and used in clinical practice and marketing authorizations from licensing bodies. A product license from such organizations as the FDA and EMEA certainly implies that the product has been subject to a high degree of scrutiny. Published data in peer-reviewed journals covering such areas as adverse events and efficacy are also important.

Plasma-derived concentrates for rare bleeding disorders

Plasma-derived concentrates of fibrinogen, FVII, FXI, and FXIII are available. Clinical data on the use of such concentrates may be limited, and not all have product licenses and thus need to be used on a named patient basis. All prothrombin complex concentrates contain factor II (prothrombin), FIX, and FX; some also contain FVII. The products containing four coagulation factors are widely used to reverse the effect of anticoagulation. They may also be used for the treatment of isolated congenital deficiencies of these factors, but it should be noted that the potency is usually assigned to the vials according to the FIX content and the amount of the other factors may be quite different. Recombinant activated FVII is being used increasingly in the treatment of congenital FVII deficiency, in preference to a plasma-derived concentrate. No concentrate containing FV is available and treatment with fresh-frozen plasma is required in such cases.

References

1 Larsson SA. Life expectancy of Swedish haemophiliacs, 1831–1980. *Br J Haematol* 1985; **59**: 593–602.
2 Darby SC, Ewart DW, Giangrande PLF, *et al*. Mortality before and after HIV infection in the complete UK population of haemophiliacs. *Nature* 1995; **377**: 79–82.
3 Darby SC, Ewart DW, Giangrande PLF, *et al*. Mortality from liver cancer and liver disease in haemophilic men and boys given blood products contaminated with hepatitis C. *Lancet* 1997; **350**: 1425–31.
4 Royal S, Schramm W, Berntorp E, *et al*. Quality-of-life differences between prophylactic and on-demand factor replacement therapy in European haemophilia patients. *Haemophilia* 2002; **8**: 44–50.
5 Giangrande PLF. Treatment of hemophilia: recombinant products only? Yes. *J Thromb Haemost* 2003; **1**: 214–15.
6 Mannucci PM: Treatment of hemophilia: recombinant products only? No. *J Thromb Haemost* 2003; **1**: 216–17.
7 Rock G, Berger R, Lange J, *et al*. A novel, concentrated method of

temperature cycling to produce cryoprecipitate. *Transfusion* 2001; **41**: 232–5.

8 Evatt BL, Austin H, Leon G, *et al.* Haemophilia therapy: assessing the cumulative risk of HIV exposure by cryoprecipitate. *Haemophilia* 1999; **5**: 295–300.

9 Kernoff PB, Durrant IJ, Rizza CR, Wright FB. Severe allergic pulmonary oedema after plasma transfusion. *Br J Haematol* 1972; **23**: 777–81.

10 Riedler GF, Haycoxx AR, Duggan AK, Dakin HA. Cost-effectiveness of solvent/detergent-treated fresh-frozen plasma. *Vox Sang* 2003 **85**: 88–95.

11 De Biasi R, Rocino A, Miraglia E, *et al.* The impact of a very high purity factor VIII concentrate on the immune system of human immunodeficiency virus-infected hemophiliacs: a randomized, prospective, two-year comparison with an intermediate purity concentrate. *Blood* 1991; **78**: 1919–22.

12 Goedert JJ, Cohen AR, Kessler CM. Risks of immunodeficiency, AIDS and death related to purity of factor VIII concentrate. Multicenter Hemophilia Cohort Study. *Lancet* 1994; **344**: 791–2.

13 Sabin C, Pasi J, Phillips A, *et al.* CD4+ counts before and after switching to monoclonally high-purity factor VIII concentrate in HIV-infected haemophilic patients. *J Thromb Haemost* 1994; **72**: 214–17.

14 Hay CR, Ludlam CA, Lowe GD, *et al.* The effect of monoclonal or ion-exchange purified factor VIII concentrate on HIV disease progression: a prospective cohort comparison. *Br J Haematol* 1998; **101**: 632–7.

15 United Kingdom Haemophilia Centre Doctors' Organisation (UKHCDO). Guidelines on the selection and use of therapeutic products to treat haemophilia and other hereditary bleeding disorders. *Haemophilia* 2003; **9**: 1–23.

16 Lusher JM: Factor VIII inhibitors with recombinant products: prospective clinical trials. *Haematologica* 2000; **85**: 2–6.

17 Mauser-Bunschoten EP, van der Bom JG, Bongers M, *et al.* Purity of factor VIII product and incidence of inhibitors in previously untreated patients with haemophilia A. *Haemophilia* 2001; **7**: 364–8.

18 Scharrer I, Bray GL, Neutzling O. Incidence of inhibitors in haemophilia A patients—a review of recent studies of recombinant and plasma-derived factor VIII concentrates. *Haemophilia* 1999; **5**: 145–54.

19 Behrmann M, Pasi J, Saint-Remy J-M, *et al.* von Willebrand factor modulates factor VIII immunogenicity: comparative study of different factor VIII concentrates in a haemophilia A mouse model. *Thromb Haemost* 2002; **88**: 221–9.

20 Auerswald G, Spranger T, Brackmann H-H. The role of plasma-derived factor VIII/von Willebrand factor concentrates in the treatment of hemophilia A patients. *Haematologica* 2003; **88** (Suppl. 9): 21–5.

21 Thomas DP, Hampton KK, Dasani H, *et al.* A cross-over pharmacokinetic and thrombogenicity study of a prothrombin complex concentrate and a purified factor IX concentrate. *Br J Haematol* 1994; **87**: 782–8.

22 Kasper CK. Thromboembolic complications. *Thrombosis et Diathesis Haemorrhagica* 1975; **33**: 640–4.

23 Conlan MG, Hoots WK. Disseminated intravascular coagulation and hemorrhage in hemophilia B following elective surgery. *Am J Hematol* 1990; **35**: 203–7.

24 Fuerth JH, Mahrer P: Myocardial infarction after factor IX therapy. *JAMA* 1981; **245**: 1455–6.

25 Horowitz MS, Rooks C, Horowitz B, Hilgartner MW. Virus safety of solvent/detergent-treated antihaemophilic factor concentrate. *Lancet* 1988; **ii**: 186–9.

26 Schimpf K, Brackmann HH, Kreuz W, *et al.* Absence of anti-human immunodeficiency virus types 1 and 2 seroconversion after the treatment of hemophilia A or von Willebrand's disease with pasteurized factor VIII concentrate. *N Engl J Med* 1989; **321**: 1148–52.

27 Rizza CR, Fletcher ML, Kernoff PB. Confirmation of viral safety of dry heated factor VIII concentrate (8Y) prepared by Bio Products Laboratory (BPL): a report on behalf of UK Haemophilia Centre Directors. *Br J Haematol* 1993; **84**: 269–72.

28 Vermylen J, Peerlinck K. Review of the hepatitis A epidemics in hemophiliacs in Europe. *Vox Sang* 1994; **67** (Suppl. 4): 8–11.

29 Soucie JM, Roberston BH, Bell BP, *et al.* Hepatitis A virus infections associated with clotting factor concentrate in the United States. *Transfusion* 1998; **38**: 573–9.

30 Yee TT, Cohen BJ, Pasi KJ, Lee CA. Transmission of symptomatic parvovirus B19 infection by clotting factor concentrate. *Br J Haematol* 1996; **93**: 457–9.

31 Azzi A, Morfini M, Mannucci PM. The transfusion-associated transmission of parvovirus B19. *Transfusion Med Rev* 1999; **13**: 194–204.

32 Farrugia A. Risk of variant Creutzfeldt-Jakob disease from factor concentrates: current perspectives. *Haemophilia* 2002; **8**: 230–5.

33 Burnouf T, Radosevich M. Nanofiltration of plasma-derived biopharmaceutical products. *Haemophilia* 2003; **9**: 24–37.

34 Makris M, Conlon CP, Watson HG. Immunization of patients with bleeding disorders. *Haemophilia* 2003; **9**: 541–6.

35 Jantsch-Plunger V, Beck G, Maurer W. PCR detection of a low viral load in a prothrombin complex concentrate that transmitted hepatitis B virus. *Vox Sang* 1995; **69**: 352–4.

36 Hubbard AR, Weller LJ, Bevan SA. A survey of one-stage and chromogenic potencies in therapeutic factor VIII concentrates. *Br J Haematol* 2002; **117**: 247–8.

37 Lee CA, Owens D, Bray G, *et al.* Pharmacokinetics of recombinant factor VIII (Recombinate) using one-stage clotting and chromogenic factor VIII assay. *Thromb Haemost* 1999; **82**: 1644–7.

38 Farrugia A. *Guide for the Assessment of Clotting Factor Concentrates for the Treatment of Hemophilia.* World Federation of Hemophilia (Montreal), 2003. Also available as a PDF file at www.wfh.org.

26 Products used to treat hemophilia: recombinant factor VIIa

Ulla Hedner

Background

Recombinant factor VIIa (rFVIIa) was developed for treatment of acute bleeding in hemophilia patients with inhibitors against factor VIII (FVIII) or FIX. Treatment of hemophilia patients with inhibitors remains a significant problem and includes treatment of acute bleeding as well as methods to induce immunologic tolerance in order to permanently eradicate the inhibitors.

Since the 1970s, prothrombin complex concentrates and activated prothrombin complex concentrates (aPCCs) have been used to treat hemophilia patients with inhibitors against FVIII or FIX. These concentrates contain all the vitamin K-dependent coagulation proteins, active forms of FIX and FX, and trace amounts of FVIII protein. The use of aPCCs has, however, been associated with a certain risk of the development of thromboembolic side-effects and the hemostatic effect in moderate to mild joint bleeds was only 50–60% [1]. One of the components in the aPCCs is activated FVII (FVIIa), which is the only activated coagulation protein that is not enzymatically active by itself. The requirement of tissue factor (TF) for FVIIa to become an active enzyme suggested that rFVIIa should be hemostatically active only at a local level, where TF is available. Using rFVIIa alone therefore should minimize the risk of inducing a systemic activation of the coagulation system and thereby the risk of systemic thromboembolic side-effects.

Mechanism of action of rFVIIa

Normal hemostasis is initiated by the complex formation between tissue factor (TF) and FVII or FVIIa. TF is expressed in a number of cells located in the deeper layers of the vessel wall and is exposed to the circulating blood only as a result of injury to the vessel wall [2]. During recent years, increasing knowledge of the whereabouts of TF has been accumulated. In the 1970s it was already being reported that platelet and platelet membranes enhanced the procoagulant activity of leukocytes [3]. A hemostatic effect of platelet membrane vesicles was demonstrated in thrombocytopenic rabbits in 1987 [4]. A transfer of TF-containing particles by monocytes and polymorphonuclear leukocytes to platelets, the process being dependent on the interaction of CD15 and P-selectin, was reported by Rauch and coworkers [5]. These authors thus showed that monocytes and possibly leukocytes may be sources of TF-containing membrane particles that are transferred to platelets. The presence in whole blood of TF-containing microparticles originating from platelets has been confirmed [6,7]. The group of Müller [6] demonstrated the presence of TF within platelets more specifically in the α-granules and the open canalicular system, an observation that has not, however, been confirmed by others [8]. As pointed out by several authors, under normal conditions the TF found on cell surfaces as well as in microvesicles is encrypted, which thus allows the circulation of such TF-containing particles to occur without generalized coagulation [5,9]. The de-encryption of TF bound to various membranes seems to require binding of the TF-containing particles to injured surfaces where hemostasis is required. Such a binding may be mediated by P-selectin and PSGL-1, CD18 integrins thereby involving both platelets and neutrophils [6,10–13]. Recently, the presence of an alternatively spliced human TF that is soluble, circulates in blood, and exhibits procoagulant activity when exposed to phospholipids was reported. This soluble TF has also been found to be incorporated into thrombi [14]. Although there are reports on the presence of TF-containing microvesicles in various situations, such as in a baboon model of lethal *Escherichia coli* sepsis [15], in patients with stable as well as unstable angina [16], and in healthy blood donors [17], the physiologic significance of all these findings is still not totally clear.

Approximately 1% of the total FVII protein mass is normally present in an activated form in the circulation. In the absence of FIX (severe hemophilia B) the amount of activated FVII (FVIIa) is significantly decreased, indicating that FIX plays a role in the initial activation of FVII [1,18]. Several coagulation proteins have been shown to be present in the extravascular compartment, and formation of FVII–TF complexes in the interstitial tissues has been demonstrated [1,18]. Such complexes may mediate the activation of the hemostatic mechanism demonstrated in normal individuals during normal circumstances, resulting in the formation of the normally occurring FIX, FX, and prothrombin activation peptides [19]. However, during normal conditions, this may not lead to the deposition of significant amounts of fibrin and would be consistent with the observation that only negligible amounts of extravascular, cross-linked fibrin were present in normal guinea-pig tissues, unless there was increased vascular permeability [1,18].

Following an injury to the vessel wall, an increased exposure of TF to the circulating blood will occur. Furthermore, von Willebrand factor (VWF) and FVIII, as well as platelets, will become available. As a result of the formation of TF–FVII complexes, FX is activated into FXa, which converts a limited amount of prothrombin into thrombin. This first phase has been called the "initiation" and is followed by the "priming" and finally the "propagation" [8].

The "priming" phase includes the activation of FVIII by the thrombin formed during the "initiation," which leads to the release of VWF. Furthermore, FXI and platelets adhering to the site of injury, partly mediated by VWF bound to collagen, will be activated by the initially formed thrombin. [8]. As pointed out by Monroe and coworkers [8], the binding to matrix proteins, especially collagen, partially activates platelets and localizes them near a site of TF exposure. A tentative synergy between the collagen and thrombin activation of platelets has been suggested [8]. On thrombin activation of the platelets, degranulation occurs and partially active FV is released from the platelet α-granules, and thrombin cleaves the FV to a fully active form. Thrombin activation of platelets also results in the exposure of negatively charged phospholipids on the platelet surface, providing the template for binding of FIXa (activated during the "initiation" by TF–FVIIa), FVIIIa, FVa, FXIa, and FXa [20] and activation of more thrombin.

During the "propagation" phase, FIXa–FVIIIa as well as FXa–FVa complexes form, and a burst of thrombin is generated on the platelet surface. FXIa bound to the platelet surface enhances further the activation of FIX into FIXa, thereby increasing the thrombin formation further. The platelet surface seems to play a central role in the regulation of thrombin generation and extends beyond the expression of phosphatidylserine on the outer surface, resulting in a negatively charged surface [8]. Increasing evidence indicates a significant variability of platelet procoagulant response in individuals [8,21].

Full thrombin generation is necessary for full hemostasis. It generates fibrin monomers by splitting off the fibrinopeptides A and B from the fibrinogen molecule. Furthermore, thrombin activates FXIII, which is required for cross-linking of the soluble fibrin monomers. A fully cross-linked fibrin plug is more resistant against premature fibrinolysis. High concentrations of thrombin are required for full activation of the so-called "thrombin activatable fibrinolytic inhibitor" (TAFI), which protects the fibrin plug from premature lysis by downregulating fibrinolysis. Full thrombin burst as well as the rate of thrombin generation are important also for the fibrin structure of the hemostatic plug [22].

Hemophilia patients have a normal "initiation" and "priming" phase of hemostasis, with a normal formation of FX and prothrombin activation peptides. The intact TF pathway results in a normal platelet activation, probably the reason for the normal bleeding time seen in hemophilia patients. However, in hemophilic dogs, in which normal initial bleeding time was observed, frequent rebleedings and the formation of larger than normal hemostatic plugs rich in channels and areas of loosely packed platelets with an incomplete fibrin cap were observed [23]. Recently, the formation of loose fibrin clots with a high permeability constant was reported in hemophilia plasma containing platelets after recalcification [22]. The fibrin permeability constant was dose dependent with regard to FVIII (hemophilia A plasma) or FIX (hemophilia B plasma). The fibrin clot structure was also found to be influenced by the concentration of prothrombin in a study showing a loose fibrin structure in the presence of prothrombin concentrations of less than 10% [24], supporting the importance of coagulation factors for the fibrin structure and thereby for the formation of stable fibrin plugs efficient in providing full and maintained hemostasis.

In hemophilia, the thrombin generation is impaired due to the lack of FVIII or FIX, which results in an impaired activation of FXIII and TAFI, as well as in the formation of a loose fibrin structure in the clots formed. It is thus obvious that the impaired hemostasis in hemophilia depends on the formation of defective hemostatic plugs that are sensitive to lysis and therefore fail to sustain hemostasis.

rFVIIa in hemophilia

In 1987 it was suggested that rFVIIa may bind not only to TF but also to phospholipids [25]. A TF-independent FVIIa activation of FX was independently suggested by others, and later FVIIa was demonstrated to bind weakly to thrombin-activated platelets in a cell-based model and enhance the FX activation on this surface, resulting in a dose-dependent enhancement of the thrombin generation. In the same model, rFVIIa was found to increase the rate and extent of platelet activation [1,26]. Also, the adhesion of platelets from a patient with Glanzmann's thrombasthenia increased independently of TF in the presence of rFVIIa [27]. Furthermore, the increased fibrin permeability seen in hemophilia plasma normalized after addition of rFVIIa in concentrations of 1.2 µg/mL and higher supports the importance of thrombin generation for the fibrin structure and clot quality [22].

In an *in vitro* system in which platelets were substituted for by synthetic phospholipid vesicles, zymogen FVII was demonstrated to prolong the lag phase of thrombin generation and it was claimed that the presence of zymogen FVII may compete with FVIIa for binding to TF and that the effect of rFVIIa in hemophilia could be explained by this mechanism [28]. However, in the platelet-containing system no such competition between zymogen FVII and FVIIa was found.

In summary, the hemostatic effect of exogenously added rFVIIa in high doses seems to be mediated by enhancing the rate of thrombin generation on thrombin-activated platelet surfaces, thereby ensuring enough thrombin formation, necessary for providing a fully stabilized fibrin plug with a tight fibrin structure that makes it resistant to premature lysis. The enhanced thrombin generation also ensures a full activation of FXIII and TAFI.

Clinical experience with rFVIIa in hemophilia patients with inhibitors

Recombinant FVIIa was developed in baby hamster kidney cells and was shown to be principally identical to the plasma-derived FVIIa. It did not induce any systemic activation of the coagulation system in several animal models [18].

Successful use of rFVIIa in major surgery, including major orthopedic surgery such as total hip replacement and bilateral knee replacement, in a number of hemophilia patients (both hemophilia A and B) has been reported [29,30]. Most patients were also given antifibrinolytic therapy (tranexamic acid), and the dose schedule recommended was 90–120 µg/kg rFVIIa given every 2 h during the first 24 h depending on type of surgery and the clinical response. Successful use of rFVIIa has also been demonstrated in minor surgery and dental surgery [30].

A prospective, double-blind, randomized trial, published in 1998, compared two doses of rFVIIa (35 and 90 µg/kg) in hemophilia patients with inhibitors who were undergoing surgery [31]. Bolus injections of rFVIIa were given every second hour for the first 48 h. Thereafter, the same dose was given every 2–6 h for an additional 3 days. The study included major surgical procedures such as synovectomies, hip arthroplasties, and knee joint replacement. A significant difference in efficacy favoring the high-dose group was observed from day 3 to day 5 with regard to maintained hemostasis, number of days of dosing required, and the number of injections. Based on the results, the investigators concluded that rFVIIa appears to be an efficacious first-line agent in surgery in hemophilia patients with inhibitors, and the 90 µg/kg dose was more effective for both minor and major procedures [31].

Continuous infusion (CI) of coagulation factor concentrates has been recommended [32] and was tried also for rFVIIa [1]. Schulman and coworkers [33] used continuous infusion of rFVIIa in two patients with hemophilia A and inhibitors, the dose following the initial bolus dose of 90 µg/kg was based on the individual clearance and varied between 15.5 µg/kg/h and 31 µg/kg/h. In a study of elective surgery in six hemophilia A patients with inhibitors and two patients with acquired hemophilia, using an initial bolus dose of 90 µg/kg followed by CI at a fixed rate of 16.5 µg/kg/h showed effective hemostasis in only one out of two minor procedures and in two of six major operations. No thrombotic events were reported [1]. Another study using a similar dose schedule of 90 µg/kg as a bolus followed by CI at a rate of 17–18 µg/kg/h showed an overall efficacy of 70% (30 out of 43 episodes effective). However, for bleedings in the oral cavity, this regimen was effective in producing hemostasis in only one of seven patients, while 27 of 37 bleedings in other parts of the body were effectively treated, thus supporting the conclusion that rFVIIa in the dose used may be less effective in bleedings associated with substantial fibrinolytic activity [34]. A somewhat modified schedule [35] for continuous infusion of rFVIIa during surgery (bolus 90–150 µg/kg; CI 20 µg/kg/h in major surgery; 17–16 µg/kg/h in minor procedures) demonstrated satisfactory hemostasis in 30 out of 35 episodes (88%), which should be compared with the 95–100% efficacy achieved with the bolus regimen (90–120 µg/kg every 2 h for the first 24 h) as described by Ingerslev and coworkers [29].

Recently, a study using an initial bolus of 90 µg/kg followed by continuous infusion of 50 µg/kg/h showed an overall efficacy of 89% [36].

Since 1988, rFVIIa also has been given to hemophilia patients suffering from *serious bleedings* in the central nervous system, intraperitoneal and retroperitoneal, as well as muscle (compartment syndrome) bleedings. Essentially, the same dose schedule as that recommended in surgery has been used. The overall effective response after 8 and 24 h in the first 55 consecutive bleeds was 91% and 90% respectively [30]. A similar efficacy (97%) was recently reported from an open-label, uncontrolled, emergency-use program including 35 bleeding episodes in 23 patients (hemophilia A and B patients or acquired hemophilia). In this program, only patients who were experiencing a limb-threatening bleeding episode and had previously failed on alternative therapy were included. The dose schedule was 90 µg/kg (a maximum of 120 µg/kg) given every 2 h. Adverse events were reported in 6 of 23 patients (26%), the majority of which (15 of 16 events; 94%) were considered to be unrelated to rFVIIa therapy. The remaining event was a treatment failure (increasing hemarthrosis during treatment with rFVIIa in a dose of 90 µg/kg) [37].

A randomized, double-blind, multicenter trial included 178 joint, muscle, and mucocutaneous bleeding episodes in 78 patients treated with two doses of rFVIIa (35 and 70 µg/kg) [38]. A substantial delay before start of treatment (8.4–10.0 h) may have contributed to the lack of significant difference in efficacy between the two groups. The effect of early treatment as well as of regular treatment several times per week in preventing the development of long-term arthropathy is well documented [39]. In order to facilitate an early initiation of treatment, rFVIIa was studied in a home treatment setting (dose of 90 µg/kg at 3-h intervals). An average of 2.3 doses was required to achieve hemostasis [40], indicating that the dose used may not have been optimal. Later studies showing an increased clearance rate of rFVIIa in children than in adults [1] also support the use of higher doses in order to achieve full effect already after one single dose of rFVIIa.

In summary, rFVIIa has been shown to induce hemostasis in severe hemophilia patients with inhibitors against FVIII or FIX both in major surgery and in serious bleedings. A dose of 90 µg/kg given every 2 h was more efficient than 35 µg/kg. Several series of major and minor surgery have been successfully performed. CI of rFVIIa (90 µg/kg followed by CI at a fixed rate of 16.5 µg/kg/h) to inhibitor patients undergoing elective surgery was not effective (hemostasis in 38%). A modified CI schedule (50 µg/kg/h) showed an efficacy rate of 89%. The improved efficacy using bolus administration may be explained by the fact that rFVIIa enhances the peak generation of thrombin on the activated platelet surface in a dose-dependent way and the rate as well as the amount of thrombin formed is essential for the formation of a tight fibrin hemostatic plug resistant against premature lysis. In a home treatment setting, hemostasis was achieved in around 90% but an average of 2.3 injections were required.

Dosing and monitoring of rFVIIa in hemophilia patients

Current experience indicates that rFVIIa given in doses of 90–120 µg/kg as a bolus every 2 h at least for the first 24 h is effective in acute bleedings and in surgery [30]. The requirement of more than one injection of 90 µg/kg in a home treatment setting indicates, however, a suboptimal dose for full hemostatic effect, at least in some individuals. In early *in vitro* experiments, normalization of the aPTT required a concentration of rFVIIa of 3.8 µg/mL. Assuming a specific activity of rFVIIa of 50 U/µg (NovoSeven package insert), this would roughly correspond to 190 U/mL of plasma of FVII:C, which would require a dose of around 320 µg/kg (recovery 47%). However, the optimal individual dose of rFVIIa may vary substantially, the key issues being a wide interindividual variation in the capacity of thrombin generation on the platelets [8], a difference in clearance especially between adults and children [1], and a substantial individual variation of recovery. The patients treated initially with rFVIIa were given lower doses than indicated by the *in vitro* experiments. Doses between 90 and 120 µg/kg also resulted in a high efficacy rate in major surgery, provided the doses were repeated every second hour. In order to achieve full hemostasis in a joint or muscle bleed by one single dose, children will probably require higher doses. Furthermore, by enlarging the population subjected to treatment with rFVIIa, any individual variations in the thrombin generation capacity on activated platelets, as well as any variation in recovery of rFVIIa, may show up as a number of patients requiring higher doses for full hemostatic effect, as indicated by reported failures.

Although only anecdotal so far, higher doses of rFVIIa given as bolus have been reported to improve the hemostatic effect in a few children [41,42]. In the patient described by Cooper and coworkers [42], daily doses of rFVIIa prevented spontaneous breakthrough bleeds during the course of mechanical traction of bilateral knee joint flexion contractures, indicating that rFVIIa may maintain clinical hemostasis with a prophylactic dose of rFVIIa given only once daily, at least in some patients. The dose given to this specific patient, with a clearance rate of about three times the adult average, was 320–240 µg/kg for almost 2 months without any signs of systemic activation of the hemostatic system or thromboembolic events. In another patient, the vicious circle of repeated bleeds in a target ankle joint was broken by daily doses of rFVIIa (90 µg/kg). No pharmacokinetic data were reported in this patient [43]. Hopefully, clinical trials will soon be performed and reported using higher doses of rFVIIa in children, as well as a study on the use of rFVIIa in prevention of joint and muscle bleedings.

Monitoring of rFVIIa therapy

The hemostatic effect of rFVIIa seems to be mediated through enhancing the thrombin generation at the site of injury on the surface of thrombin-activated platelets. The exact relation between the plasma level of FVII:C or FVIIa and this local thrombin generation is not known. Based on experience, the FVII:C levels immediately after an injection should be higher than 30 U/mL in order to ensure satisfactory thrombin generation and hemostasis. In some patients, especially children, this level should potentially be much higher.

Currently, a number of assay techniques measuring thrombin generation are undergoing development and evaluation. One of them, the modified thrombelastogram method ROTEG (Rotational Thrombelastography, Pentapharm, Munich, Germany), has been studied in hemophilia patients. The modified ROTEG analysis used includes a highly diluted TF to increase the sensitivity of the method to changes in the FVIIa concentrations [44].

Use of rFVIIa in other bleeding disorders

The hemostatic effect of rFVIIa seems to be mediated through activation of FX and thereby enhances the thrombin generation on activated platelets at the site of injury. Improved thrombin generation appears to initiate the formation of a tight fibrin hemostatic plug that is more resistant to lysis. A number of situations associated with excessive hemorrhage may have an impaired thrombin generation owing to low levels of circulating coagulation proteins, low platelet counts, and other platelet defects. Furthermore, by ensuring the formation of a tight fibrin plug resistant to fibrinolysis, rFVIIa may contribute to an improved hemostasis in situations with increased fibrinolysis. Recent data seem to suggest that rFVIIa may induce hemostasis in a broad range of such clinical situations [1,26]. Unfortunately, most of these data are still anecdotal (case reports). However, clinical trials are ongoing or planned in several of these type of patients.

Safety

In clinical data from studies of rFVIIa in hemophilia, including elective surgery, treatment of joint and muscle bleedings in a home setting [1], no serious side-effects were recorded. The overall estimated incidence of serious adverse events, including thrombotic complications, in the more than 600 patients with hemophilia A and B participating in clinical trials with rFVIIa was found to be about 1%.

Acute nonfatal myocardial infarction (AMI) has been reported in eight patients, three with congenital hemophilia and five with acquired hemophilia. All except for one patient were elderly and had known coronary artery disease. Successful and safe use of rFVIIa in patients that had previously had a myocardial infarction associated with the use of activated prothrombin complex concentrates has been reported [45].

Despite the fact that patients with proven septicemia were included in the group of patients with life- and limb-threatening bleedings treated with rFVIIa, DIC seems to be an infrequent complication during rFVIIa therapy [18,45].

References

1 Hedner U, Erhardtsen E. Potential role of rFVIIa as a hemostatic agent. *Clin Adv Hematol Oncol* 2003; **1**: 112–19.

2 Rapaport SI, Rao LVM. The tissue factor pathway: How it has become a "prima ballerina". *Thromb Haemost* 1995; **74**: 7–17.

3 Niemetz J, Marcus AJ. The stimulatory effect of platelets and platelet membranes on the procoagulant activity of leukocytes. *J Clin Invest* 1974; **54**: 1437–43.

4 McGill M, Fugman DA, Vittorio N, Darrow C. Platelet membrane vesicles reduced microvascular bleeding times in thrombocytopenic rabbits. *J Lab Clin Med* 1987; **109**: 127–33.

5 Rauch U, Bonderman D, Bohrmann B, *et al.* Transfer of tissue factor from leukocytes to platelets is mediated by CD15 and tissue factor. *Blood* 2000; **961**: 170–5.

6 Müller I, Alex M, Klocke A, *et al.* Microvesicle and platelet associated tissue factor promote intiation of coagulation. *XIX Congr Int Soc Thromb Haemost* 2003 (Abstract OC007).

7 Siddiqui FA, Desai H, Amirkhosravi A, *et al.* Tissue factor is present in platelet-derived microparticles from healthy donors. *XIX Congr Int Soc Thromb Haemost* 2003 (Abstract PO534).

8 Monroe D, Hoffman M, Roberts HR. Platelets and thrombin generation. *Arterioscler Thromb Vasc Biol* 2002; **22**: 1381–9.

9 Engelmann B, Luther T, Müller I. Intravascular tissue factor pathway — a model for rapid initiation of coagulation within the blood vessel. *Thromb Haemost* 2003; **89**: 3–8.

10 Giessen PLA, Rauch U, Bohrmann B, *et al. Blood*-borne tissue factor: another view of thrombosis. *Proc Natl Acad Sci USA* 1999; **96**: 2311–15.

11 André P, Hartwell P, Hrachovinova I, *et al.* Pro-coagulant state resulting from high levels of soluble P-selectin in blood. *Proc Natl Acad Sci USA* 2000; **97**: 13835–40.

12 Snapp KR, Heitzig CE, Kansas GS. Attachment of the PSGL-1 cytoplasmic domain to the actin cytoskeleton is essential for leukocyte rolling on P-selectin. *Blood* 2002: **99**: 4494–502.

13 Hrachovinová I, Cambien B, Hafezi-Moghadam A, *et al.* Interaction of P-selectin and PSGL-1 generates microparticles that correct hemostasis in a mouse model of hemophilia A. *Nature Med* 2003; **98**: 1020–5.

14 Bogdanov VY, Balasubramanian V, Hatchcock J, *et al.* Alternatively spliced human tissue factor: a circulating, soluble, thrombogenic protein. *Nature Med* 2003; **94**: 458–62.

15 Lupu F, Westmuckett AD, Taylor FB Jr. Cell and tissue-specific expression of tissue factor pathway proteins in a baboon model of lethal *E. coli* sepsis. *Blood* 2002; **100** (Abstract 1933).

16 Camera M, Frigerio M, Marenzi GC, *et al.* Platelet-associated tissue factor expression in patients with unstable coronary artery disease. *XIX Congr Int Soc Thromb* 2003 (Abstract OC009).

17 Siddiqui FA, Dessai H, Amirkhosravi A, *et al.* Platelet microparticles from healthy donors contain tissue factor. *Blood* 2002; **100**: Abstract 1936.

18 Hedner U, Erhardtsen E. Potential role for rFVIIa in transfusion medicine. *Transfusion* 2002; **42**: 114–24.

19 Bauer KA, Mannucci PM, Gringeri A, *et al.* Factor IXa–factor VIIIa–cell surface complex does not contribute to the basal activation of the coagulation mechanism in vivo. *Blood* 1992; **79**: 2039–47.

20 Monroe DM, Hoffman M, Oliver JA, Roberts HR. Platelet activity of high-dose factor VIIa is independent of tissue factor. *Br J Haematol* 1997; **99**: 542–7.

21 Sumner WT, Monroe DM, Hoffman M. Variability in platelet procoagulant activity in healthy volunteers. *Thromb Res* 1996; **81**: 533–43.

22 He S, Blombäck M, Jacobsson Ekman G, Hedner U. The role of recombinant factor VIIa (rFVIIa) in fibrin structure in the absence of FVIII/FIX. *J Thromb Haemost* 2003; **1**: 1215–19.

23 Hovig T, Rowsell HC, Dodds WJ, *et al.* Experimental hemostasis in normal dogs and dogs with congenital disorders of blood coagulation. *Blood* 1967; **305**: 636–68.

24 Wolberg AS, Monroe DM, Roberts HR, Hoffman M. Elevated prothrombin results in clots with an altered fiber structure: a possible mechanism of the increased thrombotic risk. *Blood* 2003; **1018**: 3008–13.

25 Hedner U. Factor VIIa in the treatment of haemophilia. *Blood Coagul Fibrinol* 1990; **1**: 307–17.

26 Allen GA, Hoffman M, Roberts HR, Monroe DM. Recombinant activated factor VII: its mechanism of action and role in the control of hemorrhage. *Can J Anesth* 2002; **49**(10): S7–S14.

27 Lisman T, Moschatsis S, Adelmeijer J, Nieuwenhuis HK, de Groot PG. Recombinant factor VIIa enhances deposition of platelets with congenital or acquired αIIbβ3 deficiency to endothelial cell matrix and collagen under conditions of flow via tissue factor-independent thrombin generation. *Blood* 2003; **101**: 1864–70.

28 van´t Veer C, Golden NJ, Mann KG. Inhibition of thrombin generation by the zymogen factor VII: Implications for the treatment of hemophilia A by factor VIIa. *Blood* 2000; **95**: 1330–5.

29 Ingerslev J, Friedman D, Gastineau D, *et al.* Major surgery in haemophilic patients with inhibitors using recombinant factor VIIa. *Haemostasis* 1996; **26**: 118–23.

30 Hedner U, Ingerslev J. Clinical use of recombinant FVIIa (rFVIIa). *Transfus Sci* 1998; **19**: 163–76.

31 Shapiro AD, Gilchrist GS, Hoots WK, *et al.* Prospective, randomized trial of two doses of rFVIIa (NovoSeven) in haemophilia patients with inhibitors undergoing surgery. *Thromb Haemost* 1998; **80**: 773–8.

32 McMillan CW, Webster WP, Roberts HR, Blythe WB. Continuous intravenous infusion of factor VIII in classic haemophilia. *Br J Haematol* 1970; **18**: 659–67.

33 Schulman S, Bech Jensen M, Varon D, *et al.* Feasibility of using recombinant factor VIIa in continuous infusion. *Thromb Haemost* 1996; **75**: 432–6.

34 Mauser-Bunschoter EP, Koopman MMW, Goede-Bolder ADE, *et al.* and the Recombinante Factor VIIa Data Collection Group. Efficacy of recombinant factor VIIa administered by continuous infusion to haemophilia patients with inhibitors. *Haemophilia* 2002; **8**: 649–56.

35 Santagostino E, Morfini M, Rocino A, *et al.* Relationship between factor VII activity and clinical efficacy of recombinant factor VIIa by continuous infusion to patients with factor VIII inhibitors. *Thromb Haemost* 2001; **86**: 954–8.

36 Ludlam CA, Smith MP, Morfini M, *et al.* A prospective study of recombinant activated factor VII administered by continuous infusion to inhibitor patients undergoing elective major orthopaedic surgery: a pharmacokinetic and efficacy evaluation. *Br J Haematol* 2003; **120**: 808–13.

37 Arkin S, Blei F, Fetten J, *et al.* Human coagulation factor FVIIa (recombinant) in the management of limb-threatening bleeds unresponsive to alternative therapies: results from the NovoSeven emergency-use programme in patients with severe haemophilia or with acquired inhibitors. *Blood Coag Fibrinol* 2000; **11**: 255–9.

38 Lusher JM, Ingersler J, Roberts HR, Hedner U. Clinical experience

with recombinant factor VIIa. A review. *Blood Coag Fibrinolysis* 1998; **9**: 119–28.

39 Nilsson IM, Berntorp E, Lofqvist T, Pettersson H. Twenty-five years' experience of prophylactic treatment in severe haemophilia A and B. *J Int Med* 1992; **232**: 25–32.

40 Key NS, Aledort LM, Beardsley D, *et al.* Home treatment of mild to moderate bleeding using recombinant factor VIIa (NovoSeven) in haemophiliacs with inhibitors. *Thromb Haemost* 1998; **80**: 912–18.

41 Kenet G, Lubetsky A, Luboshitz J, Martinowitz U. A new approach to treatment of bleeding episodes in young hemophilia patients: a single bolus megadose of recombinant activated factor VII (Novo-Seven®). *J Thromb Haemost* 2003; **1**: 450–5.

42 Cooper HA, Jones CP, Campion E, *et al.* Rationale for the use of high dose rFVIIa in a high-titre inhibitor patient with haemophilia B during major orthopaedic procedures. *Haemophilia* 2001; **7**: 517–22.

43 Saxon BR, Shanks D, Bryony Jory C, Williams V. Effective prophylaxis with daily recombinant factor VIIa (rFVIIa-Novoseven) in a child with high titre inhibitors and a target joint. *Thromb Haemost* 2001; **86**: 1126–7.

44 Friedrich U, Tengborn L, Hedner U. Assay analysis on a hemophilia A patient with inhibitors under factor VII therapy. *Ann Hematol* 2003; **82** (Suppl. 1): 26.

45 Levi M. Safety of recombinant factor VIIa. *J Thromb Haemost* 2004 (in press).

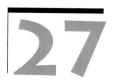

Products used to treat hemophilia: dosing

Miguel A. Escobar

The temporary correction of the coagulation defect is the mainstay of treatment in hemophilia. However, the "ideal" dose of factor VIII (FVIII) or FIX that needs to be administered to invariably achieve hemostasis without "overtreating" is unknown. To date, there are no controlled clinical trials that address this important question, mainly because of the ethical implications of reducing dosing to a threshold of bleeding symptoms. Dosing for hemophilia treatment has been arrived at by empirical assessment, essentially "trial and error" based on the pharmacokinetics of the factors and the characteristics of replacement product [1].

Historical background

Since hemarthroses constitute the most common manifestation of severe hemophilia, the prevention of this morbid clinical state has been long studied. Brinkhous and collaborators treated hemophilic dogs in the initial studies in 1947 and continued to study outcomes of therapy for more than 20 years. When plasma was given every 3.5 days to the animals, the frequency and severity of hemarthrosis decreased to where there was no evidence of joint disease when compared with the administration of small and infrequent transfusions of plasma [2,3]. Their observations were fundamental for the understanding of dosing in prophylaxis.

In the 1950s, Brinkhous and his group [4], and Biggs and Macfarlane [5], working independently, reported their observations in the treatment of bleeding in patients with hemophilia A. Their conclusion was that to maintain adequate hemostasis in these individuals, FVIII levels of at least 35% of normal are necessary for treating minor injuries and levels of around 50% of normal are required for major trauma or surgery.

In the 1960s, cryoprecipitate and a fraction of human plasma (fraction I of Cohn) became available as an alternative source of therapy for patients with hemophilia A. One of the advantages of these products was the need for smaller amounts of volume when compared with plasma [6,7]. Subsequently, several FVIII and FIX concentrates became available for the treatment of hemophilia A and B respectively, significantly facilitating the management of these diseases.

Based on the principle that moderate hemophiliacs (FVIII or FIX level above 1%) rarely develop severe disabling arthropathy [8–10], multiple studies were performed between 1967 and 1982 using low doses of factor for the treatment of acute hemarthrosis with variable results (Table 27.1).

In most cases, treatment was administered within the first few hours of onset of bleeding. It is interesting to note that even very low doses of factor replacement (less than 10 U/kg) were effective in 73–100% of cases. Possible explanations for some of these results are: (i) studies were carried out during summer camps for hemophiliacs during which close surveillance and early treatment were the norm; (ii) infusions were administered for traumatic hemarthroses only; (iii) target joints were not included; and (iv) only mild and moderate bleeds were assessed. Further studies by Aronstam *et al.* [11,12] evaluated different treatment regimens versus severity of the hemarthroses. As expected, lower doses of factor replacement were associated with higher failure rates in target joints and bleeds that were ongoing for some time prior to administration of replacement therapy.

Pharmacokinetics and dosage calculations

The appropriate dose of FVIII or FIX for replacement therapy is an amount of the relevant clotting factor that will provide satisfactory hemostasis to control a bleeding episode [13]. Regardless of the product used, the dose of FVIII or FIX should be calculated in terms of units per kilogram of body weight. All calculations should be made with the assumption that one unit of FVIII per kilogram of body weight will raise the circulating FVIII level about 0.02 U/mL, and one unit of FIX per kilogram of body weight will raise the plasma FIX by 0.01 U/mL. Much of the difference in expected recovery between FVIII and FIX is due to variable volumes of distribution. FVIII circulates almost exclusively intravascularly and FIX diffuses into the extracellular water space [14].

The dose needed to achieve hemostasis varies widely and choice of dose needs to be calculated taking into account a number of parameters: severity of the bleeding episode; pharmacologic properties of the clotting factors, which include the half-disappearance time; and the *in vivo* factor recovery based on the volume of distribution within the vascular compartments. The doses suggested in Table 27.2 serve as a guide to calculate the approximate amount required and are not based on randomized clinical trials. Therapeutic infusion of replacement factor should be administered as early as possible in an attempt to prevent permanent damage to joints and soft tissues and should continue until adequate hemostasis has been achieved or wound healing is complete. Bleeding complications in associa-

Table 27.1 Treatment of hemarthrosis with low doses of FVIII and IX.

Dose (U/kg BW)	Factor plasma level (%)	Number of treated episodes	Success rate (%)	Therapeutic material	Type of bleed	Reference
23	24–33	25	56–64	Cryo	Hemarthrosis	27
20–30	40–50	51	92	FVIII, other	Hemarthrosis	26
10		51	96	FVIII	Hemarthrosis	13
7–9		106	90	FVIII	Hemarthrosis	28
11–13		173	79			
15–17		64	94			
8–12		62	100	FVIII	Hemarthrosis, other	29
7.5–12.5	15–25	196	89	FVIII	Hemarthrosis, other	30
12.5–20	25–40	349	94			
3–7		60	100	FVIII/FIX	Hemarthrosis	31
31	53	144	99	Cryo	Hemarthrosis, other	32
7		119	73	FVIII, other	Hemarthrosis	33
14		134	75			
28		86	64			
11–16		144	78	FVIII, other	Hemarthrosis	34
7		95	89	FVIII	Hemarthrosis	35
14		106	77			

Reprinted with permission from ref. 1.

Table 27.2 Guidelines for factor replacement in severe and moderate hemophilia A and B.

Site of hemorrhage	Optimal factor level (%)	Factor VIII	Factor IX	Duration in days
Joint	30–50	15–25	30–50	1–2
Muscle	30–50	15–25	30–50	1–2
Gastrointestinal tract	40–60	30–40	40–60	7–10
Oral mucosa	30–50	15–25	30–50	Until healing
Epistaxis	30–50	15–25	30–50	Until healing
Hematuria	30–50	15–25	30–50	Until healing
Central nervous system	80–100	50	80–100	10–21
Retroperitoneal	50–100	30–50	60–100	7–14
Trauma or surgery	50–100	30–50	60–100	Until healing

Reprinted with permission and modifications from ref. 1.

tion with surgical procedures can be seen in 4–23% of cases, usually in the postoperative period rather than during the surgery [15–18].

Factor replacement can be administered by either intermittent bolus or continuous infusion. Some advantages of the latter are the following: total factor use may decrease by as much as 30% [19,20]; achievement of a faster steady state in plasma; maintenance of a constant therapeutic factor level; and avoidance of peaks and troughs, which facilitates laboratory monitoring [21] (for further details on continuous infusion see Chapter 8). Of note, when continuous infusion is started, the dose needed is often higher during the first few postoperative days because of the rapid clearance of the factor in the immediate postoperative period [22].

Ideally, for individuals who must undergo elective major sur-

gical procedures, a recovery and half-life study should be performed during a nonbleeding state with a 3–5 half-life washout period. A dose of the therapeutic product to increase the plasma level to 100% should be used and samples for factor activity should be drawn at times 0, 15, 30, 60 min, 4, 8, 12, and 24 h post infusion. For FIX additional time points at 36, 48 and 56 h should be drawn given the longer half-life [23].

Based on the pharmacokinetic study of the individual, an initial "loading" dose and subsequent doses can be calculated. For example, in an individual with FVIII deficiency and a normal recovery and half-life, factor dosing can be calculated using the following formula:

Initial loading dose = (desired FVIII level − patient baseline FVIII) × body weight (kg) × 0.5 unit/kg.

Assuming that 8–12 h after the initial bolus the plasma level will decrease by about 50%, further doses can be given of one-half of the loading dose every 8–12 h. If constant infusion is employed, the initial loading dose should be divided by 12, which is equal to the number of units per hour of FVIII concentrate. For example, to raise the FVIII level to 100% in a 70-kg individual with less than 1% activity, the initial loading dose will be 3500 units followed by boluses of 1750 units every 8–12 h. For continuous infusion, 292 units per hour will be the calculated dose in this scenario. FVIII levels should be monitored and ongoing dosing adjusted accordingly.

The dose calculations for FIX concentrates are different from those used in FVIII deficiency because the recovery of infused FIX is lower (~50%) owing to the diffusion over a larger volume. In addition, there is some evidence to suggest that FIX binds to elements on the vessel wall, more specifically to collagen type IV [24]. Thus, to raise to 100% of normal a 70-kg severely affected patient, 7000 units should be given as a bolus, followed by half this amount every 12–18 h. The continuous infusion dosing for this scenario can be calculated by dividing the loading dose by 24, i.e., approximately 292 units of FIX per hour [25].

For those individuals with a rapid initial phase decay or consumption (more than 50% decline in 6 h), a second bolus of FVIII or FIX can be given (approximately 50% of initial bolus) within 3–6 h of starting the surgery to avoid excessive intraoperative and immediate postoperative hemorrhage. Thereafter, half or more of the initial loading dose should be readministered every 12 h in order to maintain nadir factor levels greater than 50%. Factor activity should be measured daily and adjusted to maintain the desired level (see Table 27.2).

In the 1970s, home therapy was introduced as supplies of factor production became more widely available and as self-infusion was taught more commonly. This made a great impact on the treatment of hemophilia. This mode of treatment has substantially improved the quality of life of these individuals, especially those with severe hemophilia, since it reduces visits to the hospital and prevents long-term complications such as arthropathy when early treatment is initiated. As an indication for home infusion, a minimal spontaneous bleeding episode is defined as any symptom of pain or distress recognized by the patient in a joint or soft-tissue space. Minimal bleeding or hemarthrosis at an early stage may not be associated with significant edema, erythema or heat, and usually there is no known trauma [13]. Doses as small as 10 U/kg of FVIII or FIX have been proven to be effective in this type of bleeding and theoretically will lead to a plasma level of approximately 20% in FVIII or 10% in FIX activity. Such dosing proved successful in the management of 49 of 51 early joint hemorrhages in hemophilia A patients described by Abildgaard in 1975 [13]. It should be noted that this dose is not adequate for full-blown hemarthroses or for bleeding in critical anatomical areas (head and neck, throat, wrists, hand, foot, abdomen, or gastrointestinal tract).

Moderate bleeding episodes (hemarthrosis, advanced soft-tissue hemorrhage) often respond to an early infusion of 20–25 U/kg, which will correspond to a plasma level of 40–50% FVIII activity or 20–25% FIX activity. Honig et al. [26] reported successful treatment of acute hemarthrosis in 48 of 51 episodes using a single dose of 20–30 U of FVIII per kilogram of body weight. In many of these individuals, a single infusion is sufficient to control the bleeding; however, if no improvement is noted in 12–24 h or if significant symptoms persist, a second infusion should be administered.

During severe bleeding episodes (central nervous system, surgical procedures, and severe trauma) larger doses of replacement therapy are necessary. In addition, maintenance doses are needed to sustain hemostatic levels until bleeding is controlled or, if surgery is required, until the wound is well healed. This may take up to 10–20 days of replacement therapy depending on the surgery. For FVIII-deficient individuals, an initial infusion of 40–50 U/kg should be sufficient to obtain hemostasis in this context and levels should be maintained by repeated doses of at least 20–25 U/kg at approximately 12-h intervals to maintain physiologic circulating levels of the deficient clotting factor for a specified duration (see Table 27.2). Factor IX replacement should be started with an initial bolus of 80–100 U/kg followed by repeated doses of 40–50 U/kg every 18–24 h.

Treatment guidelines for specific bleeding episodes

Mouth and neck region

Bleeding from the floor of the mouth, pharynx, or epiglottic area can result in partial or complete airway obstruction. External compression of airway due to hemorrhage can also be seen after placement of neck or subclavian catheters in hemophilic individuals. Hence, such bleeding should be treated with aggressive replacement therapy of the deficient factor until complete resolution of the bleeding is established. Doses to maintain factor levels above 80% should be the goal of treatment.

Complicated joint bleeds

Hip joint or acetabular hemorrhages are of major concern because of increased intra-articular pressure from accumulated blood. The concomitant inflammation may lead to aseptic necrosis of the femoral head. Replacement therapy should start promptly. These individuals can be treated with twice-daily infusions to sustain a factor level above 30% for at least 3 days, along with enforced bed rest.

Iliopsoas hemorrhages

Iliopsoas bleeds are less frequently encountered in young children. Together with pain, common clinical manifestations of iliopsoas bleeding are upward flexion of the thigh, discomfort on passive extension, and decreased sensation over the ipsilateral thigh due to compression of the sacral plexus root of the femoral nerve. Twice-daily infusion should be administered to maintain a factor level above 20% for about 3 days. Bed rest should be enforced.

Compartment syndrome

Bleeding into closed-compartment muscle and tissue areas such as hand, wrist, forearm, and anterior or posterior tibial compartments may result in compression of nerves and blood vessels. Initial symptoms such as pain and edema can be preceded by paresthesias and loss of distal pulses. Prompt treatment with replacement factor is indicated to maintain levels of around 30–50% of normal. If replacement therapy fails to stop the progression, surgical decompression may be indicated.

Central nervous system hemorrhages

These are usually traumatic in origin and should be considered an emergency until proven otherwise by imaging studies. Factor infusion should be given immediately, even prior to imaging studies and neurologic consultation. FVIII or FIX levels should be kept at 80–100% of normal. Late bleeding after head trauma can manifest as long as 3–4 weeks after the injury. Hence, patients with head trauma should be infused immediately unless the injury is proven insignificant.

Following treatment of the acute episode, which usually is of approximately 2 weeks' duration, prophylactic treatment for about 6 months is usually indicated to decrease the possibility of a recurrent intracerebral hemorrhage. Doses of about 40 U/kg of FVIII every other day and 50 U/kg of FIX twice weekly should be given [22].

Hematuria

Gross spontaneous and asymptomatic hematuria is not uncommon in the hemophilia population. Trauma, calculi, and infections should also be considered. If the last are ruled out, treatment with increased oral or intravenous fluids, bed rest, and a short course of corticosteroids (i.e., prednisone 0.5 mg/kg/day) for 3–4 days is usually sufficient to arrest the bleeding. If symptoms persist then therapy with the deficient factor should be given at a dose to keep plasma levels of about 30–50% of normal until complete resolution of the hematuria. Antifibrinolytic agents, such as tranexamic acid or ε-aminocaproic acid, are contraindicated in individuals with hematuria because of the risk of forming clots in the urinary tract and producing obstruction.

For certain particular circumstances such as aggressive rehabilitation after orthopedic surgery, prophylactic replacement therapy is indicated. Doses of 20–30 U/kg of FVIII or 40–60 U/kg of FIX on the day of therapy should be sufficient to prevent hemorrhages.

References

1 Escobar MA. Treatment on demand—in vivo dose finding studies. *Haemophilia* 2003; **9**: 360–7.
2 Swanton MC. Hemophilic arthropathy in dogs. *Lab Invest* 1959; **8**: 1269.
3 Brinkhous KM, Swanton MC, Webster WP, Roberts HR. In: Vanderfield IR, ed. Dosing. *Hemophilic arthropathy transfusion therapy in its amelioration—canine and human studies.* The Haemophilia Society of NSW, Sydney, Australia; 1966: 18–21.
4 Brinkhous KM, Langdell RD, Penick G, *et al.* Newer approaches to the study of haemophilia and haemophilioid states. *JAMA* 1954; **154**: 481.
5 Biggs R, Macfarlane RG. Haemophilia, Christmas disease and related conditions. In: Biggs R, Macfarlane RG, eds. *Human Blood Coagulation and its Disorders*, 2nd edn. Springfield, IL: Charles C Thomas, 1957: 239–74.
6 Pool JG, Hershgold EJ, Pappenhagen AR. High-potency antihaemophilic factor concentrate prepared from cryoglobulin precipitate. *Nature (London)* 1964; **203**: 312–3.
7 McMillan CW, Diamond LK, Surgenor DM. Treatment of classic hemophilia: the use of fibrinogen rich in factor VIII for hemorrhage and for surgery. *N Engl J Med* 1961; **265**: 277.
8 Ramgren O. Haemophilia in Sweden, III. Symptomatology, with special reference to differences between haemophilia A and B. *Acta Med Scand* 1962; **171**: 237.
9 Biggs R, Macfarlane RG. Haemophilia and related conditions: a survey of 187 cases. *Br J Haematol* 1958; **4**: 1.
10 Kasper CK, Dietrich, SL, Rapaport SI. *Hemophilia Prophylaxis with AHF Concentrate.* XII Congress International Society of Hematology. New York; 1968: 176.
11 Aronstam A, Wassef M, Hamad Z *et al.* A double-blind controlled trial of two dose levels of factor VIII in the treatment of high risk haemarthroses in haemophilia A. *Clin Lab Haematol* 1983; **5**: 157–63.
12 Aronstam A. Prevention of haemophilic arthropathy. *Folia Haematol* 1990; **117**: 499–504.
13 Abildgaard CF. Current concepts in the management of hemophilia. *Semin Hematol* 1975; **12**: 223–32.
14 Berntorp E, Bjorkman S. The pharmacokinetics of clotting factor therapy. *Haemophilia* 2003; **9**: 353–9.
15 Kasper CK, Boylen AL, Ewing NP, *et al.* Hematologic management of hemophilia A for surgery. *JAMA* 1985; **253**: 1279–83.
16 Lachiewicz PF, Inglis AE, Insall JN, *et al.* Total knee arthroplasty in hemophilia. *J Bone Joint Surg Am* 1985; **67**: 1361–6.
17 Kitchens CS. Surgery in hemophilia and related disorders. A prospective study of 100 consecutive procedures. *Medicine (Baltimore)* 1986; **65**: 34–45.
18 Rudowski WJ, Scharf R, Ziemski JM. Is major surgery in hemophiliac patients safe? *World J Surg* 1987; **11**: 378–86.
19 Hathaway WE, Christian MJ, Clarke SL, Hasiba U. Comparison of continuous and intermittent Factor VIII concentrate therapy in hemophilia A. *Am J Hematol* 1984; **17**: 85–8.
20 Bona RD, Weinstein RA, Weisman SJ, Bartolomeo A, Rickles FR. The use of continuous infusion of factor concentrates in the treatment of hemophilia. *Am J Hematol* 1989; **32**: 8–13.
21 Goldsmith JC. Rationale and indications for continuous infusion of antihemophilic factor (factor VIII). *Blood Coagul Fibrinolysis* 1996; **7** (Suppl. 1): S3–6.
22 Lusher J. Hemophilia A and B. In: Lilleyman JS, Hann IM, Blanchette VS, eds. *Pediatric Hematology*, 2nd edn. London: Churchill Livingstone, 1999: 585–600.

23 Bjorkman S, Carlsson, M., Berntorp, E. Pharmacokinetics of factor IX in patients with haemophilia B. Methodological aspects and physiological interpretation. *Eur J Clin Pharmacol* 1994; **46**: 325–32.

24 Wolberg A, Stafford, DW, Erie DA. Human factor IX binds to specific sites on the collagenous domain of collagen IV. *J Biol Chem* 1997; **272**: 16717–20.

25 Roberts HR, Escobar MA. Other coagulation factor deficiencies. In: Loscalzo J, Schafer AI, eds. *Thrombosis and Hemorrhage*, 3rd edn. Philadelphia: Lippincott Williams & Wilkins, 2003: 575–98.

26 Honig GR, Forman EN, Johnston CA, *et al*. Administration of single doses of AHF (factor VIII) concentrates in the treatment of hemophilic hemarthroses. *Pediatrics* 1969; **43**: 26–33.

27 Brown DL, Hardisty RM, Kosoy MH, Bracken C. Antihaemophilic globulin: preparation by an improved cryoprecipitation method and clinical use. *BMJ* 1967; **2**: 79–85.

28 Penner JA, Kelly PE. Lower doses of factor VIII for hemophilia. *N Engl J Med* 1977; **297**: 401.

29 Ashenhurst JB, Langehannig PL, Seeler RA. Early treatment of bleeding episodes with 10 U/kg of factor VIII. *Blood* 1977; **50**: 181–2.

30 Weiss AE. Doses of Factor VIII for hemophilic bleeding. *N Engl J Med* 1977; **297**: 1237–8.

31 Ripa T, Scaraggi FA, Ciavarella N. Early treatment of hemophilia with minimal doses of factor VIII or factor IX. *Blood* 1978; **51**: 763.

32 Allain JP. Dose requirement for replacement therapy in hemophilia A. *Thromb Haemost* 1979; **42**: 825–31.

33 Aronstam A, Wasssef M, Choudhury DP, *et al*. Double-blind controlled trial of three dosage regimens in treatment of haemarthroses in haemophilia A. *Lancet* 1980; **i**: 169–71.

34 Aronstam A, Wassef M, Hamad Z, Aston DL. The identification of high-risk elbow hemorrhages in adolescents with severe hemophilia A. *J Pediatr* 1981; **98**: 776–8.

35 Aronstam A, Wassef M, Hamad Z. Low doses of factor VIII for selected ankle bleeds in severe haemophilia A. *BMJ* 1982; **284**: 790.

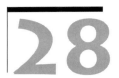

Products used to treat hemophilia: regulation

Albert Farrugia

Introduction

Hemophilia care consists of many components [1]. The provision of concentrates of the deficient coagulation factors is an essential component and their safety, quality, and efficacy need to be assured independently of the measures dictated by the market and the individual manufacturers. Over the past 20 years, this assurance has become the role of regulatory authorities. Compared with other products of pharmaceutical manufacture, the regulation of hemophilia products is a relatively recent phenomenon. The products of industrial-scale plasma fractionation have been subject to the oversight of the United States Food and Drugs Administration (FDA) since the 1940s, because of the products' status as biologics, subject to a regulatory framework that is over a century old. In Europe, the evolution of a system of harmonized and centralized approval of medicinal products in the European Union initially exempted plasma derivatives [2] and only began to incorporate them in 1989 [3]. The factors contributing to the significant heightening of this supervision over the past 20 years have been reviewed [4].

These factors have resulted in a regulatory framework in the developed world that assesses hemophilia products as medicines in the highest category of risk relative to other therapeutic agents. It is noteworthy that systems of official regulation mandating standards and other measures are now coupled with voluntary standards adopted by industry bodies as additional features of a comprehensive nexus of arrangements contributing to product quality and risk minimization [5]. While the requirements now in place in the European Union demonstrate a comprehensive range of measures in that market (Figure 28.1), they are fairly representative of the systems in place worldwide in terms of the aspects of product manufacture that they address, and the target outcomes. The principles underlying these product-related measures have been discussed [6], and while the principal focus has been on the products of industrial plasma fractionation, the lessons learned through these products are now reflected in the requirements for the products of recombinant technology.

Underpinning these measures is the unspoken but practiced concept of "zero risk" in blood product manufacture and delivery. While this is a natural outcome of past failures, it has led to a regulatory framework that appears to be detached from the standard risk management and cost-effective, evidence-based principles that shape modern healthcare delivery. While product safety is paramount, some of the measures introduced and embedded in current practice are difficult to quantify in terms of safety, while their effect on supply and delivery can be profound.

Products of local and blood bank production

The option of delivering product from local production in mainstream blood banking environments generally only exists for hemophilia A through the production of cryoprecipitate (cryo). Cryoprecipitate in blood banks may be produced in a closed system of blood bags and then lyophilized to increase its convenience [7]. The following features of the product need to be kept in mind:

• Cryo is a crude product that will not meet criteria for high-purity plasma concentrates, such as potency, purity, and solubility. However, this is not a significant problem in terms of its safety.

• The ability to characterize the product through representative batch sampling is limited. In other words, it is not possible to label a vial of freeze-dried cryo for potency.

• Viral reduction techniques are not easily applied to the manufacture of cryo. This is because they are based on technology not easily adapted to blood centers, and because the low purity of the product prevents inactivation through heat.

The issues underpinning access to cryo have been reviewed [8]. In particular, the safety aspects have been emphasized by Evatt *et al.* [9], who have shown that, in the absence of additional safety measures, the risk of HIV infection in individuals with hemophilia exposed to cryo over a lifetime is significant (Table 28.1). Enhancement of cryo safety could include the selection of donors from low-risk populations, whose plasma could be quarantined until the donor has been recalled and retested for markers of infection. All such testing should be done with the most sensitive tests possible and using intervals that allow donors to seroconvert for the transfusion-transmitted viruses in case they were infected at the time of donation. Using nucleic acid testing (NAT), the viral window period for the important viruses can be substantially decreased. Pools of dedicated plasma donors, carefully selected and repeatedly tested, can in time become a source of very safe raw material, compared with first-time donors

Some approaches to the viral inactivation of cryo have been described [10]. Any level of viral inactivation will result in a drop in factor VIII (FVIII) yield, and therefore the optimization

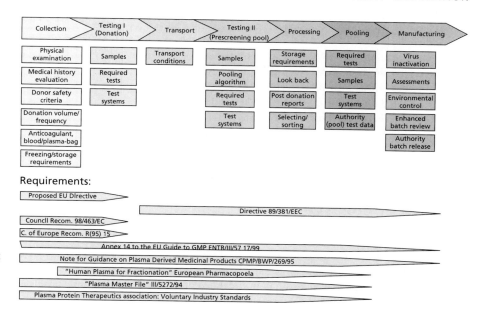

Figure 28.1 Systems of oversight for assuring product quality and safety in the plasma products sector in Europe (after J. Bult, unpublished observations).

Table 28.1 Risk (%) that a person with hemophilia in Venezuela or the USA will be exposed to HIV-contaminated blood products, based on years of treatment and risk of an HIV-infected donation. From Evatt et al. [9].

| Years of treatment | Venezuela | | | USA |
	Lower (1/25 700)*	Mid (1/21 200)*	Upper (1/17 500)*	Mid (1/545 100)*
5	3.4	4.2	5.0	0.16
10	6.8	5.1	9.8	0.33
15	10.0	12.0	14.3	0.49
20	13.1	15.6	18.6	0.66
30	19.0	22.5	26.6	0.99
40	24.4	28.8	33.7	1.3
50	29.5	34.6	40.2	1.6
60	34.3	39.9	46.0	2.0

*Estimated risk for HIV-infected donation

of yields using improved plasma handling techniques is necessary if the safety and supply of cryo are to be enhanced. The pharmacologic stimulation of donors to produce more FVIII may be worth considering as a means of improving yields [11].

The nature of the manufacturing process for cryo results in a limitation in the ability to exert many of the standard features of pharmaceutical quality control that are possible for concentrates. In particular, the absence of sizeable batches makes homogeneous batch sampling, characterization, and labeling of ingredients of interest (active and impurities) difficult. Nevertheless, the ability to impose quality system management and adherence to good manufacturing practices is nowadays considered to be universally applicable. There are several standards and regulations in the international regulatory environment, which are applied for the manufacture and characterization of cryo. The US Code of Federal Regulations (CFR) [12] includes requirements for cryoprecipitate that ensure that the measures

underpinning whole-blood transfusion safety in the USA will be reflected in cryo. These measures include NAT, which will enhance cryo safety as discussed above. In Europe, centralized oversight of blood components including cryo is under way with the recent introduction of the Blood Directive of the European Commission [13], which will replace the current national requirements for these products. This Directive will be underpinned by technical standards for safety and quality, which are currently unspecified. It is likely that standards such as those recommended by the Council of Europe [14] will be introduced. Such standards currently do not include NAT, which is not in universal use in the European environment at the blood donor level. Therefore, alignment to the evolving European regulatory framework will not, as currently perceived by this author, enhance the safety of cryo to the level found in the USA.

In summary, cryo may be subjected to a level of regulatory oversight that, while unable to assure safety and quality to the standards available for concentrates, can result in these properties being reflective of the safety of the local blood supply. Any additional measures, such as the introduction of viral inactivation for cryo, cannot be supported by the regulatory requirements for these measures for concentrates, as these demand substantial validation and extensive studies, unavailable in blood centers. Therefore, while much can be done to improve the safety of cryo as a therapeutic modality in the developing world, it can never substitute for concentrates in terms of safety and quality that can be assured by regulatory oversight.

Products of large-scale plasma fractionation

Plasma concentrates are similar to conventional pharmaceuticals in that they are produced in large batches from a homogeneous pool of starting material, through well-defined processes subject to the tenets of standard pharmaceutical quality control. However, biologic drugs such as factor concentrates cannot be considered as generic agents, and each manufacturing process requires individual assessment with full product specification. While general properties leading to quality and safety may be reflected in standards of the pharmacopeia, the range of approaches to the manufacture of FVIII and factor IX (FIX) concentrates developed over the past 40 years has resulted in significant differences between products, which require thorough evaluation for their potential effect on the factors of interest and the impurities in the products.

Regulatory agencies oversee the introduction and maintenance of factor concentrates on the market through a set of well-defined principles that are common across the developed world. These include (i) facility licensure (good manufacturing practice; GMP); (ii) premarket product assessment; and (iii) postmarket surveillance.

Facility licensure

Licensure of plasma fractionation plants is done through reference to codes of good manufacturing practice (GMP), which are generally generic documents specifying quality standards for manufacture that are common to all medicinal products. GMP seeks to ensure that manufacture is consistently carried out to high standards such that product safety, quality, and consistency are assured. Following inspections, which may identify deficiencies, the regulator and the manufacturer generally collaborate to ensure the issue of a manufacturing license, which will allow production to a high standard. Recently, the Pharmaceutical Inspectorate Convention has adopted a GMP for medicinal products that includes a chapter specifically addressing plasma-derived products [15]. The requirements of this chapter are shown in Table 28.2.

The importance of GMP in assuring product safety is recognized by the regulator and product manufacturer alike. The ability of the latter to manufacture product consistently to a similar,

Table 28.2 Principles of good manufacturing practice for plasma fractionation agencies (Pharmaceutical Inspectors Convention Scheme 2003).

Quality management
Premises and equipment
Blood and plasma collection
Traceability and post collection measures
Production and quality control
Retention of samples
Disposal of rejected blood, plasma or intermediates

predefined, and high manufacturing standard is pivotal to safety and depends on GMP. Examples of breakdowns in GMP impacting on product safety are nowadays rare owing to the high standards of manufacture evolved over the past 20 years, but such incidents have been implicated in product safety problems including viral transmission due to inadequate segregation between previral and postviral inactivation streams [16]. With viral inactivation processes, it is impossible to subject product batches to final testing to assure adequate viral elimination, and reliance on GMP for this is absolute. The whole of the manufacturing chain requires adherence to GMP, and its presence in collection and testing procedures is strictly enforced by regulators [17]. Voluntary industry standards have been introduced for ensuring that the minimal measures enforced by regulators are buttressed by additional measures for areas such as the processing of fractionation intermediates from different sources [18].

Premarket product approval

The assessment of the manufacturing process and the features of the product are done through the submission of product dossiers, which describe these in great detail. The main agencies the—FDA and the EMEA—have standard formats for the submission of data for manufacturing, preclinical and clinical assessment. The data for the description and validation of the viral inactivation steps incorporated into the manufacture are a crucial component of these submissions. The EMEA has issued detailed guidance for the performance of such studies [19]. Such guidances are a feature of the regulatory framework of all the major agencies, and provide the industry with state-of-the-art assessment and regulation of the aspects related to the safety, quality, and efficacy of plasma derivatives.

International efforts for the harmonization of regulatory procedures have included the development of standardized approaches for the collation and presentation of data for regulatory review, through the so-called Common Technical Document (CTD). The International Conference for Harmonization (ICH) has developed CTDs for the assessment of several aspects of safety, quality, and efficacy [20]. These documents provide a structured path for manufacturers to compile data in a form that is easily assessable, and their use for plasma derivatives, while still at an early stage, should contribute to further streamlining of the regulatory process.

An essential component of the premarket approval process is the demonstration of product pharmacokinetics and efficacy through the conduct of appropriate clinical trials. It is necessary to demonstrate that a product will show the established pharmacokinetic profile for the relevant coagulation factors, i.e., *in vivo* recovery and half-life. Proof of efficacy to a clinical endpoint under the various indications sought, e.g., prophylaxis, treatment of episodic bleeds, and surgery, is also needed. Clinical requirements for the assessment of adverse events such as viral transmission and inhibitor development demand patient numbers that are considerably larger than is feasible if conventional assurance based on statistical principles is to be generated. Given these limitations, the EMEA has revised its requirements for the clinical efficacy of FVIII and FIX to allow efficacy and adverse event assessment to be reviewed through lower patient numbers than previously required [21]. Similar flexibility has been shown on the need for previously untreated patients (PUPs) and nonbleeding patients, both scarce groups to access. It is still not possible, in the opinion of this author, for regulators to fully exempt plasma concentrates from the requirements of clinical studies on the basis of so-called "comparability" with similar products [22]. The level of characterization possible for these products, particularly in relation to potential predictors of efficacy and adverse events, is necessarily limited, and surrogates for clinical studies are not yet available.

While the pressure is on regulators to avoid "over-regulation," this author believes that there are still some areas of plasma product regulation where provisions could be strengthened. The European system mandates centralized—and rigorous—oversight for these products if they are manufactured using certain biotechnological techniques, e.g., monoclonal antibody affinity chromatography. Products produced with earlier technology are regulated through the "mutual recognition" procedure [23] emanating from review by one authority in a single member state. Considering that these products were developed and placed on the market prior to the modern era of stringent regulation, the maintenance, in individual European states, of hemophilia products that are not reflective of current best practice in the field, demands review if patient care and safety are to be ensured.

Postmarket surveillance

Once products are approved and on the market, it is essential that their quality, safety and efficacy are maintained throughout their market lifetime. This is achieved through postmarket activities, which include:
- maintenance of GMP through regular inspections after the introduction of the products;
- testing of batches prior to release in order to ensure conformance to specifications;
- appropriate recording and reporting mechanisms for adverse events.

The importance of these measures needs to reflect the fact that novel plasma-derived hemophilia concentrates are rare nowa-

days, and their presence on the market can be prolonged. The products introduced in the mid-1980s were developed prior to the many additional measures that were subsequently incorporated into the regulatory requirements as more problems were identified. It is therefore reasonable to maintain vigilance with these more recently identified issues in mind, particularly in relation to pathogen safety issues. Appropriate adverse event detection and reporting assists in this. Of more questionable relevance is the role of prerelease testing of all batches introduced into the market by the regulatory authority. It is pertinent that such testing cannot be applied to the primary pressure point of viral safety. Some government agencies in less developed countries attempt to assure viral safety through demanding end-product testing using serologic or molecular techniques to detect viral markers used for blood screening. This approach is scientifically worthless. However, end-product testing for potency still has a role, particularly for products newly developed and released. The vagaries of coagulation factor assay and standards in relation to hemophilia concentrates are well recognized [24] and batch release testing assists in the detection of problems, as recently exemplified by B domain-deleted recombinant FVIII (BDD-FVIII) (see below).

Issues related to hemophilia concentrates from recombinant technology

The developments in viral safety over the past 20 years have achieved plasma product safety to a large extent. The robustness of viral inactivation techniques was tested successfully when the West Nile virus (WNV) entered the North American blood supply during 2002 and infected the recipients of fresh blood components but not plasma derivatives [25]. However, the prospect of previously unknown and resistant pathogens became an acute concern in the late 1990s with the emergence of the prionic diseases as possible threats to blood safety [26]. This issue emphasized the importance of continuing to move to alternatives of blood-derived therapeutics when possible.

Essentially, all the principles specified for plasma concentrates are equally applicable and mandatory for recombinant alternatives. The importance of these principles is best demonstrated by reviewing a series of incidents involving recombinant products that demanded regulatory engagement:
- In 2001, a serious breach of GMP forced the FDA to severely restrict the production capacity of a recombinant manufacturer, affecting product supply worldwide [27]. This breach of GMP had the potential to affect product and patient safety. The importance of maintaining a GMP audit program was emphasized by this incident.
- In 2001, the EMEA restricted the use of recombinant FIX in pediatric patients when postmarket studies required as a condition of European licensure indicated a worrisome variability in the pharmacokinetics of the product in these patients [28].
- In 2003, studies performed in European medicine control laboratories indicated potency problems in a B domain-deleted re-

combinant FVIII (Refacto), as a result of a potency misalignment in the initial calibration of the standard of the product [29].

Of particular relevance is the role of prerelease potency testing in detecting the BDD-FVIII problem. This problem would have remained undetected in the absence of such testing, which has been excised from the regulatory framework of the FDA under the consideration that recombinant coagulation products represent "well-specified proteins" whose regulation does not demand the same level of depth and rigor required of plasma products.

The current generation of recombinant products is available in formulations lacking any blood or tissue excipient, and products that have this feature through their manufacture are expected imminently. The only FIX recombinant product—Benefix—is of this type, and may be described as state-of-the-art in terms of pathogen safety. This product, however, has raised other issues pertinent to the oversight of the recombinant coagulation factors. The differences in higher-order structure in this FIX compared with the wild-type molecule have been implicated in the lower *in vivo* recovery of this product [30]. The problem with this product highlights the desirability of regulators and industry reviewing the whole standardization framework for hemophilia products, traditionally derived from the concept of a "biological unit" initially defined as the amount in 1 mL of normal plasma. The lineage of the various standards used in this environment has been reviewed [31]. This author believes that, with the development of pure and recombinant variants of the plasma-derived protein, the adherence to this concept requires review. The issue is well-exemplified by the Benefix problem, where the pharmaceutical development based on the biological unit was unable to predict the lower recovery of the recombinant FIX. This author would propose that product development, including clinical development and dosage, for these products, should be based on the concept, now possible, of labeling and dosing using product mass rather than units. This would obviate problems resulting from an inappropriate alignment to concepts and standards based upon the wild-type molecule. The analogy in the area of fibrinolysis, where a truncated tissue plasminogen activator is labeled relative to its own particular standard, suggests the feasibility of developing particular standards for novel molecules. It may be argued that this concept should only be applied for a radical molecular change like deletion of the B domain in FVIII. For that product, the dangers of initially aligning the potency with the wild-type molecule standard were demonstrated by the BDD-FVIII problem referred to above [32]. The use of mass rather than unitage has been successfully applied to the use of recombinant FVIIa in the treatment of inhibitors in hemophilia [33].

Conclusions

Currently, the regulation of products for hemophilia in less developed economies relies on reference to decisions in the First

World authorities. This may not always result in optimal outcomes as most of the hemophilia care in the developing world is through local plasma and cryoprecipitate, which are not subject to the oversight of mainstream regulators. Furthermore, the emergence of companies based outside the developed world and seeking to supply the emerging economies of the developing world with hemophilia concentrates has necessitated new strategies for regulation that are independent of the established frameworks. A minimalist approach developed by the World Federation of Hemophilia is intended to address the needs of less developed countries seeking to ensure optimal outcomes under their own, more limited, circumstances [34]. Overall, the principles used by mainstream agencies and described in this chapter may be applied in all environments seeking to assure the quality of hemophilia care. Applied properly, they can contribute to maintaining the delivery of a form of therapy that is nowadays among the safest in therapeutic practice.

References

1 Hoots WK. Comprehensive care for hemophilia and related inherited bleeding disorders: why it matters. *Curr Hematol Rep* 2003; **2**: 395–401.
2 European Council Directive 75/319/EEC available on http://www.europa.eu.int.
3 European Council Directive 89/381/EEC available on http://www.europa.eu.int.
4 Farrugia A. The regulatory pendulum in transfusion medicine. *Trans Med Rev* 2002; **16**: 273–82.
5 Plasma Protein Therapeutics Association. Standards for members under the QSEAL Program. On http://www.plasmatherapeutics.org/en/qualitysafety qseal.cfm.
6 Farrugia A. Evolving perspectives in product safety for haemophilia. *Haemophilia* 2002; **8**: 236–43.
7 Lloyd S. The preparation of single donor cryoprecipitate. On http://www.wfh.org/Content_Documents/FF_Monographs/FF2_Cryo_V6.doc.
8 Srivastava A. Factor replacement for haemophilia—should cryoprecipitate be used? *Haemophilia* 1999; **5**: 301–5.
9 Evatt, Austin H, Leon G, *et al.* Haemophilia therapy: assessing the cumulative risk of HIV exposure by cryoprecipitate. *Haemophilia* 1999; **5**: 295–300.
10 Keeling DM, Luddington R, Allain JP, *et al.* Cryoprecipitate prepared from plasma virally inactivated by the solvent detergent method. *Br J Haematol* 1997; **96**: 194–7.
11 McLeod BC, Sassetti RJ, Cole ER, Scott JP. A high-potency, single-donor cryoprecipitate of known factor VIII content dispensed in vials. *Ann Intern Med* 1987; **106**: 35–40.
12 Code of Federal Regulations of the United States. Available on www.fda.gov.
13 European Commission. Directive 2002/98/EC of the European parliament and of the council of 27 January 2003 setting standards of quality and safety for the collection, testing, processing, storage and distribution of human blood and blood components and amending directive 2001/83/EC. On http://europa.eu.int/eur-lex/en/dat/2003/l_033/l_03320030208en00300040.pdf.
14 Council of Europe. Guide to the preparation, use and quality assurance of blood components—8th edition (2002). On http://book.coe.int/GB/CAT/LIV/HTM/l1838.htm

15 Pharmaceutical Inspection Convention (2003) Guide to Good Manufacturing Practice for medicinal products. Annex 14 Manufacture of products derived from human blood or human plasma. On http://www.picscheme.org/docs/pdf/PE%20009-1%20GMP%20 Guide%20September%202003.pdf#PE%20009-1.

16 Williams PE, Yap PL, Gillon J, *et al.* Transmission of non-A, non-B hepatitis by pH4-treated intravenous immunoglobulin. *Vox Sang* 1989; **57**: 15–18.

17 Therapeutic Goods Administration. Blood regulator takes action on South Australian Blood Service—Friday 12th September 2003. On http://www.health.gov.au/tga/docs/html/mediarel/mrsablood.htm.

18 Plasma Protein Therapeutics Association. Voluntary Standard for Intermediates. On http://www.pptaglobal.org/librarydocs/PPTA Intermediates Standard.pdf.

19 Committee for Proprietary Medicinal Products. Note for Guidance on Virus Validation Studies: The design, contribution and interpretation of studies validating the inactivation and removal of viruses. On http://www.emea.eu.int/pdfs/human/bwp/026895en.pdf.

20 International Conference on Harmonisation. General Information on the Common Technical Document. On http://www.ich.org/ WORD/CTD%20General%20Info.ppt.

21 Committee for Proprietary Medicinal Products. Note for Guidance on the clinical investigation of human plasma derived Factor VIII and IX products. On http://www.emea.eu.int/pdfs/human/bpwg/ 019895en.pdf.

22 Center for Biologics Evaluation and Research. Comparability Studies for Human Plasma-Derived Therapeutics—Workshop on Friday, May 31, 2002. On http://www.fda.gov/cber/minutes/plasma 053102.htm.

23 European Commission 2001. Proposal for a regulation of the European Parliament and the Council laying down Community procedures for for the authorisaton and supervision of medicinal products for human and veterinary use and establishing a European Agency for for the Evaluation of Medicinal products. On http:// europa.eu.int/eur-lex/en/com/pdf/2001/en_501PC0404_01.pdf.

24 Barrowcliffe TW, Mertens K, Preston FE, Ingerslev J. Laboratory aspects of haemophilia therapy. *Haemophilia* 2002; **8**: 244–9.

25 Pealer LN, Marfin AA, Petersen LR, *et al.* Transmission of West Nile virus through blood transfusion in the United States in 2002. *N Engl J Med* 2003; **349**: 1236–45.

26 Brown P. Creutzfeldt–Jakob disease: blood infectivity and screening tests. *Semin Hematol* 2001; **38** (4): 2–6.

27 Center for Biologics Evaluation and Research. Warning letter to Carol M. Moore, Vice President, Quality Assurance/Regulatory Affairs, Bayer Corporation, Biologics Product Division. On http://www.fda.gov/foi/warning letters/g1575d.pdf.

28 European Medicines Evaluation Agency. Public Statement on Benefix (nanacog alfa). Intensive post-marketing surveillance for all new patients—new clinical trials. 04 October 2001. On http:// www.eudra.org/humandocs/Humans/EPAR/Benefix/Benefix.htm.

29 Hubbard AR, Sands D, Sandberg E, Seitz R, Barrowcliffe TW. A multi-centre collaborative study on the potency estimation of Refacto. *Thromb Haemost* 2003; **90**: 1088–93.

30 White GC 2nd, Beebe A, Nielsen B. Recombinant factor IX. *Thromb Haemost* 1997; **78**: 261–5.

31 Barrowcliffe TW. Clotting factor concentrates in clinical practice. Standardization and assay. *Semin Thromb Haemost* 1993; **19**: 73–9.

32 Farrugia A. Potency assessment of the new generation of coagulation factor concentrates—time for a new paradigm? *Thromb Haemost* 2003; **90**: 968–70.

33 Negrier C, Lienhart A. Overall experience with NovoSeven. *Blood Coagul Fibrinolysis* 2000; **11** (Suppl. 1): S19–24.

34 Farrugia A. Guide for the assessment of clotting factor concentrates for the treatment of haemophilia 2003. On http://www.wfh.org/ Content_Documents/Other_Publications/Reg_Guide_Eng.pdf.

Joint replacement

Nicholas J. Goddard

Introduction

Hemophilia care has steadily improved over the years and especially so during the last decade. The routine use of prophylactic treatment has undoubtedly resulted in a significant improvement in the lifestyle, quality of life, and life expectancy of these hemophilic patients, and bodes well for the future. However, despite our best efforts there is still a group of young adults who have a severe degree of knee joint destruction as a result of repeated articular bleeding episodes during their early years.

Total joint replacement has transformed the quality of life for countless thousands of patients worldwide but there has been a reluctance to offer this operation to younger patients. However, the results of joint replacement in patients less than 55 years old are generally equivalent to those in the older population and our previous conservative approach was perhaps flawed.

The combined experiences of joint replacement over the past 20 years have been encouraging, with significant improvements in measurable outcome parameters, reduction in spontaneous hemarthroses, and improvements in quality of life.

We believe that total joint replacement is a safe and effective procedure in the management of hemophilic joint arthropathy. The latest techniques using continuous infusion and recombinant factor replacement have gone a long way to reducing the complications rate and to achieving results that match those of the general population.

Joint replacement surgery is never a simple undertaking in someone with hemophilia; it requires aggressive factor replacement pre and post surgery, a long hospital stay, and considerable rehabilitation. Fortunately, the majority of our patients are healthy, motivated, and well prepared for the operation that they may be facing. They are young men in the prime of their life professionally and physically, whose quality of life is affected by a single destroyed joint.

The major objective of total joint replacement is to reduce the level of pain in the affected joint. This will have beneficial effects on the adjacent joints. In addition, there is a significant reduction in the frequency and number of joint bleeds, which all adds up to an increase in both function and mobility.

It goes without saying that the operation should only take place in a recognized center with appropriate hematologic back-up. This is not surgery for the occasional operator or the faint-hearted.

At the Royal Free Hospital we now have approximately 1500 patients registered at the unit, of which some 200 are severely affected. We have adopted a team approach in the management of our patients. We hold a dedicated monthly combined clinic run by the hematologist and the orthopedic surgeon, with other key members involved being physiotherapist, nurse, and counselor. The clinic is held in a relatively open format, and thus information and experiences are traded and shared between patients, who are often valuable sources of advice, inspiration, and reassurance.

Total joint replacement now forms the bulk of our surgery. Our experience now extends to 68 total joint replacements in 54 patients. A total of 47 total knee replacements (TKRs) have been performed in 37 patients (nine bilateral and five revisions), 18 total hip replacements (THRs) in 15 patients (two bilateral and one revision), two shoulder replacements, and one elbow replacement.

Total knee replacement

The knee is the most common joint affected in hemophilia (approximately 50%), and despite our best efforts there is still a group of young adults who have a severe degree of knee joint destruction as a result of repeated articular bleeding episodes during their early years. This in turn leads to the onset of pain and significant functional disability at a time when the patient requires the best possible quality of life.

The indications for operation are primarily disabling pain that is unresponsive to medical treatment. Deformity and poor functional range of motion, particularly a severe flexion contracture of the knee, are relative indications and may in themselves justify joint replacement. However, joint contractures and flexion deformity pose various surgical challenges for the surgeon.

The main question remains as to when one should offer such surgery given the widely held belief that relative youth is a contraindication. This may in fact be true of the "normal population" with single joint involvement, whose demands and expectations may be unrealistic, but this is generally not the case in the present population of hemophilic patients, who frequently have other joint involvement. With this in mind, and armed with the knowledge of encouraging reports of excellent long-term results of total knee replacement in the <55 age group, knee replacement represents an appropriate procedure.

The early literature was full of pessimism, reporting poor results and, in particular, a high incidence of both significant bleeding episodes and deep joint infection, up to 17% in some series [1–3].

The biggest problem arose between 1979 and 1985, when some 80–90% of the hemophilic population in the developed world became infected with HIV. These patients were shown to be more susceptible to infection and in 1993 the Oxford group showed that there was a high risk of secondary infection in HIV-positive patients and that surgery should be reserved for a carefully selected group of patients [4]. Their experience was confirmed by Weidel et al. [5] and later by Ragni et al. [6], who reported a 30% incidence of infection in a series of 27 total knee arthroplasties in HIV-positive patients, in stark contrast to an infection rate of 1–2% in the nonhemophilic population, and concluded that when offering such surgery to HIV-infected patients there must be a very careful analysis of the risk–benefit ratio.

Data from the Royal Free group were, however, more encouraging, with Birch [7] and later Phillips et al. [8] reporting that there was no evidence to suggest that major surgery had any adverse effects on the rate of decline in the CD4 count, the onset of AIDS, or the mortality rate, and that the outcome of all the TKRs was excellent or good, with no acute infections.

Total joint replacement in HIV-positive patients with hemophilia carries a considerable risk. The pooled data therefore suggest that total knee arthroplasty in hemophilic patients carries with it an increased risk of postoperative infection in comparison with nonhemophilic patients. Those patients at particular risk are the HIV-positive hemophilic patients whose CD4 count is less than 200 cells/mm^3 [9,10]. We believe that, nonetheless, total knee arthroplasty is a surgical procedure that should be considered for selected cases.

The operation consists of a standard resurfacing total knee replacement combined with an adequate synovectomy. Details of the procedure are covered in other texts; however, one must appreciate that the surgery itself is not always straightforward given the high incidence of joint deformity and soft-tissue contractures and that, accordingly, some experience of revision knee replacement is a distinct advantage.

It should be borne in mind that postoperatively, these patients often require higher doses of opiates for longer periods than patients undergoing TKR for straightforward osteoarthritis.

There is little doubt that, nowadays, total knee arthroplasty represents a safe and effective procedure in the management of hemophilic joint arthropathy. The latest techniques using continuous infusion and recombinant factor replacement have gone a long way to reducing the complications rate and to achieving results that match those of a similar nonhemophilic population, especially with regard to pain relief, restoration of function, and, importantly, an improvement in the quality of life.

Rodriguez-Merchan and Wiedel [11] reported their combined experience of 37 total knee arthroplasties performed on 26 men between March 1975 and November 1995. Of this group, 17 (46%) were HIV positive, of whom nine had died from complications of acquired immunodeficiency disease (AIDS). Overall, 84% of this group was classed as good to excellent, 8% fair, and 8% poor according to their Hospital for Special Surgery (HSS) rating. Importantly, the greatest improve-

ments were with regard to pain and function, with a less marked improvement with respect to range of motion. The incidence of hemarthroses dropped from a mean of 5.5 per annum to 1.2.

The experience at the Royal Free Hospital is very similar [12]. Over the period 1983–2003, we performed 36 primary total knee replacements in 27 patients. The mean HSS scores improved from 30 preoperatively to 79.5 postoperatively, with 86% of patients being rated excellent or good, 5% fair, and 9% poor. There have been no major complications and only one case of late infection and one unusual case of prolonged postoperative bleeding, which was subsequently shown to be due to an aneurysm of the lateral inferior geniculate artery [13].

We have also undertaken seven simultaneous bilateral TKR during the past 7 years. Our results for this procedure are identical to unilateral TKR or staged bilateral TKR, with no increase in the rate of complications, or prolongation of the hospital stay. There are obvious financial advantages, since only one hospitalization is required and, significantly, the factor replacement requirements are the same as for a single procedure.

Elbow replacement

The elbow is the second most common site for arthropathy in the hemophilic patient. Destructive changes occur insidiously as it is not a classical weight-bearing joint, and early limitations of flexion and extension seldom interfere with overall function [14].

Various operations have been described in the use of elbow arthropathy associated with hemophilia. These operations include synovectomy, simple excision of the radial head combined with joint debridement, excision arthroplasty, arthrodesis, and silastic interposition arthroplasty [14–18]. Excision of the radial head combined with synovectomy has resulted in consistently good results, with reduction in pain, an increased range of motion, and a reduction in the frequency of joint bleeds.

In 1990, the group from St Thomas Hospital in London reported their experience of 13 elbows affected by severe hemophilic arthropathy and treated by silastic interposition arthroplasty [19]. The severity of pain, the frequency and severity of spontaneous hemorrhage, and the range of movement were much improved and needed less factor replacement. Three elbows were revised, one for infection and two because of fragmentation of the silastic sheet, with good restoration of function following revision.

The actual incidence of joint replacement, however, is likely to be low given that Bajekal reported that 81% of hemophiliacs suffered recurrent elbow bleeds but reported a low incidence of total joint replacement in the same group [20].

While total joint replacement has been well described for the hip, knee, and shoulder in hemophilia, there have been few reports concerning total elbow replacement. Most reports have been restricted to isolated case reports [21,22]. The first report by Luck and Kasper [23] reviewed the 20-year results of a total of 168 surgical procedures carried out for hemophilic arthropathy, but included only two total elbow replacements, one of which became infected. Kasten and Skinner [24], in their large series of total elbow replacements, described only two cases of hemophilia, one primary and a further revision, likewise Chatelot *et al.* [25].

The largest series to date was recently reported from the Oxford group and concerned seven elbow replacements in five patients with severe hemophilia A [26]. All patients demonstrated excellent relief of pain and improvement of function. There was one failure due to infection in an immunocompromised patient with HIV and hepatitis C.

The patients were followed for a minimum of 25 months and implants varied from unconstrained (Kudo or Souter–Strathclyde) to the more constrained Coonrad–Morrey joint replacements. There were three major postoperative complications: one ulnar nerve palsy, one axillary vein thrombosis, and one late infection requiring excision arthroplasty.

Overall, the results of the patients in this group were excellent in the short to medium term, and the Oxford group concluded that total elbow replacement is both feasible and useful in patients with severe hemophilic arthropathy.

Ankle replacement

The ankle joint is the third most commonly affected joint, accounting for 14.5% of recorded bleeds. The pattern of bleeding varies according to age, with the ankle most commonly affected during the second and third decades of life. Once the joint has been subjected to repeated bleeds, it becomes more vulnerable and ultimately becomes a target joint, with relentless deterioration of function and comfort in the hindfoot [27]. Surgical intervention is considered only when conservative measures have failed. In patients with synovitis and recurrent hemarthroses, and with congruent joint surfaces, synovectomy [open, arthroscopic, or chemical (synoviorthesis)] may decrease pain and prevent recurrent bleeding. In more advanced cases, joint debridement and excision of osteophytes (O'Donoghue procedure) can restore some joint motion [28], especially dorsiflexion. In our experience, though, any benefit is relatively short-lived, and further surgery will become necessary within 5 years [29,30].

Pearce *et al.* [31] reported their experience of supramalleolar varus osteotomy on seven ankles (in six patients) for hemophilic arthropathy and secondary valgus deformity. The operation reduced pain and the frequency of intra-articular bleeding while preserving joint function, for a mean of 9 years. They felt that this procedure offered an attractive alternative to the more commonly used surgical option of arthrodesis.

In patients with severe pain and end-stage arthropathy, who have failed conservative treatment, an ankle arthrodesis may be indicated. The surgery is intended to produce a more comfortable hindfoot unit, with better ambulation and a reduced bleeding tendency. There are relatively few reports of ankle arthrodesis in the literature, but our experience is that the procedure is well tolerated and success can generally be assured provided care is taken over the final position of the talus and hindfoot [17,29,30,32].

Total ankle replacement has had a checkered past and a relatively high failure rate in patients with degenerative ankle disease. I am aware of only one cited case of ankle replacement in hemophilia, by Luck [17], and, although the patient did well, the author concluded that "ankle and sub-talar joint are best treated by arthrodesis rather than by arthroplasty." This comment is appropriate and, given the good results of ankle arthrodesis at present, there is no place for ankle replacement in a hemophiliac patient.

Total hip replacement

Hemophilic arthropathy of the hip is relatively rare, accounting for only approximately 4% of patients [33]. Nonetheless, degenerative disease of the hip represents a significant volume of the workload of the orthopedic surgeon and it is therefore perhaps more pertinent to consider patients with hemophilia as having osteoarthritis of the hip rather than true hemophilic arthropathy.

However, unlike knee replacement, the results of total hip replacement (THR) in hemophilia remain relatively poor in the medium to long term. The common complications of THR are those common to the uncomplicated procedure. Deep infection remains the most significant and indeed serious complication, and it has been estimated that the incidence of infection in the hemophilic patient is approximately three times the anticipated incidence, with a high infection rate and a 33% incidence of aseptic loosening. It has been proposed that this could be related to coexisting knee and ankle involvement, resulting in a tendency for the patient to walk with a stiff-legged gait, so subjecting the hip to additional stress, which with the passage of time can cause the prosthetic hip to loosen.

Luck and Kasper [23] published the first significant series of THRs in hemophilic patients in 1989. This was a series of 13 patients over a 20-year period, with a 60% failure rate largely due to infection. The Mayo Clinic reported a series of 12 hip replacements with only six rated excellent or good at 5 years' follow-up [34]. Six hips were rated poor or failures, with four being painful with evidence of gross loosening, and infection affecting the other two.

The largest published series to date is that of Nelson *et al.* [33], who reported a series of 39 total hip replacements with a mean age of 48 years and mean follow-up of 7.6 years. Of the 22 available for review, five had already been revised and a further three were awaiting revision, representing a failure rate of at least 30%. Similar results were reported by Lofqvist [35], with five out of 13 hips having failed by 6 years, and Heeg [36] with a 33% failure rate at 9 years.

Kelly *et al.* [37] set out to determine the true incidence of hemophilic arthropathy in hip patients and performed a multicenter analysis. They looked at 34 total hip replacements in four major hemophilia centers in the USA. The mean duration of follow-up was 8 years, with a minimum of 2 years. Four patients were HIV positive. There were no early infections after 34 replacements but three late infections, possibly related to HIV. As with earlier series, though, the aseptic loosening rate was 21% of the 28 cemented femoral components and 23% of 26 cemented acetabular components.

The most encouraging data were published recently by Rodriguez-Merchan [38], reporting a 25-year experience of 22 patients undergoing THR for painful end-stage hemophilic arthropathy. Of the 19 patients available for review, there were no infections and only two had undergone revision procedures for aseptic loosening.

As with TKR, there are undoubted benefits to the patient following THR, but the objective outcome measures and the incidence of complications is higher than in the normal population. Despite the increased risks, there seems to be general agreement that total hip replacement is an appropriate operation for disabling hemophilic arthropathy.

Total shoulder replacement

The shoulder has never been considered to be a major problem in hemophilia [39]. Indeed, in a recent review article Gilbert referred to the shoulder as the "neglected joint" [40]. This could be owing to the unique anatomical arrangement of the shoulder girdle, with movement taking place at both glenohumeral and scapulothoracic levels. This double articulation will thus still permit a functional range of "shoulder" movement even in the absence of any glenohumeral motion. Nonetheless, hemophilic arthropathy is less common in the shoulder than in either the elbow or the knee but can lead to significant pain and loss of function.

The reported incidence of symptomatic hemophilic arthropathy of the shoulder is relatively rare; however, MacDonald et al. reported radiographic incidence of hemophilic arthropathy in 15 out of 41 patients [41]. They found that the incidence of hemarthrosis was much commoner than had previously been anticipated. Pettersson reported the results of two studies undertaken at the Malmö Hemophilia Centre in the early 1960s and then again in the early 1990s [39]. In the early study, incidence of symptomatic shoulder arthropathy was 13% and one-third of the patients were below the age of 30 years. In the later study, the incidence was approximately the same (16%) but no patient was below 35 years old, leading to a conclusion that isolated shoulder hemorrhages and shoulder arthropathy in hemophilic patients on prophylactic treatment was uncommon. It is likely, of course, that this pattern will be reflected in other joints now that prophylactic treatment is the norm.

Shoulder problems have traditionally been dealt with using nonoperative measures, trying to minimize the prevalence for bleeding. Radioactive or chemical synoviorthesis have been performed and synovectomy, either open or arthroscopic, is now becoming more common. Fusion of the shoulder can be effective in converting a painful, stiff joint into a painless stiff joint [23].

Total shoulder replacement is a relatively uncommon procedure undertaken in hemophilia, with sporadic case reports only. Luck and Kasper [23] reported three patients, with satisfactory results with regard to both pain relief and range of motion. Greene [42] recorded a satisfactory outcome in a single patient who underwent a total shoulder replacement but who later died of the effects of HIV. Phillips et al. [22] reported the successful outcome of a case of ipsilateral shoulder and elbow replacement in a patient with hemophilia B.

Now that prophylactic factor treatment programs are becoming more widespread, the incidence of bleeding into the shoulder and subsequent arthropathy is becoming a rare event. It is therefore likely that very few patients will present with significant shoulder symptoms and thus the demand for shoulder intervention, and shoulder replacement, in particular, will remain minimal for the foreseeable future.

Conclusions

It would therefore seem that joint replacement surgery should be the treatment of choice in hemophilic patients suffering from severe arthropathy and disability. There can be little doubt that a successful implant provides considerable benefits in the majority of hemophilic patients, with marked pain relief and improvement in function. However, the increased risk of infection and noninfective complications remains a cause for concern.

Thus, before embarking upon a potentially dangerous procedure, the orthopedic surgeon should consider the risks and benefits very carefully, taking into account the age of the patient, ambitions, life expectancy, and immunologic status. The patient should be managed in a dedicated hemophilia center, where a comprehensive team approach can be provided.

The risk of HIV infection through contaminated blood products has significantly diminished with time since coagulation factor concentrates have been subject to viricidal agents, and in the UK there have been no new HIV infections in hemophilic patients since 1986. In addition, the introduction of recombinant factor replacement in 1998 has been a major development particularly in removing the unacceptably high risk of viral transmission (HIV, hepatitis B and C).

Patients with HIV are now living longer as a result of the improvements in medication and combination therapy. There still remains a question as to the effect of combination therapy on hemostasis and there is a degree of uncertainty around the timing of withdrawing treatment prior to surgery.

For hemophilic patients in the developing world, there is accumulating evidence that better prophylaxis in childhood and adolescence is leading to a marked reduction in hemophilic arthropathy. Hopefully, therefore, the need for operative intervention will also diminish. Ultimately, of course gene therapy may cure the disease.

References

1 Lachiewicz PF, Inglis AE, Insall JN, *et al*. Total knee arthroplasty in hemophilia. *J Bone Joint Surg Am* 1985; **67**: 1361–6.

2 Karthaus RP, Novakova IR. Total knee replacement in haemophilic arthropathy. *J Bone Joint Surg Br* 1988; **70**: 382–5.

3 Thomason HC III, Wilson FC, Lachiewicz PF, Kelley SS. Knee arthroplasty in hemophilic arthropathy. *Clin Orthop* 1999; **360**: 169–73.

4 Gregg-Smith SJ, Pattison RM, Dodd CAF, Duthie RB. Septic arthritis in haemophilia. *J Bone Joint Surg Br* 1993; **75B**: 368–70.

5 Wiedel JD, Luck JV, Gilbert MS. Total knee arthroplasty in the patient with haemophilia; evaluation and long term results. In: Gilbert MS, Greene WB, eds. *Musculo-skeltal Problems in Hemophilia*, New York National: Hemophilia foundation, 1989: 152–7.

6 Ragni MV, Crossett LS, Herndon JH. Postoperative infection following orthopaedic surgery in human immunodeficiency virus-infected hemophiliacs with CD4 counts "200/mm³. *J Arthroplasty* 1995; **10**: 716–21.

7 Birch NC, Ribbans WJ, Goldman E, Lee CA. Knee replacement in haemophilia. *J Bone Joint Surg Br* 1994; **76B**: 165–6.

8 Phillips AM, Sabin CA, Ribbans WJ, Lee CA. Orthopaedic surgery in hemophilic patients with human immunodeficiency virus. *Clin Orthop* 1997; **343**: 81–7.

9 Hicks JL, Ribbans WJ, Buzzard B, *et al*. Infected joint replacements in HIV-positive patients with haemophilia. *J Bone Joint Surg Br* 2001; **83**: 1050–4.

10 Rodriguez-Merchan EC, Wiedel JD. Total knee arthroplasty in HIV-positive haemophilic patients. *Haemophilia* 2002; **8**: 387–92.

11 Rodriguez-Merchan EC, Wiedel JD. Total knee arthroplasty in haemophilia. In: Rodriguez-Merchan EC, Goddard NJ, Lee CA, eds. *Musculoskeletal Aspects of Haemophilia*. Oxford: Blackwell Science, 2000: 78–84.

12 Goddard NJ, Rodriguez-Merchan EC, Wiedel JD. Total knee replacement in haemophilia. *Haemophilia* 2002; **8**: 382–6.

13 Mann HA, Goddard NJ, Lee CA, Brown SA. Periarticular aneurysm following total knee replacement in hemophilic arthropathy. *J.Bone Joint Surg Am* 2003; **85**: 2437–40.

14 Gilbert MS, Glass KS. Hemophilic arthropathy of the elbow. *Mt Sinai J Med* 1977; **44**: 389–96.

15 Kay L, Stainsby D, Buzzard B. The role of synovectomy in the management of recurrent haemarthroses in haemophilia. *Br J Haematol* 1981; **49**: 53–60.

16 Le Balc'h T, Ebelin T, Laurian Y. Synovectomy of the elbow in young hemophilic patients. *J Bone Joint Surg Am* 1987; **69A**: 264–9.

17 Luck JV Jr. Surgical management of advanced hemophilic arthropathy. *Prog Clin Biol Res* 1990; **324**: 241–56.

18 Rodriguez-Merchan EC, Galindo E, Magallon M, *et al*. Resection of the radial head and partial open synovectomy of the elbow in the young adult with haemophilia. *Haemophilia* 1995; **1**: 262–6.

19 Butler-Manuel PA, Smith MA, Savidge GF. Silastic interposition for haemophilic arthropathy of the elbow. *J Bone Joint Surg Br* 1990; **72**: 472–4.

20 Bajekal RA, Phillips AM, Ribbans WJ. Elbow arthropathy in haemophilia. *J Bone Joint Surg Br* 1996 (Suppl. 1): 15.

21 Beeton K, Rodriguez-Merchan EC, Alltree J. Total joint arthroplasty in haemophilia. *Haemophilia* 2000; **6**: 474–81.

22 Phillips AM, Ribbans WJ, Goddard NJ. Ipsilateral total shoulder and elbow prosthetic replacement in a patient with severe haemophilia B. *Haemophilia* 1995; **1**: 270–3.

23 Luck JV, Kasper C. Surgical management of advanced haemophilic arthropathy. *Clin Orthop* 1989; **242**: 60–82.

24 Kasten MD, Skinner HB. Total elbow arthroplasty. An 18-year experience. *Clin Orthop* 1993; **290**: 177–88.

25 Chantelot C, Feugas C, Ala ET, *et al*. [Kudo non-constrained elbow prosthesis for inflammatory and hemophilic joint disease: analysis in 30 cases]. *Rev Chir Orthop Reparatrice Appar Mot* 2002; **88**: 398–405.

26 Chapman-Sheath PJ, Giangrande P, Carr AJ. Arthroplasty of the elbow in haemophilia. *J Bone Joint Surg Br* 2003; **85**: 1138–40.

27 Gamble JG, Bellah J, Rinsky LA, Glader B. Arthropathy of the ankle in hemophilia. *J Bone Joint Surg Am* 1991; **73**: 1008–15.

28 O'Donoghue DH. Impingement exostoses of the tibia and talus. *J Bone Joint Surg Am* 1957; **39A**: 835–42.

29 Ribbans WJ, Phillips AM. Hemophilic ankle arthropathy. *Clin Orthop* 1996; **328**: 39–45.

30 Goddard NJ. Haemophilic arthropathy of the ankle. In: Rodriguez-Merchan EC, ed. *The Haemaphilic Joints: New Perspectives*. Oxford: Blackwell Science, 2003: 171–5.

31 Pearce MS, Smith MA, Savidge GF. Supramalleolar tibial osteotomy for haemophilic arthropathy of the ankle. *J Bone Joint Surg Br* 1994; **76**: 947–50.

32 MacNicol MF, Ludlam CA. Does avascular necrosis cause collapse of the dome of the talus in severe haemophilia? *Haemophilia* 1999; **5**: 139–42.

33 Nelson IW, Sivamurugan S, Latham PD, *et al*. Total hip arthroplasty for hemophilic arthropathy. *Clin Orthop* 1992; **276**: 210–13.

34 Stauffer RN. Hemophilia. In: Morrey B, ed. *Joint Replacement Arthroplasty*. London: Churchill Livingstone 1991: 759–64.

35 Lofqvist T, Sanzen L, Petersson C, Nilsson IM. Total hip replacement in patients with haemophilia. *Acta Orthop Scand* 1996; **67**: 321–4.

36 Heeg M, Meyer K, Smid WM, *et al*. Total knee and hip arthroplasty in haemophilic patients. *Haemophilia* 1998; **4**: 747–51.

37 Kelley SS, Lachiewicz PF, Gilbert MS, *et al*. Hip arthroplasty in hemophilic arthropathy. *J Bone Joint Surg Am* 1995; **77**: 828–34.

38 Rodriguez-Merchan EC, Riera JA, Wiedel JD. Total hip replacement in the haemophilic patient. In: Rodriguez-Merchan EC, ed. *The Haemophilic Joints; New Perspectives*. Oxford: Blackwell Science, 2003: 111–15.

39 Petersson CJ. The hemophilic shoulder. In: Rodriguez-Merchan EC, ed. *The Haemophilic Joints; New Perspectives*. Oxford: Blackwell Science, 2003: 163–6.

40 Gilbert MS, Klepps S, Cleeman E, *et al*. The shoulder: a neglected joint. *Int Monitor Haemophilia* 2002; **10**: 3–5.

41 MacDonald PB, Locht RC, Lindsay D, Levi C. Haemophilic arthropathy of the shoulder. *J Bone Joint Surg Br* 1990; **72**: 470–1.

42 Greene WB, DeGnore L, White G. Orthopaedic procedures and prognosis in hemophilic patients who are sero-positive for human immunodeficiency virus. *J Bone Joint Surg Am* 1990; **72A**: 2–11.

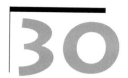

30 Synoviorthesis in hemophilia

E. Carlos Rodriguez-Merchan

Introduction

A synoviorthesis consists of the intra-articular injection of a certain material with the aim of "stabilizing" (orthesis) the synovium of a joint (synoviorthesis). There are two basic types of procedures for synovial control: medical synovectomy (or synoviorthesis) and surgical synovectomy (open or arthroscopic). It is commonly accepted today that synoviorthesis is the procedure of choice, and that surgical synovectomy should be performed only if a number of consecutive synoviortheses fail to stop or diminish the frequency of recurrent hemarthrosis [1–7]. Thus, the main indication for a synoviorthesis in a hemophilic joint is chronic hypertrophic synovitis and recurrent bleeding.

It is well known that, in hemophilia, one or several joints (elbows, knees, and ankles) tend to bleed (hemarthrosis), beginning from an early age of 2–5 years. The synovium is able to reabsorb only a small amount of intra-articular blood; if the amount of blood is excessive, the synovium will hypertrophy as a compensating mechanism, so that eventually the affected joint will show an increase in size of the synovium: so-called hypertrophic chronic hemophilic synovitis. The hypertrophic synovium is very richly vascularized, so that small injuries will easily make the joint rebleed. The final result will be the classic vicious cycle of hemarthrosis–synovitis–hemarthrosis.

If both phenomena are not controlled, they will eventually result in cartilage and bone damage visible on radiographs (chronic hemophilic arthropathy). All the aforementioned features are caused by the congenital coagulation deficiency of factor VIII (FVIII) (hemophilia A) or factor IX (FIX) (hemophilia B). Continuous prophylaxis from 2 to 18 years will significantly decrease the number of hemarthroses and, therefore, the risk of synovitis will also be diminished. On-demand treatment of hemarthroses usually does prevent the development of chronic synovitis. A very serious complication of substitutive treatment, however, is the development of an inhibitor. In such a circumstance, the frequency and severity of hemarthroses will be more intense, producing a severe degree of synovitis.

Indication of synoviorthesis

The main indication of synoviorthesis is chronic hypertrophic synovitis associated with recurrent hemarthroses that does not respond to hematologic treatment. Synoviorthesis should be performed under factor coverage to avoid the risk of rebleeding during the procedure. In patients with inhibitors, synoviorthesis can also be performed with minimal risk. In fact, the procedure is especially indicated in patients with inhibitors because of its ease of performance and low rate of complications.

When a child starts to suffer from recurrent hemarthroses that cannot be controlled with conservative treatment, he will develop hypertrophic synovitis. It is important to reach a differential diagnosis between hemarthrosis and synovitis. Acute hemarthrosis is associated with severe pain, and the joint is maintained in a position of comfort (typically in flexion). In contrast, chronic hypertrophic synovitis is not associated with as much pain. The synovium is palpable as a soft-tissue firmness whereas a hemarthrosis will have a fluid characteristic.

Before making the recommendation of a synoviorthesis, the diagnosis should be confirmed by radiographs, echography, and/or MRI. The differential diagnosis between synovitis and hemarthrosis can be determined by ultrasonography (echography) and MRI [8]. Radiographs should also be taken in order to assess the degree of hemophilic arthropathy at the time of diagnosis. In many situations, synovitis and hemarthrosis occur together. At the knee, echography is very specific and reliable.

Types of synoviorthesis

There are two basic types of synoviorthesis: chemical and radioactive. The materials most commonly used for chemical synovectomy are osmic acid, rifampicin, and oxytetracycline clorhydrate [9–12]. The radioisotopes currently used for radiation synovectomy are ^{90}Y (yttrium-90), ^{32}P (phosphorus-32) and ^{186}Rh (rhenium-186) [13–19]. Radiation synovectomy is the method of choice because it appears to be more efficacious than chemical synovectomy. Selection of the radioisotope should take into consideration the half-life, because the intensity of the inflammatory reaction is directly related to the rate of exposure, and the size of the radiocolloid: the larger the size the less tendency for the material to leak from the joint space.

The material should be a pure beta-emitting radioisotope, thereby minimizing the whole-body exposure to radiation that gamma radiation can produce. Radioactive gold (^{198}Au) should probably not be used because it does emit gamma radiation and is small in size [20]. Table 30.1 summarizes the main features of the radioisotopes most frequently used for radiosynoviorthesis in persons with hemophilia. Table 30.2 shows the clinical indications of the radioactive isotopes most frequently used for ra-

Table 30.1 Description of the radioisotopes most frequently used for radiosynoviorthesis in hemophilia.

Isotope	^{32}P	^{90}Y	^{186}Rh
Radioactive half-life (days)	14.3	2.8	3.8
Radiation	Beta	Beta	Beta and gamma
TPP (mm)	2.2	2.8	1

TPP, therapeutic penetration power.

Table 30.2 Clinical indications of the radioactive isotopes most frequently used for radiosynoviorthesis in hemophilia.

Isotope	Joint
^{90}Y and ^{32}P	Knees
^{186}Rh	Elbows, ankles

diosynoviorthesis in hemophilia patients. The recommended isotope for the knee is ^{90}Y at a dose of 185 megabecquerels (MBq). ^{186}Rh is better for elbows (56–74 MBq) and ankles (74 MBq) [21].

The current measurement unit for activity of radioisotopes is the becquerel (Bq), and the megabecquerel (MBq). However, it is still common to encounter the former measurement unit, the millicurie (mCi), in many papers. According to Coya-Viña et al. [21], the formula for the conversion of mCi into MBq is the following:

$1\,mCi = 37\,MBq$, and $1\,mCi = 3.7 \times 10^{10}$ disintegrations per second

Taking into account the concern that radioactive materials evoke, and the high cost and limited supply of these materials, it is best to schedule groups of 6–8 patients to perform radiation synovectomy. This will require some patients to wait upwards of 2–3 months until the whole group is scheduled for the procedure. If possible, patients should be maintained on continuous prophylaxis while awaiting the procedure. The aforementioned disadvantages of radiation synovectomy do not exist with rifampicin and oxytetracycline, which are very cheap and easily obtainable. Rifampicin injection can be rather painful and may have to be repeated at weekly intervals. The follow-up of oxytetracycline synoviorthesis is still very short (6 months) [12].

Age to perform synoviorthesis

Synoviorthesis can be performed at any age in the life of the hemophilic patient. Intra-articular injection in a very young child may be difficult because it requires patient cooperation, and this may require general anesthesia. The potential for radiation-induced cellular damage or chromosomal abnormalities remains a concern, particularly in the child. After more than 30

years of experience in using radiation synovectomy, neither articular nor systemic (neoplastic) damage has been reported. Regarding the maximum age for a synoviorthesis, it should be emphasized that the main consideration is that it should be performed for the correct indications, e.g., for recurrent hemarthrosis secondary to chronic synovitis. It should not be used for chronic effusions and pain secondary to degenerative disease (chronic hemophilic arthropathy).

The technique of synoviorthesis

If the procedure is performed under local anesthetic, the proposed site injection is infiltrated with up to 10 mL 1% lidocaine (lignocaine), attempting to anesthetize not only the skin but also the deeper tissues down to and including the joint capsule and synovium. For simple joint injections, a 16- or 18-gauge spinal needle is sufficient but a wider bore 12- or 14-gauge needle (Abbocath or equivalent) may be necessary in order to evacuate a viscous hemarthrosis prior to joint injection. Once the joint has been entered, all the liquid content (blood or synovial fluid) should be evacuated, and only then should the fibrosing agent be injected. Postinjection pain may be reduced by mixing the agent with a long-acting local anesthetic, e.g., bupivacaine.

Chemical synovectomy requires no additional special precautions. However, when performing a radioactive synovectomy, the needle should be withdrawn very slowly while at the same time injecting an anti-inflammatory drug (e.g., hydrocortisone acetate, triamcinolone) in order to avoid the risk of radioactive burn of the needle track or, even worse, an adjacent skin burn.

Whichever agent is employed, care must be taken to avoid extra-articular complications (radiation burn and/or inflammatory reaction) as a result of extravasation or needle track contamination. The most frequently affected joints in hemophilia are the elbows (Figure 30.1), knees (Figure 30.2), and the ankles [22].

Efficacy of synoviorthesis

On average, synoviorthesis has a 75–80% satisfactory outcome in the long term [2–7]. From the clinical standpoint, such efficacy can be measured by the decrease in the number of hemarthroses, with complete cessation for several years in some cases. In 20–25% of cases, synoviorthesis fails to control hemarthroses but it can be repeated.

It is commonly accepted that the more severe the degree of synovitis, the more difficult it will be to remove the synovium by means of a synoviorthesis. In fact, in cases where marked hypertrophy is present, it may be necessary to perform multiple consecutive synoviortheses, or even a surgical synovectomy. Synoviorthesis with rifampicin and oxytetracycline clorhydrate can be repeated many times at weekly intervals. With radiation synovectomy, no more than three synoviortheses are advised at

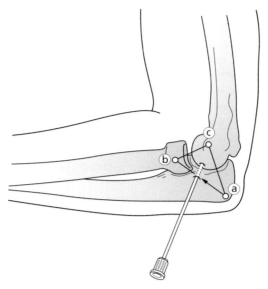

Figure 30.1 Elbow synoviorthesis; with the elbow in lateral view the needle should be inserted in the center of the triangle formed by the olecranon (a), the radial head (b), and the lateral epicondyle (c) (reprinted with permission from ref. 22).

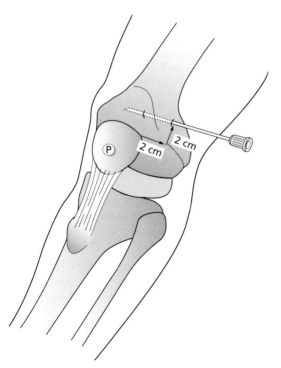

Figure 30.2 Knee synoviorthesis through the suprapatellar lateral route. The injection is made above the lateral corner of the patella (p) and directly into the suprapatellar pouch (reprinted with permission from ref. 22).

3-month intervals. When repeated synoviortheses fail, a surgical synovectomy (open or arthroscopic) may be indicated.

Complications of synoviorthesis

The main complication of radiation synovectomy is a cutaneous burn if the radioactive material is injected out of the joint. Another potential complication is an inflammatory reaction after injection; in such a case, rest and nonsteroidal anti-inflammatory drugs (NSAIDs) will control these symptoms. No malignant effects (carcinogenic) of radioactive materials have been reported after more than 30 years of their use worldwide [23].

Multiple synoviorthesis in a single session

It is well known that the individual with hemophilia commonly has more than one target joint. In such cases, it is possible to perform more than one synoviorthesis in the same session. Two injections can be performed at the same time, but it is impractical to inject the same joint bilaterally (e.g., both elbows or both knees, both ankles) or two different joints of the lower limbs of different sides (e.g., right knee and left ankle). If two joints are to be injected, the two joints should be on the same side, e.g., elbow and knee; elbow and ankle; knee and ankle. Figure 30.3 summarizes the recommended treatment algorithm for synovitis and recurrent hemarthrosis in hemophilia with synoviorthesis.

Alternatives to synoviorthesis

A study was reported to determine optimal treatment for chronic hemophilic synovitis of the knee and synovitis of the elbow [19]. This included 65 patients with synovitis affecting 65 knee joints and 40 patients who had synovitis of the elbow (44 elbows), who, despite a 3-month trial of prophylactic substitution therapy, were treated by synovectomy during 1974 to 1996. Radiation synovectomies ([198]Au synoviorthesis) were performed on 38 knees, open surgical synovectomy on 18, and nine had an arthroscopic procedure. Radioactive gold synoviorthesis was performed on 29 elbows, and 15 had a resection of the radial head and partial open synovectomy. This study concluded that synovectomy (by any method) significantly reduced bleeding episodes but did not halt the radiographic deterioration of the joints.

It is thought that radiation synovectomy is the best choice for patients with persistent synovitis of the knee and elbow unresponsive to a three-month trial of prophylactic factor replacement (Table 30.3). If two to three consecutive synoviortheses given at 3 month intervals fail, a surgical synovectomy is indicated (Figure 30.3). When chronic synovitis is allowed to persist, the membrane can hypertrophy to the point where it cannot be adequately ablated by a pure beta-emitting radiocolloid, which only penetrates between 2.2 and 2.8 mm (Table 30.1). In

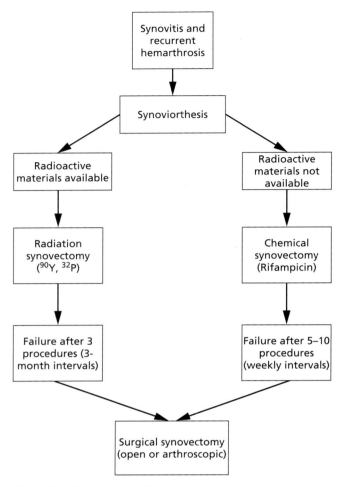

Figure 30.3 Treatment algorithm recommended by the author when treating a patient with chronic hemophilic synovitis (reprinted with permission from ref. 3).

Table 30.3 Synoviorthesis versus synovectomy.

Synoviorthesis	Surgical synovectomy
Inexpensive	Expensive
Simple	Complex
Painless	Painful
Less invasive	Invasive
Lower risk of infection	High risk of infection
No general anesthetic	General anesthetic

these cases, as well as those in which repeated radiosynoviorthesis has failed, surgical synovectomy (open or arthroscopic) is often effective [7].

Conclusions

Synoviorthesis is a very effective procedure that decreases both the frequency and the intensity of recurrent intra-articular

bleeds related to joint synovitis. Radiosynoviorthesis is currently recommended with ^{90}Y for the knees and ^{186}Rh for elbows and ankles. The procedure should be performed as soon as possible to minimize the degree of articular cartilage damage. It can also be used in patients with inhibitors with minimal risk of complications [24,25].

On average, synoviorthesis has a 75–80% satisfactory outcome in the long term. Such efficacy can be measured clinically by the decrease in the number of hemarthroses, with complete cessation for several years in some cases. In 20–25% of cases, synoviorthesis fails to control hemarthroses, but in such cases, it can be repeated [26].

Global long-term results of treatment with chemical synovectomy (osmic acid and rifampicin) seem to be less favorable than with radionuclides (^{90}Y and ^{32}P). Although the short-term results of oxytetracycline synoviorthesis are encouraging, a much longer follow-up is needed to ascertain the efficacy of such a new type of chemical synoviorthesis. In cases where the synovium is thicker than 3 mm, and hemarthroses persist following synoviorthesis, surgical synovectomy (open or arthroscopic) is indicated.

References

1 Molho P, Verrier P, Stieltjes N, *et al*. A retrospective study on chemical and radioactive synovectomy in severe haemophilia patients with recurrent haemarthrosis. *Haemophilia* 1999; 5: 115–23.
2 Salis G, Molho P, Verrier P, *et al*. Nonsurgical synovectomy in the treatment of arthropathy in Von Willebrand's Disease. *Rev Rheum Engl Ed* 1998; 65: 232–7.
3 Rodriguez-Merchan EC, Wiedel JD. General principles and indications of synoviorthesis (medical synovectomy) in haemophilia. *Haemophilia* 2001; 7 (Suppl. 2): 6–10.
4 Rodriguez-Merchan EC, Goddard NJ. Chronic haemophilic synovitis. In: Rodriguez-Merchan EC, Goddard NJ, Lee CA, eds. *Musculoskeletal Aspects of Haemophilia*. Oxford, Blackwell Science, 2000: 43–9.
5 Fernandez-Palazzi F. Treatment of acute and chronic synovitis by non-surgical means. *Haemophilia* 1998; 4: 518–23.
6 Fernandez-Palazzi F, Rivas S, Cibeira JL, *et al*. Radioactive synoviorthesis in hemophilic hemarthrosis: materials, techniques, and dangers. *Clin Orthop* 1996; 328: 14–8.
7 Rodriguez-Merchan EC, Luck JV Jr, Silva M, Quintana M. Synoviorthesis in haemophilia. In: Rodriguez-Merchan EC, ed. *The Haemophilic Joints. New Perspectives*. Oxford: Blackwell Science, 2003: 73–9.
8 Nuss R, Kilcoyne RF, Rivard GE, Murphy J. Late clinical, plain X-ray and magnetic resonance imaging findings in haemophilic joints treated with radiosynoviorthesis. *Haemophilia* 2000; 6: 658–63.
9 Caviglia HA, Fernandez-Palazzi F, Maffei E, *et al*. Chemical synoviorthesis for hemophilic synovitis. *Clin Orthop* 1997; 343: 30–6.
10 Caviglia H, Galatro G, Duhalde C, Perez-Bianco R. Haemophilic synovitis: is rifampicin an alternative? *Haemophilia* 1998; 4: 514–17.
11 Fernandez-Palazzi F, Rivas S, Viso R, *et al*. Synovectomy with rifampicin in haemophilic haemarthrosis. *Haemophilia* 2000; 6: 562–5.
12 Fernandez-Palazzi F, Viso R, Bernal R, *et al*. Oxytetracycline clorhy-

drate as a new material for chemical sinoviorthesis in haemophilia. In: Rodriguez-Merchan EC, ed. *The Haemophilic Joints. New Perspectives*. Oxford: Blackwell Science, 2003: 80–3.

13 Heim M, Horoszowski H, Lieberman L, *et al.* Methods and results of radionuclide synovectomies. In: Gilbert MS, Greene WD, eds. *Musculoskeletal Problems in Hemophilia*. New York: National Hemophilia Foundation, 1990: 98–101.

14 Rodriguez-Merchan EC. Methods to treat chronic haemophilic synovitis. *Haemophilia* 2001; 7: 1–5.

15 Mathew P, Talbut DC, Frogameni A, *et al.* Isotopic synovectomy with P-32 in paediatric patients with haemophilia. *Haemophilia* 2000; 6: 547–55.

16 Heim M, Goshen E, Amit Y, Martinowitz U. Sinoviorthesis with radioactive yttrium in haemophilia: Israel experience. *Haemophilia* 2001; 7 (Suppl. 2): 36–9.

17 Rodriguez-Merchan EC, Jimenez-Yuste V, Villar A, *et al.* Yttrium-90 synoviorthesis for chronic haemophilic synovitis: Madrid experience. *Haemophilia* 2001; 7 (Suppl. 2): 34–5.

18 Silva M, Luck JV Jr, Siegel ME. [32]P chromic phosphate radiosynovectomy for chronic haemophilic synovitis. *Haemophilia* 2001; 7 (Suppl. 2): 40–9.

19 Rodriguez-Merchan EC, Magallon M, Galindo E, Lopez-Cabarcos C. Hemophilic synovitis of the knee and the elbow. *Clin Orthop* 1997; 343: 47–53.

20 Rodriguez-Merchan EC, Magallon M, Martin-Villar J, *et al.* Long term follow up of haemophilic arthropathy treated by [198]Au radiation synovectomy. *Int Orthop* 1993; 17: 120–4.

21 Coya-Viña J, Marin-Ferrer M, Martin-Curto LM. Radioactive isotopes for radiosynoviorthesis. In: Rodríguez-Merchan EC, ed. *The Haemophilic Joints. New Perspectives*. Oxford: Blackwell Science, 2003: 68–72.

22 Rodriguez-Merchan EC, Goddard NJ. The technique of synoviorthesis. *Haemophilia* 2001; 7 (Suppl. 2): 11–15.

23 Falcon de Vargas A, Fernandez-Palazzi F. Cytogenetic studies in patients with hemophilic hemarthrosis treated by 198Au, 186Rh, and 90Y radioactive synoviorthesis. *J Pediatr Orthop B* 2000; 9: 52–4.

24 Lofqvist T, Petersson C, Nilsson IM. Radioactive synoviorthesis in patients with hemophilia with factor inhibitor. *Clin Orthop* 1997; 343: 37–41.

25 Petersson CJ, Berntorp E. Radiosynoviorthesis in patients with haemophilia and inhibitors. In: Rodriguez-Merchan EC, Lee CA, eds. *Inhibitors in Patients with Haemophilia*. Oxford: Blackwell Science, 2002: 129–31.

26 Rodriguez-Merchan EC. Radionuclide synovectomy (radiosynoviorthesis) in hemophilia: a very efficient and single procedure. *Sem Thromb Haemost* 2003; 29: 97–100.

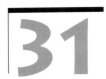

Pseudotumors in patients with hemophilia

Michael Heim and Uri Martinowitz

Introduction

Many anecdotal reports have been published in the literature regarding the development of pseudotumors in individuals with hemophilia. Historically, these reports originated mainly from countries where prophylactic replacement of the missing coagulation factor was not practiced. An assumption was thus made that there is a connection between the lack of factor replacement and pseudotumors. This suspicion has been strengthened by the reports of the occurrence of pseudotumors in patients who have developed an antibody to the missing coagulation factor. Pseudotumors are rare and the frequency is reported at about 1%.

Why is this entity called a pseudotumor and not a tumor?

There are two distinct pathologic forms that have been noted and categorized under the heading of pseudotumors. The first form occurs within the peripheral long bones and very often in the developing skeleton, while the second has a predilection particularly for the area of and around the pelvis. The former starts as an intraosseous expansion that can perforate the cortex, while the latter begins its growth in the soft tissues and may erode skeletal structures. Some authors believe that the pathology starts in the Sharpley's fibers (the tissue connecting muscles to the periosteum). Anatomically, this situation exists extensively around the pelvis and the thighs [1]. The intraosseous form is more aggressive then a simple bone cyst, for it actively expands, and yet is amenable to conservative treatment [2]. The soft-tissue masses have a distinct histologic structure [3]. The contents comprise necrotic, aseptic remnants of blood products and may also contain large quantities of blood and other liquefied tissue products. The pseudotumor has a thick capsule wherein blood vessels encase and infuse the entire pseudotumor. The mass is expansive and hence has the ability to cause pressure necrosis of the surrounding tissues, which can include the cortex of bone (Figures 31.1, 31.3, 31.4 and plate 3, facing p. 212). The pseudotumor may expand *around* structures such as the ureters, blood vessels and nerves. These structures are not *invaded* as with tumoral growth but encircled, and upon gross anatomy would appear to be within the tumor mass [4].

Clinical presentation

As stated previously, there are two forms. The peripheral pathology is generally amenable to early diagnosis in view of the anatomical deformation of fingers and toes and/or the perceivable swelling noted over the dorsum of the hand or foot. Radiographic evidence is easily obtained and treatment can then be instituted.

The second form is usually intra-abdominal and slow growing. Early diagnosis rarely occurs as the expanding mass slowly fills up the area of the abdomen and/or the pelvis and retroperitoneum. The patients may note a general discomfort but in the light of their experiences with intra-articular hemarthroses and muscle bleeds these generalized symptoms are often ignored. Radiologic plates may show a displacement of viscera and/or bone erosion and a more extensive investigation is then indicated in order to assess the extent of the pseudotumor.

Investigations required prior to planning a treatment protocol

Large pseudotumors, although, as stated earlier, usually arising in the area of the pelvis, can theoretically appear anywhere in the body. It must be appreciated that not only are the dimensions of the mass relevant, but also the contents and the anatomy of the surrounding area. The following investigations should be considered:

1 Radiologic assessment in order to ascertain the osseous extent of the damage. Regular radiographs and computerized tomography usually suffice.

2 The assessment of the structure and nature of the soft tissues and their relations to the bone can be mapped out by ultrasound and magnetic resonance imaging (MRI). Intravenous injection of gadolinium in conjunction with the MRI is suggested. This

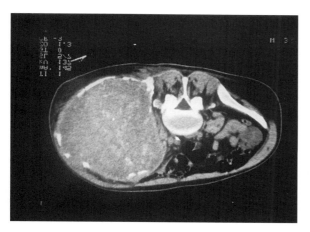

Figure 31.1 CT section through the level of the lumbar spine. A huge round pseudotumor can be noted. The pseudotumor has destroyed and fragmented the ileum and the mass almost extends to the midline.

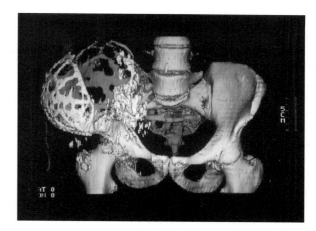

Figure 31.4 This figure clearly shows a CT reconstruction of the pseudotumor, which has fragments of the ileum surrounding the mass. Note the encroachment onto the sacrum and the destroyed sacroiliac articulation.

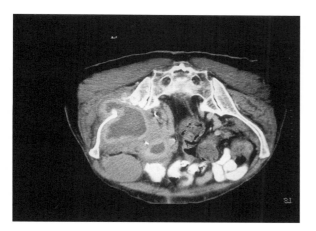

Figure 31.3 The CT section shows a large pseudotumor mass that has expanded through the ileum. The mass can clearly be seen in the destroyed bone and on both sides of the ileum.

gadolinium will assist by recording pathologic blood vessels and also help to delineate the pseudotumor capsule.

3 It is important to establish the presence of a major blood vessel in or close to the mass on arteriogram, in order to provide a safe surgical approach to the pseudotumor.

4 Intravenous pyelography should be carried out if the growth is in the region of the kidney and its draining apparatus.

5 A full and comprehensive hematologic assessment of the patients is essential. There should be a coagulation team available for the surgery and postoperative care, and provision of sufficient blood and coagulation products. The surgery can be complicated, requiring blood transfusion, and it may become necessary to provide prophylactic factor supplementation for an extended period.

6 Hemostasis can be produced not only by the intravenous infusion of the missing coagulation factor but intraoperatively by the dissemination of fibrin glue over the raw surfaces. The fibrin glue is spread over the oozing area by the use of a controlled-pressure atomizer. It is important that if the surgeon is not familiar with the technique and the instrumentation, he or she should learn these skills prior to surgery.

7 Time should be set aside for the patient and his family to meet with the team so that not only does the patient sign an informed consent but the family unit is aware of what is before them and the risks involved.

8 A date should be set aside when all the team is available and this should include competent experienced surgeons from the various disciplines.

Prior to the day of surgery

As stated previously, the pseudotumor receives its blood supply from vessels that are present within the capsule that surrounds the mass. These vessels have a number of "feeding" arteries and if they can be thrombosed the risk of massive intraoperative bleeding can be reduced [5] and the pseudotumor mass may be reduced in size. Arteries have the ability of recanalization and hence the thrombosis should be carried out 7–10 days before surgery.

Realistic aims

The intention should be the entire eradication of the pseudotumor and the reconstruction of the normal anatomy. This is not always possible for there may be destroyed bone. The displaced viscera are not usually a problem. Bony structures, for example the iliac bone, should be left in a stable condition [6], and if large bone fragments remain viable but free floating after the tumor has been excised it is suggested that fixation methods be implemented [7]. "Dead space" can be "plugged" by the insertion of the omentum [8]. Bone allografts and/or bone substitutes can be used together with fibrin glue in the reconstruction of skeletal integrity. The peripheral pseudotumors are easily treated by the opening of a bone window, the drainage and curettage of the contents and then the packing of the pseudotumor space with bone and/or bone substitutes [9] mixed with glue [10].

Total excision is the intention but is not always possible. The dissection is carried out around the capsule of the pseudotumor but, as stated previously, vital structures, although completely surrounded by the capsule, may be very deeply "embedded" within the contents of the pseudotumor. Structures such as the ureter can easily be damaged even though a catheter may have been inserted previously. It is probably safer to leave a small fragment of the pseudotumor wall attached to the vital structure then to risk damaging it. Abdominal pseudotumors may be enormous and the authors have managed a case where 6 L of liquid contents were drained out of the pseudotumor.

Complications

The complications may be divided into two groups, intra- and perioperative, and late complications. The former relates to the surgical procedure, which may require a multidisciplinary surgical team to conduct complicated surgery in a very protracted procedure. Infection is always a risk but even more so in the late recovery phase. The formation of a constantly draining sinus creates a situation wherein an open canal exists between the exterior, the bowel [11], and the abdominal cavity. This situation inevitably results in a purulent discharge and may lead to death. Another complication is the regrowth or regeneration of a pseudotumor. As stated previously, the intra-abdominal pseudotumors are usually only diagnosed at a late stage, when huge expansion and destruction has taken place. If the pseudotumor is recognized early, excision can be less complicated. Excision causes extensive alteration in the soft-tissue anatomy owing to the extensive healing fibrosis and adhesions. Postexcision follow-up is necessary in order to document and discover whether the pseudotumor has re-formed and started growing once again.

It should be stressed and noted that the hematologic control of the coagulation status of these patients may be complicated by acute hemorrhage requiring massive blood replacement, large oozing areas, and the fact that the patient may have an inhibitor to the missing coagulation factor. Factor assays should be carried out during the preoperative period and ample supplies of relevant clotting factor should be present and not just on stand-by elsewhere.

The physical rehabilitation of patients after such massive surgery requires dedication of the rehabilitation team. Initially, the patient requires intensive nursing care. The wound dressing and the general nursing guides the patient from the postoperative catabolic state into an anabolic phase and psychologic sup-port is essential for the patient and the family. Progress is slow and the physical therapist and the occupational therapist enhance joint movements and muscle strengthening. Once the wounds have healed, the patient adds to the therapeutic regime hydrotherapy and more intensive physical therapy. During this rehabilitation period, which starts initially on an inpatient basis and progresses to an ambulatory service, the authors have found it necessary from time to time to remind the patient of his status quo prior to the surgery. This reinforcement assists the patient in appreciating the improvement in the quality of life.

In conclusion, where surgery is necessary it should be carried out in a tertiary medical center by the most experienced multidisciplinary team. For more information a short list of the key references has been provided. There are many case reports in the older medical literature that have been omitted from this short list. The major issues are covered by the references.

References

1 Duthie R, Matthews J, Rizza C, Steel W. Haemophilic cysts and pseudotumours. In: Duthie R, Matthews J, Rizza C, Steel W, eds. *The Management of Musculoskeletal Problems in the Haemophilias.* Oxford: Blackwell Science, 1972: 84–98.

2 Gilbert MS, Forster A. A rational approach to the treatment of haemophilic blood cysts (pseudotumours) in patients with inhibitors. In: Rodrigues Merchan EC, Lee CA, eds. *Inhibitors in Patients with Haemophilia.* Oxford: Blackwell Science, 2002: 142–45.

3 Rodrigues Merchan EC. The haemophilia pseudotumour. *Haemophilia* 2002; 8: 12–16.

4 Heim M, Luboshitz J, Amit Y, Martinowitz U. The management of giant haemophilic pseudotumours. In: Rodrigues Merchan EC, Goddard NJ, Lee CA, eds. *Musculoskeletal Aspects of Haemophilia.* Oxford: Blackwell Science, 2000: 105–11.

5 Sevilla J, Alvarez MT, Hernandez D, *et al.* Therapeutic embolization and surgical excision of haemophilic pseudotumour. *Haemophilia.* 1999; 5: 360–63.

6 Heeg M, Van Smit M, de Meer J, Van Horn JR. Excision of a haemophilic pseudotumour of the ileum complicated by fistulation. *Haemophilia* 1998; 4: 132–5.

7 Ishiguro N, Iwahosi Y, Kato T, *et al.* The surgical treatment of haemophilic pseudotumours on an extremity: a report of three cases with pathological fractures. *Haemophilia* 1998; 4: 126–31.

8 Bellinazzo P, Silvello L, Caimi T, *et al.* Long-term evaluation of a novel surgical approach to the pseudotumour of the ileum in haemophilia: exeresis and transposition of the omentum in the residual cavity. *Haemophilia* 2000; 6: 702–4.

9 Sagarra M, Lucas M, de La Torre G, *et al.* Successful surgical treatment of haemophilic pseudotumour, filling the defect with hydroxyapatite. *Haemophilia* 2000; 6: 55–6.

10 Caviglia HA, Fernandez-Palazzi F, Galatro G, *et al.* Percutaneous treatment of haemophilic pseudotumours. In: Rodrigues-Merchan EC, Goddard NJ, Lee CA, eds. *Musculoskeletal Aspects of Haemophilia.* Oxford: Blackwell Science, 2000: 97–104.

11 Heaton D, Robertson R, Rothwell A. Iliopsoas haemophilic pseudotumour with bowel fistulation. *Haemophilia* 2000; 6: 41–3.

32

Radiology

Holger Pettersson

Diagnostic imaging has long been established as an objective tool for evaluation of musculoskeletal manifestations in hemophilia [1]. Ultrasonography, introduced for examinations of hemophilic patients in the 1970s, was used mainly for evaluation of soft-tissue bleedings, but, given modern high-tech equipment, today periarticular changes may also be examined, as well as the cartilage in some of the joints [2]. For more than 10 years, magnetic resonance imaging (MRI) has been established as the diagnostic imaging tool that can visualize in great detail both early and advanced changes in the soft tissues as well as in the skeleton. When available, it should be the method of choice [3].

This chapter will focus on X-ray examination in hemophilic arthropathy.

Indications for radiologic examination

Diagnostic imaging in hemophilia is very seldom used for diagnosis of the disease itself. The diagnosis is made and confirmed using other diagnostic tools. However, it is of great value in two particular situations:

1 For evaluation of the destruction in a specific joint, for evaluation and planning of, for instance, physiotherapy, synoviosthesis, or joint replacement.

2 For general evaluation of the joint destruction. Here, different classification methods, using evaluation of the large joints, have been used for decades. These classifications are of value for monitoring treatment, and comparing the efficacy of different treatments in respective patient groups (see below).

Hemophilic arthropathy

A spectrum of pathologic changes, which characterize the course of the disease, may be seen on radiographic examination. Most of the changes are the same in all joints, and appear in a given sequence during the course of the destruction of the joint. However, the repeated bleedings may also give rise to changes that are specific for different joints. The initial general changes, and then some of the specific changes in the different joints, are described below.

General changes

The first bleedings in a joint will appear on the radiograph as an expansion of the joint capsule, and may not be seen at all. Later, after several hemarthroses, the synovial hypertrophy with hemosiderin deposition and fibrosis will be visible as an increased density in the periarticular soft tissue (Figure 32.1). The density may be so high as to mimic calcification.

The hyperemia in the bone ends caused by the hemarthrosis will in childhood cause accelerated ossification and growth of the epiphyses, and in both children and adults the hyperemia will also cause epiphyseal osteopenia. Because of disuse of the limb, there may also be a general osteopenia, with thinning of the diaphyseal cortex.

Progressive destruction of the cartilage and later destruction of the subcartilaginous bone results in a joint space narrowing and subchondral bone irregularity. Later in the course, erosions in the joint periphery, as well as subchondral cyst formation, may be seen (Figure 32.2). The further ongoing destruction that may develop, irrespective of further bleedings, is similar to a secondary osteoarthritis, with sclerosis, and in the end severe destruction of the bone ends. The end result before the era of modern treatment could be a severe deformity, to the degree that only two destroyed bone ends were articulating toward each other (Figure 32.3), or a fibrous or bony ankylosis.

Changes typical for specific joints

Shoulder

In the early stages, growth disturbances of the humeral head may be noted; to begin with these may manifest as an enlargement, but the end result may well be a small atrophic humeral head. As the shoulder is not a weight-bearing joint, subchondral bone destruction and collapse is uncommon. On the other hand, osteophyte formation on the inferior margin of the glenohumeral joint may be pronounced.

Elbow

In the elbow, a fairly commonly affected joint, growth disturbances are common, with early appearance of the ossification center of the radial head, which in the end stages may be severely enlarged, causing incongruity (Figure 32.4). This may be followed by enlargement of the radial notch of the ulna. The distal

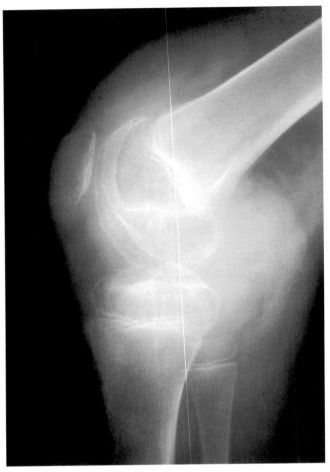

Figure 32.1 Early hemophilic arthropathy in a child. Note the pronounced expansion of the joint capsule, with increased density. There is also an overgrowth of the femoral condyles, which are osteopenic, and a squaring of the lower pole of the patella.

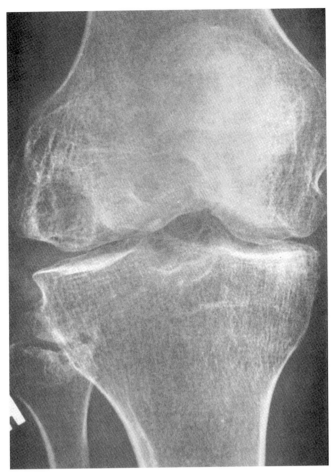

Figure 32.2 Moderately advanced hemophilic arthropathy in an adult. There is decreased joint space, subchondral irregularities, and cyst formation.

humerus is broadened and enlarged, with an olecranon fossa that is increased in size. Often, the bone wall of the fossa is resolved, producing an olecranon foramen. Subchondral cysts are more common in the elbow than in other joints, and the cysts in the ulna may be enlarged.

Wrist

Growth disturbances of the distal ulna cause luxation of the distal radioulnar joint, but generally involvement of the wrist is uncommon.

Hip

Hip arthropathy is uncommon. Most often, the changes seen are caused by a vascular necrosis of the femoral head, the end result in some cases being enlargement of the femoral head, but resorption of the femoral head is equally often seen. In the advanced stage, a central migration of the femoral head may be seen, with thinning of the medial wall of the acetabulum, resulting in a pronounced acetabular protrusion.

Knee

Early manifestations of the growth disturbances in small children will lead to an early ossification and accelerated growth of the patella. A disturbed growth pattern is typical, resulting in squaring of the lower pole (Figure 32.1). This was once thought to be pathognomonic for hemophilia, but it is commonly seen in juvenile rheumatoid arthritis, as a result of the hyperemia. Typical of hemophilic arthropathy in the knee is the overgrowth of the femoral condyles, with widening of the intercondylar notch, and also the groove between the tibial spines may be widened. These changes for a long time were also considered pathognomonic for hemophilic arthropathy but may also be seen in rheumatoid arthritis, tuberculous arthritis, and nonspecific bacterial arthritis.

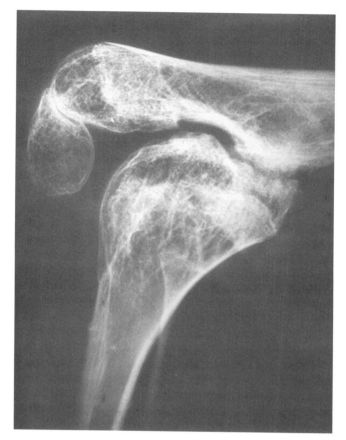

Figure 32.3 End stage of hemophilic arthropathy in a knee, with two destroyed bone ends articulating toward each other.

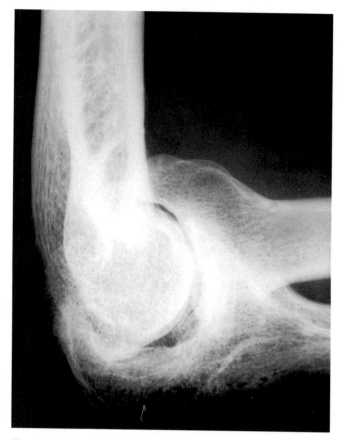

Figure 32.4 Hemophilic arthropathy of the elbow, with severe overgrowth of the radial head, decreased joint space and subchondral irregularity.

In the advanced stages, severely destroyed bone ends may be seen, with posterior subluxation of the tibia, giving malalignment involving genu valgum, fixed flexion and external rotation of the lower leg. Bony ankylosis may also be seen as an end result.

Ankle

Typical for the early changes in the ankle is narrowing of the lateral part of the tibial epiphyses concomitant with widening medially. Responding to this, the talar trochlea is often deformed, being higher in the lateral than in the medial part. This may cause valgus deformity (Figure 32.5). As in the knee joint, bone ankylosis may be seen as an end result.

Hand and foot

Hemophilic arthropathy in the hands and feet was not commonly seen, even in the days before the era of modern treatment. However, arthropathy of the metacarpophalangeal joints of the hand and the posterior subtalar joints of the foot have been described. In the foot, widening of the sinus tarsi, similar to the

widening of the intracondylar notch of the femur, as well as ankylosis of the tarsal and metatarsal joints have also been reported [1].

Classification of hemophilic arthropathy

It is obvious from the above description that the joint lesions appear in many different ways depending on both how long the destruction has been ongoing and the type of joint. Therefore, there was an early demand on radiology to find some sort of classification system, in order both to describe the natural cause of the arthropathy and to evaluate the effect of different therapeutic regimens.

In 1892, before the era of radiography, König [4] was able to distinguish between hemarthrosis, panarthritis, and a regressive stage of the disease, and later Key [5] simplified the classification to only two stages, acute hemarthrosis and chronic arthritis.

The first classification, based partly on clinical and partly on radiologic findings ,was suggested in 1956 by De Palma and Cotler [6], and in 1958 Jordan [7] presented a very similar classification, based mainly on the radiographic changes.

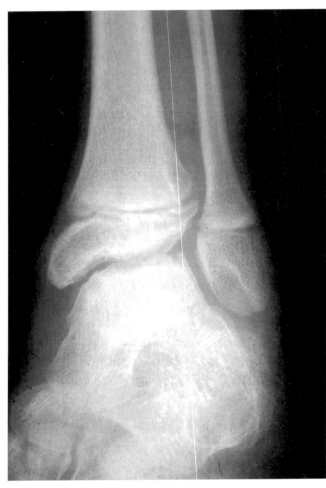

Figure 32.5 Hemophilic arthropathy of the ankle, with narrowing of the lateral part and enlargement of the medial part of the tibial epiphysis. The trochlea of the talus is deformed, with pronounced subchondral irregularity.

Table 32.1 The Arnold–Hilgartner progressive classification.

Stage I	No changes
Stage II	Osteoporosis, overgrowth
Stage III	Disorganization (cysts) — normal joint space
Stage IV	Narrowed joint
Stage V	End stage

Table 32.2 Radiologic classification recommended by the Orthopedic Advisory Committee of the World Federation of Hemophilia.

Type of change	Finding	Score (point)
Osteoporosis	Absent	0
	Present	1
Enlarged epiphysis	Absent	0
	Present	1
Irregular subchondral surface	Absent	0
	Partly involved	1
	Totally involved	2
Narrowing of joint space	Absent	0
	Joint space >1 mm	1
	Joint space <1 mm	2
Subchondral cyst formation	Absent	0
	One cyst	1
	> One cyst	2
Erosions of joint margins	Absent	0
	Present	1
Gross incongruence of articulating bone ends	Absent	0
	Slight	1
	Pronounced	2
Joint deformity (angulation and/or displacement between articulating bones)	Absent	0
	Slight	1
	Pronounced	2

Possible joint score: 0–13 points.

The classifications that have been in use for the last decades and still are in use are those of Arnold and Hilgartner, suggested in 1977 [8], and of Pettersson, suggested in 1981 [9].

The Arnold and Hilgartner classification is progressive, i.e., a certain number of stages are given (see Table 32.1), and the radiologist has to determine the most advanced stage that fits the radiographic findings. This gives a classification that is easily and quickly used.

The Pettersson classification represents a more detailed system, providing the opportunity for statistical analysis and observation of small changes from one examination to the next. It is thus an additive system, in which a number of changes are given a certain value, and the values added to give a total value for the joint. The classification uses some of the parameters mentioned above. The parameters should not be dependent on a recent bleeding episode but should describe events going on over a long period of time. It should also be easy to define and quantifi-able. The radiologic parameters used are thus osteopenia, enlargement of the epiphyses, subchondral irregularity, narrowing of the joint space, subchondral cyst formation, erosion, gross incongruence between the bone ends, and displacement and angulation. These changes are given a score from zero to 1, which means that they are either absent or present, or a score between zero and 2, with a definition of what constitutes a score of zero, 1, and 2. The possible joint score for a single joint varies between zero (normal joint), and 13 (i.e., a totally destroyed joint) (Table 32.2).

This classification has been recommended by the World Federation of Hemophilia for the last 20 years, and has proven to be of value as an objective measure of hemophilic joint destruction, as well as for describing the natural cause of the arthropathy, measuring the effect of prophylaxis, and comparing treatment regimens from hemophilic centers around the world [10]. It has been demonstrated that the intra-observer and inter-observer variation is acceptable, and experience has demonstrated that the classification can be used as an objective measure for evaluating hemophilic destruction of the joints.

However, for evaluation of early destruction, radiography is no longer the method of choice; instead MRI should be used. Thus, an MRI score of hemophilic arthropathy is being created in a worldwide project under the auspices of the World Federation of Hemophilia, and this will be presented during the World Federation of Hemophilia Congress in the fall of 2004. No doubt, the MRI score will be the most accurate for monitoring new treatment regimens, but, as mentioned above, for about 70% of the world's population, MRI will not be available in the foreseeable future, and therefore the radiographic score will still be of value.

References

1 Pettersson H, Gilbert MS. Diagnostic imaging in hemophilia. *Musculoskeletal and Other Hemorrhagic Complications.* Berlin: Springer-Verlag, 1985: 28–54.

2 Hermann G, Gilbert MS, Abdelwahab F. Hemophilia: evaluation of musculoskeletal involvement with CT, sonography, and MR imaging. *AJR* 1992; **158**: 119–23.

3 Nuss R, Kilcoyne RF, Geraghty S, *et al.* MRI findings in hemophilic joints treated with radiosynoviorthesis with development of an MRI scale of joint damage. *Haemophilia* 2000; **6**: 162–9.

4 König F. Die Gelenkerkrankungen bei Blutern mit besonderer Berücksichtigung der Diagnose. *Klin Vorträge NF* 1892; **36**: 233–43.

5 Key JA. Hemophilic arthritis. *Ann Surg* 1932; **95**: 198–225.

6 DePalma AF, Cotler J. Hemophilic arthropathy. *Clin Orthop* 1956; **8**: 163–190.

7 Jordan HH. *Hemophilic Arthropathies.* Springfield, IL: Charles C. Thomas, 1958, 12.

8 Arnold WD, Hilgartner MW. Hemophilic arthropathy: current concepts of pathogenesis and management. *J Bone Joint Surg* 1977; **59**: 287–305.

9 Pettersson H, Ahlberg Å, Nilsson IM. A radiologic classification of hemophilic arthropathy. *Clin Orthop* 1980; **149**: 153–9.

10 Aledort LM, Haschemeyer RH, Pettersson H. A longitudinal study of orthopaedic outcomes for severe factor VIII-deficient haemophiliacs. The Orthopaedic Outcome Study Group. *J Int Med* 1994; **236**: 391–9.

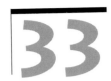

33 Magnetic resonance imaging/joint outcome assessment

Marilyn J. Manco-Johnson and Ray F. Kilcoyne

Introduction

Joint damage causes the most frequent and costly morbidity in hemophilia [1]. Ninety percent of persons with severe hemophilia suffer recurrent episodes of hemorrhage into one or more joints, resulting in degenerative arthritis [2]. Chronic pain and functional disability related to hemophilic arthropathy limit employment and recreational opportunities, decrease quality of life, drive affected individuals to expensive orthopedic surgeries, and sometimes prevent independent living. In response to the enormous human and economic burden of hemophilic arthropathy, intense efforts have been focused on factor replacement protocols and surgical procedures to prevent or limit joint damage. Joint evaluation instruments are necessary to diagnose orthopedic complications of hemophilia, to confirm efficacy of preventive regimens, to guide interventions, and to monitor the orthopedic status of a person with hemophilia over time. These scales function as the language with which we can communicate outcomes and compare populations. This chapter will describe various joint evaluation instruments, with an emphasis on the magnetic resonance imaging (MRI) scale, and discuss their use in the management of hemophilia.

Background

The pathophysiology of posthemorrhagic joint damage is probably multifactorial. There is evidence that cartilage and synovium play important and independent roles in the pathogenesis of hemophilic arthropathy [3–7]. Evidence from human and animal tissue suggests that cartilaginous fissures, decreased synthesis of cartilage matrix, and decreased chondrocyte proliferation all occur early in the course of joint bleeding and probably result from both mechanical and metabolic disruption [3–5,8]. The subchondral surface erodes, possibly caused by direct dissection of blood through cartilage [3–5]. Subchondral cysts develop and increase in size and number. Cysts can affect one or more bones contiguous to an affected joint. Cartilage changes in hemophilic joints most closely resemble osteoarthritis [6,7]. The joint space thins as cartilage is lost. Active joint range of motion becomes limited by pain. Cartilage loss has been closely related to loss of joint motion [9]. In a dog model, articular cartilage of young animals was more susceptible to blood-induced damage than that of older dogs [8].

Hemorrhage into a joint is associated with synovial hyperplasia. Iron deposition into lining and deeper layers of synovial cells is found following recurrent hemarthroses and associated with release of inflammatory cytokines, collagenases, and proteinases and local tissue damage [10–13]. Oxidant damage to synovium has been hypothesized to derive from iron released from hemoglobin. Proto-oncogene expression on synovial cell surfaces in response to contact with blood has been detected and has been invoked as a mediator of synovial proliferation [14]. Persistent synovial infection with parvovirus B19 has been suggested as a contributory cause of synovitis in patients with hemophilia [15]. Thickened synovium can be palpated around the joint by an experienced examiner. Joint fluid is increased. A weight-bearing joint will be guarded owing to pain, resulting in subtle decreases in muscle strength and bulk as well as gait abnormalities early in the course of chronic hemarthrosis. Bony overgrowth occurs proximal to the joint, secondary to hyperemia. Osteopenia develops. Loose bodies may be found free in the joint cavity. Eventually, fibrous scars contract the joint into fixed flexion deformity. As joint damage progresses, pain and scarring limit limb activity, causing more severe muscle atrophy and weakness. The number and severity of involved joints varies considerably among persons with severe hemophilia [2].

Physical examination scales

The number and frequency of bleeding episodes into a joint have been used as surrogate markers to indicate risk for structural and functional joint damage. Number of bleeding episodes has been correlated with radiologic evidence of joint damage [16]. Radiologic abnormalities, in turn, correlate with decreased functional range of motion, chronic pain, depression, and need for pain medications [9,17]. Joints with no or few clinical hemarthroses rarely show structural damage, and the risk of arthropathy increases with a greater number of bleeding events. Physical joint assessment, because it is readily available and inexpensive, has been frequently used for joint assessment. The World Federation of Hemophilia joint physical examination scale (WFH PE scale) is most widely used [18]. Tables 33.1 and 33.2 display the WFH PE and pain scale respectively.

The WFH PE scale scores swelling, atrophy, crepitus, and fixed contracture as present or absent; axial deformity, loss of range of motion, and instability are given two gradations. All points for abnormal findings are added with equal weight given to each. A score of zero denotes a normal joint. The ankles and

Table 33.1 Physical joint examination recommended by the Orthopaedic Advisory Committee of the WFH [18].

Physical finding	Score	Scoring key
Swelling	0 or 2+ (S)	0 = None
		2 = Present; (S) if chronic synovitis is present
Muscle atrophy	0–1	0 = ″ 1 cm
		1 = Present
Axial deformity (measured at knee and ankle only)		
Knee	0–2	0 = 0–7° valgus
		1 = 8–150° valgus or 0–50° varus
		2 = >150° valgus or >50° varus
Ankle	0–2	0 = No deformity
		1 = <10° valgus or <5° varus
		2 = ≥100° valgus or ≥50° varus
Crepitus on motion	0–1	0 = none
		1 = present
Range of motion (ROM)	0–2	0 = loss of <10% of total full ROM
		1 = loss of 10–33.3% of total ROM
		2 = loss of >33.3% of total ROM
Fixed contracture	0 or 2	0 = <15% fixed flexion contracture
		2 = ≥15% fixed flexion contracture at hip or knee or equinus at ankle
Instability	0–2	0 = None
		1 = Present but neither interferes with function nor requires bracing
		2 = Instability that creates a functional deficit or requires bracing
Total	0–12	Ankle or knee
	0–10	Elbow

Table 33.2 Pain instrument recommended by the Orthopaedic Advisory Committee of the World Federation for Haemophilia.

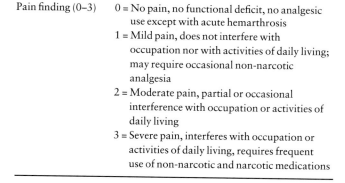

Pain finding (0–3)
0 = No pain, no functional deficit, no analgesic use except with acute hemarthrosis
1 = Mild pain, does not interfere with occupation nor with activities of daily living; may require occasional non-narcotic analgesia
2 = Moderate pain, partial or occasional interference with occupation or activities of daily living
3 = Severe pain, interferes with occupation or activities of daily living, requires frequent use of non-narcotic and narcotic medications

knees can score as high as 12 points while the elbows, because they are not subject to axial deformity, can score up to 10 points. By accepted convention, outcome studies have added the scores of six index joints, including both elbows, knees, and ankles, for a cumulative PE score. The WFH PE scale easily differentiates adults treated with primary prophylaxis (or near-complete prevention of hemorrhages) from adults who developed bleeding events and received no therapy or were treated each episode with the minimum factor replacement necessary to suppress signs and symptoms of joint hemorrhage. However, application of the WFH PE scale to young children on intensive treatment regimens has been unsatisfactory. Most young children with recurrent joint hemorrhage exhibit some degree of swelling and atrophy, with limited range of motion noted less consistently. Because the WFH scale scores very limited data, children who differ visibly in severity of physical disability to the casual observer can achieve identical WFH PE scores.

To improve sensitivity of the scale, the Denver physical examination (PE) scale added analysis of gait and strength and expanded the scores for swelling, atrophy and crepitance to a three-point scale, as shown in Table 33.3 [19]. The Denver (Colorado) scale allows greater discrimination among less-involved joints. However, though advanced arthropathy can be detected on physical examination, early physical findings indicate a risk for joint damage but are not diagnostic of such. Positive scores

Table 33.3 Colorado Young Child Instrument [18].

Physical finding	Score	Scoring key
Swelling	0–3	0 = None 1 = Joint looks slightly "puffy"; there is slight palpable swelling present; may not be any measurable difference between the joints; bony landmarks clearly visible 2 = Joint looks swollen and the swollen area feels firm on palpation; may also feel boggy; there is a measurable difference between the joints; bony landmarks are palpable but not visible 3 = Swollen and are tense to palpation; there is measurable difference between the joints and the bony landmarks are difficult to palpate
Muscle atrophy	0–3	0 = None 1 = Muscle has slightly less contour than the contralateral side 2 = Flattening of the muscle belly 3 = Severe muscle wasting and depression
Axial deformity Knee	0–2	0 = Normal; 1–7° valgus 1 = 8–15° valgus or 0–5° varus 2 = >15° valgus or >5° varus
Ankle	0–2	0 = No deformity 1 = Up to 10° valgus or 1–5° varus 2 = >10° valgus, or >5° varus
Range of motion	0–3	0 = No loss 1 = Loss of <10% of total ROM 2 = Loss of 10–33% of total ROM 3 = Loss of >33% of total ROM
Contracture (measured at knee, ankle and elbow)	0–3	0 = Normal 1 = 1–7° 2 = 8–15° 3 = >15°
Strength	0–3*	0 = Moves easily through full ROM against gravity without observable/measurable atrophy and can take additional resistance 1 = Moves through full or available ROM easily against gravity, may have observable/measurable atrophy and can take some additional muscle resistance 2 = Moves through full or available ROM against gravity, cannot take resistance 3 = Unable to move through full or available ROM against gravity due to weakness
Gait	0–2	0 = Normal walking, running, skipping, galloping, stairs 1 = Normal walking, at least one gait abnormality, e.g., foot turned out, shortened stance phase, no heel-toe pattern, decreased push-off, toe walking, etc. 2 = Abnormal walking and abnormal higher skills

The components of gait that should be assessed in each of the above skills are:

Ankle	*Knee*
1 Equal weight shift	1 Equal weight shift
2 Heel–toe pattern	2 Heel strike with full knee extension
3 Good plantar flexion push-off	3 Good knee extension on push-off
4 Steps of equal length	4 Steps of equal length
5 Steps of equal cadence	5 Steps of equal cadence
6 Toes pointed symmetrically forward	6 Toes pointed symmetrically forward

Continued

Table 33.3 *Continued*

Physical finding	Score	Scoring key
Splinting/orthotics	0–3	0 = No use of splinting/orthotics
		1 = Splinting/orthotic use required as needed after an acute hemarthrosis or for occasional support
		2= Splinting/orthotic use required regularly for high-activity sports or to prevent recurrent hemarthrosis
		3= Splinting/orthotic use required continuously
Pain with activity	0–3	Uses Faces Pain Rating Scale (Wong–Baker)
		0 = Face is very happy
		1 = Wong–Baker faces 1 and 2: hurts a little bit or a little bit more
		2 = Wong–Baker face 3: hurts even more
		3 = Wong–Baker faces 4 and 5: hurts a whole lot and as much as you can imagine
Pain without activity	0–3	Uses Faces Pain Rating Scale (Wong–Baker)
		0 = Face is very happy
		1 = Wong–Baker faces 1 and 2: hurts a little bit or a little bit more
		2 = Wong–Baker face 3: hurts even more
		3 = Wong–Baker faces 4 and 5: hurts a whole lot and as much as you can imagine
Total	0–28	Ankle or knee
	0–26	Elbow

*NB. In children under the age of 4 years, it is impossible to perform a strength break test. Functional testing is performed using skills that young children should be able to perform. See table for examples.

on joint physical scales, similar to joint bleeding number and frequency, are correlated with structural joint damage. Still, physiotherapy can improve several physical findings including swelling, strength, atrophy, and motion, without affecting structure (see Chapter 34). In addition, the convention of summing the score of six joints dilutes the impact of a single abnormal joint on the scale. Young children tend to present a single abnormal joint initially, while adults with severe hemophilia often have 2–6 abnormal joints.

Joint imaging

Plain radiography is the "gold standard" in structural assessment of hemophilic joints (see Chapter 32). Findings of hemophilic arthropathy on plain radiography include osteoporosis, widening of the epichondral notch of the knee, epiphyseal overgrowth, bone cysts, joint space irregularity and narrowing, angulation of the knee and ankle, and bony fusion. Soft-tissue swelling can be suggested but is often not clearly delineated. However, plain radiography is not sensitive to soft-tissue changes and detects primarily irreversible bone and cartilage lesions.

Two scoring systems have been developed for plain radiography of hemophilic joints, reflecting two different philosophies. The Arnold–Hilgartner scale is progressive, based upon a priori judgments regarding the evolution of joint damage in hemophilia; a modification of this scale is shown in Table 33.4 [20]. In the Arnold–Hilgartner scale, numeric score increases as radiographic findings progress to categories of abnormalities that are given greater weight. The Pettersson scale is additive, as shown in Table 33.5 [21]. Equal weight is placed upon each radiographic finding and the sum of abnormal findings is totaled. For example, findings of osteoporosis and joint narrowing are given equal weight and no presumptions are made regarding pathophysiologic progression or clinical significance of the findings. The Pettersson scale is complicated, but has been demonstrated to have high inter-observer reproducibility when used by experienced observers [22]. In addition, the Arnold–Hilgartner scale gives an initial point for soft-tissue swelling, while the Pettersson scale scores bone and cartilage changes alone and does not assess soft tissue.

Although it is controversial whether soft-tissue changes, including synovial hyperplasia and hemosiderin deposition, or chondrocyte hypoproliferation and microfissuring in persons with hemophilia occur simultaneously or sequentially, soft-tissue changes are uniformly found in persons with hemophilic arthropathy [3,6,7]. Radiographic images consistently underestimate the extent of damage to the joint surface seen at surgery [4]. Plain radiography is not sensitive for soft tissue and can, at best, only note the presence of soft-tissue swelling, in a nonspecific fashion. In order to detect the earliest evidence of joint

Table 33.4 Modified from the Arnold–Hilgartner scale of plain radiographic evaluation of joints [20].

	Ankle		Elbow		Knee	
	Left	Right	Left	Right	Left	Right
Joint findings						
Normal joint	0	0	0	0	0	0
No skeletal abnormalities; soft-tissue swelling present	I	I	I	I	I	I
Osteoporosis and overgrowth of epiphysis; no erosions; no narrowing of cartilage space	II	II	II	II	II	II
Early subchondral bone cysts; squaring of the patella; intercondylar notch of distal femur or humerus widened; preservation of cartilage space	III	III	III	III	III	III
Findings of stage III more advanced; cartilage space narrowed	IV	IV	IV	IV	IV	IV
Fibrous joint contracture; loss of joint cartilage space; marked enlargement of the epiphyses and substantial disorganization of joint	V	V	V	V	V	V
Other radiographic findings						
Pseudotumor	Absent	Absent	Absent	Absent	Absent	Absent
	Present	Present	Present	Present	Present	Present
Osteonecrosis	Absent	Absent	Absent	Absent	Absent	Absent
	Present	Present	Present	Present	Present	Present
Osteophyte	Absent	Absent	Absent	Absent	Absent	Absent
	Present	Present	Present	Present	Present	Present
Loose body	Absent	Absent	Absent	Absent	Absent	Absent
	Present	Present	Present	Present	Present	Present

inflammation, determine the natural history of hemophilic arthropathy, and compare efficacies of different preventive regimens in young children, magnetic resonance imaging (MRI) was applied to joint imaging.

Magnetic resonance imaging of hemophilic arthropathy was first described by Kulkarni and colleagues in 1986 [23]. Enhanced anatomic detail that could be detected by MRI was confirmed by several reports over the next 13 years [24–30]. The Denver scoring system for MR joint imaging was published in 2000 and is shown in Table 33.6 [31].

The Denver magnetic resonance imaging protocol

Imaging parameters must be chosen that will enhance the conspicuity of "soft-tissue" changes. On T1-weighted images, synovial fluid and most blood products will be low signal (dark). Conversely, on T2-weighted images, these structures will be high signal (bright). Various imaging methods besides conventional T1 and T2 imaging have been employed. One of the most

usual variations is "gradient echo" (GE) imaging. Values for TE (50 ms), TR (15 ms), and flip angle (30°) can be chosen that will give useful T2 information, although not as specific as true T2 imaging. (This is called "T2*" information.) GE images can be obtained more quickly than true T2 images and have better spatial resolution. The amount of time required for the examination is important when dealing with small children or patients who are in pain, and when multiple joints need to be surveyed at one time. Lastly, an artifact of GE imaging is useful in seeing synovium. In hemophilia, blood in the joint is absorbed into the synovium and becomes deposited in the form of hemosiderin. On GE imaging, hemosiderin is intensely black owing to "magnetic susceptibility artifact". This artifact makes it easier to see the abnormal synovium. Another way to enhance visibility of synovium, and to semiquantify the rate of effusion of fluid into the joint and absorption into the synovium, is by the intravenous administration of a contrast agent (gadolinium). Gadolinium travels through the circulation and is secreted into the joint along with synovial fluid [30]. Although this can give useful information about the rate of synovial fluid production and absorption, it is not routinely employed in screening examinations.

Table 33.5 Pettersson scale of plain radiographic assessment of joints [20].

Findings	Ankle		Elbow		Knee	
	Left	Right	Left	Right	Left	Right
Osteoporosis						
Absent	0	0	0	0	0	0
Present	1	1	1	1	1	1
Enlarged epiphysis						
Absent	0	0	0	0	0	0
Present	1	1	1	1	1	1
Irregular subchondral surface						
Absent	0	0	0	0	0	0
Partly involved	1	1	1	1	1	1
Totally involved	2	2	2	2	2	2
Narrowing of joint space						
Absent	0	0	0	0	0	0
Visible joint space >1 mm	1	1	1	1	1	1
Visible joint space <1 mm	2	2	2	2	2	2
Subchondral cyst formation						
Absent	0	0	0	0	0	0
One cyst	1	1	1	1	1	1
>1 cyst	2	2	2	2	2	2
Erosion of joint margins						
Absent	0	0	0	0	0	0
Present	1	1	1	1	1	1
Gross incongruence of articulating bone ends						
Absent	0	0	0	0	0	0
Slight	1	1	1	1	1	1
Pronounced	2	2	2	2	2	2
Joint deformity (angulation and/or displacement)						
Absent	0	0	0	0	0	0
Slight	1	1	1	1	1	1
Pronounced	2	2	2	2	2	2
Total score (sum all points)						

For survey purposes, GE images are obtained in coronal and sagittal planes of the knee, ankle, and elbow. In addition, axial images are obtained of the elbow owing to difficulty in positioning the elbow for true coronal and sagittal views. If the joint examination is not part of a survey protocol, additional imaging with T1 parameters in two or three planes should be obtained.

Magnetic resonance imaging findings

A small amount of increased joint fluid is easily detected. Gadolinium allows the differentiation of blood from inflammatory fluid; this distinction is rarely needed in patients with hemophlilia. In the Denver scale, joint fluid is graded small, moderate, or large.

Synovium is seen as gray soft tissue on T1, T2, and GE imaging. However, in hemophilia, the synovium usually contains hemosiderin, which is black on synovium by all parameters, most noticeably GE. The distribution of synovium and hemosiderin is often identical. Both are graded small, moderate, or large. The differentiation of synovial hyperplasia from hemosiderin deposition is rarely needed.

Subchondral cysts and erosions of the joint surface can be considered as findings on a spectrum of similar pathophysiology. Cysts are scored as a single subchondral cyst, multiple cysts, a partial joint surface erosion, or complete erosion.

Joint narrowing can be seen and is graded <50% or ≥50% of joint cartilage.

Scales for scoring magnetic resonance imaging findings in hemophilic joints

Scoring of MRI images of hemophilic joints can follow philoso-

Table 33.6 The Denver MRI scale [31].

	Ankle		Elbow		Knee	
	Left	Right	Left	Right	Left	Right
Effusion						
Absent	0	0	0	0	0	0
Small	1	1	1	1	1	1
Moderate	2	2	2	2	2	2
Large	3	3	3	3	3	3
Hemarthrosis						
Absent	0	0	0	0	0	0
Small	1	1	1	1	1	1
Moderate	2	2	2	2	2	2
Large	3	3	3	3	3	3
Synovial hyperplasia						
Absent	0	0	0	0	0	0
Small	4	4	4	4	4	4
Moderate	5	5	5	5	5	5
Large	6	6	6	6	6	6
Hemosiderin						
Absent	0	0	0	0	0	0
Small	4	4	4	4	4	4
Moderate	5	5	5	5	5	5
Large	6	6	6	6	6	6
Erosion						
Absent	0	0	0	0	0	0
Partial surface erosion	7	7	7	7	7	7
Full surface erosion	8	8	8	8	8	8
Subchondral cyst						
Absent	0	0	0	0	0	0
1 cyst	7	7	7	7	7	7
>1 cyst	8	8	8	8	8	8
Cartilage loss						
Absent	0	0	0	0	0	0
Less than 50% loss	9	9	9	9	9	9
50% or greater loss	10	10	10	10	10	10

MRI score (highest number in any category)

Other MRI findings

	Ankle		Elbow		Knee	
Pseudotumor	Absent	Absent	Absent	Absent	Absent	Absent
	Present	Present	Present	Present	Present	Present
Osteonecrosis	Absent	Absent	Absent	Absent	Absent	Absent
	Present	Present	Present	Present	Present	Present
Fibrocartilage tear	NA	NA	NA	NA	Absent	Absent
	NA	NA	NA	NA	Present	Present
Ligament tear	Absent	Absent	Absent	Absent	Absent	Absent
	Present	Present	Present	Present	Present	Present
Loose body	Absent	Absent	Absent	Absent	Absent	Absent
	Present	Present	Present	Present	Present	Present

NA, not applicable.

phies similar to those applied to plain radiography. The Denver MRI scale is progressive, similar to the Arnold–Hilgartner scale. The Denver scale presumes a pathophysiology beginning with joint hemorrhage, and progressing through synovial hypertrophy with hemosiderin deposition to subchondral cysts and erosions to narrowing of the joint space. Findings of joint fluid and synovial hypertrophy are each rated mild, moderate, or severe, whereas subchondral damage and cartilage loss are each graded on a two-point scale. Illustrated examples of the various MRI stages on the Denver scale have been recently published [32,33].

An alternative approach, modeled on the Pettersson radiographic scale, is being developed by an international working group [34]. A version of the international MRI scale currently under development and refinement is shown in Table 33.7 [34].

Ultrasound imaging in hemophilic joints

Several reports have described the use of ultrasound imaging in hemophilic joints. Ultrasound has been found useful in detection of increases in both joint fluid and synovial soft-tissue thickening, particularly in the knee [35–38]. One report additionally evaluated cartilage by ultrasound [37]. Ultrasound, in combination with plain radiography, may offer additional information, especially in settings where MRI is not available.

How are the results of various joint assessments applied to care of persons with hemophilia?

Application of assessment tools must be tailored to the clinical setting. The following scenarios illustrate the use of the various physical and imaging assessment tools to direct clinical management of joint bleeding in hemophilia, with an emphasis on newer applications of MRI.

Assessment of risk for joint damage in the infant and very young child

The onset of joint hemorrhage is currently accepted as an indication for initiation of prophylaxis in a very young child. Similarly, the occurrence of multiple hemarthroses in a child on once-weekly prophylaxis is an indication to escalate the frequency and/or dose of routine infusions. It is sometimes difficult for parents and healthcare providers to differentiate an early hemarthrosis from a soft-tissue hematoma. The Denver joint physical assessment tool, with its emphasis on subtle asymmetry of gait and limb function, can identify a joint with probable hemarthrosis. Mild joint swelling can indicate the past occurrence of hemarthroses that were not clinically suspected. Occasionally, abnormalities on physical examination are sufficiently subtle that confirmation with imaging is required to direct ther-

Table 33.7 The European MRI scale ([34]), given in the format A(e:s:h)*.

Subchondral cysts (part of A)
Present in at least one bone
Present in at least two bones
More than three cysts in at least one bone
More than three cysts in at least two bones
Largest size more than 4 mm in at least one bone
Largest size more than 4 mm in at least two bones

Irregularity/erosion of subchondral cortex (part of A)
Present in at least one bone
Present in at least two bones
Involves more than half of joint surface in at least one bone
Involves more than half of joint surface in at least two bones

Chondral destruction (part of A)
Present in at least one bone
Present in at least two bones
Full-thickness defect in at least one bone
Full-thickness defect in at least two bones
Full-thickness defect involves more than one third of joint surface in at least one bone
Full-thickness defect involves more than one third of joint surface in at least two bones

Effusion/hemarthrosis (e)
Hypertrophic synovia (s)
Hemosiderin (h)
0   Absent
1   Equivocal
2   Small
3   Moderate
4   Large

* Maximum score 16(4:4:4); explained in detail in the *Results* section.

apeutic interventions. Specifically, soft-tissue changes of synovial hyperplasia and hemosiderin deposition are routinely determined on MRI that would not be detected with plain radiography. It is possible that subchondral cysts, erosions, and cartilage damage may occur prior to, or concomitant with, synovial reaction. If so, structural abnormalities detected using MRI, including bone and cartilage damage, are similar to but consistently more extensive than those detected on radiographic images obtained at the same time. Current longitudinal studies comparing MRI and plain radiography in children with hemophilia will help determine the prevalence and clinical significance of early cartilage loss [39].

Ascertainment of more difficult diagnoses

Occasionally, an unusual presentation of pain and swelling in a person with hemophilia will require investigations beyond physical examination to assign a diagnosis. MRI has been used successfully to determine normal and abnormal anatomic structures, such as hemorrhage into a suprapatellar pouch [40] and diagnosis of a large iliopsoas hematoma in a female carrier of hemophilia [41]. Ultrasound may be applied more economically to certain differentials, for example to determine whether blood is within the hip joint or the surrounding muscles.

Determining appropriateness of therapeutic interventions

Synovial hyperplasia routinely develops in hemophilic target joints following recurrent hemarthroses. However, in advanced hemophilic arthropathy, it is a common occurrence that synovium regresses as bone and cartilage changes progress; often during this phase of hemophilic arthropathy, the pain of an acute hemorrhage is poorly distinguished from arthritic pain. MRI can be used to evaluate synovium with a high degree of sensitivity. Procedures designed to decrease joint hemorrhage, including radiosynoviorthesis and synovectomy, can be judged unlikely to improve the patient's condition on the basis of an MR image with scant synovium or hemosiderin. Figure 33.1 shows MR images of the left elbow in a 12-year-old boy with severe hemophilia A early in the course of recurrent hemarthroses and 1 year later. Joint fluid and moderate synovial hyperplasia can be seen on the initial MRI scan (as well as a minimal erosion seen on other views, not shown) in spite of normal plain radiography (Figure 33.1a). In the course of 1 year, increased hemosiderin and a large erosion are evident, whereas synovium has regressed somewhat (Figure 33.1b). MRI shows earlier signs of joint damage; an intervention at the time of the first MR study may have prevented or slowed the rapid joint deterioration.

We have used joint imaging to determine joint structure prior to institution of secondary prophylaxis or surgical synovectomy [29,42]. Hemophilic arthropathy has been detected in otherwise asymptomatic children, and determined to progress despite cessation of joint hemorrhage. In this case, MRI and, less sensitively, plain radiography, document damage prior to the institution of secondary prophylaxis. The baseline images support the need of very early prophylaxis to prevent arthropathy and can be used to plan additional local interventions concomitant with routine infusion therapy.

MRI as an outcome measure in prospective clinical trials

MRI sensitively detects early soft-tissue changes in response to joint hemorrhage. By virtue of this capability, MRI can be ideally applied to clinical trials comparing various treatments to prevent joint damage. Synovial hyperplasia with hemosiderin deposition strongly supports the occurrence of previous hemorrhage and can be used as a surrogate indicator of the success of a regimen designed to prevent joint hemorrhage long before hemophilic arthropathy can be diagnosed clinically. Currently, there are two ongoing prospective North American clinical

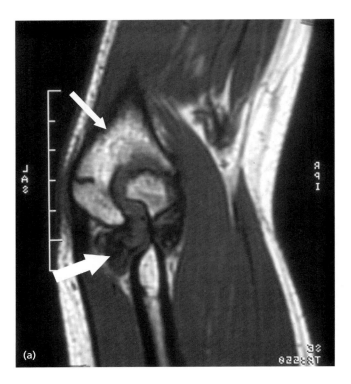

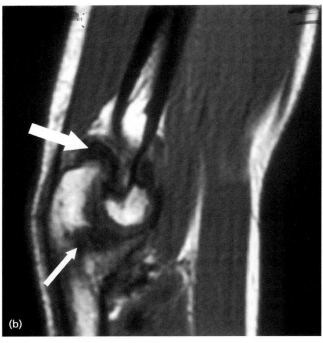

Figure 33.1 T-1 saggital images of a left elbow MRI in a boy with severe hemophilia at ages 12 and 13. (a) Early in the course of recurrent hemarthroses MRI of this elbow shows fluid and synovial hyperplasia (arrow). Concurrent radiograph was normal. (b) The same child's left elbow, 1 year later. Although synovium has regressed somewhat, there is increased hemosiderin deposition (thick arrow), and a large erosion can be seen (thin arrow).

trials of early prophylactic regimens in young children with severe hemophilia [39]. Because parental reporting of joint hemorrhage is subject to variability in individual parent assessments as well as variable clinical presentations of hemorrhage, MRI outcomes are more objective.

Clinical trials employing full or modified (e.g., escalating) prophylaxis or enhanced factor replacement therapy to prevent or treat early joint hemorrhage in young children are unlikely to need the expanded stratification of cysts and erosions offered by the new international MRI scale. However, studies of surgical interventions for adults with hemophilia or population comparisons of less intensive treatment strategies available to developing hemophilia programs may benefit from the enhanced discrimination capacity offered by the international scale.

Finally, MRI can be used to compare and validate the sensitivity and specificity of less costly outcome indicators, including bleeding frequency, joint physical examination, and plain radiography, that subsequently can be applied to clinical care as well as to future prospective clinical trials. Through application to comparison studies of outcome measures, MRI has the opportunity to benefit all persons with hemophilia, independent of their individual access to this expensive imaging modality.

References

1 Hilgartner MW. Current treatment of hemophilic arthropathy. *Curr Opin Pediatr* 2002; **14**: 46–9.

2 Aledort LM, Haschmeyer RH, Pettersson H. A longitudinal study of orthopaedic outcomes for severe factor VIII-deficient haemophiliacs. The Orthopaedic Outcome Study Group. *J Intern Med* 1994; **236**: 391–9.

3 Rippey JJ, Hill RR, Lurie A, *et al.* Articular cartilage degradation and the pathology of haemophilic arthropathy. *S Afr Med J* 1978; **54**: 345–51.

4 Speer DP. Early pathogenesis of hemophilic arthropathy. Evolution of the subchondral cyst. *Clin Orthop* 1984; **185**: 250–65.

5 Madhok R, Bennett D, Sturrock RD, Forbes CD. Mechanisms of joint damage in an experimental model of hemophilic arthritis. *Arthritis Rheum* 1988; **31**: 1148–55.

6 Roosendaal G, van Rinsum AC, Vianen ME, *et al.* Haemophilic arthropathy resembles degenerative rather than inflammatory joint disease. *Histopathology* 1999; **34**: 144–53.

7 Roosendaal G, Lafeber FP. Blood-induced joint damage in hemophilia. *Semin Thromb Haemost* 2003; **29**: 37–42.

8 Roosendaal G, Tekoppele JM, Vianen ME, *et al.* Articular cartilage is more susceptible to blood induced damage at young than at old age. *J Rheumatol* 2000; **27**: 1740–4.

9 Johnson RP, Babbitt DP. Five stages of joint disintegration compared with range of motion in hemophilia. *Clin Orthop* 1985; **201**: 36–42.

10 Ghadially FN. Overview article: the articular territory of the reticuloendothelial system. *Ultrastruct Pathol* 1980; **1**: 249–64.

11 Roosendaal G, Vianen ME, Wenting MJ, *et al.* Iron deposits and catabolic properties of synovial tissue from patients with haemophilia. *J Bone Joint Surg Br* 1998; **80**: 540–5.

12 Mainardi CL, Levine PH, Werb Z, Harris ED Jr. Proliferative synovitis in hemophilia: biochemical and morphologic observations. *Arthritis Rheum* 1978; **21**: 137–44.

13 Morris CJ, Blake DR, Wainwright AC, Steven MM. Relationship between iron deposits and tissue damage in the synovium: an ultrastructural study. *Ann Rheum Dis* 1986; **45**: 21–6.

14 Wen FQ, Jabbar AA, Chen YX, *et al.* C-myc proto-oncogene expression in hemophilic synovitis: *in vitro* studies of the effects of iron and ceramide. *Blood* 2002; **100**: 912–16.

15 Zakrzewska K, Azzi A, De Biase E, *et al.* Persistence of parvovirus B19 DNA in synovium of patients with haemophilic arthritis. *J Med Virol* 2001; **65**: 402–7.

16 Brown IS, Toolis F, Prescott RJ. Haemophilic arthropathy: a ten-year radiological and clinical study. *Scott Med J* 1982; **27**: 279–83.

17 Wallny T, Lahaye L, Brackmann HH, *et al.* Clinical and radiographic scores in haemophilic arthropathies: how well do these correlate to subjective pain status and daily activities? *Haemophilia* 2002; **8**: 802–8.

18 Gilbert MS. Prophylaxis: musculoskeletal evaluation. *Semin Hematol* 1993; **30**: 3–6.

19 Manco-Johnson MJ, Nuss R, Funk S, Murphy J. Joint evaluation instruments for children and adults with haemophilia. *Haemophilia* 2000; **6**: 649–57.

20 Arnold WD, Hilgartner MW. Hemophilic arthropathy. Current concepts of pathogenesis and management. *J Bone Joint Surg Am* 1977; **59**: 287–305.

21 Pettersson H, Ahlberg A, Nilsson IM. A radiologic classification of hemophilic arthropathy. *Clin Orthop* 1980; **149**: 153–9.

22 Erlemann R, Rosenthal H, Walthers EM, *et al.* Reproducibility of the Pettersson scoring system. An interobserver study. *Acta Radiol* 1989; **30**: 147–51.

23 Kulkarni MV, Drolshagen LF, Kaye JJ, *et al.* MR imaging of hemophilic arthropathy. *J Comput Assist Tomogr* 1986; **10**: 445–9.

24 Yulish BS, Lieberman JM, Strandjord SE, *et al.* Hemophilic arthropathy: assessment with MR imaging. *Radiology* 1987; **164**: 759–62.

25 Pettersson H, Gillespy T, Kitchens C, *et al.* Magnetic resonance imaging in hemophilic arthropathy of the knee. *Acta Radiol* 1987; **28**: 621–5.

26 Baunin C, Railhac JJ, Younes I, *et al.* MR imaging in hemophilic arthropathy. *Eur J Pediatr Surg* 1991; **1**: 358–63.

27 Hermann G, Gilbert MS, Abdelwahab IF. Hemophilia: evaluation of musculoskeletal involvement with CT, sonography and MR imaging. *AJR* 1992; **158**: 119–23.

28 Idy-Peretti I, Le Balc'h T, Yvart J, Bittoun J. MR imaging of hemophilic arthropathy of the knee: classification and evolution of the subchondral cysts. *Magn Reson Imaging* 1992; **10**: 67–75.

29 Nuss R, Kilcoyne RD, Geraghty S, *et al.* Utility of magnetic resonance imaging for management of hemophilic arthropathy in children. *J Pediatr* 1993; **123**: 388–92.

30 Rand T, Trattnig S, Male C, *et al.* Magnetic resonance imaging in hemophilic children: value of gradient echo and contrast-enhanced imaging. *Magn Reson Imaging* 1999; **17**: 199–205.

31 Nuss R, Kilcoyne RF, Geraghty S, *et al.* MRI findings in hemophilic joints treated with radiosynoviorthesis with development of an MRI scale of joint damage. *Haemophilia* 2000; **6**: 162–9.

32 Nuss R, Kilcoyne RF. *The MRI Atlas of Hemophilic Arthropathy.* New York: Professional Publishing Group, 2002.

33 Kilcoyne RF, Nuss R. Radiologic assessment of haemophilic arthropathy with emphasis on MRI findings. *Haemophilia* 2003; **9**: 57–63, discussion 63–4.

34 Lundin B, Pettersson H, Ljung R. A new magnetic resonance imaging scoring method for assessment of haemophilic arthropathy. *Haemophilia*, 2004; **10**: 383–9.

35 Wyld PJ, Dawson KP, Chisholm RJ. Ultrasound in the assessment of

synovial thickening in the hemophilic knee. *Aust N Z J Med* 1984; **14**: 678–80.

36 Wilson DJ, McLardy-Smith PD, Woodham CH, MacLarnon JC. Diagnostic ultrasound in haemophilia. *J Bone Joint Surg Br* 1987; **69**: 103–7.

37 Merchan EC, De Orbe A, Gago J. Ultrasound in the diagnosis of the early stages of hemophilic arthropathy of the knee. *Acta Orthop Belg* 1992; 122–5.

38 Klukowska A, Czyrny Z, Laguna P, *et al.* Correlation between clinical, radiological and ultrasonographical image of knee joints in children with haemophilia. *Haemophilia* 2001; **7**: 286–92.

39 Manco-Johnson MJ, Blanchette VS. North American prophylaxis studies for persons with severe haemophilia: background, rationale and design. *Haemophilia* 2003; **9**: 44–9.

40 Nuss R, Kilcoyne R, Geraghty S, *et al.* Magnetic resonance imaging visualization of hemorrhage into a superpatellar pouch in a child with hemophilia. *Am J Pediatr Hematol Oncol* 1994; **16**: 183–5.

41 Lefkowitz JB, Nuss R, Haver T, *et al.* Factor IX Denver, ASN346 → ASP mutation resulting in a dysfunctional protein with defective factor VIIIa interaction. *Thromb Haemost* 2001; **86**: 862–70.

42 Manco-Johnson MJ, Nuss R, Geraghty S, *et al.* Results of secondary prophylaxis in children with severe hemophilia. *Am J Hematol* 1994; **47**: 113–17.

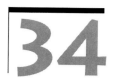

34 Physiotherapy in the management of hemophilia

Karen Beeton and Jane Tuffley

Introduction

The successful management of patients with hemophilia requires a coordinated multidisciplinary team approach that involves doctors, nurses, counselors, scientists, and physiotherapists. Good communication between team members is essential to provide optimal delivery of care, and a thorough understanding of each respective role is crucial. In the UK, the physiotherapist is an autonomous practitioner responsible for the physical health and well-being of patients and can offer assessment, treatment based on physical methods, advice, and education. Ideally, one physiotherapist should have sole responsibility for providing the service, so enabling mutual trust and understanding to develop over time between the hemophilic patient and physiotherapist. The physiotherapist must also have sound postgraduate experience because of the complex musculoskeletal problems of many of these patients. The physiotherapy service should be located in the hemophilia center or with easy access to the hemophilia team. Close links with local physiotherapy services also need to be developed for those patients who live too far away to attend the hemophilia center for physiotherapy on a regular basis.

This chapter will begin by discussing the role of the physiotherapist in the management of adults and children. Key issues relevant to the physiotherapy management of patients with inhibitors and acquired hemophilia will then be considered. The outcome measures available to evaluate physiotherapy so that robust evidence of effectiveness can be provided will be briefly discussed. Finally, the importance of regular monitoring of hemophilic patients, highlighting some of the protocols currently available, will be presented.

Adults with hemophilia

Adults with hemophilia who present with musculoskeletal problems should be referred to the physiotherapist for their opinion. Depending on local arrangements, patients may also be able to refer themselves directly to the physiotherapist. The physiotherapist will always assess the patient prior to any intervention. A detailed description of the assessment process is described by Beeton and Ryder [1]. This will help to establish baseline data regarding the patient's problem, to determine if there are any precautions and contraindications to physiotherapy, and to identify the goals of the patient and expectations from physiotherapy management.

Physiotherapy strategies

The adult with hemophilia may present with an acute joint or muscle bleed, chronic synovitis, or arthropathy, but he may also present with musculoskeletal problems, such as low back pain, which may be unrelated to hemophilia. The typical clinical presentation of acute bleeds, chronic synovitis, and arthropathy, aims of treatment and possible physiotherapy strategies for each condition are outlined in Table 34.1.

The effectiveness of factor replacement in the treatment of bleeds and the increasing use of home treatment programs means that many patients do not present to a hemophilia center when they experience a bleeding episode. However, this emphasis on self-management, with a focus often only on factor replacement, may mean that other strategies such as electrotherapy modalities and graded exercise programs are not employed. These strategies may hasten the resolution of bleeds and ensure a return to maximum functional status. The importance of physiotherapy as an integral part of the management of the acute bleeds should not be overlooked. An increase in muscle strength and endurance and proprioceptive training are being increasingly recognized as important areas to address in reducing bleeds and increasing function. There is also limited published evidence that strengthening exercises can reduce the occurrence of bleeds [2], but considerable anecdotal opinion would also support this concept. In the professional arena, there is currently debate regarding the value of ice in the management of acute bleeds [3]. Physiotherapists need to be aware of emerging research and use their clinical judgment and experience in determining whether ice is a useful modality.

Patients may also present with musculoskeletal problems unrelated to hemophilia, and it is important to keep an open mind and not assume that all dysfunction is related to hemophilia. A patient may, for example, complain of low back pain or neck pain due to poor seating at work. Another may have low back pain secondary to arthropathy involving the lower limbs that makes correct lifting difficult. The thorough assessment process by the physiotherapist aims to identify the main source of the problem as well as the contributing factors and manage these as necessary.

Classification of adult patients with hemophilia

Adults with hemophilia can be grouped into four main categories (Table 34.2), and this can have implications for their

Table 34.1 Physiotherapy management of musculoskeletal problems in hemophilia.

	Clinical presentation	Aims of physiotherapy	Possible physiotherapy strategies
Acute joint bleeds	"Aura" Pain Swelling Limitation of movement Muscle inhibition	Relieve pain Reduce swelling Restore function to prebleed status Prevent recurrence of bleeds	Advice on appropriate rest Ice Elevation Electrotherapy Graded exercise program Modification of activities Advice and education
Acute muscle bleeds	Pain on palpation and stretching muscle Limitation of movement Bruising may be evident Muscle inhibition/spasm Neural compression	Relieve pain Reduce swelling Restore function to prebleed status Prevent recurrence of bleeds	Rest Ice Elevation Electrotherapy Graded exercise program with appropriate muscle stretching Modification of activities Advice and education
Chronic synovitis	Chronic effusion and thickening of the synovial membrane Minimal pain Severe muscle atrophy Poor proprioception	Reduce swelling Increase muscle strength and endurance Improve coordination and proprioception Maximize function	Electrotherapy Supports/braces to protect joint in presence of muscle weakness Graded strengthening program and correction of muscle imbalances Proprioceptive retraining Hydrotherapy Advice and education
Arthropathy	Pain Loss of range of movement Muscle weakness Contractures Deformity Bony or fibrous ankylosis	Relieve pain Increase or maintain range of movement Increase or maintain muscle strength and endurance Maximize function	Mobilization of joints Correction of muscle imbalances Hydrotherapy Splints and braces Electrotherapy including TNS for pain relief Advice and education

Based on Beeton [9]. TNS, transcutaneous nerve stimulation.

Table 34.2 Classification of adult patients with hemophilia.

Group	Use of factor replacement	Typical physical status
1	Patients with mild/moderate hemophilia rarely have factor replacement	Few physical problems but can present late if a bleed develops as may underestimate the effect of trauma
2	Patients have been on long-term prophylaxis	Normal mobility Minimal joint dysfunction
3	Patients on prophylaxis but minimal treatment during childhood and the early years	Marked joint dysfunction involving one or two joints May require joint replacement or other orthopedic procedures
4	Minimal treatment until 20–30 years of age. Patients may or may not be on prophylaxis now, often on-demand treatment, few if any bleeds at present time	Multiple joint involvement. Pain variable, can be severe or mild but often marked stiffness, contractures, and disability. May have had joint replacements or other orthopedic procedures in past

possible clinical presentation and subsequent physiotherapy management.

Patients with mild and moderate hemophilia rarely have physical problems caused by their hemophilia and will often participate in more vigorous physical activities and sports. However, these patients generally do not have experience in the management of bleeds compared with patients who are more severely affected, and may ignore initial bleeding problems. These patients may not be able to administer their own factor replacement and may not seek help until the bleeding has become severe. The patient should be encouraged to seek advice promptly if a traumatic incident does occur. Delays in administering factor replacement can lead to long-term problems, and even pseudotumors have been reported in these patients [4]. All mildly and moderately affected patients should be reviewed at least on an annual basis by the physiotherapist to evaluate the musculoskeletal system and provide advice on appropriate physical activities.

Patients who have had long-term prophylaxis since a young age may have minimal joint dysfunction, owing to the long-term benefits of factor replacement [5]. Interestingly, like the mildly affected patients, these patients may also have limited experience of bleeds and this may promote more risk-taking behavior. These patients can have one or two target joints and may experience symptoms from time to time from acute bleeds or early arthropathy. The ankle joint rather than the knee is increasingly being identified as the joint most involved, although the reasons for this are not yet clear [6]. Physiotherapy modalities, including manual techniques and correction of lower limb biomechanics by use of custom-made inserts, have been recommended in reducing symptoms [7]. These patients may have few physical limitations but may have to restrict some activities to avoid symptoms or to prevent problems occurring. However, while the physical limitations may be minimal, the psychologic impact of "appearing normal" but being unable to be involved in all activities is unknown [8].

Patients who did not have access to factor replacement when they were younger may have marked musculoskeletal dysfunction, with one or two joints that may be severely affected due to synovitis or arthropathy. The physiotherapist has a range of treatment strategies to offer depending on the patient preferences, previous benefit from treatment, and available research evidence (see Table 34.1). Factor replacement is usually administered prior to physiotherapy. Although physiotherapy can with care be provided without factor cover, it does enhance confidence for both the patient and physiotherapist, particularly when introducing new techniques and exercise regimes. If, following physiotherapy treatment, the condition is unchanged then the patient should be referred for an orthopedic opinion. Joint clinics attended by all members of the team are very valuable in these situations as shared discussions with the patient can facilitate the most appropriate management strategy.

The final group of patients, who are often older, may have multiple joint arthropathy and demonstrate marked disability. Some patients in this situation may have severe pain and others little, if any, pain, although all patients are likely to have limited range of movement, deformity, and contractures. The joints may bleed little, if at all. The aim of treatment is focused on maximizing function and adapting to limitations with appropriate strategies such as pacing activities, protecting joints appropriately, and avoiding aggravating activities. If the limitation of movement is due to contractures, and the end feel of the joint is hard and bony, manual physiotherapy techniques may have limited benefit. Patients often learn appropriate strategies to manage their limitations and in doing so mask their disability. It is important to discuss the strategies patients use. The physiotherapist may be able to suggest other strategies and can also advise on exercise programs and appropriate activities to maintain physical fitness and cardiovascular function.

Children with hemophilia

The main aim of the physiotherapy management of children with hemophilia is to minimize the long-term musculoskeletal effects of hemophilia. This can be achieved by:
- early detection and physiotherapy treatment of bleeds;
- advising on appropriate activity and sport to reduce the risk of bleeds;
- offering sufficient care and support to enable children and their parents to have a thorough understanding of the condition.

Primary prophylaxis has been recommended by the World Federation of Hemophilia (WFH) as the optimum treatment for children [10]. However, there is no consensus on the optimal age to start prophylaxis, and 10% of children with severe hemophilia maintain normal joints without having prophylaxis [11]. Research into this area is ongoing [12].

Assessment of the child is always undertaken prior to physiotherapy. Knowledge of the patient's prophylactic regimen and his bleeding history is essential in planning effective physiotherapy management. The musculoskeletal sequelae of bleeds include pain, effusion, muscle inhibition, poor proprioception, synovitis, and eventually arthropathy [13,14]. The physiotherapist will identify the musculoskeletal dysfunctions that need to be addressed and devise an appropriate individualized exercise regime based on the goals and expectations of the child and his parents. In situations in which the expectations and goals are inappropriate, a careful explanation should be offered and, if necessary, the involvement of an experienced counselor may be required [15]. Hydrotherapy has been shown to have positive effects in reducing bleeding frequency, pain, and instability in a target joint and also in improving range of movement and muscle girth [16]. It is a stimulating environment for most children and a modality of treatment that merits further study.

The use of electrotherapy modalities, particularly ultrasound and pulsed shortwave, in children is an area of considerable controversy. It is a widely held view that it is acceptable to treat children with electrotherapy. However, there is a theoretical risk that some modalities of electrotherapy may affect the epiphyseal growth plates, and they should be avoided where there is an active bleed or the possibility of a rebleed. It is important to determine whether the theoretical risks of electrotherapy outweigh the risks of not using electrotherapy and the joint dysfunction that may ensue [17].

Physical exercise and appropriate sports should be encouraged. The benefits and risks of exercise need to be considered when advising on sport as more vigorous activity may carry a risk of trauma, but this must be balanced against the potential benefits to the musculoskeletal system [18]. It has been noted that children with hemophilia have lower muscle strength and aerobic power than age-matched groups of children without hemophilia [19]. The prescription of routine resistance exercise has been shown to decrease joint bleeding [2]. An algorithm has recently been developed that aims to provide a framework by which particular sports can be matched to fitness levels, muscle endurance and power, flexibility, and coordination in order to determine appropriate activities for children with hemophilia, so minimizing the risk of injury [20].

Regular exercise is also important in the regulation of body mass, particularly obesity and skeletal mineralization [21]. The World Health Organization has declared obesity a global epidemic and, although there is a strong relationship between poor cardiovascular fitness and obesity [22], no studies suggest that children with hemophilia are more at risk of obesity than children who do not have hemophilia. However, weight control is important in children with hemophilia as it prevents excess strains through a vulnerable musculoskeletal system.

Patients with inhibitors/ acquired hemophilia

This section will discuss some of the key issues that need to be considered when undertaking physiotherapy for patients with inhibitors and acquired hemophilia. Patients with inhibitors present a particular challenge to all the members of the multidisciplinary team [23]. It is therefore particularly important that the physiotherapist has considerable knowledge of the manifestations of hemophilia before managing these patients. It has been reported that these patients may experience more pain and disability than other patients with hemophilia owing to poor control of bleeding [24] and therefore assessment by a physiotherapist is even more important. However, concerns about the ease with which spontaneous bleeds may occur may deter members of the team from referring to the physiotherapist, and physical dysfunction that could be improved may go unmanaged.

The physiotherapist may be the first person to question whether a patient may have developed an inhibitor. Careful subjective questioning will alert the physiotherapist to the fact that the bleed is not resolving or the patient may be complaining of frequent bleeds in spite of regular and adequate factor replacement, and a medical opinion should be sought [1]. Once the patient has been diagnosed as having an inhibitor, there is much that the physiotherapist can offer. Bleeds may or may not be treated with factor replacement depending on whether the patient has a high- or low-titer inhibitor (measured in Bethesda units) and whether the patient is a low or high responder [25]. All patients must be managed with considerable care as the type of inhibitor present can change over time [25] and it is always essential to avoid causing bleeds or exacerbating further bleeding episodes.

Following an acute muscle or joint bleed, a very limited physical examination should be performed. This may include only observation of posture and extent of bruising, if any, and measurement of swelling and active pain-free movement. For the treatment of bleeds, synovitis, and arthropathy, similar techniques and modalities as used for adult patients and children with hemophilia can be employed for patients with inhibitors, provided that there is no active bleeding, all movements are pain free and exercises are progressed cautiously. The key issue in physiotherapy management for the patient with inhibitors is to avoid exacerbating the bleeding, therefore:

• It is particularly important to ensure the bleeding has stopped before starting physiotherapy.

• Electrotherapy modalities should be used with care only when bleeding has ceased [17].

• A very controlled, graded exercise program should be followed, starting with isometric exercises with low repetitions and progressing carefully based on response to exercises and patient comfort.

- High-resistance and high-impact exercises are contraindicated [23].

Many patients with long-term inhibitor problems will have multiple joint arthropathy due to uncontrolled bleeds in the past. Surgery may not be a possibility for some of these patients, and conservative measures may be the only option in relieving symptoms and maximizing function. Advice and education are essential to help the patient develop strategies to minimize stress on joints and control pain. Simple exercise regimes to build up muscle strength and maintain, and if possible increase, mobility should be provided. Hydrotherapy can be a particularly useful adjunct as the buoyancy of the water can relieve weight bearing and enable the patient to move more freely. It is essential that patients do not overexercise in the hydrotherapy pool, particularly in the early stages of rehabilitation, as the warm water and weightlessness can promote overconfidence. It is important that the patient has an appropriate lifestyle. Physical activities need to be chosen with care. Sports such as t'ai chi may still be enjoyed facilitating muscle strength, control and good posture as well as promoting the psychological benefits of exercise [26].

Patients with acquired inhibitors may develop severe bleeds often affecting the muscles. Left untreated, these muscle hematomas can lead to contractures and compartment syndromes [23]. The acquired inhibitor may have occurred secondary to other medical conditions such as rheumatoid arthritis. These additional medical problems need to be considered when planning treatment. Patients may be very frightened and anxious about the bleeding problem and require a great deal of reassurance and appropriate explanations. Treatment is focused on reducing symptoms due to bleeds using the strategies as described above and providing advice on avoiding or minimizing problems in the future.

Outcome measures

It is important that an appropriate tool is chosen to evaluate the impact of physiotherapy in order to demonstrate the effectiveness of the care. In most situations, the evaluation should be undertaken before and after the intervention to monitor any changes. As a result, it is essential that the measures used are reliable, valid, and sensitive to change [27]. Three main types of outcome measure are available. These are impairment measures, functional measures and quality-of-life measures.

Impairment measures

Measures of impairment include the evaluation of a range of physical testing procedures including posture, range of movement, and muscle strength. The advantage of using an impairment measure to evaluate outcome is that these measures are relatively easy and quick to perform. The disadvantages of these measures are the poor reliability of measurements, especially between different raters [28]. Changes in measures may also not correspond to changes in the function or quality of life of the pa-

tient. These measures are also measures of relevance to the healthcare professional but do not involve the perspective of the patient.

Functional measures

These measures can be used to provide information on the functional health status of a patient. The advantage of functional measures is that they assess the ability to undertake tasks of daily living that is usually of relevance to the patient as well as the physiotherapist. They do not, however, consider other aspects of health, such as psychological and social factors, that may also be changed as a result of physiotherapy interventions. The Health Assessment Questionnaire (HAQ) was developed for patients with arthritis and has been used as an outcome measure to demonstrate effectiveness of physiotherapy for patients with hemophilia [29].

Quality-of-life measures

There has been an emerging interest in recent years in evaluating the effect of hemophilia on quality of life (QoL). A number of published studies over the last 10 years have investigated the impact of hemophilia on QoL [30], although none has specifically evaluated physiotherapy interventions. Most studies have used standardized questionnaires, in particular the Medical Outcomes Study SF36 (SF36), which is a well-known example of a generic standardized questionnaire. The reliability and validity of the SF36 has been extensively evaluated for patients with a variety of conditions [31], although the reliability and sensitivity of the SF36 have not been specifically evaluated for patients with hemophilia.

The results of published studies have generally demonstrated that QoL scores are lower in patients with hemophilia than in the normal population. However, a number of authors have suggested that scores would be expected to be even lower than those achieved [32–34]. A number of reasons were proposed to explain this, including adapting to condition, re-evaluating priorities, and coping strategies. The relevance of these issues needs to be evaluated in the hemophilia population, but we suggest caution in the use of standardized QoL questionnaires in isolation.

Annual monitoring of children and adults with hemophilia

It is recommended that the musculoskeletal system is monitored over time for all patients with hemophilia. Ideally, a 6-month or, at the minimum, yearly review of the patient to evaluate the status of the musculoskeletal system should be undertaken [35]. Physical impairment measures can be useful when evaluating the progression of hemophilic arthropathy. If a deterioration in range of movement or strength is noted, physiotherapy intervention can be instigated to improve this. A number of standardized assessment forms are available [36,37]. The WFH scoring system does not appear to be sensitive enough to detect the more minor changes that tend to occur in younger patients [38,39] and other assessment protocols have recently been devised [38,40]. However, clinical assessment and even plain radiographs may not identify early joint abnormalities in children [41]. The European Paediatric Network for Hemophilia Management is also developing pediatric orthopedic and MRI scoring systems [40]. MRI has been shown to be more beneficial than radiography for detecting early joint damage, chronic synovitis, iron deposits, and joint changes as pathologic alterations can be picked up with greater sensitivity [42] (see Chapter 33).

Summary

The physiotherapist needs to use problem-solving skills, clinical reasoning, and reflection on practice when managing musculoskeletal dysfunction for patients with hemophilia. Patients with a chronic condition such as hemophilia are often experts, and there is much to learn from listening and talking to the patient and developing appropriate treatment strategies based on mutually agreed goals. Not all patients will necessarily have experience of the potential manifestations of hemophilia, such as patients with mild hemophilia, or those who have recently developed an inhibitor or acquired hemophilia. Other patients may have denied their hemophilia and continued to adopt an inappropriate lifestyle. These patients need careful explanations, encouragement, and regular monitoring of their problems. Finally, a valid, reliable, and sensitive outcome measure must be used in order to provide an objective measure of the effectiveness of the physiotherapy treatment. Physiotherapists should be encouraged to publish the outcomes of their interventions, so enhancing the evidence base and promotion of best practice in the physiotherapy management of hemophilia.

References

1 Beeton K, Ryder D. Principles of assessment in haemophilia. In: Buzzard B, Beeton K, eds. *Physiotherapy Management of Haemophilia*. Oxford: Blackwell Science, 2000: 1–13.

2 Titinsky R, Falk B, Heim M, *et al*. The effect of resistance training on the frequency of bleeding in haemophilia patients: a pilot study. *Haemophilia* 2003; 8: 22–7.

3 Zourikian N. Ice: is it really effective when used as a means of reducing haemorrhage and/or oedema following an acute musculoskeletal injury? *Haemophilia* 2002; 8: 484 (abstract).

4 Buzzard B. Trauma induced pseudotumours in two brothers with moderate factor IX deficiency. In: *Proceedings of the 4th Musculoskeletal Congress of the World Federation of Haemophilia*, Madrid, 1997.

5 Liesner R, Khair K, Hann I. The impact of prophyalctic treatment on children with severe haemophilia. *Br J Haematol* 1996; 92: 973–8.

6 Betsy M, Gilbert M. Haemophilic haemarthrosis. In: Rodriguez-Merchan EC, ed. *The Haemophilic Joints: New Perspectives*. Oxford: Blackwell Publishing, 2003: 17–19.

7 Stephensen D. Biomechanics of the lower limb in haemophilia. In:

8 Schoenmakers M, Gulmans V, Helders P, *et al*. Motor performance and disability in Dutch children with haemophilia: a comparison with their healthy peers. *Haemophilia* 2001; 7: 293–8.

9 Beeton K. Physiotherapy for adult patients with haemophilia In: Rodriguez-Merchan EC, Goddard NJ, Lee CA, eds. *Musculoskeletal Aspects of Haemophilia*. Oxford: Blackwell Science, 2000: 177–86.

10 Ljung R. Aspects of haemophilia prophylaxis in Sweden. *Haemophilia* 2002; 8: 34–7.

11 Aledort L, Haschmeyer R, Pettersson H, *et al*. A longitudinal study of orthopaedic outcomes for severe factor-VIII-deficient haemophiliacs. *J Intern Med* 1994; 236: 391–9.

12 Brown S, Aledort L, Lee CA. Optimal treatment regimens for patients with bleeding disorders. *Haemophilia* 2001; 7: 113–20.

13 Buzzard B. Physiotherapy management of haemophilia in children. In: Rodriguez-Merchan EC, Goddard N, Lee CA, eds. *Musculoskeletal Aspects of Haemophilia*. Oxford: Blackwell Science, 2000: 169–76.

14 Heijnen L, Helders P. Prevention and treatment of joint problems in children with haemophilia. In: Rodriguez-Merchan EC, ed. *The Haemophilic Joints: New Perspectives*. Oxford: Blackwell Science, 2003: 133–7.

15 Miller R, Beeton K, Goldman E, *et al*. Counselling guidelines for managing musculoskeletal problems in haemophilia in the 1990s. *Haemophilia* 1997; 3: 9–13.

16 Higginbottom M. Hydrotherapy for haemophilia. *Haemophilia* 1998; 4: 223 (abstract).

17 Watson T. Current concepts in electrotherapy. *Haemophilia* 2002; 8: 413–8.

18 Froberg K. Lammert O. *Exercise and Fitness — Benefits and Risks in Children and Exercise XVIII*. Odense: Odense University Press, 1997.

19 Falk B, Portal S, Titinsky R, *et al*. Muscle strength and aerobic power in young haemophiliac patients. *Haemophilia* 1998; 4: 220 (abstract).

20 Seuser A, Wallny T, Schumpe G, *et al*. How to advise young haemophiliacs to find the right sport? A new and safe algorithm! In: *8th Musculoskeletal Committee Conference of the World Federation of Hemophilia*. Bonn, Germany, 2003.

21 Malina R. Growth and maturation: do regular physical activity and training for sport have a significant influence? In: Armstrong N, van Mechelen W, eds. *Paediatric Exercise, Science and Medicine*. Oxford: Oxford University Press, 2000: 209–27.

22 Boreham C, Strain JJ, Twisk J, *et al*. Aerobic fitness, physical activity and body fatness in adolescents In: Armstrong N, Kirby B, Welsman J, eds. *Children and Exercise. XIX*, London: E & FN Spon, 1997: 69–74.

23 Beeton K, Buzzard B. Physiotherapy in the management of patients with inhibitors. In: Rodriguez-Merchan EC, Lee CA, eds. *Inhibitors in Patients with Haemophilia*. Oxford: Blackwell Science, 2002.

24 Roberts H. Inhibitors and their management. In: Rizza C, Lowe G, eds. *Haemophilia and Other Inherited Bleeding Disorders*. London: W.B. Saunders, 1997: 365–89.

25 Dimichele D. Inhibitors in haemophilia: a primer. *Haemophilia* 2000; 6 (Suppl. 1): 38–40.

26 Danusantoso H, Heijnen L. Tai Chi Chuan for persons with haemophilia. *Haemophilia* 2001; 7: 437–8 (correspondence).

27 Fitzpatrick R, Davey C, Buxton M, *et al*. Evaluating patient-based outcome measures for use in clinical trials. *Health Technology Assessment* 1998; 2: 1–73.

28 Rodriguez-Merchan EC. Orthopaedic assessment in haemophilia. *Haemophilia* 2003; 9: 65–74.

29 Cornwall J. Disability and outcome measures in patients with haemophilia. In: Buzzard B, Beeton K, eds. *Physiotherapy Management of Haemophilia*. Oxford: Blackwell Science, 2000: 101–9.

30 Fischer K, van der Bom J, van den Berg H. Health-related quality of life as outcome parameter in haemophilia treatment. *Haemophilia* 2003; **9**: 75–82.

31 Bowling A. *Measuring Health. A Review of Quality of Life Measurement Scales*, 2nd edn. Buckingham: Open University Press, 1997.

32 Rosendaal F, Smit C, Varekamp I, *et al.* Modern haemophilia treatment: medical improvements and quality of life. *J Intern Med* 1990; **228**: 633–40.

33 Djulbegovic B, Goldsmith G, Vaughn D, *et al.* Comparison of the quality of life between HIV-positive haemophilia patients and HIV-negative haemophilia patients. *Haemophilia* 1996; **2**: 166–72.

34 Miners A, Sabin C, Tolley K, *et al.* Assessing health-related quality-of-life in individuals with haemophilia. *Haemophilia* 1999; **5**: 378–85.

35 Haemophilia Alliance. *A National Service Specification for Haemophilia and Related Conditions*, London, 2001.

36 Haemophilia Chartered Physiotherapists Association. *Standards for Haemophilia*. London: Chartered Society of Physiotherapy, 1996.

37 Pettersson H, Gilbert M. *Diagnostic Imaging in Haemophilia*. Berlin: Springer-Verlag, 1985.

38 Ljung R. Paediatric care of the child with haemophilia. *Haemophilia* 2003; **8**: 178–82.

39 Yee TT, Beeton K, Griffioen A, *et al.* Experience of prophylaxis treatment in children with severe haemophilia. *Haemophilia* 2002; **8**: 76–82.

40 Manco-Johnson M, Nuss R, Funk S, *et al.* Joint evaluation instruments for children and adults with haemophilia. *Haemophilia* 2000; **6**: 649–57.

41 Arnold W, Hilgartner M. Haemophilic arthropathy, current concepts of pathogenesis and management. *J Bone Joint Surg* 1977; **59**: 287–305.

42 Nuss R, Kilcoyne R, Geraghty S, *et al.* Utility of magnetic resonance imaging for management of haemophilic arthropathy in children. *J Paediatr* 1993; **123**: 388–92.

Transfusion-transmitted disease: history of epidemics (focus on HIV)

W. Keith Hoots

The association between transfusion-transmitted disease and the receipt of untreated clotting factor concentrates

The realization that individuals with hemophilia who are treated with replacement clotting factor concentrates (CFCs) were at particular risk for transfusion-associated infection from this treatment antedated the theoretical earliest date for widespread exposure to human immunodeficiency virus (HIV). From the late 1960s, it was recognized that people with hemophilia treated with the newly introduced CFCs made from cryoprecipitates for factor VIII (FVIII) and fresh-frozen plasma for factor IX (FIX)] were highly exposed to blood-borne infectious agents. The identification of the Australian antigen as a protein marker of hepatitis B provided the first capacity to identify "pathogen contaminants" in the large plasma pools (ranging in size from 15 000 to >30 000 donors per batch or lot) that were processed into CFCs by physical separation technology [1].

This testing for Australian antigen (renamed hepatitis B surface antigen; HBV) [2] and the serologic response to this HBV capsular protein (HB$_s$ antibody) in the plasma of CFC-exposed people with hemophilia revealed that at least one more hepatitis pathogen was ubiquitous in CFCs. Since no antigenic or serologic identifiers were yet available to identify this second pathogen, it was referred to as non-A, non-B hepatitis (NANB), and transient or sustained elevation of transaminases in previously normal hemophilic individuals following single or recurrent treatment with CFCs became a surrogate for identifying this blood-borne pathogen. As definitive identification of NANB by molecular virologic techniques would not occur until 1989, the nearly universal mild to severe elevation in transaminases in the serum of individuals with hemophilia A and B became a surrogate for viral hepatitis infection [3].

Early efforts to attenuate the pathogen risk from CFC use focused on efforts to heat the lyophilized CFCs. However, the exquisite sensitivity of FVIII, in particular to denaturation, stalled the early efforts in producing virus-attenuated CFCs. Further, the latency of clinical symptoms of HCV contributed to a false sense of security about the morbid risks associated with the regular infusion of CFCs [4].

The early HIV epidemic in hemophilia populations receiving clotting factor concentrates

Against this backdrop, acquired immune deficiency syndrome (AIDS) became recognized as a severe new clinical disease in 1979–1980 in the USA and elsewhere [5]. It was characterized epidemiologically by its primary target population of homosexual men and clinically by its extraordinarily rapid destruction of the host immune system, predisposing to opportunistic infections such as *Pneumocystis carinii* (PCP). The first suspicions that it might be other than a sexually transmitted pathogen arose in July 1982 when the US Center for Disease Control (CDC) reported three requests for compassionate use of the investigational drug pentamidine for PCP in hemophilia A individuals widely separated geographically [6]. By the end of 1982, the number of such requests increased to eight [7]. None of these individuals was felt to have other risk factors for AIDS besides their hemophilia.

Aggressive surveillance for immune dysfunction in both children and adults with hemophilia was undertaken in 1983 at several hemophilia treatment centers (HTCs) in the USA, Canada, and Europe as more individuals with hemophilia A (and subsequently B) became immune suppressed and as the death rate from AIDS rose. These reports confirmed findings from other AIDS cohorts of marked lymphopenia with particular reduction in T4 subsets [2,8–11]. CD8 subsets were variable. Lymphadenopathy and splenomegaly, previously rare in hemophilia, became commonplace among patients in HTCs [12]. The individuals with the most profound depression in their T4 count (the terminology was later changed to CD4$^+$ lymphocytes) often were experiencing wasting and recurrent opportunistic infections such as PCP, atypical mycobacterial infections (such as *Mycobacterium avium intracellulare* — MAI), and central nervous system varicella infections [13].

In 1983, Montagnier isolated (with the assistance of Gallo) the human T-cell leukemia virus III (HTLV-III), and implicated the retrovirus as the cause of AIDS [14,15]. Serologic testing of blood and blood components for HTLV-III by both enzyme-linked immunosorbent assay (ELISA) and Western blot became possible with these definitive viral genomic sequences [16]. In this way, the profound implications for the hemophilia populations who had been treated with CFCs began to be documented for the first time. Eyster *et al.* [17], in a study conducted in one

HTC in Hershey, Pennsylvania, found an HTLV-III (HIV) infection rate among the population of patients with *severe* hemophilia A approaching 90% and reported that the percentage infected (based on analyses of stored serum specimens from the 1970s into the early 1980s) had increased exponentially between 1981 and late 1983 (Figure 35.1) . Other reports and ongoing Centers for Disease Control (CDC) surveillance in the USA as well as reports from UK, France, Italy, and Spain confirmed that the majority of individuals with moderate or severe hemophilia A receiving lyophilized CFCs were infected by the middle of the decade and that a sizable percentage of hemophilia B patients were also infected [9,18–20].

As the above epidemiologic reports imply, the impact of HIV on the mean lifespan of individuals with hemophilia was immediate and profound. Prior to 1960, the median lifespan of a person with hemophilia was ~42 years, with bleeding complications constituting the highest prevalence cause of death. By 1980, lifespan had risen to approximately 69 years from better therapy for bleeding. Figure 35.2 [21] details the dramatic decline in this enhanced survival over the years following the unforeseen introduction of HIV into the population. It would take nearly a decade and a half [following the introduction of highly active antiretroviral therapy (HAART) therapy as effective HIV

treatment in 1996 — see discussion below] before there would be significant mitigation in this trend. Fortunately, as the following section discusses, efforts to eliminate HIV from its infectious source (CFCs) in this population fairly rapidly insured that children born with hemophilia and those fortunate enough to have avoided infection with former exposure to HIV-infected CFCs did not, by and large, become accompanying casualties to the epidemic in this population.

Technological improvements for enhancing the safety of clotting factor concentrates

Early efforts to attenuate the risk for hepatitis, HIV and other blood-borne pathogens resulted in a licensed heat-treated FVIII concentrate (Hemofil T™) for the USA in April 1983 with licensure in Europe and elsewhere over the following year or two. To overcome the FVIII yield loss from heating in the lyophilized state, stabilizers were added. Over subsequent years, this resulted in achieving a yield of approximately 60% when compared with nonheated FVIII concentrate [22]. More importantly, however, *ex vivo* work at the CDC and elsewhere in 1984 indicated that HTLV-III (HIV) is exquisitely sensitive to heating, resulting in large log kill with heating in either the wet or dry preparation phase. Subsequently, epidemiologic studies showed that previously HIV-uninfected hemophilic individuals who were infused exclusively with heat-treated FVIII CFCs *remained* uninfected [23]. Unfortunately, the capacity of heating (in particular dry-heating) to eradicate non-A, non-B hepatitis was not nearly so successful [24].

Fortunately, other technological advances were being pursued for the attenuation of all lipid envelope viruses. Specifically, solvents such as tri-*n*-butyl phosphate, when combined with detergent compounds such as Tween™ or polysorbate 80, disrupt the viral capsid of most known lipid-enveloped viruses (including HIV, HBV, and HCV) [25,26]. For optimal viral attenuation, the solvent/detergent (SD) needs to be applied without the presence of protein aggregates, often necessitating prior filtration

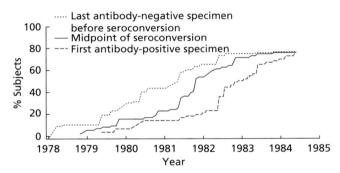

Figure 35.1 Prevalence of human T-cell lymphotropic virus antibodies in a cohort of recipients of factor VIII concentrates. The data are shown as three Kaplan–Meier plots depicting range of time over which seroconversion could have occurred.

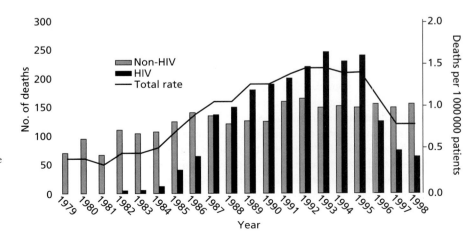

Figure 35.2 The impact of HIV infection in the United States, 1979–98. Annual mortality among patients with hemophilia A, with and without HIV-related disease, and overall age-adjusted death rate. From Chorba *et al.* [21].

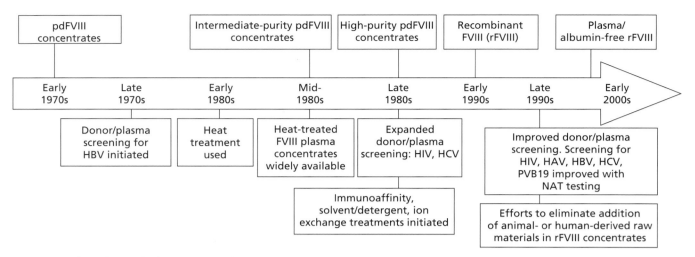

Figure 35.3 The evolution of safety measures in factor VIII replacement therapy.

before SD treatment [22]. Applied accordingly, CFCs processed with SD treatment have not been implicated in the transmission of lipid-enveloped pathogens to an individual with hemophilia A or B. Unfortunately, SD treatment is ineffectual for attenuation or killing of nonlipid enveloped viruses [27] (Figure 35.3 [24]).

Treatment of all CFCs that have undergone either heating (in wet or dry state) or SD treatment resulted in (by approximately 1985 for FVIII and 1986 for FIV) very few previously uninfected individuals with hemophilia becoming infected with HIV thereafter. Hence, the horrific epidemic summarized above became, for the first time, circumscribed with regards to overall risk to treated individuals with hemophilia. This profound advance unfortunately came too late for many thousands of people with hemophilia worldwide. In addition, comparable elimination of hepatitis C (non-A, non-B) would require universal application of either SD treatment or combination of newer techniques of CFC purification such as monoclonal technology before CFCs made from source (donated for CFCs) or recovered plasma (salvaged from single donor units) was accomplished [28]. Later-evolving technologies, in particular the development of FVIII and FIX CFCs afforded by recombinant technology, added a similar level of security against nonlipid-enveloped viruses (e.g., human parvovirus B19) as well.

The advent of ultrahigh-purity FVIII and FIX concentrates (CFCs purified using monoclonal or recombinant technologies) also brought about a degree of immune stabilization in HIV-infected individuals with hemophilia. Several studies demonstrated and confirmed that these ultrapure CFCs resulted in significant stabilization of CD4+ lymphocyte counts in controlled, randomly selected cohorts when compared with comparable control cohorts receiving intermediate purity CFCs [29–31]. However, no clearly reproducible cause for this effect has been demonstrated, although biochemical contaminants of intermediate-purity CFCs (e.g., cytokines, β_2-microglobulin,

fragments of proteins residual after purification techniques are applied, etc.) have been proposed [32].

The contributions of hemophilic cohorts to understanding the pathogenesis of HIV infection

From the inception of the HIV epidemic in hemophilia, the unfortunate individuals with bleeding disorders who were unwittingly infected volunteered early and often to participate in scientific studies about HIV and the associated complications. Particularly in European countries and the USA, cohorts of variable size were assembled first to study the natural history of HIV and other pathogens (e.g., the hepatitides B, C, and D) and, once therapeutic options such as AZT were developed, to participate in early phase clinical trials. Large hemophilic HIV cohort studies such as the Multinational Multicenter Cohort Study [33] and the UK HTC Directors and studies from France, Germany, and Japan helped to provide important seminal information such as the following: (i) relative risk factors for opportunistic infections (e.g., high prevalence of *Mycobacterium avium intracellulare* infection) [34]; (ii) the virtual nonexistence of Kaposi's sarcoma (now recognized to derive from coinfection with HHV-8) [35]; (iii) the importance of age at the time of infection on outcome in HIV-infected hemophilia populations [18,36]; (iv) the utility of HIV-RNA levels in assessing time to development of AIDS [37]; (v) the influence of HLA on susceptibility for AIDS development [38]; and (vi) the recognition that a very rapid downward clinical spiral did not inevitably occur in everyone infected with HIV — even in the era preceding effective antiretroviral therapy. Unlike other HIV-infected populations, a substantial percentage of the hemophilia population survived for more than 15 years before the advent of highly active antiretroviral therapy [39–41]. Aggressive use of HAART in this select population now permits consideration that HIV may be a chronic, rather than a universally fatal, disease.

Hemophilic HIV cohorts, when combined with large homosexual and intravenous drug-abusing HIV cohorts, enabled investigators to identify mutant receptors and ligand alleles on immune cells (particularly HIV-targeted CD4 lymphocytes) by population genomic analyses. These mutations in CCR5, CCR2, CXCR4, SDF1, and others help to explain why certain HIV-exposed individuals do not become infected [25,42–44]. Longitudinal studies that compared HIV-infected hemophilic adolescents and children, age-matched uninfected hemophilic boys, and nonhemophilic siblings helped to delineate chronic effects of HIV on growth and development and to assess the subtle morbidities of chronic HIV on children. These provided among the first observations that HIV could delay puberty [45], cause subtle anatomic and pathophysiologic abnormalities in older children and adolescents [46], induce subtle, but measurable neurologic and neuropsychologic abnormalities distinct from hemophilia-induced causes [47,48], and, in most severe manifestations, confound the musculoskeletal pathology of hemophilia itself [49].

Most recently, studies of long-term hemophilic survivors with HIV, who are coinfected with HCV (most of whom have been infected for more than two decades and who are doing well clinically on highly active antiretroviral therapy), have provided insights into the greater morbidity of HCV liver disease in individuals chronically immune suppressed from HIV (see below). In this instance and in those cited above and elsewhere, the uniqueness of the hemophilic cohort and the willingness of HIV-infected individuals with hemophilia to participate in clinical research has contributed significantly to the medical knowledge about HIV.

HIV and hemophilia in the twenty-first century

According to data from the Universal Data Collection sponsored by the Centers for Disease Control and Prevention in the USA, approximately half of the estimated 9200 hemophilic individuals in the USA who were HIV-infected are alive with HIV (due in part to the improved therapy with HAART, discussed below) in 2004 [50]. As Eyster et al. [13], and others, have shown, however, nearly all of them have coinfection with HCV and liver failure has surpassed AIDS-related causes as the leading cause of mortality. Matched for age, genotype, and infection duration, progression to cirrhosis and chronic liver failure is more prevalent in coinfected hemophilia individuals than in those infected with HCV alone. This higher rate of liver disease progression and reduced HCV clearance appears to persist even in those individuals who have had no detectable HIV viral load for more than 7 years and who have maintained stable CD4 cell counts [51].

This greater hepatic damage in coinfected individuals has led to high morbidity from complications such as bleeding, wherein hemorrhage from esophageal varices is complicated by both low FVIII/IX and decreased levels of other clotting proteins (in particular the vitamin K-dependent proteins II, VII, IX and X). In coinfected individuals, cholestasis is an additional prognostic marker for survival that may reflect both impaired systemic immune function and defective hepatic homeostasis [52]. Further, the potential for toxicity from many of the HAART regimens (the pharmaceutical variety of which is beyond the scope of this discussion) is enhanced by the remarkably reduced hepatocellular function.

Antiretroviral therapy

Although a thorough discussion of the many advances made in the treatment of HIV in recent years (most notably the advent of multidrug HAART therapy) is beyond the scope of this chapter, a perusal of particular aspects relevant to hemophilia is not only appropriate, but critical to the discussion of HIV impact on people with hemophilia. For example, early on, following the introduction of protease inhibitors as the "third leg" of the HAART "stool," it was reported that a number of hemophilia individuals receiving these drugs were experiencing greater spontaneous hemorrhage. These observations were confirmed in several countries. Investigations to elucidate the exact etiology were undertaken but a single explanation was elusive. Possibilities included platelet dysfunction and negative impact on liver synthetic function [53,54]. Despite these observations and reports that some individuals have needed more frequent infusions of CFCs, protease inhibitors remain a mainstay of HAART therapy for individuals with HIV and hemophilia. Their use has resulted in long periods of nondetectable HIV in plasma in many of them [55]. To maximize the benefits of these drug regimens, therapeutic drug monitoring (TPM) has been suggested to optimize the response to HAART therapy. Its routine use will require further clinical research [56].

Reference was made above to the transition of HIV infection from a universally fatal disease to a chronic one (particularly among long-term hemophilic survivors). Unfortunately, this improvement in outcome prospects has been somewhat more problematic in other groups, typically more recently infected populations. Greater development of drug resistance to HAART drugs may account for some of these differences since the HIV genotypes of long-surviving hemophilic individuals may be less prone to rapid mutation than the multiple quasispecies of HIV more characteristic of recently infected cohorts. Nonetheless, as noted above, the long-term coinfection of HIV and HCV in the surviving hemophilic individuals partially counterbalances these possible HIV survival advantages among persons with hemophilia. Other confounders for the management of hemophilia, HIV, and HCV are the sometimes observed symptomatic lactic acidosis (secondary to nucleoside reverse transcriptase inhibitors) and the more commonly observed dyslipidemias seen with protease inhibitor use [57,58]. Clinical management of the complications requires the expertise of the HIV infectious disease specialist, the gastroenterologist, and the hemophilia specialist. Close involvement of the last is needed for the complex management of hemophilia, other decreased procoagulation from liver failure, and, often, bleeding esophageal varices.

The rise in death from liver failure among the HIV-infected hemophilic population provides new challenges not only to reduce the HIV viral load to undetectable levels and to continue to target the reservoirs of residual viral replication, but also to eradicate HCV (if possible) with aggressive therapy with ribavirin and alpha-interferon (or pegylated alpha-interferon). The enhancement of HCV-induced hepatocellular destruction among coinfected individuals has, on occasion, necessitated extraordinary interventions in efforts to preserve metabolic function and to prolong life — particularly in individuals for whom HAART therapy has provided an asymptomatic course for their HIV disease.

Once end-stage liver disease is reached in coinfected hemophilic individuals, the only option is orthotopic liver transplantation. Despite the paucity of donor livers for patients with liver failure from any etiology, Ragni and colleagues have described successful cadaveric liver transplantation in candidate individuals with HIV, HCV, *and* hemophilia. Reports confirm the expected cure of the hemophilic bleeding diathesis, restoration of liver function with improvement in morbidity related to portal hypertension (e.g., esophageal varices), improvement in Karnofsky performance status, and maintenance of undetectable HIV viremia [59].

The role of hemophilia treatment centers in caring for hemophilic patients with HIV disease

HIV impacted hemophilia treatment centers (HTCs) in ways that previously had been unthinkable. As the mortality rate among hemophilics rose exponentially and severely debilitated patients again became common, by exigency HTCs were forced to assume responsibility for preventive strategies against the spread of this lethal disease [41]. Psychosocial professionals in HTCs adapted risk reduction strategies from the social science literature to educate sexually active, HIV-infected hemophilia individuals about their risk of spreading the disease to a sexual partner. A body of medical literature evolved that established hemophilia and HTCs as leaders in the early phase of developmental programs of risk reduction among heterosexual populations [60]. By 1987, 48 of 72 hemophilia centers in the USA, as well as many in Europe, Canada, and Australia, were using formal pre- and posteducation knowledge testing with their patients. The patients' sexual partners were invited to participate in many instances. In addition, innovative risk reduction programs were designed and implemented specifically by HTC psychologists for adolescents with hemophilia. These were aimed at both teaching prevention of the spread of HIV and exploring in a nonthreatening way human sexuality and intimacy [41,61,62].

Fortunately for HTCs, the scourge of HIV did not accelerate following the advent of CFC purification techniques (e.g., heat treatment, solvent/detergent). Nonetheless, this decade-long commitment by HTCs to the care of people with HIV (and to their family members who might be at risk because they were sexual partners of the hemophilia patient) had a profound influence on the evolution of hemophilia care in Europe, the USA, Canada, Australia, and elsewhere. It demonstrated tangibly the capacity of this multidisciplinary model to adapt to even the most catastrophic of medical challenges and harnessed the educational creativity of dedicated professionals, the latter ultimately benefiting all patients (with or without pathogenic complication) who receive care from HTCs. Now, the health professionals in HTCs have the added commitment of insuring that HIV-infected survivors with hemophilia receive the support, care, and compassion needed in adhering to complex drug regimens with myriad toxicities while trying to maintain normal lives. Managing their bleeding while helping their adherence to the other treatment strategies will continue to offer challenges to HTCs for years to come.

Conclusion

HIV infection has had catastrophic consequences for people with hemophilia born before 1985. Widespread use of CFCs produced in the USA and Europe prior to the advent of effective antipathogen donor screening and technologic advances in viral attenuation of large pools of human plasma used to produce CFCs resulted in a majority of exposed hemophilia individuals (in countries using these products) becoming infected between 1979 and 1985. Unfortunately, many died prematurely in the following years. Further, untoward suffering from HIV-associated complications dramatically impaired the quality of life of many who survived these early years of the epidemic.

A complex interplay of determinants such as viral genetics, host genetics, early access to antiretroviral therapy, excellent supportive care, and other as yet undefined factors resulted in long-term survival for many of these hemophilic individuals for whom the early prospects were grim. With the advent of HAART, these prospects have, in the intervening two decades, brightened considerably, despite the added burden created by concomitant HCV infection. It is hoped that new advances in eradicating *both* pathogens completely (including the occult reservoirs of HIV) will convert this now chronic disease into a historical one for these long-term survivors. Coupled with the advent of new virally safe recombinant CFCs (and the predecessor CFCs, which eliminated HIV infection since the 1980s), the chapter of HIV and hemophilia might then finally be closed.

References

1 Nordenfelt E, Kjellen L. Presence and persistence of Australian antigen in a Swedish hepatitis series. *Acta Pathol Microbiol Scand* 1969; 77: 489–94.

2 Abe T. Clinical, immunological, and virological aspects in Japanese hemophiliacs and AIDS patients. *AIDS Res* 1986; **2**: S141–6.

3 Norkrans G, Widell A, Teger-Nilsson AC, *et al.* Acute hepatitis non-A, non-B following administration of factor VIII concentrates. *Vox Sang* 1981; **41**: 129–33.

4 Hoots WK. Safety issues affecting hemophilia products. *Transfus Med Rev* 2001; **15**: 11–19.

5 Shilts R. *And the Band Played On: Politics, People, and the AIDS Epidemic*. New York: St. Martin's Press; 1987.

6 Centers for Disease Control. Epidemiologic notes and reports: *Pneumocystis carinii* pneumonia among persons with hemophilia A. *MMWR Weekly* 1982; **31**: 365–7.

7 Centers for Disease Control. Update on acquired immune deficiency syndrome (AIDS) among patients with hemophilia A. *MMWR Weekly* 1982; **31**: 644–6; 652.

8 Group CHCD. Effect of using safer blood products on prevalence of HIV infection in haemophilic Canadians. *BMJ* 1993; **306**: 306–7.

9 Berntorp E, Jarevi G, Wedback A, *et al.* Natural history of HIV infection in Swedish haemophiliacs. *Eur J Haematol* 1989; **42**: 254–8.

10 Garsia RJ, Gatenby PA, Basten A, *et al.* Australian hemophiliac recipients of voluntary donor blood products longitudinally evaluated for AIDS. A clinical and laboratory study, 1983–1986. *Aust NZ J Med* 1987; **17**: 371–8.

11 Weimer R, Schweighoffer T, Schimpf K, Opelz G. Helper and suppressor T-cell function in HIV-infected hemophilia patients. *Blood* 1989; **74**: 298–302.

12 Daul CB, deShazo RD, Andes WA. Human immunodeficiency virus infection in hemophiliac patients. A three-year prospective evaluation. *Am J Med* 1988; **84**: 801–9.

13 Eyster ME, Gail MH, Ballard JO, *et al.* Natural history of human immunodeficiency virus infections in hemophiliacs: effects of T-cell subsets, platelet counts, and age. *Ann Intern Med* 1987; **107**: 1–6.

14 Montagnier L RW, Vèzinet-Brun F, Rouzious C, *et al.* Isolation of a T-Lymphotropic retrovirus from a patient at risk for acquired immune deficiency syndrome (AIDS). *Science* 1983; **220**: 868–71.

15 Goedert JJ, Gallo RC. Epidemiological evidence that HTLV-III is the AIDS agent. *Eur J Epidemiol* 1985; **1**: 155–9.

16 Gallo RC, Montagnier L. The discovery of HIV as the cause of AIDS. *N Engl J Med* 2003; **349**: 2283–5.

17 Eyster ME, Goedert JJ, Sarngadharan MG, *et al.* Development and early natural history of HTLV-III antibodies in persons with hemophilia. *JAMA* 1985; **253**: 2219–23.

18 Darby SC, Rizza CR, Doll R, *et al.* Incidence of AIDS and excess of mortality associated with HIV in haemophiliacs in the United Kingdom: report on behalf of the directors of haemophilia centres in the United Kingdom. *BMJ* 1989; **298**: 1064–8.

19 Brettler DB, Brewster F, Levine PH, *et al.* Immunologic aberrations, HIV seropositivity and seroconversion rates in patients with hemophilia B. *Blood* 1987; **70**: 276–81.

20 Sjamsoedin-Visser LJ, Heijnen CJ, Zegers BJ, Stoop JW. Defective T suppressor-inducer cell function in human immune deficiency virus-seropositive hemophilia patients. *Blood* 1988; **72**: 1474–7.

21 Chorba TL, Holman RC, Clarke MJ, Evatt BL. Effects of HIV infection on age and cause of death for persons with hemophilia A in the United States. *Am J Hematol* 2001; **66**: 229–40.

22 Fischer G, Hoots WK, Abrams C. Viral reduction techniques: types and purpose. *Transfus Med Rev* 2001; **15**: 27–39.

23 Ramsey RB, Evatt BL, McDougal JS, *et al.* Antibody to human immunodeficiency virus in factor-deficient plasma. Effect of heat treatment on lyophilized plasma. *Am J Clin Pathol* 1987; **87**: 263–6.

24 Hoots WK. History of plasma-product safety. *Transfus Med Rev* 2001; **15**: 3–10.

25 Daar ES, Lynn H, Donfield S, Gomperts E, *et al.* Effects of plasma HIV RNA, CD4+ T lymphocytes, and the chemokine receptors CCR5 and CCR2b on HIV disease progression in hemophiliacs. Hemophilia Growth and Development Study. *J Acquir Immune Defic Syndr* 1999; **21**: 317–25.

26 Horowitz MS, Rooks C, Horowitz B, Hilgartner MW. Virus safety of solvent/detergent-treated antihaemophilic factor concentrate. *Lancet* 1988; **ii**: 186–9.

27 Solheim BG, Rollag H, Svennevig JL, *et al.* Viral safety of solvent/detergent-treated plasma. *Transfusion* 2000; **40**: 84–90.

28 Brettler DB, Forsberg AD, Levine PH, *et al.* Factor VIII:C concentrate purified from plasma using monoclonal antibodies: human studies. *Blood* 1989; **73**: 1859–63.

29 de Biasi R, Rocino A, Miraglia E, *et al.* The impact of a very high purity factor VIII concentrate on the immune system of human immunodeficiency virus-infected hemophiliacs: a randomized, prospective, two-year comparison with an intermediate purity concentrate. *Blood* 1991; **78**: 1919–22.

30 Seremetis SV, Aledort LM, Bergman GE, *et al.* Three-year randomised study of high-purity or intermediate-purity factor VIII concentrates in symptom-free HIV-seropositive haemophiliacs: effects on immune status. *Lancet* 1993; **342**: 700–3.

31 Teitel JM, Card R, Strawczynski H. Laboratory and clinical markers of HIV infection in a national haemophilia cohort treated with recombinant factor VIII concentrate. The Association of Hemophilia Clinic Directors of Canada. *Haemophilia* 1998; **4**: 731–8.

32 Hoots K, Canty D. Clotting factor concentrates and immune function in haemophilic patients. *Haemophilia* 1998; **4**: 704–13.

33 Goedert JJ, Kessler CM, Aledort LM, *et al.* A prospective study of human immunodeficiency virus type 1 infection and the development of AIDS in subjects with hemophilia. *N Engl J Med* 1989; **321**: 1141–8.

34 Ragni MV, Winkelstein A, Kingsley L, *et al.* 1986 update of HIV seroprevalence, seroconversion, AIDS incidence, and immunologic correlates of HIV infection in patients with hemophilia A and B. *Blood* 1987; **70**: 786–90.

35 Rabkin CS, Goedert JJ, Biggar RJ, *et al.* Kaposi's sarcoma in three HIV-1-infected cohorts. *J Acquir Immune Defic Syndr* 1990; **3** (Suppl. 1): S38–43.

36 Phillips AN, Lee CA, Elford J, *et al.* More rapid progression to AIDS in older HIV-infected people: the role of CD4+ T-cell counts. *J Acquir Immune Defic Syndr* 1991; **4**: 970–5.

37 O'Brien TR, Blattner WA, Waters D, *et al.* Serum HIV-1 RNA levels and time to development of AIDS in the Multicenter Hemophilia Cohort Study. *JAMA* 1996; **276**: 105–10.

38 Kroner BL, Goedert JJ, Blattner WA, *et al.* Concordance of human leukocyte antigen haplotype-sharing, CD4 decline and AIDS in hemophilic siblings. Multicenter Hemophilia Cohort and Hemophilia Growth and Development Studies. *Aids* 1995; **9**: 275–80.

39 Ghirardini A, Schinaia N, Chiarotti F, *et al.* Epidemiology of hemophilia and of HIV infection in Italy. GICC. Gruppo Italiano Coagulopatie Congenite. *J Clin Epidemiol* 1994; **47**: 1297–306.

40 Lee CA, Phillips AN, Elford J, *et al.* Progression of HIV disease in a haemophilic cohort followed for 11 years and the effect of treatment. *BMJ* 1991; **303**: 1093–6.

41 Kasper CK, Mannucci PM, Bulyzhenkov V, *et al.* Hemophilia in the 1990s: principles of management and improved access to care. *Semin Thromb Haemost* 1992; **18**: 1–10.

42 Dean M, Carrington M, Winkler C, *et al.* Genetic restriction of HIV-1 infection and progression to AIDS by a deletion allele of the CKR5 structural gene. Hemophilia Growth and Development Study, Multicenter AIDS Cohort Study, Multicenter Hemophilia Cohort Study, San Francisco City Cohort, ALIVE Study. *Science* 1996; **273**: 1856–62.

43 Winkler C, Modi W, Smith MW, *et al.* Genetic restriction of AIDS pathogenesis by an SDF-1 chemokine gene variant. ALIVE Study, Hemophilia Growth and Development Study (HGDS), Multicenter AIDS Cohort Study (MACS), Multicenter Hemophilia Cohort Study (MHCS), San Francisco City Cohort (SFCC). *Science* 1998; **279**: 389–93.

44 Smith MW, Dean M, Carrington M, *et al.* Contrasting genetic influence of CCR2 and CCR5 variants on HIV-1 infection and disease progression. Hemophilia Growth and Development Study (HGDS), Multicenter AIDS Cohort Study (MACS), Multicenter Hemophilia Cohort Study (MHCS), San Francisco City Cohort (SFCC), ALIVE Study. *Science* 1997; **277**: 959–65.

45 Mahoney EM, Donfield SM, Howard C, *et al.* HIV- associated immune dysfunction and delayed pubertal development in a cohort of young hemophiliacs. Hemophilia Growth and Development Study. *J Acquir Immune Defic Syndr* 1999; **21**: 333–7.

46 Ratner Kaufman F, Gertner JM, Sleeper LA, Donfield SM. Growth hormone secretion in HIV-positive versus HIV-negative hemophilic males with abnormal growth and pubertal development. The Hemophilia Growth and Development Study. *J Acquir Immune Defic Syndr Hum Retrovirol* 1997; **15**: 137–44.

47 Mitchell WG, Lynn H, Bale JF, Jr., *et al.* Longitudinal neurological follow-up of a group of HIV-seropositive and HIV-seronegative hemophiliacs: results from the hemophilia growth and development study. *Pediatrics* 1997; **100**: 817–24.

48 Loveland KA, Stehbens JA, Mahoney EM, *et al.* Declining immune function in children and adolescents with hemophilia and HIV infection: effects on neuropsychological performance. Hemophilia Growth and Development Study. *J Pediatr Psychol* 2000; **25**: 309–22.

49 Hoots WK, Mahoney E, Donfield S, *et al.* Are there clinical and laboratory predictors of 5-year mortality in HIV-infected children and adolescents with hemophilia? *J Acquir Immune Defic Syndr Hum Retrovirol* 1998; **18**: 349–57.

50 Kontorinis N, Dieterich D. Hepatotoxicity of antiretroviral therapy. *AIDS Rev* 2003; **5**: 36–43.

51 Daar ES, Lynn H, Donfield S, *et al.* Relation between HIV-1 and hepatitis C viral load in patients with hemophilia. *J Acquir Immune Defic Syndr* 2001; **26**: 466–72.

52 Rockstroh JK, Spengler U, Sudhop T, *et al.* Immunosuppression may lead to progression of hepatitis C virus-associated liver disease in hemophiliacs coinfected with HIV. *Am J Gastroenterol* 1996; **91**: 2563–8.

53 Pollmann HRH, Jurgens H. Platelet dysfunction as the cause of spontaneous bleeding in two haemophilic patients taking HIV protease inhibitors. *Thromb Haemost* 1998; **79**: 1213–14.

54 Teitel J. A side-effect of protease inhibitors. *Canadian Medical Association Journal* 1998; **158**: 1129–30.

55 Daniel V, Susal C, Melk A, *et al.* Reduction of viral load and immune complex load on CD4⁺ lymphocytes as a consequence of highly active antiretroviral treatment (HAART) in HIV-infected hemophilia patients. *Immunol Lett* 1999; **69**: 283–9.

56 Aarnoutse RE, Schapiro JM, Boucher CA, *et al.* Therapeutic drug monitoring: an aid to optimizing response to antiretroviral drugs? *Drugs* 2003; **63**: 741–53.

57 Claessens YE, Chiche JD, Mira JP, Cariou A. Bench-to-bedside review: severe lactic acidosis in HIV patients treated with nucleoside analogue reverse transcriptase inhibitors. *Crit Care* 2003; **7**: 226–32.

58 Clotet B, Negredo E. HIV protease inhibitors and dyslipidemia. *AIDS Rev* 2003; **5**: 19–24.

59 Ragni MV, Bontempo FA, Lewis JH. Organ transplantation in HIV-positive patients with hemophilia. *N Engl J Med* 1990; **322**: 1886–7.

60 Hoots WK. Comprehensive care for hemophilia and related inherited bleeding disorders: why it matters. *Curr Hematol Rep* 2003; **2**: 395–401.

61 Mason PJ, Olson RA, Parish KL. AIDS, hemophilia, and prevention efforts within a comprehensive care program. *Am Psychol* 1988; **43**: 971–6.

62 Winter M. The practical management of haemophilia. *Blood Rev* 1992; **6**: 174–81.

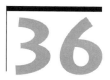

36 Transfusion-transmitted disease: hepatitis C virus infection and liver transplantation

Margaret V. Ragni

Introduction

Hepatitis C virus (HCV) infection is the leading cause of chronic hepatitis in the United States [1] and, among those with hemophilia, it is the major comorbid complication of treatment and the second leading cause of death [2]. Despite the virtual elimination of HCV in concentrates through viral inactivation and recombinant technologies, over 80% of adults with hemophilia are infected with HCV [3]. After 20 or more years of HCV infection in this group, most have chronic liver disease, and some develop end-stage liver disease, especially those with HIV coinfection or alcohol use [4]. Liver transplantation may be life-saving and curative for hemophilia but is complicated by HCV recurrence, underscoring the need for better HCV treatment.

Epidemiology of hepatitis C in hemophilia

Transfusion-induced hepatitis C-associated liver disease is the major comorbid condition in hemophilia, arising as an unexpected complication of exposure to pooled plasma concentrates, which could be infused outside the hospital, at home, school, or the workplace. Clotting factor concentrate improved the lifespan of individuals with hemophilia to normal in the early 1970s. However, chronic liver disease developed in those exposed following exposure to hepatitis C in the clotting factor concentrate, becoming the second leading cause of death in this population [5]. In contrast to other high-risk populations, e.g., transfusion recipients or injectable drug users, individuals with hemophilia were exposed to HCV (non-A, non-B) early in life, becoming infected through their first exposure to a noninactivated clotting factor concentrate [6] (Table 36.1). Over 90% of those with hemophilia treated with plasma-derived clotting factor concentrates during the 1970s and 1980s became infected with HCV [7], nearly all of whom were determined by polymerase chain reaction (PCR) to be HCV RNA positive, consistent with the detection of HCV in untreated clotting factor concentrates [8]. With 20 or more years since first exposure, 95% of hemophiliacs with HCV infection are over 18 (mean 30) [3]. Not only did HCV infection occur at a younger age than in other risk groups [1,6], but it preceded HIV exposure, which

peaked in 1982–1983 [4] (Table 36.2). Second, through the chronic use of clotting factor concentrates for recurrent bleeds, individuals with hemophilia were also infected with numerous other transmissible agents, including hepatitis A, B, D, and E [9], which may independently increase the severity of hepatitis C liver disease and lead to defects in B-cell and T-cell function, down-regulation of monocyte function, and depressed natural killer cell activity, CD4+ number, mitogen-induced B-cell responses, and antibody response to vaccine [10,11].

Clinical manifestations of HCV infection in hemophilia

Clinically, hepatitis C infection is asymptomatic. Over 60% of patients will develop abnormal liver function, 30% extrahepatic manifestations, 20% cirrhosis, and 5% end-stage liver disease (ESLD) [1,5,12]. Standard tests to assess HCV effect, including alanine aminotransferase (ALT), serum HCV RNA, and HCV genotype, are poor predictors of liver pathology [13], suggesting the importance of histopathologic diagnosis. The onset of ESLD may be associated with nonspecific fatigue, disruption of the sleep–wake cycle, and progressive evidence of portal hypertension, including ascites, edema, hepatic encephalopathy, varices, and gastrointestinal bleeding. Laboratory tests may reveal slowly worsening thrombocytopenia due to hypersplenism, nonspecific platelet dysfunction, and prolonged prothrombin time (PT) and activated partial thromboplastin time (aPTT), reflecting coagulation factor deficiency due to hepatic synthetic dysfunction, although these tests do not correlate with bleeding tendency [14]. Factor VIII (FVIII) or FIX deficiency of hemophilia, when superimposed on the factor deficiencies from failed liver synthesis and thrombocytopenia, may increase the risk of bleeding. Typical symptoms of the coagulopathy of liver disease may include epistaxis or gastrointestinal, oral, or central nervous system bleeding. If unrecognized and untreated in an individual with hemophilia, the high protein load of a gastrointestinal bleed may quickly precipitate hepatic encephalopathy. Heightened surveillance for this complication is crucial, and prophylactic factor replacement considered for platelet counts ″50 000/μL.

Table 36.1 Natural history studies of hepatitis C infection.

Study	Number of subjects	Duration (years)	Liver disease (%)	Cirrhosis (%)	Death (%)
Transfusion recipients [1]	400	14	13	20	3
Blood donors [1]	248	15	17	5	–
Postpartum anti-D recipients [1]	50 000	17	40	2	–
Military recruits [6]	8568	48	11.8	–	5.9
Hemophilic men [5]	157	20	60	11.4 (ESLD)	10.2

Table 36.2 Characteristics of HCV infection in hemophilia.

HCV infection
<1% of HCV+ in USA
Exposure to HCV early in life
Infection with first clotting factor exposure
90% of exposed became HCV+
Repeated exposure to multiple hepatitis viruses
Nearly all HCV RNA PCR +
HCV detected in clotting factor
Higher liver disease mortality
Second leading cause of death

HIV/HCV coinfection
40% of HCV+ are coinfected with HIV
95% are > 18 years of age
Increased HCV replication
Upregulated cytokine production
Impaired host immune response to HCV
Accelerated fibrosis, disease progression
Reduced response to HCV antiviral agents
Increased hepatotoxicity with antiretroviral agents

Host immune response and HCV viral factors

The hepatitis C virus is a unique pathogen. It is a heterogeneous virus with a high mutation rate and immunologically distinct quasispecies that escape immune response [15]. The cytotoxic T lymphocyte response (CTL) is suboptimal [15], resulting in no protective immunity and in reactivation, reinfection, and viral persistence [15]. It is also known that, although HCV-specific CTLs may mediate the hepatocyte repair response, they may also mediate liver cell damage through the production of cytokines, e.g., interferon gamma (IFN-γ), tumor necrosis factor alpha (TNF-α), interleukin 6 (IL-6), IL-10, and transforming growth factor beta (TGF-β) (Figure 36.1a–c) [16]. These cytokines may lyse HCV-infected hepatocytes and contribute to the pathogenesis of chronic liver disease. Among those with HIV coinfection, HIV may further up-regulate cytokine production, increasing the risk of progression to ESLD [16,17] (Table 36.3 and Figure 36.1b).

HCV liver disease progression

A number of host, viral, and immune factors may worsen the severity of hepatocyte inflammation or accelerate HCV liver disease progression (Table 36.4). These include age at exposure, coinfection with HBV, alcohol, smoking, environmental hepatotoxins, analgesics, immunosuppression, the dose of virus at infection, and the presence and level of quasispecies in early HCV infection [3,5]. Individuals with hemophilia, however, differ in important ways from transfusion recipients. In contrast to transfusion recipients, individuals with hemophilia are younger at HCV exposure [4,6,7]; are repeatedly exposed to multiple hepatitis viruses, i.e., HAV, HBV, HDV, HBe, and HGV; and develop chronic immunosuppression related to chronic factor treatment [10,11]. Liver disease mortality is higher in those with hemophilia [2,5] and, in addition, many became infected with human immunodeficiency virus (HIV) [4]. HIV coinfection appears to hasten HCV liver disease progression [16,17].

The role of HIV coinfection

HIV infection is associated with a progressive decline in CD4+ T-helper lymphocyte number and function, defective CD4+ proliferation, and CD4+ apoptosis [17]. HCV/HIV coinfection is associated with greater HCV replication, higher HCV RNA levels, and more aggressive histologic changes and greater degrees of liver fibrosis and necrosis than HCV alone [16,18] (Table 36.2). A greater proportion of coinfected hemophiliacs have elevated alanine aminotransferase (ALT) levels, more rapid liver disease progression [5,16], and higher liver-related mortality than those with HCV alone [2,5]. Although the precise proportion of HCV/HIV-coinfected hemophiliacs who develop cirrhosis is unknown, data from several studies suggest that the rate of progression to cirrhosis in those with HCV infection is several-fold higher among HIV-positive than HIV-negative patients. Without definitive histopathology, these figures may underestimate the proportion with cirrhosis.

In one study of HCV natural history in 157 individuals with hemophilia, 85 of whom were HIV positive, the relative risk (RR) of ESLD, adjusting for age, HBsAg, and alcohol abuse, was 3.72 [5] (Table 36.5). The adjusted relative risk for death due to ESLD was 3.81, with the risk increasing with each decade of HCV infection (RR = 2.26), and with each decade of HIV infec-

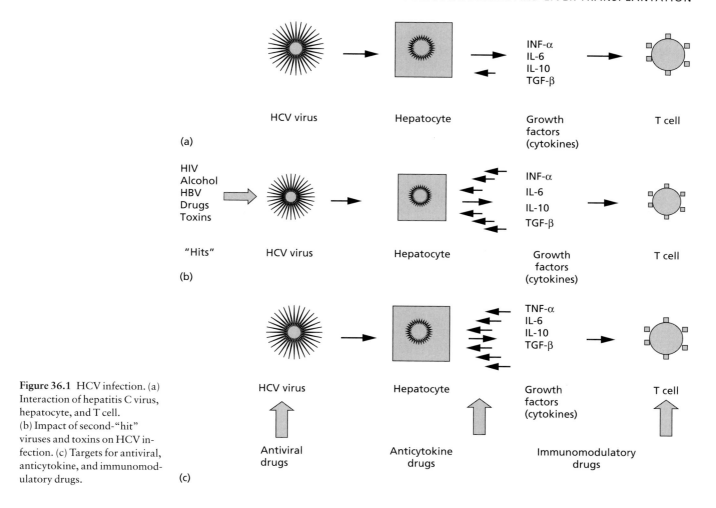

Figure 36.1 HCV infection. (a) Interaction of hepatitis C virus, hepatocyte, and T cell. (b) Impact of second-"hit" viruses and toxins on HCV infection. (c) Targets for antiviral, anticytokine, and immunomodulatory drugs.

Table 36.3 Survival after liver transplantation in HCV end-stage liver disease.

	HIV+/HCV+ (%)	HIV−/HCV+ (%)
Time after liver transplant		
12 months	90.9	87.6
24 months	75.9	83.3
36 months	75.9	80.3

Data from ref. 41.

tion (RR = 2.18) [5]. These data support the hypothesis that HIV accelerates HCV disease progression.

The role of host immune response and cytokines

In individuals with concomitant HIV infection, the immune response to HCV may be poorer and the liver damage greater than in those with HCV infection alone. HIV infection in an individual with HCV infection may weaken the already limited immune response to HCV infection (Figure 36.1b and Table 36.2).

Table 36.4 Factors affecting severity of hepatitis C infection.

Host factors
Age at exposure
Alcohol use
Smoking
Hepatotoxins
Analgesics
Hepatitis B infection
Immunosuppression
HIV infection

Viral factors
Heterogeneous
Six major genotypes
High mutation rate
Immunologically distinct quasispecies

Immune response
Suboptimal cytotoxic T-cell (CTL) response
Lack of protective immunity
Reactivation, reinfection
Viral persistence
Liver cell proliferation, fibrosis (cytokine elaboration)

Table 36.5 Impact of risk factors on risk of HCV progression.

Risk factor for end-stage liver disease	Relative risk
Age	1.5-fold risk
HBsAg	3-fold risk
HIV infection	3.7-fold risk
Alcohol	4-fold risk

Data from ref. 5.

The CD4$^+$ lymphocyte controls cell-mediated immune responses, and the fall in CD4 with HIV infection may further reduce virus-specific CTL responses, therefore leading to increased HCV replication [16–18]. The detection of HIV in the hepatocyte and macrophage Kupffer cell [19], and the detection of a tat-binding motif, similar to the HIV *tat* gene, which upregulates HIV gene expression [20], further suggest that HIV also directly up-regulates HCV replication. Moreover, HIV is also a potent activator of the immune response through upregulation of cytokine production [20], including specifically IL-6 [21] and TGF-β [22], which may further contribute to the pathogenesis of HCV liver cell damage.

Both IL-6 and TGF-β are growth factors not only for cells of the immune system, but also for the liver. Both cytokines are secreted in response to liver injury and contribute to the immunopathology of hepatitis C liver disease [23]. IL-6 is a proinflammatory cytokine that mediates inflammatory and immune responses to infection and injury, and is also a hepatocyte growth factor stimulating bile duct proliferation, a precursor of cirrhosis [23]. TGF-β is an anti-inflammatory cytokine that suppresses humoral and cellular immune response [23], and regulates hepatic extracellular matrix protein production and fibrosis [22,23]. Levels of IL-6 and TGF-β, elevated in chronic hepatitis C, correlate with the level of fibrosis and histologic progression [23]. Anti-cytokine therapies have been introduceed to prevent fibrosis in hepatitis C (Figure 36.1c) (see below).

Clinical management of HCV and liver biopsy in hemophilia

The management of chronic hepatitis C liver disease in hemophilia is best accomplished in collaboration with a hepatologist. In general, liver function tests, including α-fetoprotein every 6 months, and amylase levels if on HIV medications, along with liver function tests and CBC are routine [24]. A hepatitis C genotype should be obtained. Qualitative hepatitis C viral load, HCV RNA PCR, may be used to confirm a diagnosis of hepatitis C, but quantitative HCV RNA PCR does not correlate with severity of liver disease: liver biopsy remains the gold standard for determining the severity of liver disease [24]. A number of noninvasive markers of liver disease progression are currently under study, including genetic polymorphisms and cytokine promoter

Table 36.6 Management of hepatitis C infection in hemophilia.

Liver biopsy in hemophilia [27,29]
Indications
Persistently abnormal liver function tests
Hepatomegaly
Suspected liver cancer
Over 20 years of HCV infection

Approach
Transjugular biopsy preferred

Risk of transjugular biopsy procedure
<1% Overall complications
<1% Bleeding complications

Management of liver biopsy in hemophilia [28]
Prior to biopsy
Check PT, platelet count, inhibitor titer
Review medications, especially nonsteroidal anti-inflammatory drugs, platelet inhibitors
Correct vitamin K deficiency — vitamin K
Correct thrombocytopenia — platelets
Correct prolonged PT — fresh-frozen plasma
Immediately prebiopsy, infuse 100% dose clotting factor

Postprocedure
Monitor vital signs, blood loss, hemoglobin
Continue factor replacement at 4 and 24 h, or more

genotypes [25]. In addition, some investigators have proposed the use of an index, or a combination of noninvasive markers, specifically the platelet count, asparagine aminotransferase (AST), and alkaline phosphatase: together, these markers are able to accurately predict cirrhosis in up to 80% [26].

Symptoms of liver disease progression may include fatigue, reduced mental acuity, disrupted sleep–wake pattern, edema, increasing abdominal girth, and side-effects with medications. Hepatotoxicity with drugs metabolized through the liver is not uncommon in this group, and alcohol and analgesics may contribute. Generally, acetaminophey is contraindicated as, in the quantities required to reduce the pain associated with hemophilic arthropathy, there is potential for hepatotoxicity. Alcohol use should be strongly discouraged, given its additive effects on HCV liver disease progression. Mental status change should be carefully assessed, as recurrent encephalopathy in an individual with hemophilia may suggest ongoing slow blood loss, such as from portal hypertension-related variceal bleeding, gum or mouth bleeding, epistaxis, or even CNS oozing. Once the platelet count has fallen below 60 000/μL, chronic prophylaxis should be initiated, either 50 U/kg every other day, or 25 U/kg daily, to avoid CNS, GI, oral, or other mucosal bleeding [27].

A physical examination should be carried out at least every 4–6 months and should include evaluation for hepatosplenomegaly, spider angioma, muscle wasting, ascites, edema, and splenomegaly (Table 36.6). If there is evidence of portal hypertension (ascites, edema, varices, splenomegaly, encephalopathy), a sonar or computed tomography (CT) scan of the liver should be performed and followed yearly. A liver biopsy should be considered in any patient with chronic hepatitis C over 20 years provided there is no contraindication, e.g., inhibitor, as this is considered standard of care [24] (Table 36.6). Liver biopsies are invasive, costly, and may cause bleeding complications [24], and less than 50% of physicians request biopsies in hemophilia patients with chronic hepatitis [3]. Indications for biopsy include persistently abnormal liver function tests, hepatomegaly, or suspected liver cancer. Transjugular liver biopsy is less invasive than the percutaneous route [28,29] and, therefore, it may be the preferred procedure in hemophilic patients. Prior to performing liver biopsy, the PT, international normalized ratio (INR), platelet count, and inhibitor titer should be obtained [28] (Table 36.6). The presence of an inhibitor is considered a contraindication to liver biopsy. All medications should be reviewed, and NSAIDs should be discontinued at least 48 h prior to biopsy. Prolongation of the PT/INR, thrombocytopenia, and/or vitamin K deficiency should be corrected within several hours prior to the biopsy. Individuals with hemophilia should receive a 100% dose (50 U/kg FVIII or 75 U/kg FIX) immediately prior to transjugular liver biopsy, followed by a 50% dose (25 U/kg FVIII or 37 U/kg FIX) at 4 h and again at 24 h after the procedure. Fresh-frozen plasma, vitamin K, and platelets should be used as needed [28]. When liver biopsy is performed with factor concentrate, the risk of bleeding in hemophilic patients, in the absence of inhibitors or thrombocytopenia, is less than 1% [27].

Advances in HCV treatment and prevention

Current antiviral treatment of hepatitis C infection is suboptimal, with significant toxicity and poor response rate in the majority of HCV-infected individuals. The current most effective treatment for hepatitis C is a combination of interferon and ribavirin, but this combination, even using the pegylated interferon, clears HCV infection, at best, in only 55% of those with the most common HCV genotype, type 1 [30]. Among individuals with hemophilia, the response is even lower, with only 29% achieving a sustained viral response [31], and, among

HIV/HCV-coinfected hemophiliacs, preliminary data show an even poorer sustained response [32] (Table 36.7).

New approaches to treatment of hepatitis C fall into three categories: antiviral drugs, anticytokine drugs, and immunomodulatory drugs (Figure 36.1c). A number of these drugs, among which are inhibitors of the HCV helicase and of the HCV protease, inhibit liver fibrosis. One potent HCV protease inhibitor, BILN 2061, with antiviral activity in subjects with liver fibrosis, appears to be well tolerated in early phase clinical trials [33].

Anti-cytokine drugs may also have potential anti-HCV effect. For example, inhibitors of IL-6 and TGF-β might be expected to reverse fibrosis. An inhibitor of TGF-β soluble receptor that inhibits fibrosis in a mouse model is in early human clinical trials [34]. Hepatocyte growth factor (HGF), a potent inhibitor of TGF-β, reverses fibrosis in the rat model of cirrhosis and, in HCV-positive patients with renal disease, elevated levels following dialysis appear to be protective against fibrosis and liver disease progression [35]. These findings have increased interest in the role of inhibitors of interleukins and cytokines in the treatment of disorders associated with fibrosis, including treatment of HCV-associated hepatic fibrosis.

The establishment of a mouse model of chronic hepatitis C, by orthotopic engraftment of transplanted human hepatocytes into a severe combined immunodeficient (SCID) mouse followed by inoculation with HCV-infected human serum [36] may assist in future HCV drug development. This model develops a high HCV viral load with viral persistence, with 50% replacement of mouse cells by human liver cells. Thus, this mouse model provides a mechanism to accomplish antiviral drug testing.

Vaccines to prevent hepatitis C have been difficult to develop because HCV escapes the host immune response and mutates during the course of infection. However, recent studies suggest that immunity to hepatitis C may be possible. In one study, previously HCV-infected injecting drug users were 50% less likely to develop HCV infection than previously HCV-naive users [37], suggesting that protection against persistent hepatitis C infection and its complications, cirrhosis and liver cancer, may be possible. An immunogen studied in chimpanzees, which induces antibodies to HCV gpE1 and gpE2 proteins, has been found to protect against persistent HCV infection [38]. Other candidate vaccines may enhance the immune response to existing HCV infection: for example, DNA and polypeptide vaccines that induce HCV-specific cellular immune (CD4, CD8) responses are currently in phase I clinical trials in humans.

Table 36.7 Treatment of hepatitis C infection in hemophilia.

Study	No.	Subjects	Treatment	24-week response	P-value
Fried [31]	113	HCV+	IFN	7% SVR (4 of 57)	
			IFN + RBV	29% SVR (16 of 56)	$P = 0.27$
Sauleda [32]	18	HIV+/HCV+	IFN + RBV + HAART	32% VR (6 of 18)	

SVR, sustained viral response; VR, viral response by HCV RNA PCR; IFN, interferon; RBV, ribavirin; HAART, highly active antiretroviral therapy.

Liver transplantation in hemophilia

Transplantation is the treatment of choice for decompensated ESLD, e.g., intractable ascites, recurrent variceal bleeding, and encephalopathy. It also cures hemophilia [39], by providing functional hepatocytes capable of producing FVIII or FIX. However, many HCV-infected hemophiliacs are also coinfected with HIV, and as HIV has been an absolute contraindication for transplantation, treatment of ESLD has been limited. The improvement in survival and immune function by highly active antiretroviral therapy (HAART) [40], however, suggested that orthotopic liver transplantation (OLTX) might be possible in those with HIV.

In a pilot study of 24 HIV-positive individuals with ESLD undergoing OLTX, cumulative survival in HIV-positive OLTX recipients was shown to be similar to that in age- and race-matched HIV-negative OLTX recipients [41] (Table 36.7), suggesting that HIV should no longer be a contraindication to OLTX. Although survival is poorer in subjects with post-OLTX CD4 < 200/μL, and post-OLTX HIV viral load >400 copies/mL, it was not associated with pretransplant CD4 or HIV viral load, suggesting that limitations for accepting candidates for OLTX based on inability to tolerate HAART therapy are unjustified [42]. A prospective multicenter study of OLTX in HIV infection is ongoing. The optimal time for OLTX in HIV-positive subjects with ESLD remains unknown. For this reason, it is recommended that individuals with ESLD be evaluated for OLTX early, preferably at the first signs of ESLD.

It is important to recognize that those with decompensated end-stage disease may have impaired metabolism of antiviral drugs, leading to worsening hepatotoxicity and inability to tolerate HAART. Increasing duration of HIV infection is an independent marker for liver disease progression [5], and therefore ESLD is likely to continue to be a growing problem among a significant number of coinfected individuals.

A new approach in transplantation is the concept of hematopoietic stem cell repopulation of damaged livers, leading to hepatocyte regeneration and return of biochemical function. When bone marrow is transplanted in fumarylacetoacetate hydrolase deficient (Fah–/–) mice, the model for tyrosinemia type I, donor bone marrow cells fuse with recipient Fah–/– hepatocytes and repopulate the liver and regenerating nodules, normalizing liver function [42]. Stem cells are being investigated as adjuvant therapy to routine antirejection immunosuppression in liver transplant recipients. Finally, a recent study suggests that reduction in antirejection immunosuppression following OLTX may safely reduce potential post-transplant infections, accomplished in some subjects [43].

Acknowledgment

We thank Ms Karen Saban for secretarial assistance and for help in preparation of the manuscript.

References

1 Liang TJ, Rehermann B, Seeff LB, Hoofnagle JH. Pathogenesis, natural history, treatment and prevention of hepatitis C. *Ann Intern Med* 2000; **134**: 296–305.
2 Darby SC, Ewart DW, Giangrande PLF, *et al.* Mortality before and after HIV infection in the complete UK population of hemophiliacs. *Nature* 1995; **377**: 79–82.
3 Ewenstein B, Koerper M. *Survey of Diagnostic and Treatment Practices of Chronic Hepatitis C in Federally-funded Hemophilia Treatment Centers.* Medical and Scientific Advisory Council, National Hemophilia Foundation, Orlando, FL, October, 1998.
4 Ragni MV, Winkelstein A, Kingsley LA, *et al.* 1986 Update of HIV seroprevalence, seroconversion, AIDS incidence, and immunologic correlates of HIV infection in hemophiliacs. *Blood* 1987; **70**: 786–90.
5 Ragni MV, Belle SH. Impact of human immunodeficiency virus (HIV) on progression to end-stage liver disease in individuals with hemophilia and hepatitis C. *J Infect Dis* 2001; **183**; 1112–15.
6 Seeff LB, Miller RN, Rabkin CS, *et al.* 45-Year followup of hepatitis C virus infection in healthy young adults. *Ann Intern Med* 2000; **132**: 105–11.
7 Kasper CK, Kipnis SA. Hepatitis and clotting-factor concentrates. *JAMA* 1972; **221**: 510.
8 Makris M, Garson JA, Ring CJA, *et al.* Hepatitis C viral RNA in clotting factor concentrates and the development of hepatitis in recipients. *Blood* 1993; **81**: 1898–1902.
9 Troisi CL, Hollinger FB, Contant C, *et al.* A multicenter study of viral hepatitis in a United States hemophilic population. *Blood* 1993; **81**: 412–18.
10 Kaplan J, Sarnaik J, Gitlin J, Lusher J. Diminished helper/suppressor lymphocyte ratios and natural killer activity in recipients of repeated blood transfusions. *Blood* 1984: **64**: 308–10.
11 Ragni MV, Ruben RL, Winkelstein A, *et al.* Antibody response to immunization in patients with haemophilia with and without evidence of HTLV-III infection. *J Lab Clin Med* 1987; **109**: 545–9.
12 Hay CRM, Preston FE, Triger DR, Underwood JCE. Progressive liver disease in hemophilia: an understated problem? *Lancet* 1985; **1**: 1495–8.
13 McCormick SE, Goodman ZD, Maydonovitch CL, Sjogren MH. Evaluation of liver histology, ALT elevation and HCV RNA titer in patients with chronic hepatitis. *Am J Gastroenterol* 1996; **91**: 1516–22.
14 Ragni MV, Lewis JH, Spero JA, Hasiba U. Bleeding and coagulation abnormalities in alcoholic cirrhotic liver disease. *Alcoholism: Clin Exp Res* 1982; **6**: 267–74.
15 Farci P, Alter HJ, Govindarajan S, *et al.* Lack of protective immunity against reinfection with hepatitis C virus. *Science* 1992; **258**: 135–40.
16 Rockstroh JK, Spengler U, Sudhop T, *et al.* Immunosuppression may lead to progression of hepatitis C virus-associated liver disease in hemophiliacs co-infected with HIV. *Am J Gastroenterol* 1996; **91**: 2563–73.
17 Pantaleo G, Graziosi C, Fauci AS. New concepts in the immunopathogenesis of human immunodeficiency virus infection. *N Engl J Med* 1993; **328**: 327–35.
18 Ragni MV, Bontempo FA, Faruki H. Increase in hepatitis C viral load in hemophiliacs treated with highly-active antiretroviral therapy. *J Infect Dis* 1999; **180**: 2027–9.
19 Housset C, Lamas E, Courngnaud V, *et al.* Presence of HIV-1 in human parenchymal and non-parenchymal liver cells in vivo. *J Hepatol* 1993; **19**: 252–8.

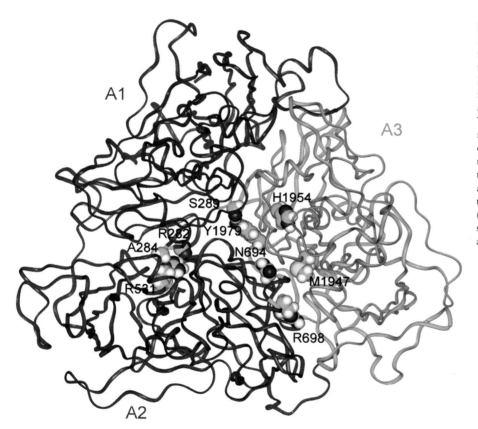

Plate 1 Molecular graphics image showing the interdomain positions of nine hemophilic mutations associated with circulating dysfunctional FVIII (factor VIII) and similar laboratory phenotypes. The mutations result in decreased affinity of the A2 domain for A1 and A3, increasing the rate of A2 dissociation. The triplicated A domains are shown as Cα ribbons (A1, red; A2, blue; A3, green) viewed down the pseudo-threefold axis, from a homology model [10] based on the crystal structure of ceruloplasmin. Sidechains of residues altered in hemophilia are shown as CPK (creatine phosphokinase) spheres, colored by atom (carbon, green; nitrogen, blue; oxygen, red; sulfur, yellow; hydrogen, white). Image generated by Insight II (Accelrys, Cambridge, UK).

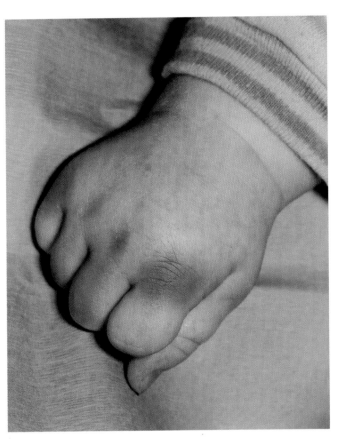

Plate 2 Bruising secondary to hand being held firmly for venipuncture in a neonate with severe hemophilia.

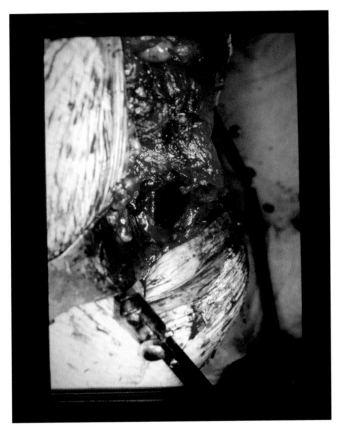

Plate 3 The intra-operative view demonstrates clearly a large hole in the ileum where the pseudotumor penetrated the cortex.

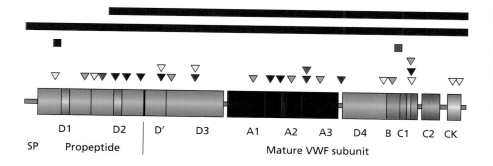

Plate 4 VWD (von Willebrand disease) type 3 mutations in Germany. The two large and two small boxes show the localization of large and small deletions. The triangles show the position of single nucleotide changes: green, nonsense mutations; blue, deletions; red, insertions; purple, splice-site mutations; yellow, missense mutations.

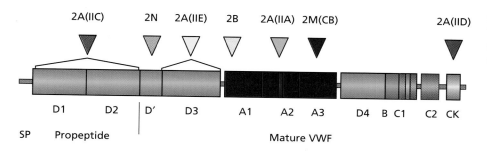

Plate 5 Clustered distribution of VWF (von Willebrand factor) mutations causing specific subtypes of VWD type 2. The box shows the pre-pro-VWF with its domains.

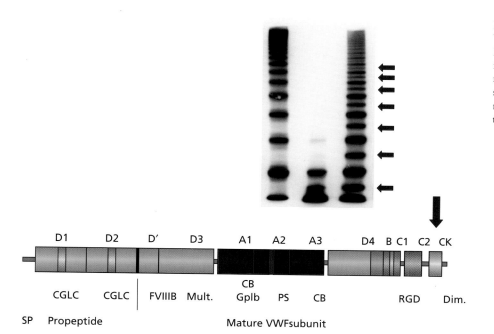

Plate 6 Recombinant expression of mutant VWF 2A, subtype IID displaying a severe lack of VWF multimers in the homozygous form and a relative loss of the large multimers in its heterozygous form. The arrows show the minor intervening bands (odd-numbered oligomers). Recombinant wild-typeVWF is shown for comparison.

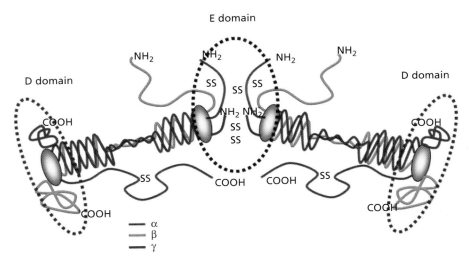

E domain

NH₂

D domain

NH₂   NH₂   NH₂

SS   SS   SS

NH₂ NH₂

COOH

SS

SS

SS

COOH

SS   COOH   COOH   SS

COOH

D domain

NH₂

COOH

COOH

—— α
≡ β
— γ

Plate 7 A schematic representation of the fibrinogen molecule. NH_2 and COOH denote the amino and carboxy termini, respectively, of the α-chain (red), β-chain (blue), and γ-chain (green). The free carboxy terminus of the α-chain is referred to as Cα. The varian γ' chain extends from the carboxy terminus of the γ-chain (not shown). SS identifies disulfide bonds. The E domain is located in the central region of the molecule and is roughly composed of amino acids 1–49 of the α-chain, 1–80 of the β-chain, and 1–23 of the γ-chain. The E domain is flanked by two D domains roughly composed of amino acids 111–197 of the α-chain, 134–461 of the β-chain, and 88–406 of the γ-chain (from Roberts: *Br J Haematol* 2001; **114**: 249–57).

20 Vogel J, Hinrichs SH, Reynolds RK, *et al.* The HIV tat gene induces dermal lesions resembling Kaposi's sarcoma in transgenic mice. *Nature* 1988; **335**: 606–11.

21 Clerici M, Hakim FT, Venzon DJ, *et al.* Changes in interleukin-2 and interleukin-4 production in asymptomatic, human immunodeficiency virus-seropositive individuals. *J Clin Invest* 1993; **91**: 759–65.

22 Kekow J, Wachsman W, McCutchan JA, *et al.* Transforming growth factor-β and non-cytopathic mechanisms of immunodeficiency in human immunodeficiency virus infection. *Proc Natl Acad Sci USA* 1990; **87**: 8321–5.

23 Matsumoto K, Fuji H, Michalopoulis G, *et al.* Human biliary epithelial cells secrete and respond to cytokines and hepatocyte growth factors: IL-6, HGF, and EGF promote DNA synthesis *in vitro. Hepatology* 1994; **20**: 376–82.

24 Perrillo RP. The role of liver biopsy in hepatitis C. *Hepatology* 1997; **26** (Suppl. 1): 57S–61S.

25 Bataller R, North KE, Brenner DA. Genetic polymorphisms and the progression of liver fibrosis: a critical appraisal. *Hepatology* 2003; **37**: 493–503.

26 Wai CT, Greenson JK, Fontana RJ, *et al.* A simple noninvasive index can predict both significant fibrosis and cirrhosis in patients with hepatitis C. *Hepatology* 2003; **38**: 518–26.

27 Wong VS, Baglin T, Beacham E, *et al.* The role for liver biopsy in haemophiliacs infected with the hepatitis C virus. *Br J Haematol* 1997; **97**: 343–7.

28 NHF Medical and Scientific Advisory Committee. Recommendations on Liver Biopsy in Individuals with Hemophilia, #98, June, 2000.

29 Little AF, Zajko AB, Orons PD. Transjugular liver biopsy: a prospective study in 43 patients with the Quick-Core biopsy needle. *JVIR* 1996; **7**: 127–31.

30 Fried MW, Shiffman ML, Reddy KR, *et al.* Peg-interferon alfa-2a plus ribavirin for chronic hepatitis C virus infection. *N Engl J Med* 2002; **347**: 975–82.

31 Fried MW, Peter J, Hoots K, *et al.* Hepatitis C in adults and adolescents with hemophilia: a randomized, controlled trial of interferon alfa-2b and ribavirin. *Hepatology* 2002; **36**: 967–72

32 Sauleda S, Juarez A, Esteban JI. Treatment of chronic hepatitis C in patients with HIV co-infection. *Gastroenterol Hepatol* 2002; **25**: 337–41.

33 Benhamou Y, Hinrichsen H, Sentjens R, *et al.* Safety, tolerability, and antiviral effect of BILN 2061, a novel HCV serine protease inhibitor, after oral treatment over 2 days in patients with chronic hepatitis C, genotype 1, with advanced liver fibrosis. *Hepatology* 2002; **304A**: 563.

34 Yata Y, Gotwals P, Koteliansky V, Rockey DC. Dose-dependent inhibition of hepatic fibrosis in mice by a TGF-β soluble receptor: implications for antifibrotic therapy. *Hepatology* 2002; **35**: 1022–30.

35 Rampino T, Arbustini E, Gregorini M, *et al.* Hemodialysis prevents liver disease caused by hepatitis C virus: role of hepatocyte growth factor. *Kidney Intl* 1999; **56**: 2286–91.

36 Mercer DF, Schiller D, Elliott E, *et al.* Hepatitis C virus replication in mice with chimeric human livers. *Nature Med* 2001; **7**: 927–33.

37 Mehta SH, Cox A, Hoover DR, *et al.* Protection against persistence of hepatitis C. *Lancet* 2002; **359**: 1478–83.

38 Houghton M. *Prospects for Vaccination against the Hepatitis C Virus.* Eleventh International Symposium on Viral Hepatitis & Liver Disease, no. 4, Sydney, 2003.

39 Bontempo FA, Lewis JH, Gorenc TJ, *et al.* Liver transplantation in hemophilia A. *Blood* 1987; **69**: 1721–4.

40 Palella FJ, Delaney KM, Moorman AC, *et al.* Declining morbidity and mortality among patients with advanced human immunodeficiency virus infection. *N Engl J Med* 1998; **338**: 853–60.

41 Ragni MV, Belle SH, Im K, *et al.* Survival in HIV-infected liver transplant recipients. *J Infect Dis* 2003; **118**: 1412–20.

42 Lagasse E, Connors H, Al-Shalimy M, *et al.* Purified hematopoietic stem cells can differentiate into hepatocytes in vivo. *Nature Med* 2000; **6**: 1229–34.

43 Starzl TE, Murase N, Abu-Elmagd K, *et al.* Tolerogenic immunosuppression for organ transplantation. *Lancet* 2003; **361**: 1502–10.

37 Gene therapy: introduction and overview

Gilbert C. White II and R. Jude Samulski

Traditionally, hemophilia A has been treated by replacing the missing coagulation factor, factor VIII (FVIII). Current products used to replace FVIII are effective and remarkably safe. Recombinant FVIII (rFVIII) concentrates are essentially devoid of all plasma-derived components, obviating any risk of blood-borne diseases, but even plasma-derived products have been deemed safe based on over a decade of clinical experience with no evidence of transmission of blood-borne diseases. While these products have once again restored hemophiliacs' confidence in treatment, they are expensive and, cost aside, require intermittent intravenous administration, which complicates attempts at prophylaxis.

Gene therapy offers the potential for sustained correction of the coagulation defect in hemophilia A. Partial correction of clotting factor levels for even as short a time as 1–2 months would change the way patients treat themselves and would have the potential almost to eliminate spontaneous joint and other bleeds. The initial clinical trials of gene transfer in hemophilia have been completed and, although the results have, perhaps, fallen short of what was hoped for, they, along with the results of similar trials in hemophilia B, demonstrate that gene therapy is feasible and that continued efforts to develop gene-based treatment are worthwhile.

Gene transfer vectors

Viral vectors

The idea of using viruses as vectors for transferring DNA into cells has been around almost since the beginning of gene therapy. Viruses have evolved highly efficient mechanisms for entering cells and using the DNA/RNA replication machinery of the cell to produce viral products [1]. By replacing viral coding sequences with, for example, the cDNA for FVIII, one could use the virus as a vector to gain entry to the cell and drive expression of the FVIII transgene. The obvious advantage of using viruses as vectors is their native ability to get into cells; the general disadvantage is the toxicity of viruses.

Retrovirus vectors

Retroviruses are enveloped RNA viruses that use reverse transcriptase to convert virion RNA into double-stranded DNA; the DNA is subsequently integrated into the genome of the cell. The surface of retroviruses consists of a lipid bilayer with protruding membrane proteins, GP41 and GP120, both encoded by the *env* gene. The tropism of the virus, e.g. the cells targeted by the virus, is determined by these surface proteins. For example, for human immunodeficiency virus 1 (HIV-1), GP120 mediates the interaction of HIV-1 with CD4 lymphocytes. For gene therapy vectors, it is common to replace the retroviral *env* gene with other sequences that change the tropism of the vector. This can be done either to target a particular tissue or cell or to broaden the tropism of the vector in order to increase the number of cells that are transduced. Two sequences that are frequently used to broaden the tropism of retrovirus vectors are the amphotropic envelope gene of murine leukemia viruses, which is able to interact with a widely expressed phosphate transporter on human cells, and the G glycoprotein of vesicular stomatitis virus (VSV-G), which interacts with a ubiquitous receptor on cells. Retroviral vector production is through a three-part packaging system, consisting of a genome vector that contains the packaging signal and the cDNA of interest, an expression vector that contains the pseudotyped envelope glycoprotein, and an expression vector that expresses the viral *gag* and *pol* genes. These are assembled into vector particles in a packaging cell. The retroviral packaging systems in current use appear safe and are designed to prevent the generation of replication-competent virus. In addition, sufficient modifications are made in the viral sequence to minimize the possibility of homologous recombination with retroviral sequences in target cells. Self-inactivating ("sin") vectors are ones in which the long terminal repeats (LTRs) have been removed to prevent activation of downstream cellular genes.

Vectors derived from the Moloney strain of murine leukemia virus (MoMLV) were the first retroviral vectors used for gene transfer. MoMLV has a 9-kb cDNA expression cassette and is therefore able to accept the entire 7.1-kb FVIII cDNA. Although MoMLV could be produced in large quantities and was able to efficiently gain entry into cells, it only transduces dividing cells [2], a disadvantage for many tissues, such as liver, where the rate of cell replication is low. Strategies for inducing cell division in the liver using partial hepatectomy [3], chemical injury [4], or hepatocyte growth factor [5] have been proposed to increase retrovirus-mediated transduction.

More recently, vectors derived from lentiviruses, including HIV-1, have been developed [6]. Members of this family of retroviruses include feline immunodeficiency virus (FIV), simian immunodeficiency virus (SIV), and equine infectious anemia virus (EIAV) [7,8]. Like MoMLV, lentiviral vectors have a 9-kb cDNA expression cassette. These vectors retain some of the attractive features of the Moloney-based retroviral vectors, such as stable integration into the host chromosome and targeted cellular uptake though coat proteins, and they are able to infect non-dividing as well as dividing cells [9]. More recent observations provide greater understanding of the mechanisms of nuclear import by lentiviruses and may lead to improvements in cell transduction. During reverse transcription of HIV-1, a three-stranded DNA flap is formed, which is composed of the central polypurine tract (cPPT) from the *pol* gene and central termination sequences (CTS). This flap functions as a cis-acting element to enhance nuclear import and improve gene transduction in non-dividing cells [10,11]. Other cis-acting DNA elements that enhance transgene expression, perhaps through a mechanism like the DNA flap described above, have been identified, including the matrix attachment region from immunoglobulin κ [12] or from β-interferon [13].

Although retroviral integration is not sequence specific, there is increasing evidence that it is also not completely random. The ability of retroviruses to successfully replicate themselves depends on integration of the viral DNA into transcriptionally active areas of the host cell chromosome. Integration into silent areas would prevent expression of viral proteins and inhibit replication. Studies to map the site of retrovirus integration demonstrate that active genes are preferential integration targets, especially genes that are activated by infection of the cell by the retrovirus [14,15]. Regional hotspots also exist [14]. Whether the predilection for active genes results from increased chromatin accessibility, locally bound transcription factors, or some other influence is not clear.

Because of their integrating properties, insertional mutagenesis is a concern with retroviruses. Integration of retroviral sequences near proto-oncogenes has long been known to be capable of activating their expression, contributing to tumorigenesis in animal models [16]. A recent report of T-cell leukemia in two subjects with X-linked severe combined immunodeficiency syndrome treated by retrovirus-mediated gene transfer [17] shows that insertional mutation occurs in humans. The two subjects were among 10 receiving *ex vivo* retrovirus-mediated gene transfer into autologous CD34 bone marrow cells. Approximately 3 years after treatment, the subjects developed acute T-cell lymphocytic leukemia. The leukemic T-cells showed evidence for retroviral insertion near the *LMO2* proto-oncogene promoter. Because of the survival advantage of the cells expressing the retroviral γc transgene over the normal T cells, it has been suggested that the insertional mutation in the *LMO2* promoter region results in uncontrolled clonal expansion of the corrected T-cells, initially correcting the severe combined immunodeficiency then resulting in T-cell leukemia.

Adenovirus vectors

Adenoviruses are linear, double-stranded DNA viruses that infect a wide variety of human cells, both dividing and non-dividing, including lung, liver, heart, and brain. The 36-kb viral genome consists of a number of early and late genes. Transcription and translation of the early genes modulates cell function to facilitate replication of the viral DNA while the late genes are involved in the structural aspects of viral replication. The icosahedral adenoviral capsid is composed of three major components: the hexon, penton base, and knobbed fiber. Viral entry into cells is accomplished through an initial high-affinity interaction between the knobbed fiber [18] and a widely expressed, 46-kDa coxsackie–adenovirus receptor (CAR) on the surface of cells [19]. After the initial interaction with CAR, entry of the virus into the cell proceeds through clathrin-mediated endocytosis, which proceeds through an interaction between the penton base and αvβ3 and αvβ5 integrins on the cell surface. Disruption of the viral capsid occurs in the endocytic vesicle and the viral genome enters the nucleus through nuclear pores. In the nucleus, the adenoviral genome does not integrate into the chromosomes of the host cell, functioning instead from an extrachromosomal or episomal template.

Adenoviral vectors characteristically elicit an intense inflammatory response. This is due in part to capsid proteins, which provoke a brisk humoral and cellular immune response [20]. At the same time, adenovirus is designed to evade the immune response that it elicits [21]. Products of the *E1A* gene interfere with nuclear factor κB (NF-κB), which is a key regulator of the innate antiviral response by cells. Products of the *E3* gene are also known to subvert the host immune response. Other gene products also play a role. One of the goals in the generation of adenoviral vectors is to retain the high degree of efficiency that these vectors have with respect to cell infection while moderating or eliminating the immune response. First-generation adenoviral vectors were deleted in *E1* and *E3*, removing some of the primary mediators of the immune response while increasing the expression cassette to 6.5 kb. The *E2* genes were removed in the second-generation vectors and, in recent vectors, all of the viral coding sequences have been removed, rendering the vector "gutless" [22]. Although preclinical studies indicate that removing these proteins may reduce the cellular immune response [23], there is also evidence that the virion shell alone elicits significant cellular responses [24].

There are at least 47 different adenoviral serotypes, each immunologically distinct. The development of an immune response to one vector serotype generally precludes readministration of that vector. Adenoviral vectors for gene transfer are primarily Ad2 or Ad5.

The only death directly attributable to a gene transfer trial occurred with an adenoviral vector in an 18-year-old subject with ornithine transcarbamylase (OTC) deficiency [25]. The second-generation vector was based on human adenovirus type 5 and was deleted in *E1* and *E4*. Following administration of the vector in the right hepatic artery, altered mental status and jaundice were noted 18 h later and the patient's subsequent clinical course was marked by a systemic inflammatory response syndrome with high levels of interleukin 6 (IL-6) and IL-10, biochemically detectable disseminated intravascular coagulation, and multiple organ system failure, leading to death 98 h following gene transfer. The story of Jessie Gelsinger has been well chronicled in the news media [26].

Adeno-associated virus (AAV) vectors

Adeno-associated viruses are small, non-enveloped, single-stranded DNA viruses that require helper virus to facilitate efficient replication. In the absence of helper virus-mediated replication, the wild-type virus persists in the host cell in a latent state. The 4.7-kb genome of AAV consists of two inverted terminal repeats (ITRs) and two open reading frames that code for the rep and cap proteins. There are four rep proteins, which function in regulating AAV replication, and three cap proteins, which form the protein coat of the virus. AAV stably integrates into the host genome at the AAVS1 region of chromosome 19q13.3–qter. Two of the rep gene products, rep68 and rep78, are believed to direct integration to the AAVS1 site on chromosome 19. Nine different serotypes have been identified, AAV1–9, each with distinct differences in tissue tropism. AAV8 targets primarily liver, while AAV1 and AAV7 transduce muscle with high efficiency. The cellular receptor for AAV2, the serotype most commonly used for gene transfer studies, is heparan sulfate, a glycosaminoglycan that is variably present on the surface of most cells [27]. Slow-twitch (slow myosin-expressing) skeletal muscle fibers have higher concentrations of heparan sulfate proteoglycan on their surface and are better transduced by AAV2 than fast-twitch fibers [28]. Interestingly, AAVS1, the site of integration, is closely linked to the slow skeletal troponin T gene, *TNNT1* [29], raising an interesting correlate with the preference of AAV for slow myofibers. The integrin αvβ5 and fibroblast growth factor receptor 1 are co-receptors for AAV2 (30,31). AAVs are not associated with any known disease and are not pathogenic [32].

Typical AAV gene transfer vectors have been derived from AAV2. The ITRs are retained but the rest (96%) of the viral genome has been removed, including the rep gene. As a result, AAV vectors currently in general use are unable to integrate into the host chromosome in a site-specific manner, and persistence as integrated sequences appears to be a low-frequency event, if it occurs at all. Efforts to quantify *in vivo* integration in skeletal muscle and liver suggest that at least 99.5% (skeletal muscle) and at least 90% (liver) of persisting AAV vector DNA was episomal, present in large concatemers [33,34].

The AAV expression cassette is approximately 5 kb, too small to accommodate the whole FVIII cDNA. However, several groups have separately packaged FVIII light- and heavy-chain sequences under the control of minimal transcriptional regulatory elements into AAV vectors and demonstrated expression *in vivo* after coinfection [35,36].

Based on the nonpathogenicity of AAV for humans, the toxicity associated with AAV has been expected to be low. In preclinical studies, AAV has been well tolerated with no effects on hematopoiesis, liver function, or other organs. Reports of late tumors in mice treated with AAV vectors [37] have not been confirmed, and the chromosomal breaks that have been observed in

cells following AAV integration [38] are of uncertain significance, especially since integration by AAV vectors lacking the rep gene is infrequent. However, in liver-directed human trials in hemophilia B, transient liver enzyme abnormalities have been reported and were associated with loss of transgene expression [39]. Interestingly, the liver enzyme abnormalities occurred 4 weeks after vector administration, in contrast to the effects of adenoviral vectors, which occur within 24–48 h.

Plasmid vectors

Nonviral approaches for delivering therapeutic genes as naked plasmid DNA are attractive because plasmid DNA is relatively simple and inexpensive to produce, does not engender cell-mediated immune responses, and does not result in humoral immune responses against the DNA vehicle that would limit the opportunity for repeated delivery. Until recently, most plasmid DNA applications have resulted in short-lived (days to weeks) transgene expression. Recent attempts to use electrical [40] or hydrodynamic [41] approaches to augment target cell uptake of plasmid DNA have resulted in expression of clotting factors lasting months after delivery. By rapidly treating mice via the tail vein with FVIII expression sequences under the control of transcriptional regulatory elements optimized for liver expression, in large fluid volumes, supraphysiologic FVIII levels were obtained [41]. Despite the attractive features of nonviral approaches, current technical limitations reduce the likelihood of human use in the near future.

Chimeraplasty

Cells contain DNA repair mechanisms that can detect and replace incorrect nucleotides that occur during the process of DNA replication. Kmiec and coworkers have utilized these natural mismatch repair mechanisms to develop a strategy for repair of small mutations [42]. The overall approach is to employ a chemically stable chimeraplast, a double-stranded DNA-RNA chimeric oligonucleotide that contains the correct DNA sequence, to drive a nucleotide exchange reaction using the natural DNA repair mechanisms of the cell. The oligonucleotide is typically 70–80 nucleotides in length and is designed with a homologous targeting sequence composed of a complementary DNA region flanked by RNA residues (the chimeric strand), an all-DNA second strand, thymidine hairpin caps, and a double-stranded GC clamp region. The double-hairpin configuration of the chimeraplast reduces nuclease digestion and the concatenation of double-stranded molecules that occurs in mammalian cells and thereby facilitates the stability of the molecule. Because of the sequence complementarity with the genomic target, the chimeraplast aligns in perfect register with the target DNA except for the designed single basepair mismatch, which is recognized and corrected by harnessing the cell's endogenous DNA repair system.

Chimeraplasty can be used to repair single nucleotide mutations or even several nucleotide deletions, but would not be applicable to larger defects or to inversion mutations that are associated with some cases of hemophilia A. This approach has been used both *in vitro* and *in vivo* to effect single nucleotide changes in genes, including inducing a hemophilic mutation in the liver of a mouse [43]. There are over 600 different single base substitutions leading to hemophilia A, with all 26 exons affected, so that a large library of specific FVIII chimeraplasts would be required to treat the population. Nevertheless, it is attractive to view chimeraplasty as a true "gene cure," rather than gene replacement, of the hemophilic individual's specific inherited defect.

Spliceosome-mediated pre-mRNA trans-splicing

Another specific repair mechanism that may be especially applicable to the common inversion mutations that cause nearly 30% of hemophilia A cases is an approach termed *spliceosome-mediated mRNA trans-splicing*, or SmaRT [44]. This is a method used to repair messenger RNA, rather than DNA. In the final steps of transcription, the introns are removed and exons are spliced together to form mature, functional mRNA. The site of splicing is directed by 30–40 nucleotides at each end of the intron that form consensus binding sites for the spliceosome, a large ribonucleoprotein complex composed of small nuclear ribonucleoprotein particles (snRNPs) that catalyzes the splicing reaction. Spliceosome-mediated pre-mRNA trans-splicing takes advantage of this normal cellular process to effect RNA repair. The method involves synthesis of a pre-trans-splicing molecule (PTM) that contains the corrected mRNA fused to a 30–40 nucleotide sequence that targets a specific pre-mRNA. The PTM binds to the pre-mRNA, allowing specific trans-splicing of the corrected mRNA through normal mechanisms.

Chao and coworkers used a SmaRT approach to correct the hemophilic defect in FVIII knock-out mice [45]. The repair PTM consisted of a 125-nucleotide binding domain that was complementary to intron 15 of the gene, a spacer sequence, and a strong 3′ splice acceptor site, linked to exons 16–26 for the mouse FVIII cDNA. Correctly trans-spliced FVIII was detectable genetically and functionally in the treated mice, with up to 17% FVIII activity observed. It was conservatively estimated that between 1.6% and 6.3% of mutant transcripts were being repaired.

Gene transfer approaches

Gene therapy involves the transfer to human tissues of therapeutic genes that are competent to express the product of the gene to produce a therapeutic benefit. In the case of monogenic disorders like hemophilia, the strategy may be to (i) repair the defective gene *in situ*, using, for example, a chimeraplast approach, or (ii) insert a normal gene somewhere else in the

genome. This may be done *in vitro*, by removing cells from the individual, correcting the gene defect in tissue culture, and returning the cells to the individual. This *in vitro* approach has an inherent safety in that only the cells targeted for gene transfer are exposed to the transfer vector. Gene transfer may also be done through an *in vivo* approach, with administration of the therapeutic gene to the intact individual. The advantage of an *in vivo* approach is that more cells may be exposed to the transferred gene, but the safety concerns may be more complex.

Gene transfer may be targeted to a particular tissue or cell or it may be untargeted. Targeting may be by direct injection of a vector into a tissue, for example into muscle or liver. Targeting may also be through the vector. For example, an asialoglycoprotein placed on the surface of a vector might be used to target the vector to the asialoglycoprotein receptor on liver cells. Another way to target gene expression is through the use of tissue-specific promoters. Using liver again as an example, the albumin promoter or the α_1-antitrypsin promoter might be used to restrict gene expression to the liver. It may be important to target a gene or gene expression to a tissue if post-translational modifications important for the function of the gene product can only be accomplished in that tissue or if expression in other tissues is detrimental to the tissue. FVIII undergoes extensive post-translational modification, with the addition of N- and O-linked carbohydrates and sulfation of tyrosine residues that are important for thrombin cleavage of FVIII. Levels of expression may be affected by targeting strategies. Targeting to a specific tissue limits the number of cells that can take up and express the gene. The use of tissue-specific promoters may affect expression levels since these promoters may be weaker than more general promoters and this may affect the levels of gene expression.

DNA that is transferred to cells must gain access to the nucleus in order to be expressed. Depending on the vector used, the DNA may integrate into the host cell genome or may exist in an extrachromosomal or episomal location. The nuclear localization of the DNA has important consequences. Integrated DNA is passed onto daughter cells when cellular division occurs, whereas episomal DNA is usually lost during cell division. As a result, vectors that are nonintegrating, such as adenoviral vectors, can be expected to have less durable effects than vectors that are integrating, such as retrovirus vectors. Integration may be random or positional and may be within functional genes or in nonfunctional intervening sequences. When integration occurs in existing genes, there is a risk of insertional mutagenesis. When integration is in a tumor promoter gene, the resulting mutagenesis may, in theory, be beneficial for the cell. When integration occurs in a tumor suppressor gene, there may be an increased risk of tumorigenesis. Despite the lack of mutagenesis complications in previous gene transfer trials [46], reports of T-cell leukemia in children with X-linked severe combined immunodeficiency syndrome (SCID-X1) treated with *ex vivo* retrovirus-mediated gene transfer [17], as discussed above, demonstrate that insertional mutagenesis can occur.

References

1 Kay MA, Glorioso JC, Naldini L. Viral vectors for gene therapy: the art of turning infectious agents into vehicles of therapeutics. *Nature Med* 2001; 7: 33–40.

2 Miller DG, Adam MA, Miller AD. Gene transfer by retrovirus vectors occurs only in cells that are actively replicating at the time of infection. *Mol Cell Biol* 1990; 10: 4239–42.

3 Kay MA, Rothenberg S, Landen CN, *et al*. In vivo gene therapy of hemophilia B: sustained partial correction in factor IX-deficient dogs. *Science* 1993; 262: 117–9.

4 Kaleko M, Garcia JV, Miller AD. Persistent gene expression after retroviral gene transfer into liver cells in vivo. *Hum Gene Ther* 1991; 2: 27–32.

5 Gao C, Jokerst R, Gondipalli P, *et al*. Intramuscular injection of an adenoviral vector expressing hepatocyte growth factor facilitates hepatic transduction with a retroviral vector in mice. *Hum Gene Ther* 1999; 10: 911–22.

7 Olsen JC. Gene transfer vectors derived from equine infectious anemia virus. *Gene Ther* 1998; 5: 1481–7.

8 Curran MA, Kaiser SM, Achacoso PL, Nolan GP. Efficient transduction of nondividing cells by optimized feline immunodeficiency virus vectors. *Mol Ther* 2000; 1: 31–8.

9 Russell DW, Miller AD. Foamy virus vectors. *J Virol* 1996; 70: 217–22.

10 Zennou V, Serguera C, Sarkis C, *et al*. The HIV-1 DNA flap stimulates HIV vector-mediated cell transduction in the brain. *Nature Biotechnol* 2001; 19: 446–50.

11 Follenzi A, Sabatino G, Lombardo A, *et al*. Efficient gene delivery and targeted expression to hepatocytes in vivo by improved lentiviral vectors. *Hum Gene Ther* 2002; 13: 243–60.

12 Park F, Kay MA. Modified HIV-1 based lentiviral vectors have an effect on viral transduction efficiency and gene expression in vitro and in vivo. *Mol Ther* 2001; 4: 164–73.

13 Dang Q, Auten J, Plavec I. Human beta interferon scaffold attachment region inhibits de novo methylation and confers long-term, copy number-dependent expression to a retroviral vector. *J Virol* 2000; 74: 2671–8.

14 Schroder AR, Shinn P, Chen H, *et al*. HIV-1 integration in the human genome favors active genes and local hotspots. *Cell* 2002; 110: 521–9.

15 Wu X, Li Y, Crise B, Burgess SM. Transcription start regions in the human genome are favored targets for MLV integration. *Science* 2003; 300: 1749–51.

16 Li Z, Dullmann J, Schiedlmeier B, *et al*. Murine leukemia induced by retroviral gene marking. *Science* 2002; 296: 497.

17 Hacein-Bey-Abina S, Von Kalle C, Schmidt M, *et al*. LMO2-associated clonal T cell proliferation in two patients after gene therapy for SCID-X1. *Science* 2003; 302: 415–9.

18 Kirby I, Davison E, Beavil AJ, *et al*. Identification of contact residues and definition of the CAR-binding site of adenovirus type 5 fiber protein. *J Virol* 2000; 74: 2804–13.

19 Bergelson JM, Cunningham JA, Droguett G, *et al*. Isolation of a common receptor for Coxsackie B viruses and adenoviruses 2 and 5. *Science* 1997; 275: 1320–3.

20 Schnell MA, Zhang Y, Tazelaar J, *et al*. Activation of innate immunity in nonhuman primates following intraportal administration of adenoviral vectors. *Mol Ther* 2001; 3: 708–22.

21 Burgert HG, Ruzsics Z, Obermeier S, *et al*. Subversion of host defense mechanisms by adenoviruses. *Curr Top Microbiol Immunol* 2002; 269: 273–318.

22 Morsy MA, Gu M, Motzel S, *et al*. An adenoviral vector deleted for all viral coding sequences results in enhanced safety and extended expression of a leptin transgene. *Proc Natl Acad Sci USA* 1998; 95: 7866–71.

23 Balague C, Zhou J, Dai Y, *et al*. Sustained high-level expression of full-length human factor VIII and restoration of clotting activity in hemophilic mice using a minimal adenovirus vector. *Blood* 2000; 95: 820–8.

24 Stilwell JL, McCarty DM, Negishi A, Superfine R, Samulski RJ. Development and characterization of novel empty adenovirus capsids and their impact on cellular gene expression. *J Virol* 2003; 77: 12881–5.

25 Raper SE, Chirmule N, Lee FS, *et al*. Fatal systemic inflammatory response syndrome in a ornithine transcarbamylase deficient patient following adenoviral gene transfer. *Mol Genet Metab* 2003; 80: 148–58.

26 Weiss R, Nelson D. Teen dies undergoing experimental gene therapy. In: *The Washington Post*. Washington, DC; 1999: p. A01.

27 Summerford C, Samulski RJ. Membrane-associated heparan sulfate proteoglycan is a receptor for adeno-associated virus type 2 virions. *J Virol* 1998; 72: 1438–45.

28 Pruchnic R, Cao B, Peterson ZQ, *et al*. The use of adeno-associated virus to circumvent the maturation- dependent viral transduction of muscle fibers. *Hum Gene Ther* 2000; 11: 521–36.

29 Dutheil N, Shi F, Dupressoir T, Linden RM. Adeno-associated virus site-specifically integrates into a muscle- specific DNA region. *Proc Natl Acad Sci USA* 2000; 97: 4862–6.

30 Summerford C, Bartlett JS, Samulski RJ. AlphaVbeta5 integrin: A co-receptor for adeno-associated virus type 2 infection. *Nature Med* 1999; 5: 78–82.

31 Qing K, Mah C, Hansen J, *et al*. Human fibroblast growth factor receptor 1 is a co-receptor for infection by adeno-associated virus 2. *Nature Med* 1999; 5: 71–7.

32 Monahan PE, Jooss K, Sands MS. Safety of adeno-associated virus gene therapy vectors: a current evaluation. *Expert Opin Drug Saf* 2002; 1: 79–91.

33 Nakai H, Yant SR, Storm TA, *et al*. Extrachromosomal recombinant adeno-associated virus vector genomes are primarily responsible for stable liver transduction in vivo. *J Virol* 2001; 75: 6969–76.

34 Schnepp BC, Clark KR, Klemanski DL, *et al*. Genetic fate of recombinant adeno-associated virus vector genomes in muscle. *J Virol* 2003; 77: 3495–504.

35 Scallan CD, Liu T, Parker AE, *et al*. Phenotypic correction of a mouse model of hemophilia A using AAV2 vectors encoding the heavy and light chains of FVIII. *Blood* 2003; 102: 3919–26.

36 Sarkar R, Tetreault R, Gao G, *et al*. Total correction of hemophilia A mice with canine FVIII using an AAV 8 serotype. *Blood* 2004; 103: 1253–60. Epub 2003 Oct 9.

37 Donsante A, Vogler C, Muzyczka N, *et al*. Observed incidence of tumorigenesis in long-term rodent studies of rAAV vectors. *Gene Ther* 2001; 8: 1343–6.

38 Miller DG, Rutledge EA, Russell DW. Chromosomal effects of adeno-associated virus vector integration. *Nature Genet* 2002; 30: 147–8.

39 High KA, Manno CS, Sabatino DE, *et al*. Immune responses to AAV and to factor IX in a phase I study of AAV-mediated liver-directed gene transfer for hemophilia B. *Blood* 2003; 102: abstract 532.

40 Fewell JG, MacLaughlin F, Mehta V, *et al*. Gene therapy for the treatment of hemophilia B using PINC-formulated plasmid delivered to muscle with electroporation. *Mol Ther* 2001; 3: 574–83.

41 Miao CH, Ye X, Thompson AR. High-level factor VIII gene expres-

sion in vivo achieved by nonviral liver-specific gene therapy vectors. *Hum Gene Ther* 2003; **14**: 1297–305.

42 Kmiec EB. Targeted gene repair — in the arena. *J Clin Invest* 2003; **112**: 632–6.

43 Kren BT, Bandyopadhyay P, Steer CJ. In vivo site-directed mutagenesis of the factor IX gene by chimeric RNA/DNA oligonucleotides. *Nature Med* 1998; **4**: 285–90.

44 Puttaraju M, Jamison SF, Mansfield SG, Garcia-Blanco MA,

Mitchell LG. Spliceosome-mediated RNA trans-splicing as a tool for gene therapy. *Nature Biotechnol* 1999; **17**: 246–52.

45 Chao H, Mansfield SG, Bartel RC, *et al*. Phenotype correction of hemophilia A mice by spliceosome-mediated RNA trans-splicing. *Nature Med* 2003; **9**: 1015–9.

46 Bonini C, Grez M, Traversari C, *et al*. Safety of retroviral gene marking with a truncated NGF receptor. *Nature Med* 2003; **9**: 367–9.

38 Gene therapy for hemophilia B

Katherine P. Ponder

Introduction

Hemophilia B is a sex-linked disorder due to deficiency of factor IX (FIX) activity, which affects 1:30 000 males [1]. Gene therapy for hemophilia B refers to a treatment in which a FIX gene is delivered to cells in the body, which results in the continuous secretion of FIX into blood, and complete or partial correction of the bleeding manifestations. Achieving >50% of normal activity (>2.5 µg/mL) should be fully therapeutic, as it should prevent most spontaneous bleeds. Obtaining 1% (0.05 µg/mL) to 10% (0.5 µg/mL) of normal activity should be partially therapeutic, as it should reduce, but not prevent, bleeding.

Target cells for gene therapy for hemophilia B

Several cell types are reasonable targets for gene therapy for hemophilia B, as most cells can perform the γ-carboxylation of FIX that is necessary for its biologic activity. Furthermore, the relatively small 50-kDa FIX protein can diffuse into blood from cells outside the vasculature such as muscle cells or fibroblasts in the peritoneum. The liver has been a popular target for gene therapy, as genes can be delivered to the liver after intravenous injection of viral or plasmid vectors, the liver is the normal site of synthesis of FIX, and hepatocytes have direct contact with the blood. Other targets have included the muscle, which can be modified after intramuscular injection, or fibroblasts, which can be implanted into the peritoneum or other sites.

Vectors for gene therapy for hemophilia B

The DNA that encodes the FIX gene needs to be transferred into a cell to be expressed. Most approaches administer a vector *in vivo*, which can involve localized injection or injection into a blood vessel. Viral vectors are usually the most efficient, as they use elements from viruses that allow them to efficiently transfer their genetic information into a cell [2]. Viral vectors are generated by deleting some or all of the coding sequences of the virus, and replacing them with a promoter that directs transcription in the appropriate cell type, and the FIX coding sequence. Figure 38.1 shows how retroviral, adeno-associated viral (AAV), and adenoviral vectors are cloned and produced.

Retroviral vectors integrate into the host-cell chromosome, which results in long-term expression, but has some risk of insertional mutagenesis. The gamma-retroviral vectors transfer genes only into dividing cells, which poses a problem for transducing cells that are not replicating. However, this may provide a measure of safety with *in vivo* delivery procedures, as irrelevant nonreplicating cells would not be transduced. Gamma-retroviral vectors can be efficiently delivered to the liver by injection into newborns whose hepatocytes are replicating, or by injection into adults who were pretreated with a hepatic growth factor [3]. The lenti-retroviral vectors can transduce nondividing cells, and thus do not require induction of replication for gene transfer [4]. Similarly, both AAV and adenoviral vectors can be transferred into nondividing cells. However, since they are usually maintained as an episome, the transferred gene can be lost over time. Different serotypes of AAV and adenoviral vectors encode different capsid proteins, which can affect the cell types that are infected. For example, AAV1 appears to be more efficient in the muscle than is AAV2 [5], whereas AAV8 appears to be more efficient in liver than is AAV2 [6]. The serotype can also affect the likelihood that patients will have antibodies that block infection *in vivo*.

Plasmid vectors have also been used to transfer genes into cells for gene therapy. This can involve *ex vivo* delivery, which involves *in vitro* transfection followed by genetic selection and transplantation of modified cells, or *in vivo* delivery. *In vivo* delivery requires some stimulus to allow the DNA to enter the cell, such as electroporation of muscle or high-pressure injection into liver. Although the latter approach is quite efficient at transferring genes into hepatocytes, it is associated with toxicity that would likely preclude its use in humans. Once inside the cell, plasmids tend to be lost from a cell over time. However, some enhancer elements seem to promote long-term maintenance of plasmid DNA [7], whereas transfer of a plasmid with the appropriate target sequence along with a protein that promotes integration allows the plasmid to integrate into the host chromosome, which leads to prolonged expression [8,9]. Alternatively, maintenance of plasmids can be stabilized with elements from the Epstein–Barr virus [10].

Efficacy of gene therapy for hemophilia B in animal models

There has been recent success in using hepatic gene therapy to express therapeutic levels of FIX in both small and large ani-

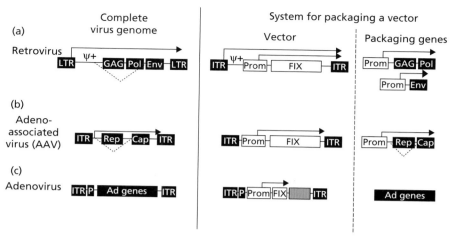

Figure 38.1 Commonly used vectors for gene therapy. The viral vectors that are most commonly used for gene therapy for hemophilia B are depicted. Sequences that are normally present in the infectious virus are shown on the left and appear as black boxes. The term 'vector' refers to sequences that are transferred into a new cell for gene therapy, as shown in the middle. Promoter (Prom) and FIX coding sequences are indicated by white boxes. Other sequences necessary for expression, such as polyadenylation sites, are also present but are not shown. In order to package the vector, mammalian cells that contain the vector must also express the packaging genes, which are shown on the right as black boxes. Promoters that direct the expression of the packaging genes are usually derived from a different source and are indicated by white boxes. Packaging cells accumulate viral particles intracellularly or secrete them into the media, after which the particles can be purified for use for gene therapy. (a) Retroviral vectors. Retroviral vectors have a single-stranded RNA genome of 5–7 kb that is copied into double-stranded DNA, which inserts into the chromosome. These include the gamma-retroviral vectors and the lenti-retroviral vectors. The vector contains the long terminal repeats (LTRs) at both ends and the packaging signal (ψ^+). The coding sequences include the group-specific antigens (GAG), polymerase (Pol), and envelope (Env) genes. The LTR directs transcription of the genomic RNA (indicated by an arrow), which can be spliced to form an RNA that encodes the envelope protein as indicated by the dotted line. (b) AAV vectors. AAV vectors have a single-stranded DNA genome of ~4.5 kb. The inverted terminal repeats (ITRs) are present at both ends. The coding sequences include the replication (Rep) and capsid (Cap) genes. Production of AAV vectors also requires expression of some helper functions from another virus such as adenovirus (not shown in the figure). (c) Adenoviral vector. Adenoviral vectors have a 36-kb linear double-stranded DNA genome. The vector contains ITRs at both ends and the packaging signal (P). The numerous adenoviral genes (Ad genes) are indicated by a single black box. Early-generation adenoviral vectors inserted the therapeutic gene into the E1 region but still contained most of the adenoviral genes. The helper-dependent adenoviral vectors are devoid of all adenoviral coding sequences and contain irrelevant stuffer sequence to maintain the appropriate size of the genome for packaging. Other adenoviral genes or stuffer sequences in the vector are indicated by the striped box.

mals. Factors that are important include the vector and its subclass, the promoter, the age at which gene therapy is performed, the route of administration, and the dose given. The key features in evaluating success are the level and longevity of expression, and an absence of adverse effects. The highest levels of expression achieved with different vectors with gene therapy for hemophilia B in mice are shown in Table 38.1. There are also several excellent recent reviews that summarize these results more extensively [11–15]. Delivery of retroviral [3] or AAV [16] vectors to the liver resulted in almost fully therapeutic (>35% of normal) and stable levels of expression. Delivery of AAV vectors to the muscle resulted in partially therapeutic (1% to 6% of normal) levels in most studies [17], although one investigation that used an AAV1 vector achieved fully therapeutic levels (100% of normal) [5]. Adenoviral vectors have directed fully therapeutic levels of expression after delivery to liver [18] or muscle [19], but expression usually falls over time and these vectors can induce inflammatory responses. Although plasmids can result in fully therapeutic expression from the liver after high-pressure injection [9,10], identification of a less toxic method for achieving gene transfer will be necessary. *Ex vivo* approaches, which involve transplantation of genetically modified fibroblasts [20],

myoblasts [21], or bone marrow-derived stromal cells [22], have resulted in partially therapeutic levels of expression (<12% of normal activity), which usually declines over time.

Results with gene therapy in large animals may be more predictive of success in humans than experiments in mice. Gene therapy in large animals has generally been less efficacious than in mice. In some cases, lower expression was obtained despite using a similar dose of vector per body weight as was used in mice, although in other cases lower expression could be attributed at least in part to giving a lower relative dose of vector. Table 38.2 summarizes the highest levels of expression that have been obtained with different vectors in large animal models. Recent reviews summarize these results more extensively [11–15]. Delivery of a retroviral [3] or AAV [23] vector to the liver of hemophilia B dogs or an AAV vector to the liver of normal rhesus macaques [24] resulted in partially therapeutic levels of expression (6–10% of normal activity). In contrast to results in mice, in which an AAV1 vector was much more effective than an AAV2 vector in the muscle, both AAV2 [25] and AAV1 [26] vectors resulted in relatively low levels of expression, at 1–2% of normal, after injection into muscle of hemophilia B dogs. Adenoviral vectors delivered to the liver directed expression of almost

Table 38.1 Summary of results of gene therapy in mice.

Vector	Subclass of vector	Target organ	Promoter*	Plasma FIX† (% normal)	Comments‡
Retroviral	Gamma [3]	Liver	hAAT	200	Neonatal; i.v.
				35	Adult; i.v.; after HGF
	Lenti [4]		CMV	6	Adult; PV
AAV	AAV1, AAV2, and AAV6 [16]	Liver	ApoE–hAAT	2000	Adult; PV
	AAV2 [17]	Muscle	CMV–β-actin	6	Adult; i.m.
	AAV1 [5]		CMV	1000	Adult; i.m.
Adenoviral	E1/E3-deleted and helper dependent [18]	Liver	ApoE–hAAT	400; 20% at 1 year	Adult; i.v.
	E1/E3-deleted [19]	Muscle	CK–CMV	100; 20% at 1 year	Adult; i.m.
Plasmid	No additional sequence [7]	Liver	ApoE–hAAT	30	Adult; i.v.; high-pressure injection
	Coinject transposase [8]		EF1α	5	
	Coinject integrase [9]		ApoE–hAAT	80	
	With EBV elements and EBNA1 [10]		ApoE–hAAT	100	
Modified fibroblasts	Ex vivo modification with plasmid [20]	Peritoneum	β-Actin	0.6; transient	Implanted i.p.
Modified myoblasts	Ex vivo modification with plasmid [21]	Peritoneum	CK–β-actin	12	Implanted i.p.; tumors developed
Modified bone marrow stromal cells	Ex vivo modification with plasmid [22]	Subcutaneous	Long terminal repeats	5; fell to 1% at 4 months	Implanted s.c.

*The promoter used to direct expression of FIX is shown.
†The level of long-term expression of FIX is shown unless otherwise indicated.
‡The age and the route of gene transfer are indicated.
ApoE, apolipoprotein E enhancer; CMV, cytomegalovirus promoter; CK, muscle creatine kinase enhancer; EF1α, elongation factor 1α promoter; hAAT, human α₁-antitrypsin promoter; HGF, hepatocyte growth factor; i.m., intramuscular; i.p., intraperitoneal; i.v., intravenous; PV, portal vein; s.c., subcutaneous.

fully therapeutic levels at >30% of normal in hemophilia B dogs [27,28] and normal rhesus macaques [29]. However, expression has been transient. Relatively low levels of expression (1% of normal) were transient after electroporation of muscle from hemophilia B dogs with plasmid [30].

Efficacy of gene therapy for hemophilia B in human patients

Results from these animal studies have led to two phase I clinical trials of gene therapy for hemophilia B in humans. Intramuscular injection of an AAV2 vector expressing hFIX may have caused a slight (<1%) increase in FIX functional activity and a modest (<50%) decrease in factor usage in some patients, but this may represent assay variation and a placebo effect respectively [31]. The second trial involves hepatic artery injection of an AAV2 vector [32]. One of two patients who received the highest dose achieved ~10% of normal FIX levels for a few weeks,

but expression fell thereafter in conjunction with a moderate elevation in transaminase levels. The hypothesis is that transduced cells were destroyed by a cytotoxic T-lymphocyte response against either the viral capsid proteins or the de novo expression of the wild-type human FIX gene, although this has not yet been proven. Thus, there is not yet unequivocal evidence of success with gene therapy for hemophilia B in human patients.

Risks of gene therapy

There are several potential risks of gene therapy that must be carefully evaluated prior to the routine use for hemophilia B. Inhibitors are antibodies that reduce the activity of a coagulation factor. Inhibitor induction is a major concern for gene therapy for congenital hemophilia B with FIX genes, as these patients do not express normal FIX protein. The risk of inhibitor formation after gene therapy is affected by the specific mutation, the route

Table 38.2 Summary of results of gene therapy experiments in large animals and humans.

Vector	Subclass of vector	Target organ	Promoter	Plasma FIX (% normal)	Comments
Results in dogs					
Retrovirus	Gamma [3]	Liver	hAAT	10	Neonates; i.v.; no inhibitors
AAV	AAV2 [23]	Liver	ApoE–hAAT	10	Adult; PV; few developed inhibitors
	AAV2 [25]	Muscle	CMV	1	Adult; i.m.; many developed inhibitors
	AAV1 [26]			2	Adult; i.m.; all developed inhibitors
Adenovirus	E1/E3-deleted [27]	Liver	RSV	270; fell to <0.1% at 3 months	Adult; i.v.; no inhibitors
	Helper-dependent [28]		ApoE–hAAT	30; fell to <0.2% at 2 months	Adult; i.v.; no inhibitors
Plasmid	No additional sequences [30]	Muscle	CMV	1; fell to 0 at 1 month	Adult; electroporation into muscle; inhibitors developed
Results in rhesus macaques					
AAV	AAV2 [24]	Liver	CMV–β-actin	6	Adult; PV or HA; 1 of 5 developed inhibitors
Adenovirus	E1/E3-deleted [29]	Liver	CMV	80; fell to 0 at 1 month	Adult; i.v.; all developed inhibitors
Results in human patients					
AAV	AAV2 [31]	Muscle	CMV	<1	Adult; i.m.; no inhibitors
	AAV2 [32]	Liver	ApoE–hAAT	10; fell to 0 at 2 months	Adult; HA; no inhibitors; transient increase LFTs

AAV, adeno-associated viral vector; CMV, cytomegalovirus promoter; HA, hepatic artery; hAAT, human α_1-antitrypsin promoter; PV, pulmonary vein; LFT, liver function test; RSV, Rous sarcoma virus promoter.

and age of administration, and the level of expression. Inhibitors are more common after gene therapy in mice [33] and dogs [23] with null mutations than in animals with single amino acid changes. These data are consistent with the fact that patients with large deletions or stop codons are more prone to produce inhibitors than are patients with missense mutations [34]. Administration of AAV vector to the liver is less likely to induce inhibitor formation than is delivery to the muscle in both mice [35] and dogs [23,25,26,36] for reasons that are unclear. Inhibitors have not developed in mice and dogs that received gene therapy at birth with a retroviral vector expressing the highly immunogenic human FIX protein [37], suggesting that early transfer might allow inhibitors to be avoided. However, it remains unclear if neonatal tolerance will be effective in humans, whose immune system may be more mature at birth relative to these other species. Finally, relatively high levels of expression reduce the chance of inhibitor formation in mice relative to that observed with low expression [33]. These data are consistent with the fact that the most effective treatment for inhibitors is administration of high doses of the protein using immune tolerance induction protocols [34]. Fortunately, inhibitors have not developed in any of the human patients who received gene therapy. However, only patients with multiple exposures to FIX without a history of inhibitor development have received gene therapy thus far, and these patients are probably at relatively low risk of inhibitor formation. Thus, it may be necessary to use transient immuno-

suppression at the time of gene therapy to prevent inhibitor development in those that are at high risk.

There are other potential risks of gene therapy. High doses of adenoviral vectors induce systemic inflammatory responses [18,29], which were probably responsible for the death of one human patient with a urea cycle disorder who received adenoviral vector-mediated gene therapy [38]. It will therefore be necessary to identify a dose of vector that does not induce significant amounts of inflammation, as was recently done with a helper-dependent adenoviral vector with a strong liver promoter [18].

A third concern is that insertional mutagenesis will result in cancer. This concern has been heightened by the recent development of leukemia in 2 out of 10 children in whom a retroviral vector integrated into an oncogene locus after gene therapy for severe combined immunodeficiency [39]. Although the therapeutic gene and the genetic disease likely contributed to the development of leukemia, it will be necessary to obtain long-term evaluation of gene therapy approaches in large animal models prior to the routine use in humans. Cancer development is also a concern using *ex vivo* procedures in which modified cells are transplanted, as the *in vitro* amplification of a clone with high expression can select for cells with a growth advantage. Indeed, tumors developed with high frequency after transplantation of genetically modified myoblasts [21].

A final concern is that gene therapy might result in germline transmission. Regulatory agencies are quite concerned about this possibility, as it could result in modification of the human genome. However, this has not been observed in either animal models or humans, and the risk appears to be low owing to the barriers that prevent viral particles or DNA from reaching germ cells in postnatal animals with intact blood vessels.

Summary

Gene therapy has the potential to permanently reduce or eliminate the bleeding manifestations of hemophilia B. Mice have achieved fully therapeutic levels of FIX with a variety of approaches. Large animals have achieved partially therapeutic levels of FIX activity with AAV and retroviral vectors introduced into the liver, and lower levels with AAV vectors introduced into the muscle. However, administration of AAV vectors to muscle or liver has not yet resulted in long-term expression in patients. Nevertheless, there is considerable optimism that this approach will be successful in the near future.

References

1 Lozier JN, Kessler CM. Clinical aspects and therapy of hemophilia. In: Hoffman R, Benz EJ, Shattil SJ, *et al.*, eds. *Hematology: Basic Principles and Practice*. New York: Churchill Livingstone, 2000: 1883–904.

2 Kay MA, Glorioso JC, Naldini L. Viral vectors for gene therapy: the art of turning infectious agents into vehicles of therapeutics. *Nature Med* 2001; 7: 33–40.

3 Xu L, Gao C, Sands MS, *et al.* Neonatal or hepatocyte growth factor-potentiated adult gene therapy with a retroviral vector results in therapeutic levels of canine factor IX for hemophilia B. *Blood* 2003; 101: 3924–32.

4 Follenzi A, Sabatino G, Lombardo A, *et al.* Efficient gene delivery and targeted expression to hepatocytes in vivo by improved lentiviral vectors. *Hum Gene Ther* 2002; 13: 243–60.

5 Chao H, Liu Y, Rabinowitz J, *et al.* Several log increase in therapeutic transgene delivery by distinct adeno-associated viral serotype vectors. *Mol Ther* 2000; 2: 619–23.

6 Sarkar R, Tetreault R, Gao G, *et al.* Total correction of hemophilia A mice with canine FVIII using an AAV8 serotype. *Blood* 2004; 103: 1253–60.

7 Ye X, Loeb KR, Stafford DW, *et al.* Complete and sustained phenotypic correction of hemophilia B in mice following hepatic gene transfer of a high-expressing human factor IX plasmid. *J Thromb Haemost* 2003; 1: 103–11.

8 Mikkelsen JG, Yant SR, Meuse L, *et al.* Helper-Independent Sleeping Beauty transposon-transposase vectors for efficient nonviral gene delivery and persistent gene expression in vivo. *Mol Ther* 2003; 8: 654–65.

9 Olivares EC, Hollis RP, Chalberg TW, *et al.* Site-specific genomic integration produces therapeutic Factor IX levels in mice. *Nat Biotechnol* 2002; 20: 1124–8.

10 Sclimenti CR, Neviaser AS, Baba EJ, *et al.* Epstein–Barr virus vectors provide prolonged robust factor IX expression in mice. *Biotechnol Prog* 2003; 19: 144–51.

11 VandenDriessche T, Collen D, Chuah MK. Viral vector-mediated gene therapy for hemophilia. Gene therapy for the hemophilias. *J Thromb Haemost* 2003; 1: 1550–8.

12 High KA. Gene transfer as an approach to treating hemophilia. *Semin Thromb Haemost* 2003; 29: 107–20.

13 Monahan PE, White GC II. Hemophilia gene therapy: update. *Curr Opin Hematol* 2002; 9: 430–6.

14 Nathwani AC, Nienhuis AW, Davidoff AM. Current status of gene therapy for hemophilia. *Curr Hematol Rep* 2003; 2: 319–27.

15 Walsh CE. Gene therapy progress and prospects: gene therapy for the hemophilias. *Gene Ther* 2003; 10: 999–1003.

16 Grimm D, Zhou S, Nakai H, *et al.* Preclinical in vivo evaluation of pseudotyped adeno-associated virus vectors for liver gene therapy. *Blood* 2003; 102: 2412–19.

17 Hagstrom JN, Couto LB, Scallan C, *et al.* Improved muscle-derived expression of human coagulation factor IX from a skeletal actin/CMV hybrid enhancer/promoter. *Blood* 2000; 95: 2536–42.

18 Ehrhardt A, Kay MA. A new adenoviral helper-dependent vector results in long-term therapeutic levels of human coagulation factor IX at low doses in vivo. *Blood* 2002; 99: 3923–30.

19 Dai Y, Schwarz EM, Gu D, *et al.* Cellular and humoral immune responses to adenoviral vectors containing factor IX gene: tolerization of factor IX and vector antigens allows for long-term expression. *Proc Natl Acad Sci USA* 1995; 92: 1401–5.

20 Van Raamsdonk JM, Ross CJ, Potter MA, *et al.* Treatment of hemophilia B in mice with nonautologous somatic gene therapeutics. *J Lab Clin Med* 2002; 139: 35–42.

21 Hortelano G, Wang L, Xu N, Ofosu FA. Sustained and therapeutic delivery of factor IX in nude haemophilia B mice by encapsulated C2C12 myoblasts: concurrent tumourigenesis. *Haemophilia* 2001; 7: 207–14.

22 Krebsbach PH, Zhang K, Malik AK, Kurachi K. Bone marrow stromal cells as a genetic platform for systemic delivery of therapeutic proteins in vivo: human factor IX model. *J Gene Med* 2003; 5: 11–17.

23 Mount JD, Herzog RW, Tillson DM, *et al.* Sustained phenotypic correction of hemophilia B dogs with a factor IX null mutation by liver-directed gene therapy. *Blood* 2002; 99: 2670–6.

24 Nathwani AC, Davidoff AM, Hanawa H, *et al.* Sustained high-level expression of human factor IX (hFIX) after liver-targeted delivery of recombinant adeno-associated virus encoding the hFIX gene in rhesus macaques. *Blood* 2002; 100: 1662–9.

25 Herzog RW, Yang EY, Couto LB, *et al.* Long-term correction of canine hemophilia B by gene transfer of blood coagulation factor IX mediated by adeno-associated viral vector. *Nature Med* 1999; 5: 56–63.

26 Arruda VR, Schuettrumpf J, Herzog RW, *et al.* Safety and efficacy of factor IX gene transfer to skeletal muscle in murine and canine hemophilia B models by adeno-associated viral vector serotype 1. *Blood* 2004; 103: 85–92.

27 Kay MA, Landen CN, Rothenberg SR, *et al.* In vivo hepatic gene therapy: complete albeit transient correction of factor IX deficiency in hemophilia B dogs. *Proc Natl Acad Sci USA* 1994; 91: 2353–7.

28 Ehrhardt A, Xu H, Dillow AM, *et al.* A gene-deleted adenoviral vector results in phenotypic correction of canine hemophilia B without liver toxicity or thrombocytopenia. *Blood* 2003; 102: 2403–11.

29 Lozier JN, Metzger ME, Donahue RE, Morgan RA. Adenovirus-mediated expression of human coagulation factor IX in the rhesus macaque is associated with dose-limiting toxicity. *Blood* 1999; 94: 3968–75.

30 Fewell JG, MacLaughlin F, Mehta V, *et al.* Gene therapy for the treatment of hemophilia B using PINC-formulated plasmid delivered to muscle with electroporation. *Mol Ther* 2001; 3: 574–83.

31 Manno CS, Chew AJ, Hutchison S, *et al.* AAV-mediated factor IX gene transfer to skeletal muscle in patients with severe hemophilia B. *Blood* 2003; 101: 2963–72.

32 High KA, Manno CS, Sabatino DE, *et al*. Immune responses to AAV and to factor IX in a phase I study of AAV-mediated, liver-directed gene transfer for hemophilia B. *Blood* 2003; **102**: 154a.

33 Mingozzi F, Liu YL, Dobrzynski E, *et al*. Induction of immune tolerance to coagulation factor IX antigen by in vivo hepatic gene transfer. *J Clin Invest* 2003; **111**: 1347–56.

34 Lusher JM. Inhibitor antibodies to factor VIII and factor IX: management. *Semin Thromb Haemost* 2000; **26**: 179–88.

35 Nathwani AC, Davidoff A, Hanawa H, *et al*. Factors influencing in vivo transduction by recombinant adeno-associated viral vectors expressing the human factor IX cDNA. *Blood* 2001; **97**: 1258–1265.

36 Herzog RW, Mount JD, Arruda VR, *et al*. Muscle-directed gene transfer and transient immune suppression result in sustained par-tial correction of canine hemophilia B caused by a null mutation. *Mol Ther* 2001; **4**: 192–200.

37 Zhang J, Xu L, Haskins ME, Ponder KP. Neonatal gene transfer with a retroviral vector results in tolerance to human factor IX in mice and dogs. *Blood* 2004; **103**: 143–51.

38 Raper SE, Chirmule N, Lee FS, *et al*. Fatal systemic inflammatory response syndrome in a ornithine transcarbamylase deficient patient following adenoviral gene transfer. *Mol Genet Metab* 2003; **80**: 148–58.

39 Hacein-Bey-Abina S, Von Kalle C, Schmidt M, *et al*. LMO2-associated clonal T cell proliferation in two patients after gene therapy for SCID-X1. *Science* 2003; **302**: 415–19.

39 Gene therapy for hemophilia A

Gilbert C. White II and Paul E. Monahan

Clinical trials in hemophilia A

Before gene transfer trials can be carried out in humans, clinical-grade vectors — viral, plasmid, or naked DNA — must undergo rigorous testing. Vectors driving expression of factor VIII (FVIII) are first tested in tissue culture systems, then in small animal models, usually mice, in large animal models, usually dogs or monkeys, and in FVIII-deficient models, usually knock-out mice or hemophilic dogs. These studies test the safety and efficacy of the vectors. Current guidelines for gene transfer trials are provided by the US National Institutes of Health (NIH) (www4.od.nih.gov/oba/rac/guidelines/guidelines.html), the US Food and Drug Administration (FDA) (www.fda.gov/cber/genetherapy/gtpubs.htm), and the European Agency for the Evaluation of Medicinal Products (EMEA) (www.emea.eu.int/index/indexh1.htm). Safety must be rigorously demonstrated before initiating human trials.

Three clinical trials in hemophilia A have been undertaken and completed.

Transkaryotic Therapy, Inc. (TKT) trial in hemophilia A

The TKT trial was a phase I, open-label, dose escalation study that was carried out from 1998 until 2002. The trial employed an *ex vivo* approach [1], similar to that employed in the initial Chinese trial in hemophilia B [2], except that the TKT trial utilized a nonviral, plasmid vector and the vector contained the cDNA for the B domain-deleted form of human FVIII under control of the cytomegalovirus (CMV) promoter [3].

A total of 12 subjects, ranging in age from 19 to 71 years, were studied, nine in a dose escalation trial and three in a comparison of sites of intraperitoneal injection. Seven of the 12 were HIV seropositive without AIDS and all were HCV seropositive with stable liver function. Dermal fibroblasts obtained from the subjects by excisional skin biopsy were electroporated with the plasmid containing the B domain-deleted human FVIII cDNA. Fibroblasts expressing the FVIII gene were clonally expanded, characterized for the stability of the integrated gene sequences and production of FVIII, and administered by laparoscopic intraperitoneal injection, either into the fat of the greater omentum or into the fibrofatty tissue that bounds the lesser omentum. Laparoscopy was performed under general anesthesia. A total of 100, 400, or 800 million autologous clonal cells were injected in three cohorts of three subjects per cohort. Follow-up was up to 24 months. There were no serious adverse events related to the study material, the skin biopsy, or the intraperitoneal injection. No inhibitors to FVIII were reported. Seven of the 12 subjects demonstrated a decreased bleeding frequency and/or FVIII use following cell transfer, with low levels of FVIII detected transiently in plasma, up to 1–2% of normal, with a maximum of 4%. Injection of cells into the lesser omentum appeared to be less effective than injection into the greater omentum. The first six subjects in this study were reported by Roth and coworkers [3].

Chiron trial

This was an open-label, multi-institution, single-dose, dose escalation, phase I trial in volunteers with severe hemophilia A utilizing a replication-deficient Moloney murine leukemia virus (MoMLV)-derived vector to deliver B domain-deleted human FVIII cDNA [hFVIII(V)] [4]. Administration of hFVIII(V) was by peripheral vein infusion, providing delivery of vector to essentially all tissues. The production of B domain-deleted FVIII was tissue nonspecific, under the control of the retroviral long terminal repeats (LTRs). Preclinical studies in rabbits, normal dogs, and hemophiliac dogs demonstrated the safety of the retroviral vector, showed persistence of FVIII antigen levels for as long as 65 weeks after gene transfer, and supported the initiation of clinical trials in humans [5].

A total of 13 subjects were enrolled, three at each of the first four doses [2.8×10^7, 9.2×10^7, 2.2×10^8, and 4.4×10^8 transduction units (TU)/kg] and one at the highest dose (8.8×10^8 TU/kg). In general, the administration of hFVIII(V) was well tolerated, with no serious infusion-related events. Liver function tests and complete blood counts showed no significant changes from baseline, and no acceleration of chronic HIV or HCV disease was apparent over the study observation period. All tests for replication-competent retrovirus (RCR) were negative. No FVIII inhibitor activity was detected by either Bethesda assay or FVIII recovery and pharmacokinetic studies. The only study-related serious adverse event was a single, transient, low-level polymerase chain reeaction (PCR)-positive vector signal that was detected in 1 of 10 replicates from a week 9 semen sample from one subject who received 4.4×10^8 TU/kg; all preceding samples and four subsequent samples in the subject were negative. It was not possible to determine whether the signal was from the sperm or the white blood cell fraction of the semen. While no subject had sustained levels >1%, six patients showed FVIII >1% on at least two occasions 5 or more days after infusion of exogenous FVIII. Most elevated levels were in the range of 1.0–1.8%, although isolated levels of 2.3, 3.0, 4.3, and 6.2 were reported for three subjects. Elevated levels of FVIII were detected as early as 8 days following treatment. Peripheral blood mononuclear cells (PBMCs) demonstrated the presence of vector gene sequences by PCR testing to 6 months in all 10 subjects tested and to 1 year in three of four subjects tested. All of the four subjects tested at 1 year were in the two lowest dose groups, indicating persistence of vector sequences even at the lowest dose. Pharmacokinetic examination following the infusion of exogenous FVIII 13 weeks after vector infusion showed a statistically increased half-life ($t_{1/2}$) and area under the curve (AUC) compared with pre-study values (18.4±4.7 vs. 15.5±3.1 for $t_{1/2}$ and 49±17 vs. 43±14 for AUC). Bleeding frequency was decreased in six subjects compared with historical rates.

Genstar trial in hemophilia A

The Genstar trial was a phase I trial in severe hemophilia A using MaxAdFVIII, a "gutless" adenovirus vector derived from type 5 adenovirus (Ad5) [6]. MaxAdFVIII was devoid of all viral genes and carried a 27-kb expression cassette that contained the full-length FVIII cDNA under the control of the human 12.5-kb albumin promoter. Vector production was accomplished through a three-part packaging system that consisted of a plasmid containing the FVIII cDNA, an ancillary Ad vector designed to support replication of the maxAd genome, and an AdE1 complementing cell line (A549E1) derived from A549 lung carcinoma cells. This was the first clinical trial of any type using a "gutless" adenovirus. This was also the first clinical trial in hemophilia in which clotting factor expression was genetically targeted to a specific tissue, the liver. One of the advantages of the "gutless" vector was the increased size of the expression cassette, which permitted incorporation of sequences such as the highly liver-specific albumin promoter. In addition to driving expression of FVIII in the liver, one of its natural sites of synthesis, restriction of expression to the liver was expected to increase the efficiency of expression while reducing expression in antigen-presenting cells, further reducing the immune response.

Preclinical studies with MaxAdFVIII in mice showed high-level expression of FVIII [7]. Interestingly, although adenoviral vectors are nonintegrating, expression of FVIII was observed for up to a year from a single intravenous infusion. Mouse liver enzymes were maintained within normal limits following administration of MaxAdFVIII. In subsequent studies, cynomolgus monkeys were administered 4.3 × 10¹¹, 1.4 × 10¹², and 4.3 × 10¹² virus particles (vp)/kg [8]. Expression of functional FVIII in primate plasma was determined using a novel "capture" assay combined with a chromogenic assay. At all three vector doses, FVIII was detected at levels ranging from 28 to 88 mU/mL. No significant adverse effects were detected in the two lower dosage groups that resulted in the expression of therapeutic hFVIII levels. In the highest-dose group, thrombocytopenia and minimal elevation in liver transaminase levels were transient and similar to those previously observed in mice.

A single individual was enrolled in the clinical trial and received an infusion of 4.3 × 10¹¹ vp/kg MaxAdFVIII. The administration was associated with the development of fever to 39.2°C, chills, and generalized myalgias 4 h after injection that lasted approximately 14 h. There was an increase in neutrophil count to 10 260/mL. There was an approximately 50% decrease in platelet count, starting post-treatment day 1, with a return to normal by day 7, and a 10-fold increase in alanine aminotransferase (ALT) starting on post-treatment day 2 and returning to normal by about day 11. There was evidence for diffuse intravascular coagulation with an increase in plasma levels of prothrombin fragment 1 + 2, thrombin–antithrombin (TAT) complexes, and D-dimer. Coagulation factor VII levels fell to 9% of normal. There was a marked increase in interleukin 6, with peak levels at 8 h postinfusion. Tumor necrosis factor (TNF-α) levels were also increased by 24 h and returned to baseline by 48–72 h. The subject had no reduction in his requirement for FVIII and there was no increase in his measurable FVIII following gene transfer. Because of the grade 3 toxicity, the trial was placed on temporary hold by the FDA, pending an evaluation of the findings. The study was reopened for enrollment, but at a log lower dose in individuals with low pretreatment anti-adenovirus type 5 antibodies, but was subsequently closed by the investigators.

Clinical trials summary

The clinical trials that have been performed in hemophilia A demonstrate a breadth of approaches — from *ex vivo* to tissue-targeted approaches, from plasmid to viral vectors, and from DNA-integrating to non-integrating viruses.

From a safety perspective, the results of the three trials show somewhat variable results but raise some important questions. The TKT study showed that *ex vivo*, nonviral gene transfer is safe. The implantation procedure was well tolerated with no serious adverse events, although the laparoscopic administration of cells required general anesthesia and was an invasive procedure. The Genstar study was at the opposite end of the spectrum, with significant toxicity directly associated with the administration of the adenoviral vector. The observed toxicity was similar to changes observed in previous adenovirus-mediated gene transfer studies, but was perhaps unexpected with a "gutted" adenovirus. In retrospect, the study subject had high levels of antibody against adenovirus type 5, the parental strain from which the vector was derived. This may have contributed somewhat to the immune response that was observed. The development of an immune response to the "gutless" adenovirus vector indicates that adenoviral toxicity is due at least in part to coat proteins, in addition to expression of viral proteins.

There has been no evidence for inhibitor formation in these initial trials even though there were concerns about inhibitor development based on some of the results from animal models [9–11].

As described above, insertional mutagenesis is a serious concern with integrating vectors such as retrovirus. No evidence for insertional mutagenesis has been observed clinically in any of the individuals on the Chiron study, but observation of the subjects is ongoing.

Another concern with integrating vectors is the possibility of germline transmission. The ability to integrate into the human genome raises concerns that DNA might reach gonadal tissue and insert into the germ cell genome, causing possible transmission to subsequent generations. Semen samples were examined at regular intervals during the Chiron study to assess for germline integration. Vector sequences were detected by PCR. Kazazian has estimated that the natural rate of endogenous insertional mutagenesis in man is about one in 10–100; that is, approximately one individual in every 10–100 will carry a mutational insertion, a number much larger than the calculated rate for gene therapy [12]. There is no evidence for germline transmission with hFVIII(V) in rabbits [13].

None of the trials achieved curative levels of protein expression, but in two of the three, the *ex vivo* TKT study and the Chiron study, there were clinical improvements and increased FVIII levels in some subjects. Neither study demonstrated a clear dose response. In the Chiron study, which used a MoMLV-derived vector, efficient transduction required dividing cells and a potential explanation for the failure to see a dose response may relate to the limited number of dividing cells in the liver.

Conclusions

In summary, the initial trials of gene therapy in hemophilia A have been completed. The results of these initial studies indicate that gene transfer is generally safe in hemophilia in the doses and routes of administration used. Low levels of expression of clotting factor have been observed in two of the clinical trials and the expression of clotting factor has been associated with some clinical improvement. The challenge now is to increase clotting factor expression without increasing toxicity. Concerns about insertional mutagenesis, always a theoretical concern with integrating vectors, are real and will shape the future of gene therapy [14]. As pointed out by Verma [15], focused efforts to better understand the basic biology of gene therapy are critical to continued advances and to the further development of gene transfer as a treatment for hemophilia and other inborn genetic disorders. These initial clinical trials are our first important steps in the process.

References

1 Selden RF, Skoskiewicz MJ, Howie KB, *et al.* Implantation of genetically engineered fibroblasts into mice: implications for gene therapy. *Science* 1987; **236**: 714–8.
2 Qiu X, Lu D, Zhou J, *et al.* Implantation of autologous skin fibroblast genetically modified to secrete clotting factor IX partially corrects the hemorrhagic tendencies in two hemophilia B patients. *Chin Med J* 1996; **109**: 832–9.
3 Roth DA, Tawa NE, O'Brien J, *et al.* Non-viral transfer of the gene encoding coagulation factor VIII in patients with severe hemophilia A. *New Engl J Med* 2001; **344**: 1735–42.
4 Powell JS, Ragni MV, White GC, II, *et al.* Phase 1 trial of FVIII gene transfer for severe hemophilia A using a retroviral construct administered by peripheral intravenous infusion. *Blood* 2003; **102**: 2038–45.
5 Greengard JS, Jolly DJ. Animal testing of retroviral-mediated gene therapy for factor VIII deficiency. *Thromb Haemost* 1999; **82**: 555–61.
6 Zhang WW, Josephs SF, Zhou J, *et al.* Development and application of a minimal-adenoviral vector system for gene therapy of hemophilia A. *Thromb Haemost* 1999; **82**: 562–71.
7 Balague C, Zhou J, Dai Y, *et al.* Sustained high-level expression of full-length human factor VIII and restoration of dotting activity in hemophilic mice using a minimal adenovirus vector. *Blood* 2000; **95**: 820–8.
8 Fang X, Zhang W-W, Sobol RE, *et al.* Studies in non-human primate and hemophilic dog models of a "gutless" adenovirus vector for treatment of hemophilia A. *Blood* 2000; **96**: 428a.
9 Herzog RW, Yang EY, Couto LB, *et al.* Long-term correction of canine hemophilia B by gene transfer of blood coagulation factor IX mediated by adeno-associated viral vector. *Nature Med* 1999; **5**: 56–63.
10 Lozier JN, Metzger ME, Donahue RE, Morgan RA. Adenovirus-mediated expression of human coagulation factor IX in the rhesus macaque is associated with dose-limiting toxicity. *Blood* 1999; **94**: 3968–75.
11 Gallo-Penn AM, Shirley PS, Andrews JL, *et al.* Systemic delivery of an adenoviral vector encoding canine factor VIII results in short-term phenotypic correction, inhibitor development, and biphasic liver toxicity in hemophilia A dogs. *Blood* 2001; **97**: 107–13.
12 Kazazian HH, Jr. An estimated frequency of endogenous insertional mutations in humans. *Nature Genet* 1999; **22**: 130.
13 Roehl HH, Leibbrandt ME, Greengard JS, *et al.* Analysis of testes and semen from rabbits treated by intravenous injection with a retroviral vector encoding the human factor VIII gene: No evidence of germ line transduction. *Hum Gene Ther* 2000; **11**: 2529–40.
14 Cavazzana-Calvo M, Thrasher A, Mavilio F. The future of gene therapy. *Nature* 2004; **427**: 779–81.
15 Verma IM. Gene therapy: the need for basic science. *Mol Ther* 2000; **2**: 531.

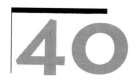

40 Gene therapy: molecular engineering of factor VIII and factor IX

David Lillicrap

Background

As we move ever closer to the era of genetic treatment for hemophilia, a number of challenges remain to be overcome before we can claim success with these novel therapeutic approaches. Although significant progress has been made in terms of preclinical trials of hemophilia gene therapy, with the successful long-term treatment of many hemophilic mice and some hemophilic dogs, no sustained phenotypic recovery has yet been accomplished in human hemophilia. Two major obstacles continue to plague the field: the lack of a system in which long-term therapeutic levels of clotting factor are expressed from the transgene, and the potential of inciting an immune response against the transgene product.

General strategies to improve hemophilia gene therapy outcomes

Despite the fact that the concept of substitutive gene therapy is simple, there are, not surprisingly, many complexities related to the effective delivery and expression of clotting factor transgenes. Thus, while this chapter will emphasize the potential benefits of modifying the transgene product itself, other approaches to enhancing the efficacy and safety of hemophilia gene therapy are also being developed (Table 40.1). These include the investigation of several different viral and nonviral delivery systems, the assessment of different viral serotypes to improve transduction efficiencies [1,2], and the generation of novel transgene expression cassettes to enhance transgene expression and restrict expression to a limited selection of tissues [3,4]. While all of these approaches have a common goal of improving transgene expression levels, and limiting the immunologic response to the transgene product, there is growing evidence to indicate that each combination of vector, expression cassette, and transgene may have its own distinct set of advantages and limitations.

New factors for gene therapy and recombinant protein production

Although the possibility of enhancing hemophilia gene therapy through the development of novel factor VIII (FVIII) and FIX molecules has become a feasible and exciting goal, it is important to recognize that these same molecules may find their initial utilization as recombinant proteins for routine replacement therapy. The recent development of recombinant clotting factor concentrates that have no contact with other human-derived proteins, either during the cell culture expression or in the final formulation, has essentially removed even the "virtual" risk of infectious agent transmission that continued to exist with the first- and second-generation recombinant concentrates. Thus, with the availability of very safe and pure concentrates, the next biotechnological challenge has been to improve on nature's work and develop clotting factor molecules with enhanced biologic and pharmacokinetic characteristics [5,6]. There is every reason to believe that the development of these proteins will proceed in parallel for use in both exogenous protein replacement and gene therapy protocols.

Features of the perfect clotting factor molecule

Just as the development of recombinant FVIII represented one of the earliest triumphs of recombinant DNA technology, there is now growing optimism that genetic engineering can improve on the therapeutic potential of native clotting factors. To begin to develop clotting proteins with enhanced biologic properties assumes that we understand enough about the structure–function relationships of these proteins to know how to engineer improved structures. Certainly, our knowledge of FVIII and FIX structure–function has progressed remarkably in the past two decades, but we are still some way from a complete understanding of the structural details of these proteins. There is as yet no complete crystal structure for FVIII, the role of the FVIII B domain (if any exists) remains unclear, and the precise cofactor function provided by FVIII in the intrinsic tenase complex is still unresolved. Thus, while some rational attempts can be made to improve on the synthesis and hemostatic properties of these proteins, there are still some complexities of structure that elude our understanding.

Improved biosynthetic efficiency

The first area where efforts have been made to improve these proteins relates to changes that might enhance the efficiency of clotting factor biosynthesis. Both FVIII and FIX undergo complex post-translational processing steps following initial synthe-

Table 40.1 Strategies for enhancing hemophilia gene therapy.

Viral vector engineering
Site-specific genomic integration
Cell-specific vector targeting
Enhanced transduction efficiency
Transgene cassette engineering
Enhanced transcriptional regulatory elements
Tissue-specific promoters
Stabilizing 3′ noncoding sequences
Intronic elements
Biologically enhanced transgene cDNAs

sis, and there is good evidence to indicate that the efficiency and accuracy of this processing is essential for optimal protein function. Furthermore, while modifications such as the sulfation of FVIII are required for full functional activity, interactions of the nascent protein with chaperone molecules in the endoplasmic reticulum regulate protein secretion in an as yet incompletely understood fashion. Generating cell lines that facilitate these processes or engineering recombinant molecules that have more efficient biosynthetic qualities are biotechnological approaches that have already been pursued with some success.

Enhanced specific activity

The second functional characteristic that has attracted biotechnological attention is the potential of generating molecules with enhanced procoagulant activity. There are a variety of approaches to pursuing such a goal, but two of the more efficient would appear to be the potential of comparing protein sequences from other species in which enhanced hemostatic activity is observed (i.e., canine FVIII in which plasma FVIII activity is approximately eightfold higher than in humans [7]) or a strategy of substituting homologous domains or residues from related proteins [8,9].

Improved protein stability

A significant problem in delivering adequate levels of FVIII for a therapeutic effect is the extreme instability of the protein. Thus, strategies to stabilize the circulating FVIII structure, and to inhibit its clearance through protein C-mediated proteolysis, have received recent attention in attempts to prolong its plasma half-life.

Prolonged intravascular survival

The average circulating half-lives of FVIII and FIX are 12 and 24 h respectively. Thus, effective prophylactic regimens of FVIII infusion have been thought, until very recently, to require the ad-

ministration of treatments three times each week. FIX prophylaxis can be administered twice weekly. However, the potential to extend the natural half-lives of the proteins would provide the opportunity for less frequent protein infusions or, in the context of gene therapy, result in a lesser requirement for transgene expression [10]. This concept has been significantly aided by the recent elucidation of a clearance mechanism for FVIII involving two widely expressed cell-surface proteins, the low-density lipoprotein receptor-related protein [11,12] and heparan sulfate proteoglycans [13]. Interference with this catabolic pathway, which is also responsible for clearing FIXa, has been shown to extend the circulating half-life of FVIII in experimental animals, and thus provides a potential strategy for improving FVIII delivery protocols.

Reduced immunogenicity

The development of neutralizing antibodies to FVIII in approximately 25% of treated patients continues to represent a critical challenge to the safe and effective treatment of hemophilia A. The incidence of inhibitors in the hemophilia B population is significantly less, at approximately 3%. The molecular basis for these immunologic events is discussed in detail elsewhere in this book, but it is sufficient to say that the inhibitors appear to represent oligoclonal responses to multiple epitopes within specific domains of the FVIII protein [14]. Over time, the pattern of reactivity against these epitopes may change [15]. Given this information, efforts have been made to reduce the immunogenicity of FVIII through the substitution of regions or residues of the native protein that appear to be immunodominant epitopes.

Biotechnological enhancements of factor VIII

Currently available "novel" factor VIII proteins

The first genetically altered FVIII protein, ReFacto, has now been in widespread clinical use for several years [16,17]. This product has been generated without the central B domain of FVIII, a region of the protein that is functionally dispensable, at least as far as FVIII cofactor activity is concerned [18,19]. Removal of the B domain provides a biosynthetic advantage to this form of the molecule owing to enhancements of FVIII mRNA expression and, to a much lesser extent, to improved protein secretion. After extensive clinical evaluation, there is every indication that this molecule functions normally as a procoagulant cofactor, and that it is no more immunogenic than the full-length FVIII molecule. However, the B domain-deleted (BDD) molecule does produce different results in *in vitro* assays of FVIII functional activity [20,21], a phenomenon that has caused significant confusion in the clinical setting. One-stage assay results with the BDD FVIII can be as low as 50% of those obtained with the chromogenic FVIII assay. While the mechanism for this discrepancy remains unresolved, the phospholipid content of the one-stage assay is one of the influential factors.

To date, most gene therapy studies have utilized the BDD form of FVIII to take advantage of both the improved biosynthetic efficiency associated with this molecule and the ease of packaging of the smaller FVIII cDNA. However, more recent studies suggest that complete deletion of the B domain may not be the most effective means for optimizing FVIII secretion, and molecules are currently being generated that have partial B domain deletions combined with mutations that interfere with the binding of FVIII to chaperones such as the immunoglobulin-binding protein (BiP) [22].

Enhancement of factor VIII's specific cofactor activity

While the precise details of the procoagulant cofactor function of FVIII remain to be elucidated, the product of this activity can be evaluated adequately with the currently available FVIII functional assays. Using these assays and a measurement of FVIII antigen, the specific cofactor activity of FVIII derived from some other species, such as dogs, can be documented to be several-fold higher than human FVIII. This observation provides the potential, through sequence comparisons, to develop FVIII molecules with enhanced hemostatic function. However, without more precise structural knowledge of the cofactor function of the protein, this strategy will likely take a considerable amount of time and effort to be productive.

Improved factor VIII stability

After proteolytic activation by thrombin, the FVIIIa A1–A2–A3/C1/C2 heterotrimer is rapidly inactivated through two distinct processes: a spontaneous dissociation of the A2 domain and the proteolytic cleavage of FVIIIa by activated protein C. In light of the instability of FVIIIa, attempts have been made to generate stable molecules that maintain cofactor activity for sustained periods of time. To date, two such molecules have been produced and evaluated (Figure 40.1).

The first inactivation-resistant form of FVIII (referred to as the IR8 molecule), involves deletion of residues 794–1689, so that the A2 domain is covalently attached to the light chain, thus prohibiting spontaneous A2 dissociation [23]. The IR8 molecule also contains missense mutations at thrombin and activated protein C cleavage sites to inhibit proteolytic inactivation. After expression in COS-1 cells, the specific activity of IR8 was fivefold higher than wild-type FVIII, and IR8 retained 38% of peak cofactor activity 4 h after thrombin exposure *in vitro*, in contrast to the wild-type protein, which was inactivated after 10 min [23]. Unfortunately, whereas spontaneous A2 dissociation is prohibited by the IR8 construct and proteolytic inactivation significantly delayed, this molecule also demonstrates 10-fold reduced binding to von Willebrand factor unless a light chain-specific anti-FVIII antibody is introduced into the system.

The second stabilized form of FVIII to have been generated again involves the covalent attachment of the A2 domain to the FVIII light chain. In this instance, a FVIII molecule containing cysteine 664 and cysteine 1826 was generated to link the A2 and A3 domains via a disulfide bond [24]. This molecule is activated normally by thrombin *in vitro*, and retains >90% of its cofactor function at a time when wild-type FVIII shows <10% activity.

Prolonging the intravascular survival of factor VIII

Studies reported in 1999 by two laboratories have shown that FVIII catabolism is mediated, at least in part, by the removal of the protein through an interaction with the low-density lipoprotein receptor-related protein (LRP) [11,12], an interaction that is facilitated by cell-surface heparan sulfate proteoglycans (HSPGs) [13]. The characterization of LRP as a catabolic receptor for FVIII represents the first documentation of a factor VIII clearance pathway and, although LRP also acts as a receptor for many other ligands, there is already *in vivo* evidence to support a physiologic role for the receptor in FVIII clearance [25]. With this information as background, there are now projects in progress to develop FVIII molecules that evade this interaction with LRP and thus achieve a prolonged circulation time for the protein (Figure 40.2).

Three LRP binding sites have been documented to date in the FVIII molecule: a region in the A2 domain between residues 484 and 509, a second site between residues 1811 and 1818 in the A3 domain, and a third region at the extreme C-terminus of the C2 domain between residues 2303 and 2332. A single site for HSPG binding has been documented in the A2 domain. While blocking the interaction of FVIII with LRP has already been shown to prolong the circulating FVIII half-life, the generation of novel FVIII variants in which LRP interactions are blocked will prove challenging, not least because the LRP binding sites overlap with regions of the protein that bind other physiologically critical ligands including FIXa, von Willebrand factor, and phospholipid. Finally, depending upon the success of this strategy, another potential long-term complication of this approach could be the generation of chronically elevated plasma levels of FVIII [26], a phenomenon now recognized as a risk factor for venous thromboembolic disease [27].

Reducing the immunogenicity of factor VIII

General comments concerning factor VIII immunogenicity

The development of neutralizing inhibitors to FVIII in approximately 25% of treated hemophilia A patients is the consequence of a number of factors, some of which are fairly well understood and some of which continue to elude us. There is now very good evidence to indicate that FVIII null genotypes are associated with a higher risk of inhibitor generation, and that there is also

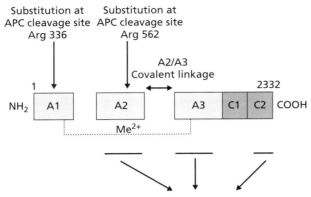

Figure 40.1 Strategies for stabilizing FVIII and reducing FVIII antigenicity. The FVIIIa heterotrimer is stabilized through a divalent metal ion linkage between the A1 and A3 domains, and weak electrostatic interactions between the A2 domain and the factor VIII A3/C1/C2 light chain. Strategies for stabilizing the factor VIIIa heterotrimer have included generating covalent linkages between the A2 and A3 domains, and substituting residues at the activated protein C cleavage sites at arginine 336 and arginine 562. Attempts to reduce the antigenicity of factor VIII have involved the insertion of multiple substitutions into the immunodominant A2, A3 and C2 domains.

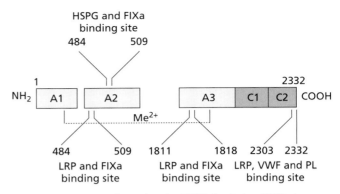

Figure 40.2 Strategies for prolonging FVIII circulation. FVIIIa is cleared from plasma through interactions with the low-density lipoprotein receptor-related protein (LRP) and cell-surface heparan sulfate proteoglycans (HSPGs) located in the A2, A3, and C2 domains of factor VIII. Substitutions in these binding regions may inhibit binding to LRP and HSPGs but may also interfere with binding to the physiologic ligands, factor IXa (FIXa), von Willebrand factor (VWF), and phospholipid (PL).

an influence from a number of treatment-related factors, including the type of FVIII concentrate, the intensity of treatment, and the coexistence of an inflammatory state. Most pertinent to this discussion is the potential for altering the immunogenicity of FVIII through the introduction of novel sequence changes. There are already precedents for an increased incidence of inhibitor development in patients treated with different forms of plasma-derived FVIII concentrate [28], and, although there has not been a clear difference between the immunogenicity of most plasma-derived and recombinant concentrates, there is still some debate about this issue [29]. The incidence of inhibitor development with the B domain-deleted concentrate, ReFacto, appears very similar to all other FVIII products.

With this background, it is clear that the use of biotechnology to create new forms of FVIII can result in three very different immunologic outcomes: a FVIII protein with a similar antigenic profile to the wild-type protein or a novel protein with either enhanced or suppressed antigenicity. Indeed, whereas some of the enhanced functional characteristics of a bioengineered FVIII may be relatively easy to evaluate, the potential for these novel protein structures to incite inhibitor formation may be considerably more difficult to assess.

Development of factor VIII molecules with reduced immunogenicity

A considerable amount has been learnt about the details of the immunologic response to FVIII over the past two decades. Most importantly, from the point of view of generating molecules

with reduced immunogenicity, we now have extensive information relating to the B-cell epitopes on the FVIII molecule [30–33]. The major immunodominant epitopes appear to be localized to the A2 and C2 domains of the protein, with the antibodies binding to these sites neutralizing FVIII through mechanisms that include the inhibition of binding to FIXa and phospholipid. A third, somewhat less immunoreactive, region of the protein exists in the A3 domain.

The basic strategy for reducing the immunogenicity to FVIII has been to introduce sequences derived from FVIII of another species (pig), which do not adversely affect cofactor function but appear to be less antigenic than the corresponding human residues (Figure 40.1) [31,34]. However, while these molecules demonstrate reduced cross-reactivity with many human FVIII alloantibodies, it is still unclear how well they will be tolerated by the human immune system *in vivo*.

Aside from the potential of using novel engineered forms of FVIII to reduce immunogenicity to this protein, there is already some evidence to suggest that FVIII gene therapy in itself could be an effective means of inducing immunologic tolerance to FVIII [35]. The success of this approach will likely depend upon a number of factors, including the site and magnitude of transgene expression, but at this stage of hemophilia gene therapy development, there is reason to be optimistic that this strategy will ultimately provide an alternative to the currently available protocols of tolerance induction.

Biotechnological enhancements of factor IX

Perhaps because of the reduced prevalence of hemophilia B, and the more robust expression, longer plasma half-life, and relatively minimal immunogenicity of FIX, attempts to enhance the production and biologic function of this protein have been limited.

Extensive clinical experience with the recombinant FIX concentrate, BeneFix, has shown that alterations to the post-translational modification of the protein can have significant consequences for the pharmacokinetic profile of the protein [36,37]. Thus, expression of FIX transgenes from cells other than hepatocytes may be associated with similar limitations, and require modifications to the transgene protein to overcome an inherent biosynthetic disadvantage [38,39].

The delivery of FIX transgenes to skeletal muscle has been compromised, to some extent, by binding of the secreted protein to collagen IV in the surrounding tissues [38]. The recent generation of two FIX mutants, at codon 5 (lysine to alanine) and 10 (valine to lysine), with reduced binding to collagen IV has resulted, in a hemophilic mouse model, in fivefold increased levels of circulating FIX and, unexpectedly, a twofold increase in specific activity [40]. Similarly, adeno-associated viral vector (AAV)-mediated hepatic delivery of a FIX transgene containing the codon 338, arginine to alanine, substitution has been shown to result in a protein with sevenfold higher specific activity. Of note, none of these variant forms of FIX elicited an inhibitor response in transgenic mice tolerant to wild-type human FIX.

The future of coagulation factor biotechnology

There is every indication that the development of recombinant wild-type FVIII and FIX, and B domain-deleted FVIII, represents only the beginning of an era in which we will see further attempts to improve upon hemostatic proteins found in nature. These novel coagulation proteins will very likely see a parallel course of development for use in routine exogenous protein replacement as well as in trials of gene therapy. It is in this setting that the biosynthetic and functional advantages of new, bioengineered forms of FVIII and FIX may be of greatest benefit as an answer to the longstanding problem of inadequate levels of transgene expression in hemophilia gene therapy studies. Finally, however, as the native protein structures are altered to achieve enhanced biological function, systems to assess the potential immunogenicity of these novel molecules will become critically important if we are to avoid an increased incidence of inhibitor generation.

References

1 Mingozzi F, Schuttrumpf J, Arruda VR, *et al.* Improved hepatic gene transfer by using an adeno-associated virus serotype 5 vector. *J Virol* 2002; **76**: 10497–502.

2 Chao H, Liu Y, Rabinowitz J, *et al.* Several log increase in therapeutic transgene delivery by distinct adeno-associated viral serotype vectors. *Mol Ther* 2000; **2**: 619–23.

3 Hagstrom JN, Couto LB, Scallan C, *et al.* Improved muscle-derived expression of human coagulation factor IX from a skeletal actin/CMV hybrid enhancer/promoter. *Blood* 2000; **95**: 2536–42.

4 Notley C, Killoran A, Cameron C, *et al.* The canine factor VIII 3′-untranslated region and a concatemeric hepatocyte nuclear factor 1 regulatory element enhance factor VIII transgene expression in vivo. *Hum Gene Ther* 2002; **13**: 1583–93.

5 Kaufman RJ, Pipe SW. Can we improve on nature? "Super molecules" of factor VIII. *Haemophilia* 1998; **4**: 370–9.

6 Saenko EL, Ananyeva NM, Shima M, *et al.* The future of recombinant coagulation factors. *J Thromb Haemost* 2003; **1**: 922–30.

7 Cameron C, Notley C, Hoyle S, *et al.* The canine factor VIII cDNA and 5′ flanking sequence. *Thromb Haemost* 1998; **79**: 317–22.

8 Chang JY, Monroe DM, Stafford DW, *et al.* Replacing the first epidermal growth factor-like domain of factor IX with that of factor VII enhances activity in vitro and in canine hemophilia B. *J Clin Invest* 1997; **100**: 886–92.

9 Chang J, Jin J, Lollar P, *et al.* Changing residue 338 in human factor IX from arginine to alanine causes an increase in catalytic activity. *J Biol Chem* 1998; **273**: 12089–94.

10 Ananyeva NM, Kouiavskaia DV, Shima M, Saenko EL. Catabolism of the coagulation factor VIII: can we prolong lifetime of f VIII in circulation? *Trends Cardiovasc Med* 2001; **11**: 251–7.

11 Saenko EL, Yakhyaev AV, Mikhailenko I, *et al.* Role of the low density lipoprotein-related protein receptor in mediation of factor VIII catabolism. *J Biol Chem* 1999; **274**: 37685–92.

12 Lenting PJ, Neels JG, van den Berg BM, *et al.* The light chain of factor VIII comprises a binding site for low density lipoprotein receptor-related protein. *J Biol Chem* 1999; **274**: 23734–9.

13 Sarafanov AG, Ananyeva NM, Shima M, Saenko EL. Cell surface heparan sulfate proteoglycans participate in factor VIII catabolism mediated by low density lipoprotein receptor-related protein. *J Biol Chem* 2001; **276**: 11970–9.

14 Scandella DH. Properties of anti-factor VIII inhibitor antibodies in hemophilia A patients. *Semin Thromb Haemost* 2000; **26**: 137–42.

15 Scandella D, Mondorf W, Klinge J. The natural history of the immune response to exogenous factor VIII in severe haemophilia A. *Haemophilia* 1998; **4**: 546–51.

16 Fijnvandraat K, Berntorp E, ten Cate JW, *et al.* Recombinant, B-domain deleted factor VIII (r-VIII SQ): pharmacokinetics and initial safety aspects in hemophilia A patients. *Thromb Haemost* 1997; **77**: 298–302.

17 Berntorp E. Second generation, B-domain deleted recombinant factor VIII. *Thromb Haemost* 1997; **78**: 256–60.

18 Sandberg H, Almstedt A, Brandt J, *et al.* Structural and functional characterization of B-domain deleted recombinant factor VIII. *Semin Hematol* 2001; **38**: 4–12.

19 Pittman DD, Alderman EM, Tomkinson KN, *et al.* Biochemical, immunological, and in vivo functional characterization of B-domain-deleted factor VIII. *Blood* 1993; **81**: 2925–35.

20 Mikaelsson M, Oswaldsson U, Jankowski MA. Measurement of factor VIII activity of B-domain deleted recombinant factor VIII. *Semin Hematol* 2001; **38**: 13–23.

21 Mikaelsson M, Oswaldsson U. Assaying the circulating factor VIII activity in hemophilia A patients treated with recombinant factor VIII products. *Semin Thromb Haemost* 2002; **28**: 257–64.

22 Pipe SW, Miao H, Tendulkar R, Kaufman RJ. Asparagine-linked glycosylation sites within the B domain of coagulation factor VIII improve secretion efficiency. *Blood* 2001; **98**: 705a.

23 Pipe SW, Kaufman RJ. Characterization of a genetically engineered inactivation-resistant coagulation factor VIIIa. *Proc Natl Acad Sci USA* 1997; **94**: 11851–6.

24 Gale AJ, Pellequer JL. An engineered interdomain disulfide bond stabilizes human blood coagulation factor VIIIa. *J Thromb Haemost* 2003; **1**: 1966–71.

25 Lenting PJ, Van Mourik JA, Mertens K. The life cycle of coagulation

factor VIII in view of its structure and function. *Blood* 1998; **92**: 3983–96.

26 Bovenschen N, Herz J, Grimbergen JM, *et al.* Elevated plasma factor VIII in a mouse model of low-density lipoprotein receptor-related protein deficiency. *Blood* 2003; **101**: 3933–9.

27 Kamphuisen PW, Eikenboom JC, Bertina RM. Elevated factor VIII levels and the risk of thrombosis. *Arterioscler Thromb Vasc Biol* 2001; **21**: 731–8.

28 Peerlinck K, Arnout J, Gilles JG, *et al.* A higher than expected incidence of factor VIII inhibitors in multitransfused haemophilia A patients treated with an intermediate purity pasteurized factor VIII concentrate. *Thromb Haemost* 1993; **69**: 115–18.

29 Rothschild C, Goudemand J, Demiguel V, *et al.* Effect of type of treatment (recombinant vs plasmatic) on FVIII inhibitor incidence according to known risk factors in previously untreated severe hemophilia A patients (PUPs). *J Thromb Haemost* 2003; Suppl: 215 (Abstract).

30 Scandella D. Human anti-factor VIII antibodies: epitope localization and inhibitory function. *Vox Sang* 1996; **70**: 9–14.

31 Lollar P. Mapping factor VIII inhibitor epitopes using hybrid human/porcine factor VIII molecules. *Haematologica* 2000; **85**: 26–8.

32 Healey JF, Barrow RT, Tamim HM, *et al.* Residues Glu2181–Val2243 contain a major determinant of the inhibitory epitope in the C2 domain of human factor VIII. *Blood* 1998; **92**: 3701–9.

33 Healey JF, Lubin IM, Nakai H, *et al.* Residues 484–508 contain a major determinant of the inhibitory epitope in the A2 domain of human factor VIII. *J Biol Chem* 1995; **270**: 14505–9.

34 Barrow RT, Healey JF, Gailani D, *et al.* Reduction of the antigenicity of factor VIII toward complex inhibitory antibody plasmas using multiply-substituted hybrid human/porcine factor VIII molecules. *Blood* 2000; **95**: 564–8.

35 Chao H, Walsh CE. Induction of tolerance to human factor VIII in mice. *Blood* 2001; **97**: 3311–12.

36. White GC, Beebe A, Nielsen B. Recombinant factor IX. *Thromb Haemost* 1997; **78**: 261–5.

37. Poon MC, Lillicrap D, Hensman C, *et al.* Recombinant factor IX recovery and inhibitor safety: a Canadian post-licensure surveillance study. *Thromb Haemost* 2002; **87**: 431–5.

38 Arruda VR, Hagstrom JN, Deitch J, *et al.* Posttranslational modifications of recombinant myotube-synthesized human factor IX. *Blood* 2001; **97**: 130–8.

39 Wolberg AS, Stafford DW, Erie DA. Human factor IX binds to specific sites on the collagenous domain of collagen IV. *J Biol Chem* 1997; **272**: 16717–20.

40 Schuettrumpf J, Herzog RW, Kaufhold A, *et al.* Improving efficacy of gene therapy of hemophilia B by the use of mutant FIX variants. *J Thromb Haemost* 2003; Suppl.: 44 (Abstract).

Laboratory assays in hemophilia

Jørgen Ingerslev

Introduction

During the coagulation process, factor VIII (FVIII) and FIX provide their natural support of the conversion of FX into FXa, thereby creating the biochemical basis for generation of thrombin, which catalyzes the production of a fibrin clot. In hemophilia, the lack of FVIII or FIX dramatically reduces the capacity of this intrinsic Xase reaction and, in consequence, there is a significantly delayed formation of insufficient amounts of fragile fibrin strands, which are unable to provide robust hemostasis.

In a hemophilic patient who receives infusions of factor concentrate sufficient to restore incrementally the factor level to 100% of normal, hemostasis should be similar to that in a non-hemophilic individual. An unresolved issue in the management of hemophilia is lack of evidence for a critical factor level that determines the arrest of bleeding and maintains hemostasis. Instead, weight-based dosage guidelines for various of types of bleed and surgery are quite commonplace in hemophilia management today, despite the fact that a heterogeneic response to treatment among patients is well recognized. The obvious lack of evidence from larger randomized controlled clinical trials creates a huge demand for laboratory monitoring of treatment in patients.

The assays commonly used in hemophilia laboratory services for diagnosis, classification, and therapy monitoring will be addressed and discussed here, and some general comments on their utility will be given. Since manufacturers of coagulation instruments and reagents provide consumers with complete protocols for recording of coagulation factors, individual assay protocols will not be considered.

The fundamentals of biometry of FVIII and FIX have previously been reported in detail in an excellent monograph, dated 1984 [1–4].

About factor VIII and IX

The FVIII molecule is undoubtedly one of the most unstable of the frequently recorded coagulation factors. FVIII displays a great ability to absorb onto foreign surfaces, and it degrades quickly when exposed to ambient temperature, if the pH value falls outside a rather narrow range, and if the FVIII molecule is exposed to natural proteolytic plasma enzymes that irreversibly inactivate FVIII. Contributing to accuracy problems, samples may give different results with different reagents and instruments.

In most of these respects, the FIX molecule is less sensitive to storage and assay conditions.

Laboratory work-up for the diagnosis of hemophilia

Table 41.1 lists analytical procedures commonly used to establish the diagnosis of hemophilia, simultaneously ruling out related bleeding disorders.

The activated partial thromboplastin time (aPTT)

In most instances, a prolonged aPTT detected in an otherwise healthy male suffering an increased tendency to bleeding is the hallmark of a deficiency state of a coagulation factor belonging to the contact pathway of coagulation, raising the suspicion of hemophilia. A multitude of different aPTT reagents are available on the market. Variance in response is related to the nature of the activating substance as well as to the type and composition of phospholipids. In most instances, protocols are provided by the manufacturer for their use with various kinds of coagulation instruments. When selecting a particular aPTT reagent for routine use in hemophilia management, there are two main points to consider: (i) the sensitivity of the reagent to detect all severity classes of hemophilia (severe, moderate, and mild) and (ii) the suitability of the reagent in assays of single coagulation factor determination. In the daily routine, most laboratories find it most practical to use the same aPTT reagent for screening and activity determination of factors in order to avoid performance errors.

Further, the content and composition of the aPTT phospholipids reagent may be an important determinant for accurate assessment of recombinant FVIII in (postinfusion) hemophilic plasma samples [5]. The assay procedure should follow the guidelines specified by the manufacturer, in particular the proposed time for preactivation prior to addition of calcium.

Keeping in mind the successes achieved with the widely adopted international normalized ratio (INR) system used for control of vitamin K antagonist treatment, several proposals have been made for standardized principles for estimation of the aPTT. However, the multitude of phospholipids and activators of various aPTT reagents have proved major obstacles in stan-

Table 41.1 Laboratory procedures commonly used in the diagnosis of hemophilia.

Platelet count	Platelet aggregation
	Agonists: collagen, ADP, ristocetin
aPTT	Activated partial thromboplastin time
PT	Prothrombin time
Factor VIII:C	Factor VIII procoagulant function (one-stage and/or chromogenic substrate method)
Factor VIII:Ag	Factor VIII antigenic determination
vWF: RCo	von Willebrand factor ristocetin cofactor
vWF:Ag	von Willebrand factor antigen
vWF:FVIIIB	von Willebrand factor/FVIII-binding capacity
Fibrinogen	Functional assay for fibrinogen
Factor XIII	Enzymatic factor XIII assay

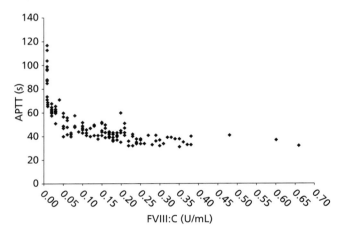

Figure 41.1 The relationship between factor VIII:C levels and aPTT in 140 plasma samples from patients with hemophilia A and five from patients with a reduced level of FVIII:C. The aPTT reagent was Platelin Excel (Organon Teknika, Turnhout, Belgium) and the aPTT and FVIII:C assays were carried out by the one-stage technique.

dardization, and as of today no recommended standard procedure exists.

Which kind of information does the crude aPTT really provide in practical use in hemophilia? Figure 41.1 illustrates graphically a large number of raw aPTT results determined in hemophilia A patients and a few people with a reduced FVIII plotted against the corresponding one-stage FVIII:C value recorded in the same sample. As shown, and as is well known to many physicians, severely affected hemophilia patients display a huge inter-patient variation in the aPTT time. In moderate and mild hemophilia A, there is a quite useful correlation with FVIII:C levels from around 0.02 U/mL, but the aPTT itself is a rather poor predictor of the correct diagnostic class or the outcome of the FVIII:C level recording.

Factor VIII activity (FVIII:C) measured by the one-stage technique

The assay for recording of FVIII:C in plasma by the one-stage assay represents an extension of the aPTT assay. It relies on the assumption that the time of clotting is a function of the level of FVIII:C in a reaction system where FVIII is the only variable, whereas all other plasma coagulation factors are constant and normal. The test base is severe hemophilia A plasma (SHP) and the primary standard should be the current international standard for plasma FVIII. Secondary standards (in-house plasma pool or commercial standard) are used in the daily routine assays following local recalibration against the international standard or other well-documented standard material. Calibration is recommended when analytical conditions change (i.e., shift of batch of aPTT reagent, change of secondary standard, shift of pool of SHP, etc.).

Deficiency plasmas

In the routine laboratory, severe hemophilia plasma (SHP) is best obtained from a well-characterized patient with severe hemophilia A (residual FVIII:C level <0.01 IU/mL, FVIII:Ag <0.01 IU/mL, and no detectable inhibitors) who has not received FVIII concentrate for 2 weeks or more. Owing to frequent treatment or prophylaxis, such material may be difficult to obtain today, and concern about laboratory operator safety often limits the use of plasma derived from patients. Commercial FVIII-deficient plasmas are usually produced by immunodepletion techniques or other principles, which may not completely remove FVIII molecules from the (healthy donor) raw plasma. The presence of tiny amounts of residual FVIII:C activity or FVIII:Ag may compromise the classification of the unknown hemophilia A patient, hamper the recording of postinfusion values of FVIII:C following administration of highly purified FVIII concentrates, and reduce the sensitivity of an assay for inhibitors against FVIII. Among commercial FVIII deficiency plasmas, some are also depleted in von Willebrand factor, which may increase the risk of accuracy problems in estimation of postdosage FVIII by the one-stage techniques following infusion of recombinant FVIII concentrates.

Calibration of the assay

Analytical variance is a major issue in FVIII:C recording. The automated instruments used today often have a memory function that saves calibration curves for various lengths of time. While such systems may save money and time for procedures recording several other components, they are not well chosen for FVIII measurements.

The calibration procedure is critical in recording of FVIII:C by the one-stage assay. A freshly prepared standard curve made up by several dilution steps of standard in SHP should be used in every series of FVIII:C measurements carried out. Double determinations are essential, and unknown sample material should preferably be tested at two or more different dilution steps.

Factor VIII:C measured by two-stage assays

In the past, the two-stage technique was often employed for its more accurate measurement of FVIII:C. This method is based on the activation of FX aided by activated FVIII and excess activated FIX, FVIIIa being the rate-limiting factor in the assay. In the second step, the function of FXa is recorded. A newer version of the two-stage assay, called the chromogenic substrate assay or peptide amidolytic assay, has replaced the traditional two-stage assay that was used in most clinical laboratories several years ago.

The principal reaction steps of the chromogenic assay are outlined in Figure 41.2.

The chromogenic assay methods record the enzymatic activity of activated FX (FXa), which is formed by the concerted action of FVIII (thrombin-) activated into FVIIIa and a preformed excess of FIXa in an environment containing phospholipids. Similar to the traditional two-stage assay, FVIIIa is the rate-limiting factor in the chromogenic reaction.

In certain respects, the critical requirements in the chromogenic assay are similar to those of the one-stage assay. A multiple dilution point standard curve should be used. If very low levels of FVIII:C are expected, a separate calibration curve should be adopted for recordings at the lower end of the dynamic measurement range (below 0.20 IU/mL of FVIII:C). Manufacturers' recommended preactivation time (activation of FVIII to FVIIIa) should be followed strictly. The principles for standardization and calibration of the chromogenic assay are similar to those mentioned for the one-stage assay. A clear advantage of the chromogenic assay is improved precision; often the coefficient of variation (CV, %) is half of that obtained with the one-stage assay, as reported in several publications.

Quality control systems in the hemostasis laboratory

In addition to the use of in-assay control procedures, which are mandatory in coagulometry, as in all other laboratory proce-

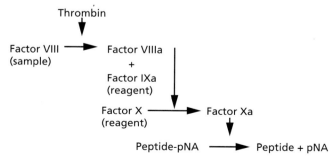

Figure 41.2 Reaction scheme steps in the chromogenic substrate method for measurement of factor VIII:C. The release of yellow free pNA molecules depends on the amount of FVIII in the sample.

dures, participation in national and international proficiency programs is very useful. Two major nonprofit organizations exist to serve laboratories on a multinational basis. In Europe, the ECAT Foundation (www.ecat.nl) annually distributes four sets of samples for proficiency testing of hemostasis components as well as a broad-based thrombophilia program. In North America, a collaborating sister organization, NASCOLA (www.nascola.org), offers a similar program. These quality assessment programs are highly valuable and of great benefit to participants.

Assay discrepancy

With some patient sample material, inconsistent results are found when comparing results of recordings of FVIII:C by the one-stage assay with those obtained with the chromogenic assay. This difference is often referred to using the term "assay discrepancy." The most likely explanation for the assay discrepancy phenomenon is differences in the way in which FVIII is activated with the two types of assays.

The FVIII activation during the course of the aPTT-based one-stage assay most likely depends on the endogenous formation of thrombin in the reaction mixture, while the chromogenic assay reagents contain exogenous thrombin that directly activates FVIII, and further thrombin formation is quenched through the use of a specific thrombin inhibitor.

Assay discrepancy has predominantly been observed in samples from certain subsets of mild hemophilia A patients, in high-purity FVIII concentrates, and in postinfusion samples from hemophilia patients undergoing treatment with FVIII concentrates purified by monoclonal antibody techniques and, in particular, recombinant FVIII concentrates.

Assay discrepancy in mild hemophilia

The assay discrepancy phenomenon in mild hemophilia was initially reported with the traditional two-stage assay for FVIII:C [6,7]. This phenomenon is probably more prevalent than previously thought. Figure 41.3 illustrates the assay discrepancy phenomenon in mild hemophilia. Plasma samples from 69 nonrecently infused patients with mild hemophilia A from 43 families were recorded by the one-stage assay and a chromogenic assay. The figure is a differential plot in which the difference between the one-stage FVIII:C result and the corresponding chromogenic FVIII:C value is plotted. If results are concordant, data should be located close to the zero line of the plot. However, a majority of patients display a significant difference between the two. In one of our families, as well as in numerous families worldwide, the assay discrepancy phenomenon in mild hemophilia was found to be associated with missense mutations causing a premature disruption of the A2 domain when exposed to thrombin [8,9]. In these examples, the one-stage assay gave a higher FVIII:C activity compared with the chromogenic assay, but cases have also been identified with the

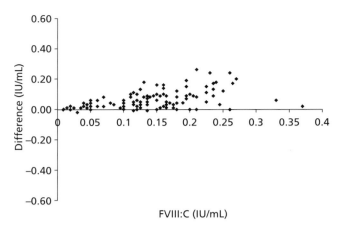

Figure 41.3 Differential plot of FVIII:C assay recorded by the one-stage method and by the chromogenic substrate method in 69 patients with moderate and mild hemophilia A from 43 Danish families. In each case, the chromogenic method result is subtracted from the one-stage result.

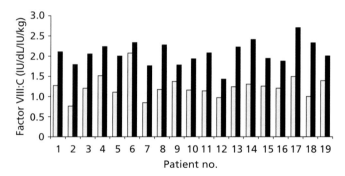

Figure 41.4 Assay discrepancy in plasma from each of 19 hemophilia A patients. The sample was collected 15 min after infusion of around 25 IU/kg of a BDD recombinant FVIII product. Gray bars: FVIII:C incremental value determined by a one-stage FVIII:C assay; black bars: FVIII:C incremental value determined by a chromogenic substrate assay for FVIII:C. The expected incremental value is around 2.00.

opposite finding, and a normal chromogenic FVIII:C result [10].

Assay discrepancy in postinfusion samples following concentrate administration

In clinical practice, assay discrepancy has been reported in hemophilia A patients undergoing treatment with recombinant FVIII products. In general, the assay discrepancy reported is in the range of 10–30%, the one-stage assay persistently giving the lowest result [11,12]. Most markedly discrepant results have been found with a B domain-depleted (BDD) recombinant FVIII concentrate. An illustration of this is found in Figure 41.4,

which shows a series of 19 patients with hemophilia in whom we routinely assessed the recovery of FVIII following infusion of a dose of around 25 IU/kg of BDD recombinant FVIII. The response was calculated as the incremental rise in IU/dL divided by IU/kg b.w. (body weight) as measured by a one-stage assay as well as by a chromogenic substrate assay. The common standard was a plasma pool previously calibrated against the 4th International Standard for FVIII in plasma. As shown, discrepant results were observed in all cases comparing the two types of assay, and the mean response was 1.27 IU/mL for the one-stage and 2.07 IU/mL for the chromogenic substrate assay. Overall, the mean ratio of one-stage FVIII:C/chromogenic FVIII:C was 0.61. Moreover, as can be seen from Figure 41.4, the assay discrepancy appears to vary substantially between patients. The assay discrepancy phenomenon with BDD recombinant FVIII can more or less be abolished using modified one-stage assays in which phospholipids are changed in composition or concentration [13,14].

When recording FVIII in postinfusion samples, the biologic effects of concentrate are similar to those of diluting concentrate in FVIII-deficient plasma *in vitro*, and the coagulometric response is expected to be similar to that obtained by adding concentrate to SHP *ex vivo*. Therefore, when recording the response to infusion of recombinant BDD FVIII, the International Society on Thrombosis and Hemostasis (ISTH) has recommended the use of the "like-versus-like" principle in which a concentrate standard of the same manufacture is used for calibration of the one-stage assay employed. A multilaboratory field study has demonstrated that the assay discrepancy phenomenon is abolished when the aforementioned strategy is adopted [15]. In contrast, since the chromogenic assay is not influenced by the type of concentrate infused when recorded against a plasma FVIII standard, the chromogenic analysis principle performs well with a plasma-based FVIII calibrator. For full-length recombinant FVIII concentrates, no recommendations have been endorsed on the use of concentrate-specific standard material at this time.

For accurate determination of FVIII in all kinds of biologic materials, it would be highly desirable to have a common assay that is unaffected by the purity of FVIII or FIX in concentrates and that is also unaffected by matrix effects. Such a system has recently been developed and tested for its suitability in recording of FVIII of varying purity and composition [16].

Factor IX:C measurements

In recording FIX:C, the fundamental principles of the assay system are the same as those governing the measurement of FVIII:C: the use of the international standard for plasma FIX:C as the primary standard for calibration of the assay, the need for a well-controlled severely FIX:C-deficient plasma test base, and the use of controls.

Chromogenic peptide assay systems do exist for recording of FIX:C, but such assays have not been challenged in formal standardization procedures and assays of this kind and they are not widely used in clinical hemostasis laboratories.

Models for studying the entire process of coagulation

In daily laboratory practice, determination of hemophilia is based on the use of citrated plasma, and the initial signal of coagulation is utilized in all methods based on the global aPTT and PT assays, the endpoint of the analysis being determined by a change in light transmission or in viscoelastic mechanical resistance. When measuring FVIII and FIX activities using clotting assays, the same endpoint principles are utilized. For around half a century, researchers have speculated whether surveillance of the entire process of coagulation might provide more information on the pathology of coagulation in various hemorrhagic disorders. An early finding was that a considerable amount of thrombin activity is generated in plasma over a period of several minutes after the initial signs of fibrin formation [17] demonstrable in continuously collected subsamples from the reaction mixture. Another early method (the thrombelastograph) characterizes the course of coagulation by means of the mechanical elasticity changes occurring in whole blood during fibrin polymerization. Although these assays differ in one respect, one being based on diluted and defibrinated plasma with or without platelets and the other using undiluted whole blood, the general characteristics of the courses of thrombin generation and fibrin formation appear to be quite similar in healthy subjects. Recent developments have led to the development of a fully automated method for study of thrombin generation [18,19]. Although not routinely utilized in the study of hemophilia, this method has considerable potential to be used in clinical research into these bleeding disorders.

A recent development of the thrombelastographic method has shown that severe hemophilia A appears to be highly heterogeneous in its pattern of fibrin formation, and that the response to *ex vivo* substitution with FVIII is highly variable among patients [20].

In the study of hemophilia and the response to treatment with these methods, research is only in its infancy. However, the adoption of study of continuous formation of thrombin or fibrin would appear to be a promising avenue in hemophilia research.

Determination of the antigens of factor VIII and factor IX

Estimation of the antigenic concentration of the coagulation factor lacking in patients' blood has several advantages, especially for phenotyping. A CRM– (cross-reacting material negative) status (low or no recordable antigen) is most often associated with a severe bleeding condition and linkage to a genetic defect that may predict a high-risk inhibitor formation, whereas a CRM+ condition (excess of antigen over activity) is

rarely found in patients with severe hemophilia but is often seen in milder cases.

For several years, immunoradiometric assays or ELISAs have existed for quantitation of FVIII antigenic concentration, and antibodies derived from patients with inhibitors were most often used in such assays. Since ultra-pure FVIII was difficult to obtain and immunization of animals often resulted in antibodies with cross-reactivity to other plasma proteins, only a few laboratories were capable of recording FVIII:Ag. Today, homemade as well as commercial ELISA systems are more widely available for quantitation of FVIII:Ag (see, e.g., ref. 21).

FIX:Ag is quite easily recorded by ELISA-based methods, and commercial kits and home-made methods are in widespread use.

Inhibitors to factor VIII and factor IX

The Bethesda assay and the Nijmegen modified assay variants

The classical test system for determination of inhibitors against FVIII and FIX is the Bethesda assay, which was published in 1975. In principle, this recording system is based on the well-known principle that inhibitors inactivate the FVIII or FIX molecules of normal plasma. In practice, several different dilutions of patient's plasma are added to a normal plasma sample and incubated for 2 h at 37°C, at the end of which all samples are recorded for their residual content of FVIII:C or FIX:C. A positive result is noted when a sample causes a significant loss of FVIII:C or FIX:C of normal plasma at 50% of the content of the control sample. Dilutions and residual FVIII:C are plotted against each other and the inhibitor titer is obtained by linear regression. This system was unchanged for 20 years until a modified assay was published in which the natural instability of FVIII and the change of pH occurring during the rather lengthy incubation period were compensated for by the use of buffered normal plasma, and by including SHP in the control mixture [22,23]. Using this assay, a number of false-positive inhibitors could largely be excluded. Later, it was found that SHP could be replaced by a 4% albumin solution [24]. Since then, the Nijmegen modification of the Bethesda assay has been increasingly adopted in clinical laboratory work. Two major problems remain unresolved: the low accuracy of inhibitor assays in general and the lack of consensus in terms of the low detection limit of inhibitors by functional methods (most often referred to as 0.6 Bethesda units per mL). The accuracy problem is tightly linked with the inherent imprecision of the one-stage FVIII assay.

In order to overcome this problem to some extent, attempts have been made to record inhibitors using a chromogenic substrate assay for FVIII. No larger series of patient samples have as yet been published on the chromogenic method. In a smaller study, inhibitor titers were lower when measured with the chromogenic assay as compared with the one-stage assay result (S. Raut, personal communication).

Detecting inhibitors using immunologic methods

Among physicians it is generally well known that the Bethesda assay is insensitive to weakly reacting inhibitors, the presence of which may be observed only by a reduced *in vivo* recovery of infused concentrate or a shortened *in vivo* half-life of concentrate administered. Two principal methods of detecting such nonmeasurable inhibitors have been introduced. In some cases, patient antibodies may be detected by their capacity to immunoprecipitate FVIII. However, in a series of patients from Germany, the immunoprecipitation method did not detect inhibitors that were undetectable by the Bethesda assay [25].

Second, various ELISAs have been developed demonstrating increased sensitivity to weakly titered antibodies [26–28]. In interpreting the results of both of the aforementioned assays, noninhibitory antibodies against FVIII cannot be distinguished from inhibiting antibodies. Several investigators have shown that noninhibiting antibodies against FVIII are a quite frequent and harmless finding in healthy individuals. This means that detection of an antibody against FVIII using immunologic methods in hemophilia patients could raise suspicion of an inhibitor, but the specificity of the results is dubious and their predictive value questionable.

Concluding remarks

Although, today, sufficient amounts of concentrates with a high safety profile are available for the treatment of hemophilia, the hemostasis laboratory still has an important role to play in correctly determining the phenotype of patients with a hemorrhagic disorder and in ensuring optimal substitution treatment. There is an urgent need for appropriate point-of-care methods in hemophilia to help tailor individualized treatment protocols.

References

1 Over J. Methodology of the one-stage assay of factor VIII (VIII:C). *Scand J Haematol* 1984; **33**: 13–24.

2 Barrowcliffe T. Methodology of the two-stage assays of factor VIII. *Scand J Haematol* 1984; **33**: 25–38.

3 Barrowcliffe T. Comparisons of one-stage and two-stage assays of factor VIII:C. *Scand J Haematol* 1984; **33**: 39–54.

4 Curtis A. The statistical evaluation of factor VIII clotting assays. *Scand J Haematol* 1984; **33**: 55–70.

5 Mikaelsson M, Oswaldsson U, Sandberg H. Influence of phospholipids on the assessment of factor VIII activity. *Haemophilia* 1998; **4**: 646–50.

6 Parquet-Gernez A, Mazurier C, Goudemand M. Functional and immunological assays of F VIII in 133 haemophiliacs — characterization of a subgroup of patients with mild haemophilia A and discrepancy in 1- and 2-stage assays. *Thromb Haemost* 1988; **59**: 202–6.

7 Rudzki Z, Duncan EM, Casey GJ, *et al.* Mutations in a subgroup of patients with mild haemophilia A and discrepancy between the one-stage and two-stage factor VIII:C methods. *Br Haematol* 1996; **94**: 400–6.

8 Pipe SW, Eickhorst AN, McKinley SH, *et al.* Mild hemophilia A caused by increased rate of factor VIII A2 subunit dissociation: evidence for nonproteolytic inactivation of factor VIII in vivo. *Blood* 1999; **93**: 176–83.

9 Schwaab R, Oldenburg J, Kemball-Cook G, *et al.* Assay discrepancy in mild haemophilia A due to a factor VIII missense mutation (Asn694Ile) in a large Danish family. *Br J Haematol* 2000; **109**: 523–8.

10 Mumford AD, Laffan M, O'Donnell J, *et al.* A Tyr346 → Cys substitution in the interdomain acidic region a1 of factor VIII in an individual with factor VIII:C assay discrepancy. *Br J Haematol* 2002; **118**: 589–94.

11 Lee CA, Owens D, Bray G, *et al.* Pharmacokinetics of recombinant factor VIII (Recombinate) using one-stage clotting and chromogenic factor VIII assay. *Thromb Haemost* 1999; **82**: 1644–7.

12 Morfini M, Cinotti S, Belatreccia A, *et al.* A multicenter pharmacokinetic study of the B-domain deleted recombinant factor VIII concentrate using different assays and standards. *J Thromb Haemost* 2003; **1**: 2283–9.

13 Mikaelsson M, Oswaldsson U, Sandberg H. Influence of phospholipids on the assessment of factor VIII activity. *Haemophilia* 1998; **4**: 646–50.

14 Caron C, Dautzenberg M-D, Delahousse B, *et al.* A blinded *in vitro* study with Refacto mock plasma samples: similar F VIII results between the chromogenic assay and a one-stage assay using higher cephalin dilution. *Haemophilia* 2002; **8**: 639–43.

15 Ingerslev J, Jankowski MJ, Weston SB, *et al.* collaborative field study on the utility of a BDD Factor VIII concentrate standard in the estimation of BDD Factor VIII:C activity in hemophilic plasma using one-stage clotting assays. *J Thromb Haemost* 2004; **2**: 623–8.

16 Eich S, Kusch M, Grundmann C, *et al.* Factor VIII determination in patients' plasma and concentrates: a novel test equally suited for both matrices. *Blood Coagul Fibrinol* 2003; **14**: 347–53.

17 MacFarlane RG, Biggs R. A thrombin generation test; the application in haemophilia and thrombocytopenia. *J Clin Pathol* 1953; **6**: 3–8.

18 Hemker HC, Beguin S. Thrombin generation in plasma: its assessment via the endogenous thrombin potential. *Thromb Haemost* 1995; **74**: 1388.

19 Hemker HC, Giesen P, Al Dieri R, *et al.* Calibrated automated thrombin generation measurement in clotting plasma. *Pathophysiol Haemostasis Thromb* 2003; **33**: 4–15.

20 Ingerslev J, Poulsen LH, Sørensen B. Potential role of the dynamic properties of whole blood coagulation in assessment of dosage requirements in haemophilia. *Haemophilia* 2003; **9**: 348–52.

21 Girma J-P, Fressinaud E, Houllier A, *et al.* Assay of factor VIII antigen (VIII:CAg) in 294 haemophilia A patients by a new commercial ELISA using monoclonal antibodies. *Haemophilia* 1998; **4**: 98–103.

22 Verbrugen B, Novakova I, Wessels H, *et al.* The Nijmegen modification of the Bethesda assay for factor VIII:C inhibitors: improved specificity and reliability. *Thromb Haemost* 1995; **73**:247–51.

23 Giles AR, Verbruggen B, Rivard GE, *et al.* A detailed comparison of the performance of the standard versus the Nijmegen modification of the Bethesda assay in detecting factor VIII:C inhibitors in the haemophilia A population of Canada. Association of Hemophilia Centre Directors of Canada. Factor VIII/IX Subcommittee of Scientific and Standardization Committee of International Society on Thrombosis and Hemostasis. *Thromb Haemost* 1998; **79**: 872–5.

24 Verbruggen B, van Heerde W, Novakova I, *et al.* A 4% solution of bovine serum albumin may be used in place of factor VIII:C deficient

plasma in the control sample in the Nijmegen Modification of the Bethesda factor VIII:C inhibitor assay. *Thromb Haemost* 2002; **88**: 362–4.

25 Mondorf W, Klinge J, Luban NL, *et al*. Low factor VIII recovery in haemophilia A patients without inhibitor titre is not due to the presence of anti-factor VIII antibodies undetectable by the Bethesda assay. *Haemophilia* 2001; **7**: 3–9.

26 Mondorf W, Ehrenforth S, Vigh Z, *et al*. Screening of F.VIII:C anti-

bodies by an enzyme-linked immunosorbent assay. *Vox Sang* 1994; **66**: 8–13.

27 Lindgren A, Wadenvik H, Tengborn L. Characterization of inhibitors to F VIII with an ELISA in congenital and acquired haemophilia A. *Haemophilia* 2002; **8**: 644–8.

28 Shetty S, Ghosh K, Mohanty D. ELISA for factor VIII antibodies: does it detect antibodies much before the conventional Bethesda assay? *Haemophilia* 2003; **9**: 654.

42 Standardization of assays

Trevor W. Barrowcliffe

Introduction

The aim of standardization in general is to ensure that assays carried out on a sample in one laboratory at any one time will give the same results when carried out in the same laboratory at a different time, or in a different laboratory. In this chapter, the principles and practice of standardization as applied to assays of coagulation factors will be described; the main emphasis is on factor VIII (FVIII) assays, which are the most frequently performed and present the most problems, but assays of FIX, von Willebrand factor (VWF), and factors of the rarer coagulation deficiencies are also covered.

Principles of biological standardization

Comparative bioassay

Coagulation factor assays are based on the principle of comparative bioassay, in which the observed results on test samples are compared with those of a standard of known potency. By testing different dilutions of the standard, a "dose–response" curve (usually converted to a straight line by mathematical manipulation) can be constructed, and the potency of the test sample can then be obtained by interpolation. The basic assumption implicit in this method is that the test sample behaves exactly like a dilution of the standard. In order to test this assumption, results for the test sample should be obtained at different dilutions. Ideally, at least three dilutions of both standard and test sample should be measured; when concentrations are expressed on a log scale, the lines for test and standard should then be parallel, and the potency can be determined from the distance between the lines. Because of possible errors in dilution and measurement, and the intrinsic biological variability of the assay system, both the dilutions and the measurements should be repeated, and the results subjected to statistical analysis. A full treatise on statistical analysis of bioassays is given by Finney [1], and a simple computer program for coagulation factor assays is described by Kirkwood and Snape [2].

Assays of concentrates by manufacturers and control laboratories usually follow the above principles, with several independent assays in order to maximize precision. However, many clinical laboratories only test patients' samples at a single dilution, a practice encouraged by the software on modern coagulometers. This practice can give only an imprecise estimate of potency and is to be deplored. All clinical samples should be tested with at least two different dilutions, and each dilution should be repeated, giving a minimum of four observations for each test sample; wherever possible, at least three dilutions should be tested and parallel line analysis should be performed.

Standards and units

The unit of activity for almost all coagulation factors was originally defined as the amount in 1 mL of "average normal plasma." This has the great advantage of clinical convenience, but it is clear that "average normal plasma" collected in different laboratories and at different times is unlikely to be the same. Indeed, when the first international collaborative study on FVIII was carried out, samples of pooled normal plasma in the 20 laboratories differed by up to a factor of 2 [3]. The only way that measurements in different laboratories can be standardized is for the various local or commercial standards used in the assays to be calibrated against stable reference standards with a fixed value.

The establishment of a range of international standards for measurements of biological activity began as long ago as 1925 with insulin — the first coagulation-related standard was that for heparin, in 1942. The first international standard for a coagulation factor (FVIII) was established in 1971 [3], and subsequently, international standards have been established for all the major coagulation factors (Table 42.1).

Establishment of international standards is the responsibility of the World Health Organization (WHO), and the work on preparation, maintenance and distribution of these standards is carried out by NIBSC (with the exception of a few standards that are held and distributed by CLB-Sanquin, Amsterdam). Because of the need to conserve stocks over a long time period, these standards cannot be used routinely in assays; they are intended to calibrate local and manufacturers' standards. For FVIII and FIX concentrates, working standards, calibrated against the WHO standards, are available from the Food and Drug Administration Center for Biologics Evaluation and Research (FDA/CBER) and the European Pharmacopoeia (EP). In the UK, working concentrate standards are available for FVII, FVIII, FIX, FX, and working plasma standards for fibrinogen, FII, FVII, FVIII, FIX, FX, VWF, antithrombin, protein C and protein S; these are provided by the National Institute for Biological Standards and Control (NIBSC).

Table 42.1 International and British standards for coagulation factors.

Factor	Type of standard		Type of material			Code
	IS	BS	Pl	Co	Pu	
II	✓		✓			99/826
	✓			✓		98/590
		✓		✓		02/162
VII	✓		✓			99/826
	✓			✓		97/592
		✓	✓			01/618
VIIa	✓				✓	89/688
VIII	✓		✓			02/150
	✓			✓		99/678
		✓	✓			00/586
		✓		✓		02/122
IX	✓		✓			99/826
	✓			✓		96/854
		✓	✓			01/618
		✓	✓			02/162
X	✓		✓			99/826
	✓			✓		98/590
		✓		✓		02/162
Thrombin	✓				✓	01/580
Fibrinogen	✓		✓			98/612
	✓			✓		98/614
		✓	✓			01/618
Antithrombin	✓		✓			93/768
	✓			✓		96/520
		✓	✓			01/618
Protein C	✓		✓			86/622
		✓	✓			01/618
Protein S	✓		✓			93/590
		✓	✓			01/618
VWF	✓		✓			02/150
	✓			✓		00/514
		✓	✓			01/618

Standards for factors V, XI, XII, and XIII are under development.
IS, International Standards; BS, British Standards; Pl, Plasma; Co, Concentrate; Pu, Purified.

"Like versus like"

The reason why there are separate plasma and concentrate standards for most coagulation factors is that, as in all biological assays, variability is minimized when the standard and test are of similar composition. This is not just a theoretical principle, it has been shown to work best in practice. Thus, when FVIII concentrates have been assayed against plasma, or vice versa, variability between laboratories has always been higher than for plasma versus plasma and concentrate versus concentrate assays [4,5].

There are two situations in which this principle is difficult to maintain. First, as is the case with FVIII, there may be a wide diversity of concentrates manufactured, so that even with a concentrate standard there may be substantial differences in composition between test and standard. Second, although postinfusion samples, being plasma from patients, are normally assayed against a plasma standard, in composition they resemble concentrates "diluted" in the patients' plasma, so there may be an argument for using concentrate standards instead. These points are dealt with more fully in subsequent sections.

Standardization of factor VIII assays

Assay methods for FVIII

The three methods that are used to assay FVIII are the one-stage and two-stage assays, both of which are coagulation assays, and the chromogenic method. The principles and practice of these methods were reviewed in detail in Chapter 41.

Although the one-stage method has always been preferred by clinical laboratories because of its simplicity and ease of automation, the two-stage method has been used extensively by manufacturers in the past because of its high precision and independence of supply of deficient plasma. At present, however, the two-stage method is used hardly at all in clinical laboratories and by only a few manufacturers, but the chromogenic method, which is based on the same principle as the two-stage assay, is being adopted increasingly for assays of concentrates. The reference method for concentrates in the European Pharmacopoeia was the two-stage assay, but in 1995 this was replaced with the chromogenic method, which is also the method recommended by the International Society on Thrombosis and Haemostasis (ISTH).

The one-stage method suffers from an extreme diversity in the reagents and assay conditions used; for instance, in clinical laboratories in the UK, 25 different aPTT reagents, 20 different deficient plasmas, 13 different reference plasmas, and 11 different instruments are used [source: UK National External Quality Assessment Scheme (NEQAS) data]. The chromogenic method has less variety, with only five different kits from four manufacturers being available. General comparisons between the methods have been reviewed extensively elsewhere [6,7].

Currently, most European manufacturers of concentrates use the chromogenic method to label their products, whereas most US concentrates, including the two full-length recombinant products, are assayed by the one-stage method. The B domain-deleted (BDD) recombinant product, ReFacto, is assayed by the chromogenic method.

Assays of concentrates

Potencies of FVIII concentrates are measured in International Units (IU), which are defined by the International Standard. As indicated in Table 42.2, the WHO standard has been replaced at approximately 5-year intervals. This is partly because of high demand, but also because of changes in the methods of production of clinical concentrates over time, and the need for the WHO standard to be representative of current concentrates. Although the previous (sixth) WHO standard was a recombinant product, the new (seventh) standard is a plasma-derived material; this is because of the large numbers of different plasma-derived products still manufactured and the relatively high variability when some of these products were assayed against the recombinant standard.

The large differences in composition among current plasma-derived and recombinant products has meant that the "like vs. like" principle is increasingly difficult to apply and, despite the universal use of the WHO standard as the primary reference material for concentrates, discrepancies between methods, and between different laboratories using the same method, still occur. However, the reasons for some of these discrepancies have been established, and recommendations developed.

In initial studies, the inter-laboratory variability for the very high-purity plasma-derived and recombinant concentrates was high, with geometric coefficients of variation (gCVs) ranging from 19% to over 100% for the three methods [8]. However, subsequent research identified a number of technical factors that had a particular influence on high-purity concentrates, especially recombinant, and therefore required standardization. These were:

1 FVIII-deficient plasma: the use of hemophilic plasma, or deficient plasma with a normal VWF level, was found to be essential to give full potency in one-stage assays.

2 Assay buffers: it was found that albumin at a concentration of 1% (w/v) was necessary in all assay buffers in order to obtain reproducible results.

3 Predilution: predilution with hemophilic plasma, or its equivalent, was necessary for assay of all recombinant and high-purity plasma-derived products, whichever assay method was used.

In a subsequent collaborative study by the same laboratories, using these simple modifications, the results showed a marked improvement, with gCVs for the two recombinant concentrates ranging from 3% to 10.7%; similar good inter-laboratory agreement was found for the other concentrates. Subsequently, these requirements for assay of recombinant and high-purity plasma-derived products were published as recommendations of the FVIII and FIX Subcommittee of the Scientific and Standardization Committee (SSC) of the ISTH [9].

These recommended assay conditions were used in an international collaborative study to calibrate the sixth WHO concentrate standard, a recombinant material, and the inter-laboratory gCVs overall were 9–10% [5]. Thus, it is clear from these studies that, provided certain technical requirements are adhered to, recombinant FVIII concentrates can be assayed sat-

Table 42.2 WHO factor VIII concentrate standards.

Number	Purity and type	Year established	Calibrated against
1	Low (PD)	1971	"Normal plasma"
2	Low (PD)	1978	Ist IS
3	Intermediate (PD)	1983	2nd IS
4	Intermediate (PD)	1989	3rd IS
5	High (PD)	1994	4th IS
6	Recombinant	1999	5th IS concentrate and 4th IS plasma
7	High (PD)	2003	5th and 6th IS concentrates, and EP2 and US mega 1 concentrate standard

PD, plasma derived; IS, international standard.

isfactorily against plasma-derived concentrate standards, and there is no need for separate standards for the two types of products. The question of whether plasma-derived products can be assayed satisfactorily against a recombinant FVIII standard was addressed in a study by Abertengo et al. [10]. In that study, nine different plasma-derived products were assayed against both the fifth (plasma-derived) and sixth (recombinant) WHO standards. There were no significant differences in potencies using the two standards, indicating that a recombinant standard can be satisfactory for calibration of a wide variety of plasma-derived concentrates.

Comparison of methods on concentrates

The use of concentrate standards for assay of therapeutic concentrates follows the "like vs. like" principle, and should theoretically result in potencies that are similar by the three different FVIII methods. Although this was broadly the case in the 1970s and early 1980s, developments in viral inactivation methods and the introduction of high-purity plasma-derived and recombinant products increased the diversity of composition of concentrates, and this has led to discrepancies between methods, even though concentrate standards are used. A survey of 13 different concentrates in 1990 [11] showed substantial discrepancies between the results of one-stage and two-stage assays, the one-stage potencies being higher than the two-stage for several plasma-derived products, by up to 40%. A more recent survey compared potency estimates by the one-stage and chromogenic methods in 10 different concentrates (seven plasma-derived and three recombinant) [12]. The largest discrepancies were associated with a plasma-derived immunopurified concentrate, where the mean one-stage potency exceeded the chromogenic potency by 33%, and with a BDD recombinant product, where the chromogenic potency exceeded the one-stage potency by 28%.

Comparisons of methods on full-length recombinant products have given varied results. As shown in Table 42.3, when several batches of each product were assayed at NIBSC against the WHO standard (fifth standard, a plasma-derived concentrate) using ISTH/SSC recommended methodology, there were no major differences between potencies with the three different methods; for product A the two-stage potencies were 8% lower than the chromogenic ($P < 0.05$), but none of the other comparisons was statistically significant.

Table 42.4 summarizes the data on potencies of recombinant concentrates from three "controlled" collaborative studies in which a common standard, defined protocol, and central calculation of results were used. It can be seen that, for five of the six data sets, the chromogenic assays gave mean potencies higher than those obtained using the one-stage method, by amounts ranging from 10% to 18%. It should be borne in mind that, at the time of the first two of these studies, the chromogenic method had only recently been introduced for the assay of concentrates in several laboratories, and data from the most recent study may be more relevant to the current situation.

Overall, it appears that, particularly if SSC-recommended methodology is used, the differences in potency of full-length recombinant products between one-stage and chromogenic methods are less than 10% and are unlikely to be clinically significant.

Table 42.3 Comparison of methods on full-length recombinant concentrates (data from NIBSC).

Product	No. of batches	Potency (percent of label)		
		One-stage	Two-stage	Chromogenic
A	10	95	91	99
B	6	112	105	106

NIBSC assays were performed with the WHO fifth concentrate standard and ISTH/SSC recommended methodology.

Manufacturers used the one-stage method against the US mega standard.

The situation with the BDD concentrate ReFacto is, however, less satisfactory. Mikaelsson *et al.* [13] found that, even when using the WHO concentrate standard and ISTH/SSC-recommended methodology, the potency of this concentrate was substantially higher by the chromogenic method than by the one-stage method, by up to a factor of 2 depending on the reagents used. Further studies showed that this discrepancy was a result of the type and concentration of phospholipid reagent used in the one-stage method, and comparison with assays in the presence of platelets, and with *in vivo* recovery data, showed that the chromogenic potency was the appropriate value. The chromogenic method is therefore used by the manufacturers to label this product. Recent studies have shown that, in assays of ReFacto against concentrate standards, either plasma-derived or full-length recombinant, differences of up to 20% may be found between results with different chromogenic kits [14]. These results emphasize the need to pay careful attention to methodology when assaying FVIII concentrates with different molecular composition to that of normal FVIII.

In the survey by Hubbard *et al.* [12], the largest discrepancies between one-stage and chromogenic methods were found for two products manufactured by the "Method M" monoclonal antibody process. It has been suggested that differences in thrombin activation between the two methods may play a role in these types of discrepancies, and evidence for this has been found in recent studies by Hubbard *et al.* [15].

Assays of plasma

The establishment of plasma standards has been more straightforward than for concentrates. Here, the main issue has been to maintain the link between the international unit and the "normal plasma unit"; this has been done by incorporating samples of normal plasma pools in the calibration studies for each successive international standard, and adjusting the potencies where necessary to minimize the difference between the IU and "1 mL average normal plasma" (e.g., in the calibration of the 4th international standard for FVIII/VWF plasma [16]).

Table 42.4 Comparison of methods on recombinant concentrates: data from controlled collaborative studies.

Study date	Reference standard	Test sample	Potency percent		
			One-stage	Two-stage	Chromogenic
1992	WHO 4th IS	1	100 (9)	99.7 (5)	114.6 (10)
		2	100 (9)	91.2 (5)	98.5 (10)
1994	WHO 4th IS	3	100 (17)	104.1 (6)	110.6 (18)
	WHO 5th IS	3	100 (17)	101.5 (6)	118.3 (18
1998	WHO 5th IS	4	100 (21)	94.7 (6)	110.7 (25)
		5	100 (21)	97.8 (6)	110.5 (25)

Samples 1–5 are different ampouled preparations of the two full-length recombinant concentrates (Kogenate and Recombinate).

Figures in brackets are numbers of laboratories performing each method. Potencies have been calculated as a percentage of those with the one-stage method.

All participants used SSC recommended methodology and data were analyzed centrally.

Despite the widespread use of the WHO standard to calibrate local and commercial working standards, the variability in FVIII assays among clinical laboratories in the UK has remained disappointingly high, with CVs of up to 35% in successive NEQAS surveys. This is probably due to the great variety of reagents and methodology in the different laboratories, as referred to earlier; the widespread practice of using only single dilutions may also be a contributory factor.

Postinfusion plasma

The assay of concentrates against plasma standards has been a long-standing problem because of wide variability between laboratories and a basic difference between assay methods, and for this reason two separate WHO standards for plasma and concentrates were developed. However, although such comparisons are avoided in routine assays, they are relevant to manufacturers of plasma-derived concentrates, and especially to clinicians measuring *in vivo* recovery. In the latter situation, patients' postinfusion samples, which essentially consist of concentrates "diluted" in the patient's hemophilic plasma, are assayed against a plasma standard.

It was first found in 1978 [4] that when concentrates were assayed against plasma, the potencies were higher by the two-stage method than by one-stage assays; the average discrepancy from a number of collaborative studies at this time was 20%. Since then, the same trend has been found in almost every collaborative study, although the size of the discrepancy varies from study to study, and possibly with different types of concentrates.

Figure 42.1 summarizes the data from several collaborative studies over a period of 15 years, and the consistency of the trend is clearly seen, with only one of 10 data sets giving no discrepancy. In recent years, the chromogenic method has largely re-placed the two-stage method for assay of concentrates, and not surprisingly it also gives higher results than the one-stage method, being based on the same principles as the two-stage. Despite considerable investigation, the basic causes of this discrepancy remain unknown, although it is thought that the extensive processing applied to both plasma-derived and recombinant concentrates could lead to differences in their rates of activation and inactivation in the two method types from the FVIII in normal plasma; there is some evidence for this from recent studies [17]. For largely historical reasons, when the WHO concentrate and plasma FVIII standards are compared against each other, the values are approximately equivalent by one-stage assays but not by two-stage or chromogenic methods, as shown in Figure 42.1.

There is some evidence that the discrepancy is greater for recombinant concentrates than for plasma-derived products. In assays at NIBSC, the ratio of chromogenic to one-stage potencies for the two full-length recombinant concentrates, assayed against the British Plasma Standard, was 1.53 and 1.44. In the collaborative study to calibrate the 5th International Standard, which included both the WHO plasma standard and a recombinant concentrate, the ratio of chromogenic to one-stage potencies was 1.48, and in the 6th International Standard study [5] it was 1.26.

These figures help to explain the large discrepancies between chromogenic and one-stage potencies found in patients' samples after infusion of recombinant concentrates [18]. It appears that, after infusion, the recombinant products are behaving in an essentially similar manner in these assays to samples produced by diluting them *in vitro* in hemophilic plasma.

The situation with plasma-derived products is variable, dependent on the nature of the product and the test systems used. For instance, in a study by Lee *et al.* [19], Hemofil M was found to give a 20% discrepancy in postinfusion plasmas between one-stage and chromogenic methods, whereas in a study of similar products performed at CLB there was no difference between the methods. Equivalence between the methods was also found in a UK NEQAS study on a postinfusion sample from a different type of plasma-derived concentrate.

A resolution of this problem is only possible when the exact causes of the discrepancy are discovered; it may then be possible to adjust one or both of the methods to give similar values. In the meantime, a practical solution that has been discussed by the FVIII/FIX Subcommittee of ISTH/SSC is to regard the postinfusion samples as concentrates, "diluted" in a patient's plasma, which is essentially what they are, and use a concentrate standard, diluted in hemophilic plasma, instead of a plasma standard, to construct the standard curve. Considering the close agreement between assay methods on recombinant concentrates when concentrate standards are used (see previous section), this should provide good agreement on *in vivo* recoveries of recombinant concentrates when measured by chromogenic and one-stage methods. This approach has recently been tested in an *in vivo* recovery study, in which patients' samples after infusion of Recombinate were assayed against both a plasma stan-

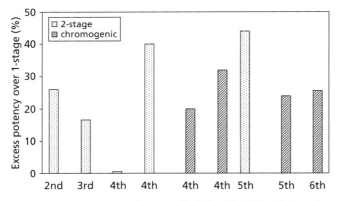

Figure 42.1 Comparisons of assay methods for World Health Organization (WHO) concentrate standards assayed against WHO plasma standards. Data are means from large international collaborative studies and potencies with the two-stage and chromogenic methods are calculated as percentages of the one-stage potencies. Results are plotted as percentage differences, e.g., 20% for the chromogenic method means that the potency by that method is 120% of the one-stage potency.

dard and a concentrate standard consisting of Recombinate itself [18]. The results showed that the 25% discrepancy between one-stage and chromogenic methods using the plasma standard was completely abolished with the concentrate standard. In a field study, the use of a Refacto concentrate standard was similarly associated with a reduced variability between laboratories and an abolition of the discrepancy between one-stage and chromogenic assays [20].

Standardization of factor IX assays

Standardization of FIX assays has presented fewer problems than that of FVIII. This is because there is only a single assay method, the one-stage clotting assay, used for both plasma and concentrates. As for FVIII, a concentrate standard was the first to be established by WHO, for therapeutic materials, and this consisted of a prothrombin complex concentrate (PCC) [21]. The recent switch to high-purity single FIX concentrates as the mainstay of therapy does not appear to have caused any problems in assay standardization; it appears that PCCs and single FIX concentrates can be assayed satisfactorily against each other. The current WHO standard is a single FIX concentrate, and the same material also serves as the FDA and EP standards.

As for FVIII, it was found that predilution of concentrates in FIX-deficient plasma was necessary to obtain optimum and reproducible potency when assaying concentrates against a concentrate standard, and also when comparing concentrates against plasma [22]. An international plasma standard for FIX, together with the other vitamin K-dependent factors, II, VII, and X, was established by WHO in 1987 [23], and most local and commercial plasma standards are now calibrated in International Units. However, UK NEQAS surveys continue to show wide variability between laboratories, probably due to the multiplicity of aPTT reagents and deficient plasmas used. As with FVIII, artificially depleted plasmas have become the main type of FIX-deficient reagent used, but there has been no systematic study of their performance compared with hemophilia B plasma.

Standardization of von Willebrand factor (VWF) assays

Assays for VWF

As described in Chapter 41, the ristocetin cofactor method has continued to be the mainstay of assays of VWF, but it suffers from very high variability, both within and between laboratories. There are difficulties also with preparation and stability of the platelet reagent, and the assay is labor intensive and difficult to automate. Because of these problems, alternative methods of measuring VWF function have been sought, and the collagen-binding method, which is much easier to perform and more reproducible, was introduced by Favorolo and colleagues

[24]. Although there has been some controversy over its clinical applicability, it is used in a number of clinical laboratories in conjunction with other methods such as multimer analysis, and is being considered also as a possible EP reference method for concentrates (see below). The measurement of VWF antigen is also useful as an adjunct to the functional measurements; the original "rocket" electrophoresis method of Laurell has now been largely replaced by ELISA assays.

Standards for VWF

The course of standardization of VWF differed from that of FVIII and FIX in that, when the 1st International Standard for FVIII, plasma, was established in 1982, the same plasma was calibrated (against normal pools) for VWF [8]. Thus, a plasma standard was established before a concentrate standard, and in fact a separate concentrate international standard for VWF was established only recently [25]. The reason for this is the relatively slow development and licensing of VWF concentrates, with cryoprecipitate and FFP continuing to be used for many patients for many years.

A British Standard for VWF, plasma, is available from NIBSC; it is calibrated for ristocetin cofactor, collagen binding, and antigen parameters.

Standardization of assays of other coagulation factors

Assays of other coagulation factors are carried out only rarely in the context of congenital deficiencies, although they are performed more frequently in relation to acquired defects, population surveys, and by manufacturers of concentrates. In general, the same principles apply, as for FVIII and FIX, with plasma standards being used for plasma samples, and concentrate standards for assay of therapeutic concentrates (see Table 42.1).

References

1 Finney D. *Statistical Method in Biological Assay*. London: Charles Griffin, 1978.
2 Kirkwood TBL, Snape TJ. Biometric principles in clotting and clot lysis assays. *Clin Lab Haematol* 1980; 2: 155–67.
3 Bangham DR, Biggs R, Brozovic M, *et al*. A biological standard for measurement of blood coagulation factor VIII activity. *Bull WHO* 1971; 45: 337–51.
4 Kirkwood TBL, Barrowcliffe TW. Discrepancy between 1-stage and 2-stage assay of factor VIII:C. *Br J Haematol* 1978; 40: 333–8.
5 Raut S, Heath A, Barrowcliffe TW. Establishment of the 6th International Standard for FVIII concentrate. *Thromb Haemost* 2001; 85: 1071–8.
6 Barrowcliffe TW. The one-stage versus the two-stage factor VIII assay. In: Triplett DA, ed. *Advances in Coagulation Testing*. Skokie, IL: College of American Pathologists, 1986; 47–62.
7 Hubbard AR, Curtis AD, Barrowcliffe TW, *et al*. Assay of factor VIII

concentrates: comparison of chromogenic and 2-stage clotting assays. *Thrombosis Res* 1986; **44**: 887–91.

8 Barrowcliffe TW. Standardization and assay. *Semin Thromb Haemost* 1993; **19**: 73–9.

9 Barrowcliffe TW. Factor VIII and Factor IX Sub-committee. Recommendations for the assay of high-purity factor VIII concentrates. *Thromb Haemost* 1993; **70**: 876–7.

10 Albertengo ME, Barrowcliffe TW, Oliva L, *et al.* New recombinant standard for FVIII concentrate gives same results as previous plasma derived standards on a range of FVIII products. *Thromb Haemost* 2000; **83**: 789–90.

11 Barrowcliffe TW, Watton J, Tubbs JE, *et al.* Potency of high purity factor VIII concentrates (Letter). *Lancet* 1990; **ii**: 124.

12 Hubbard AR, Weller LJ, Bevan SA. A Survey of one-stage and chromogenic potencies in therapeutic FVIII concentrates. *Br J Haematol* 2002; **117**: 247–8.

13 Mikaelsson M, Oswaldsson U, Sandberg H. Influence of phospholipids on the assessment of factor VIII activity. *Haemophilia* 1998; **4**: 646–50.

14 Hubbard AR, Sands D, Sandberg E, *et al.* A multi-centre collaborative study on the potency estimation of ReFacto. *Thromb Haemost* 2003; **90**: 1088–93.

15 Hubbard AR, Weller LJ, Bevan SA. Activation profiles of FVIII in concentrates reflect one-stage/chromogenic potency discrepancies. *Br J Haematol* 2002; **117**: 957–60.

16 Hubbard AR, Rigsby P, Barrowcliffe TW. Standardisation of Factor VIII and von Willebrand Factor in plasma: Calibration of the 4th International Standard (97/586). *Thromb Haemost* 2001: **85**: 634–8.

17 Hubbard AR, Bevan SA, Weller LJ. Potency estimation of recombinant factor VIII: effect of assay method and standard. *Br J Haematol* 2001; **113**: 533–6.

18 Lee CA, Owens D, Bray G, *et al.* Pharmacokinetics of recombinant factor VIII (Recombinate) using one-stage clotting and chromogenic factor VIII assay. *Thromb Haemost* 1999; **82**: 1644–7.

19 Lee CA, Barrowcliffe TW, Bray G, *et al.* Pharmacokinetic in vivo comparison using 1-stage and chromogenic substrate assays with two formulations of Hemofil-M. *Thromb Haemost* 1996; **76**: 950–6.

20 Ingerslev J, Jankowski, M, Weston SB, Charles LA. Collaborative field study on the utility of a BDD factor VIII concentrate standard in the estimation of BDD factor VIII:C activity in hemophilic plasma using one-stage clotting assays. *J Thromb Haemost* 2004; **2**: 623–8.

21 Brozovic M, Bangham DR. Study of a proposed International Standard for factor IX. *Thromb Haemost* 1976; **35**: 222–36.

22 Barrowcliffe TW, Tydeman MS, Kirkwood TBL. Major effect of prediluent in factor IX clotting assay. *Lancet* 1979; **ii**: 192.

23 Barrowcliffe TW. Standardisation of factors II, VII, IX, and X in plasma and concentrates. *Thromb Haemost* 1987; **59**: 334.

24 Favorolo EJ. Collagen binding assay for von Willebrand factor (vWF:CBA): detection of von Willebrand's disease (vWD) and discrimination of vWD subtypes, depends on collagen source. *Thromb Haemost* 2000; **83**: 127–35.

25 Hubbard AR, Sands, Chang A, Mazurier C. Standardisation of von Willebrand factor in therapeutic concentrates: calibration of the 1st International Standard for von Willebrand factor concentrate (00/514). *Thromb Haemost* 2002; **88**: 380–6.

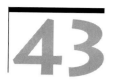

Obstetrics and gynecology: hemophilia

Rezan Kadir and Christine A. Lee

Introduction

Hemophilia A and B are X-linked recessive bleeding disorders caused by deficiency of factor VIII (FVIII) or FIX respectively. Because of the mode of inheritance, hemophilia A and B mostly affect males, and females are carriers. Thus, the clotting factor level is expected to be around 50% normal in carriers, who have only one affected chromosome. However, a wide range of values (22–116 IU/dL) has been reported [1] as a result of random inactivation of one of the two X chromosomes, the process called lyonization [2]. A significant number of hemophilia carriers may have very low factor levels as a result of extreme lyonization. In addition, women are exposed to regular hemostatic challenges during their life owing to monthly menstruation as well as childbirth, and are therefore at risk of bleeding complications such as menorrhagia and postpartum hemorrhage even with a mild degree of clotting factor deficiency.

Management of obstetric and gynecologic problems in carriers of hemophilia requires a close collaboration between gynecologists and the hemophilia center. Ideally, these women should be managed in a combined clinic, where expertise and facilities are available to provide comprehensive assessment of their bleeding disorders and obstetric and gynecologic problems as well as to provide a management plan. Advice from the hemophilia team is invaluable for arrangement and interpretation of blood tests and arrangement of prophylactic or replacement treatment, especially when there are bleeding complications.

Gynecology

Menorrhagia

Menorrhagia is defined subjectively as an excessive menstrual loss and objectively as menstrual loss of more than 80 mL per period [3]. Menorrhagia may have a local or systemic cause. It has always been presumed that bleeding disorders are a rare cause of menorrhagia, especially in adults. However, with increasing research interest and clinical awareness in this area, bleeding disorders are now recognized as an important systemic cause. Using a pictorial blood assessment chart (Figure 43.1) [4], menstrual loss was assessed in 30 carriers of hemophilia. The median menstrual score was 113 in carriers of hemophilia, sig-

nificantly higher than in the age-matched control group (73). The incidence of menorrhagia, as defined by a score of more than 100, was 57% compared with 29% in the control group [5]. In addition to heavy menstruation, carriers of hemophilia may also suffer prolonged menstruation with episodes of flooding and passage of clots [5].

Lack of awareness of the high incidence of menorrhagia and underestimation of menstrual loss in these women may lead to chronic iron deficiency anemia as well as inappropriate management and unnecessary surgical intervention, including hysterectomy at an early reproductive age [5]. Carriers of hemophilia may consider heavy menstruation as the norm and may not seek medical advice because menorrhagia usually starts at menarche. In addition, other female family members may also be carriers and have excessive menstrual blood loss. One study reported that carriers of hemophilia did not consider their menstrual loss to be greater than that of other women [6]. Thus, these women should regularly be asked about their periods and menstrual loss should be assessed.

Subjective estimation of menstrual blood loss is inaccurate, with a poor correlation between the patient's perception of blood and actual volume of blood loss as measured objectively. Therefore, objective assessment is helpful for initial assessment and monitoring response to treatment. A pictorial blood assessment chart, using a special scoring system (Figure 43.1), is useful in clinical practice. It is a simple nonlaboratory method and provides a semiquantitative measure of menstrual blood loss with reasonable accuracy compared with the available sophisticated and costly methods.

Quality of life

Menorrhagia and dysmenorrhea adversely affect quality of life and may have a major influence on women's lifestyle and employment. Quality of life during menstruation is significantly worse in hemophilia carriers than in control subjects, being lowest among those who pass clots and suffer flooding and prolonged menstruation. Between 39% and 46% of such patients have to take time off work [7,8]. They also accomplish less at work and experience difficulties performing their work. A strong relationship was found between gynecological history and psychologic problems among 181 women with von Willebrand disease (VWD) [9], and 28% of the patients in the same study met the criteria for anxiety disorders.

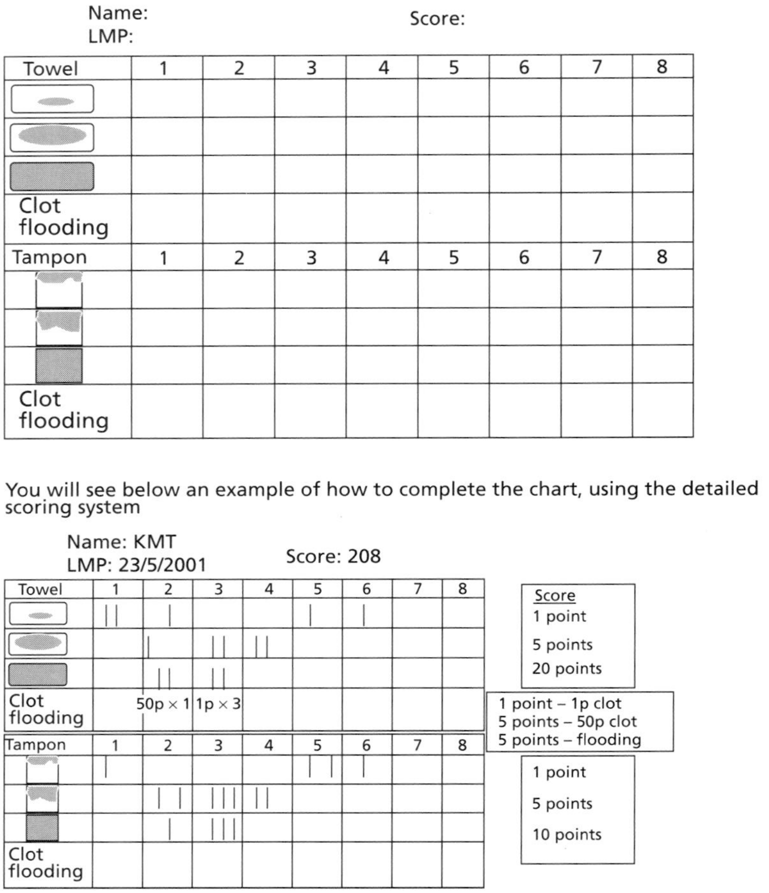

Name: Score:
LMP:

Towel	1	2	3	4	5	6	7	8
⬭								
⬭								
▭								
Clot flooding								
Tampon	1	2	3	4	5	6	7	8
Clot flooding								

You will see below an example of how to complete the chart, using the detailed scoring system

Name: KMT
LMP: 23/5/2001   Score: 208

Towel	1	2	3	4	5	6	7	8		Score	
⬭	II	I			I	I				1 point	
⬭		I	II	II						5 points	
▭		II	II							20 points	
Clot flooding	50p × 1	1p × 3								1 point – 1p clot	
										5 points – 50p clot	
Tampon	1	2	3	4	5	6	7	8		5 points – flooding	
	I				III	I				1 point	
		II	I	IIII	II					5 points	
		I	IIII							10 points	
Clot flooding											

Figure 43.1 Pictorial blood assessment chart and scoring system for assessment of menstrual blood loss.

Management of menorrhagia

Menorrhagia in carriers of hemophilia is most likely to be, but not necessarily, due to their clotting factor deficiency. Thus, each individual should be appropriately assessed and local causes excluded, especially the possibility of malignancy in older women. The treatment of menorrhagia is usually medical, and the most commonly used first-line options are tranexamic acid, combined oral contraceptive pills, or desmopressin (DDAVP, self-administered by subcutaneous injection or as intranasal spray). The choice is dependent on the age of the patient and her reproductive status, the availability of the medications, and the clinician's experience and preference.

In a recent study [10], the levonorgestrel intrauterine system Mirena (LNG IUS) was shown to be highly effective in reducing menstrual loss and was well tolerated in women with bleeding disorders who did not respond to treatment with tranexamic acid, combined oral contraceptive pills, or desmopressin. The main problem with the Mirena is a high discontinuation rate (20% in randomized controlled trials and 17% in case series reviewed by Stewart *et al.* [11]) because of irregular bleeding during the first 3–6 months and the progestogenic side-effects. Counseling and patient education may increase tolerance. The levonorgestrel intrauterine system is a very effective and re-

versible method of contraception, which is an added advantage, especially in women who wish to preserve their fertility. In women with bleeding disorders, this method should be considered prior to any surgical management.

Surgical intervention is sometimes required in patients unresponsive to medical treatment. Surgical procedures, even relatively minor operations, can be complicated by hemorrhage in some carriers of hemophilia. Therefore, good liaison between the local hemophilia center and the surgical/anesthetic team is essential. Adequate hemostatic cover should be provided with the aim of maintaining the clotting factor > 50 IU/dL until healing is complete. The treatment may need to be continued postoperatively, sometimes for up to 10 days, to reduce the development of secondary bleeding and hematomas. Surgery should be performed by expert gynecologists, choosing a technique with least risk of bleeding complication.

Other gynecologic problems

These include dysmenorrhea, intermenstrual bleedings, and mid-cycle pain. Mid-cycle pain probably arises from ovulation with subsequent hemorrhage into the corpus luteum or from peritoneal irritation due to bleeding from edges of a recently formed corpus luteum. Acute abdomen due to hemoperitoneum as well as extension of bleeding into the broad ligament with spontaneous rupture of corpus luteum has been reported in carriers of hemophilia [12]. Although this is a rare complication, it must be considered in these patients before embarking on any surgical intervention, as conservative management with factor replacement is usually effective and obviates the need for surgery.

Genetics

Genetic counseling and carrier detection in hemophilia

The purpose of genetic counseling is to provide the potential carrier and her parents or partner with adequate information to reach decisions regarding carrier testing and prenatal diagnosis and to provide support throughout the process. Genetic counseling should be provided by a good communicator who has a detailed knowledge of hemophilia, genetics, molecular biology, and prenatal diagnostic procedures. Counseling is a way of addressing the implications of the information given and of reaching a better understanding between the healthcare worker and patient about the full range of issues. Genetic counseling in hemophilia focuses on facts about the medical condition (what it is, how it is treated, and how it is passed from generation to generation), personal and relationship concerns related to hemophilia, and beliefs and wishes about the person discussing the inheritance, as well as those who might be affected [13]. Ethical considerations include human rights, issues surrounding consent, and those relating to confidentiality. However, the best interests of the person with hemophilia and the partner, sister, or child of a carrier can be in conflict, and therefore genetic counseling needs to address and consider these very issues. In the healthcare setting, responsible care involves obtaining informed consent for the treatment, genetic testing or screening offered (Table 43.1).

The first step in carrier detection is to study the pedigree. Thus, all daughters of a man with hemophilia will be carriers; sons of a carrier have a 50% chance of having hemophilia; daughters of a carrier have a 50% chance of being a carrier. However, in many countries, more than 50% of newly diagnosed cases are sporadic [14].

Conventional clotting factor levels may reveal carriership [1]. However, genotypic assessment based on direct identification of the pathogenic mutation is the most reliable method of carrier detection. Once a mutation in a specific family has been identified, it is possible to offer carrier and prenatal diagnosis at any time in the future by obtaining a blood sample from the individual concerned. In severe hemophilia A, almost 50% of families carry an inversion — a rearrangement in the long arm of the X chromosome [15]. These inversions can be demonstrated by using relatively simple laboratory methods. If the index case in the family does not carry the inversion, the specific mutation must be identified, and such mutations of FVIII are listed on the

Table 43.1 Counseling and consent for genetic testing and hemophilia.

Establish that hemophilia is present in the family and determine its type and severity
Establish a family pedigree (tree) to exclude carriers and identify possible or definite (obligate) carriers
Provide a full explanation of the potential clinical effects of being a hemophilia carrier or affected male
Provide a full explanation of the mode of inheritance of hemophilia
Discuss the rationale for identifying the genetic defect in patients with hemophilia
Outline the means by which carrier status is assessed
Discuss what is involved in genetic testing: sample collection, transfer/storage of data, research projects on stored material, insurance issues and risk of error
If appropriate, advise on the techniques for antenatal testing
Provide an opportunity to ask questions
Provide an opportunity for the individual being consulted to present her understanding of the information that has been discussed
Provide patient information sheet and an opportunity for a follow-up appointment

HAMSTeRS database (http://europium.csc.mrc.ac.uk). In hemophilia B, almost every family has a unique mutation [167]. It is important to establish that the causative mutation causes hemophilia, as neutral mutations causing no detrimental change have been described. Also, there is the possibility of mosaicism, a mixture of normal and mutation-carrying cells, in the mother of a sporadic case. Thus, even if the mutation is not found in the patient, it cannot be excluded.

It is essential to determine maternal carriership of hemophilia A or B before embarking on prenatal diagnosis. The available methods for prenatal diagnosis and their risks and implications should be discussed. The maternal clotting factor should be checked prior to any invasive prenatal procedure, and prophylactic treatment should be arranged when factor levels are less than 50 IU/dL to prevent bleeding complications. Recombinant FVIII or FIX should be used to avoid any risk of virus transmission, particularly parvovirus. Carriers who opt for invasive prenatal diagnosis must also be counseled and offered the option of testing for chromosomal abnormality from the chorionic or amniotic fluid sample.

Pregnancy and carriers of hemophilia

Prenatal diagnosis

Carrier testing and prenatal diagnosis of hemophilia, in particular the utilization and psychological consequences, have been reviewed [17]. The question arises as to whether prenatal diagnosis of hemophilia is still necessary in a time when the condition can be successfully managed with regular, albeit expensive, prophylactic treatment. The answer may be "Yes" for many carriers of hemophilia, especially those who have grown up with a hemophilic father or brother with complicated disease; those who belong to a family with inhibitor problems; those who have seen the consequences of HIV/hepatitis C virus and may be frightened of other viral or prion diseases; or those who have had some other tragic experience with the condition.

Prenatal diagnosis of hemophilia has been available for 20 years and carrier testing for an even longer period. Attitudes to prenatal diagnosis and abortion vary widely, among countries, religions, cultures, and over time. Economic factors may also influence the use of these techniques.

Thus, the uptake of prenatal diagnosis and termination of affected pregnancies have been reported to be low in several studies. It seems that many carriers of hemophilia do not consider hemophilia to be a sufficiently serious disease to justify an abortion [18,19]. There are several methods available for prenatal diagnosis of hemophilia. The choice depends on the information available about the family, whether the causative mutation has been identified, and the plans of the couple for the pregnancy, as well as their attitude toward invasive prenatal testing and termination of an affected pregnancy.

Invasive methods

Chorionic villus sampling (CVS) is the most widely used method for prenatal diagnosis of hemophilia. The procedure is performed at 11–14 weeks under ultrasound guidance (Figure 43.2). The chorionic villus sample is first used to assess fetal sex. If the fetus is male, then hemophilia status is determined by direct gene analysis (sequencing of the causative mutation). The procedure carries an approximate 1% risk of miscarriage [20]. Limb abnormalities have been reported in association with CVS performed prior to 10 weeks' gestation [21]. However, a review of 138 996 pregnancies exposed to CVS after 10 weeks' gestation did not show any increased risk of limb defects [22]. CVS has the advantage that termination of pregnancy, if opted for, can be performed during the first trimester, which is probably less traumatic and more acceptable to the patient. The disadvan-

tage of CVS is that female fetuses cannot be excluded and are exposed to CVS, as fetal sex cannot be determined by ultrasound with 100% accuracy in the first trimester. However, with the recent advances and availability of noninvasive methods of fetal sex determination in the first trimester (discussed later in the chapter), this problem will be overcome in the near future.

Amniocentesis can also be used for prenatal diagnosis. However, it is performed in the second trimester (15–20 weeks' gestation). In addition, it has been argued that it may not be possible to obtain adequate DNA for analysis with amniocentesis. However, this is less likely to be a problem nowadays with the availability of polymerase chain reaction (PCR) and fluorescence in situ hybridization (FISH) techniques. The last method of specific prenatal diagnosis is clotting factor assay of a fetal blood sample at cordocentesis. This procedure is performed at 18–20 weeks of gestation and is suitable for carriers whose DNA analysis is noninformative. The procedure is reported to have a 1.25% risk of procedure-related fetal loss when performed for nonchromosomal indications and by an experienced operator [23].

Noninvasive method

Fetal sex determination is the only noninvasive prenatal method available for hemophilia. Fetal sex can be accurately determined by ultrasound at 20 weeks' gestation; however, earlier diagnosis has required fetal karyotyping by invasive testing [24,25]. Ultrasound determination of fetal sex in the first trimester is difficult as embryologic development of the external genitalia is not complete and the phallus is of similar length in all fetuses before 14 weeks' gestation. Recently, the plane of development of the phallus has been used to assess fetal sex between 11 and 14 weeks' gestation. In mid-sagittal section, the phallus is parallel (pointing caudally) and perpendicular (pointing anteriorly) to the axis of lumbosacral spines in female and male fetuses respectively [25]. The sensitivity of this technique is limited, especially at 11–12 weeks' gestation, and in a study by Whitlow *et al.* [26] fetal sex could not be assigned in 41% and 13% of fetuses at 11 and 12 weeks of gestation respectively. An alternative noninvasive method for determining fetal sex is by assessing free fetal DNA in the maternal circulation for the presence or the absence of *SRY* loci. This method achieved 100% accuracy in 12 pregnancies at risk of hemophilia (seven males and five females) between 10 and 14 weeks of gestation [27].

Fetal sex determination is helpful in several situations. If a fetus is identified as female, then the mother can be reassured and the parents have the option of avoiding invasive testing in 50% of cases. Knowledge that the fetus is female can also be very reassuring when specific prenatal diagnosis for hemophilia is not possible, e.g., a carrier mother is not informative on DNA analysis and when a woman is unsure of her feelings about termination of pregnancy. Finally, knowledge of fetal sex is very helpful to the attending obstetrician for labor management of carrier mothers who have not undergone specific prenatal diagnostic tests. In these situations, the risks of traumatic hemorrhage to a male fetus can be minimized by avoiding invasive

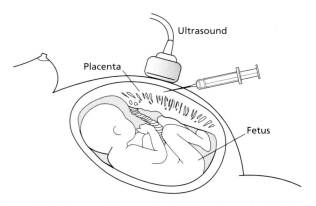

Figure 43.2 Chorionic villus sampling (CVS), performed at 11–14 weeks by the transabdominal approach under local anesthetic and ultrasound monitoring.

monitoring techniques, vacuum extraction, or difficult forceps deliveries (see Labor and delivery below).

Antenatal management

Serum FVIII levels have been shown to increase significantly in carriers of hemophilia A during pregnancy. Although the majority of patients develop levels within the normal range, the rise is variable, and a small proportion of them may still have low levels at term [12,28]. In contrast, FIX levels do not rise in carriers of hemophilia B (Figure 43.3). The risk of bleeding in early pregnancy and miscarriage is unknown in carriers of hemophilia, but there is evidence that the risk of antepartum hemorrhage (bleeding after 24 weeks' gestation) is not increased [12,28]. Women are exposed to various hemostatic challenges during pregnancy, e.g., prenatal diagnostic techniques, termination of pregnancy, or spontaneous miscarriage, which may be complicated by excessive or prolonged hemorrhage. Therefore, it is recommended that the FVIII or FIX levels are checked at booking, and at 28 and 34 weeks of gestation. This is especially important in patients with low prepregnancy levels. Monitoring during the third trimester is essential as management of labor can be planned and prophylactic treatment can be arranged to decrease the risk of postpartum hemorrhage.

Administration of desmopressin (1-deamino-8-arginine vasopressin; DDAVP) is useful for prevention and treatment of bleeding in mild or moderate hemophilia A. Its use during pregnancy has been controversial because of the risk of DDAVP causing uterine contractions and preterm labor. However, DDAVP is very specific to V2 receptors and has little effect on uterine smooth muscle V1 receptors. Desmopressin may cross the placenta, and there is a potential risk of neonatal hyponatremia if given immediately before birth. The other concern regarding antenatal use of this drug is decreasing blood flow from the placenta causing intrauterine growth retardation. However, its vasopressor effect is very weak. Recently, the use of antepartum DDAVP for the management of diabetes insipidus, in a smaller dose than is required for hemostatic purposes, was reviewed in 53 cases, and DDAVP was shown that it was not associated with prematurity, low birthweight, or any serious adverse effect on maternal health or neonatal well-being [29]. There is a need for a multicenter trial to address the safety of antepartum use of DDAVP in carriers with hemophilia A. Meanwhile, DDAVP can be used during labor and the postpartum period.

Plasma-derived clotting factor concentrates, treated with the currently available viricidal methods, carry a negligible risk of transmitting hepatitis B and C virus. However, they may not be effective against hepatitis A and parvovirus B19 [30]. The latter is of particular importance in pregnant women as it can cause severe fetal infection and hydrops fetalis. Thus, recombinant FVIII and FIX should be used in pregnant mothers when administration of this factor is indicated.

Labor and delivery

Carriers of hemophilia and their fetuses are exposed to various hemostatic challenges during labor and delivery. Invasive methods are commonly used in labor for intrapartum monitoring, e.g., fetal scalp electrode and fetal blood sampling. Affected male fetuses are potentially at risk of scalp hemorrhage from the use of these techniques. Although there is lack of published data to support this, it is advisable to avoid their use in fetuses at risk.

Affected fetuses are also at risk of serious head bleeding, including cephalohematoma, subgaleal hematoma, and intracranial hemorrhage, from the process of birth. The safest method of delivery for fetuses at risk is controversial. In one survey, cesarean section was routinely recommended in 14.4% of hemophilia centers [31]. In another survey, 11% of obstetricians preferred to deliver pregnant carriers of hemophilia by cesarean section [32]. In a review of 117 children with moderate to severe hemophilia born between 1970 and 1990, 23 neonatal bleedings were reported in association with delivery. The type of bleeding and mode of delivery is shown in Table 43.2. It was concluded that the risk of serious bleeding during normal vaginal delivery is small and that delivery of all fetuses at risk of hemophilia by cesarean section does not eliminate the risk. However, the risk is significantly increased by the use of vacuum extraction or forceps, or after a prolonged second stage of labor and prolonged pushing [28,33,34]. Thus, prolonged labor (especially prolonged second stage) and delivery by vacuum extraction and mid-cavity or rotational forceps should be avoided in affected male fetuses or in fetuses whose coagulation status is unknown. Delivery should be achieved by the least traumatic method and early recourse to cesarean section should be considered.

The use of regional block in patients with bleeding disorders is controversial because of the potential risk of spinal cord bleeding and hematoma during insertion and withdrawal of epidural catheter or spinal anesthesia in the presence of a coagulation defect. However, provided that the coagulation status is normal and FVIII or FIX levels are maintained at more than 50 IU/dL, there is no contraindication to a regional block. It may sometimes be difficult to assess factor levels when patients present in

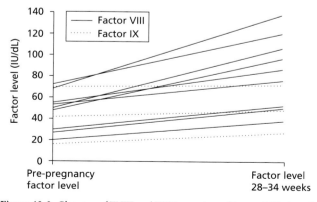

Figure 43.3 Changes of FVIII and FIX in carriers of hemophilia A and B during pregnancy.

Table 43.2 Neonatal bleeding and mode of delivery [33].

Type of bleeding	Normal vaginal delivery ($n = 87$)	Vacuum extraction ($n = 17$)	Cesarean section ($n = 13$)	Total ($n = 117$)
Subgaleal/cephalohematoma	1	10	1	12
Intracranial	2	1	1	4
Umbilical	3		1	4
Retro-orbital	1			1
Oral	1			1
Hematuria	1			1
Total	9 (10.3%)	11 (64.7%)	3 (23%)	23 (19.7%)

advanced labor. In this situation, provided that factor levels were more than 50 IU/dL during the third trimester, it is sufficient to assess platelet count, activated partial thromboplastin time (aPTT), and prothrombin time (PT). However, it is particularly important to check factor levels prior to removal of the epidural catheter because the pregnancy-induced increase in factor levels may be quickly reversed after birth and bleeding in the spinal canal may then arise. Regional block in carriers of hemophilia should be performed by an expert anesthesiologist with the help of a specialized hematologist for assessment of coagulation status and arrangement of treatment when needed.

Third stage of labor and puerperium

Carriers of hemophilia, especially those with low factor levels, are at risk of postpartum hemorrhage (PPH). Greer *et al.* [12] reported five postpartum hemorrhages and a large perineal hematoma among 43% of pregnancies in hemophilia carriers. In a review of 50 ongoing pregnancies among 32 hemophilia carriers, an increased incidence (22%) [28] of primary PPH was also demonstrated compared with the general obstetric population (5%) [35]. The incidence of secondary PPH was also increased (11%). The incidence of secondary PPH in a general obstetric population is reported to be 0.7% [36]. The risk of bleeding as well as PPH is related to plasma FVIII or FIX activity in hemophilia carriers [6,28], and most of the significant incidences of PPH have been reported in carriers with factor levels lower than 50 IU/dL. To minimize the risk of primary and secondary PPH, it is essential that factor levels are checked daily and maintained above 50 IU/dL for at least 3–4 days, or 4–5 days if cesarean section has been performed [37]. The risk of primary PPH can be further reduced by active management of the third stage of labor and minimizing maternal genital and perineal trauma.

In addition to the process of labor and delivery, the neonate is also at risk of bleeding from puncture sites, surgical interventions, (the commonest of which is circumcision), and spontaneous bleedings, such as bruising or organ and joint bleeding. In a review of bleeding episodes in 349 newborns with hemophilia in 66 publications, there were 366 bleeding episodes and head bleeding was commonest, with intracranial bleeding and subgaleal/cephalohematomas accounting for 27% and 13% of all

Table 43.3 Management of pregnancy in carriers of hemophilia.

Prepregnancy counseling
Multidisciplinary team approach
Sexing — prenatal diagnosis or 18-week anomaly scan
Clotting factor level — booking, 28 and 34 weeks
Clotting factor level in labor — if <50 IU/dL treatment
Unknown or male sex — avoid fetal monitoring and instrumental delivery
Epidural analgesia inadvisable (controversial); regional block if level >50 IU/dL
Clotting factor level of cord blood
Vitamin K by mouth if hemophilic baby or status unknown
Register hemophilic baby at hemophilia center

Adapted from ref. 28.

bleeding episodes respectively [38]. The second commonest was bleeding after circumcision, the majority occurring before 1970. It seems that, with better awareness and good communication among families and care-givers, this bleeding can be prevented.

Cord blood should be collected from all male offspring of carrier mothers to assess FVIII or FIX levels for identification and early management of newborns at risk. Signs of intracranial hemorrhage may not be apparent in the few days of life. Thus, head ultrasound/computed tomography (CT) scans should be arranged for all male fetuses at risk, and recombinant FVIII is administered if there is any suspicion of bleeding or when the delivery has been instrumental or traumatic, to raise plasma factor levels to 100 IU/dL [38]. Intramuscular injections, venepunctures, and heelsticks can cause bleeding, and should be avoided. Vitamin K should be given orally and the routine immunizations should be administered carefully intradermally or subcutaneously [37]. Circumcision should be delayed until the newborn's coagulation status is known and appropriate management planning is arranged by the hemophilia center.

Repeat blood samples may sometimes be necessary to confirm the diagnosis; this may be best performed at 6 months of age. The results of the tests should be conveyed to the parents by the person most involved in counseling, usually a member of staff from the hemophilia center. Parents should be given instruction

Table 43.4 Rare bleeding disorders.

Deficient factor	Estimated prevalence	Gene on chromosome	Plasma half-life	Recommended therapy (in order of priority)
Fibrinogen	1:1 000 000	4	2–4 days	Solvent/detergent (SD) plasma (15–20 mL/kg)
				Fibrinogen concentrate (20–30 mg/kg)
Prothrombin	1:2 000 000	11	2–3 days	SD plasma (15–20 mL/kg)
				FIX complex concentrate (20–30 U/kg)
Factor V	1:1 000 000	1	36 h	SD plasma (15–20 mL/kg)
Combined FV				
and FVIII	1:1 000 000	18	–	As for FV
Factor VII	1:500 000	13	4–6 h	FVII concentrate (30–40 U/kg every 12 h)
FX	1:1 000 000	13	40 h	SD plasma (15–20 mL/kg)
				FIX complex concentrate (20–30 U/kg)
FXI	1:1 000 000	4	60 h	SD plasma (15–20 mL/kg)
				FXI concentrates (15–20 U/kg)
FXIII	1:2 000 000	6,1	11–14 days	SD plasma (15–20 mL/kg)
				FXIII concentrates (10–20 U/kg every 5–6 weeks for prophylaxis) once

Adapted from ref. 39.

about the possibility of bleeding and signs of intracranial bleeding. Hemophilic babies should be registered with and reviewed regularly by the hemophilia center. In female offspring of carriers of hemophilia, clotting factor assay should be performed prior to any surgical intervention or when there are any signs of bleeding. At the age of informed consent and after proper counseling, carrier testing with DNA probes should be offered. This is preferably completed before these potential carriers become pregnant.

The management of pregnancy in carriers of hemophilia is summarized in Table 43.3.

Rare bleeding disorders

Other inherited deficiencies of coagulation factors that may result in bleeding include afibrinogenemia, hypoprothrombinemia, and deficiencies of factor V, combined V and VIII, FVII, FX, FXI, and FXIII. These deficiencies are inherited as autosomal recessive traits and are generally more rare than hemophilia A and B [39]. However, in countries where consanguineous marriages are frequent, such as Muslim countries and southern India, recessively inherited coagulation deficiencies are more frequent. Clinically, they are expressed in homozygotes or compound heterozygotes. General recommendations on treatment of patients with rare coagulation disorders are summarized in Table 43.4.

Menorrhagia is a common symptom in women with rare inherited coagulation disorders and should be managed in a similar way as in carriers of hemophilia A and B who have this problem.

In general, a mutation in the DNA can be identified in the genes encoding the relevant coagulation factors. For each coagulation defect, there are multiple mutations, but these are unique for any given family. Prevention of rare coagulation disorders through prenatal diagnosis of the underlying mutation is possible in couples who may present with an affected child. Primary prevention could be achieved by discouraging consanguineous marriages. However, the cultural, religious, and economic roots of this practice are deep in various communities.

The general principles of management of pregnancy and delivery in carriers of rare bleeding disorders are similar to those in carriers of hemophilia A and B. However, the available therapies are limited (Table 43.4) and are plasma derived with the exception of recombinant FVIIa, which may be used to treat FVII deficiency. Factor XI deficiency is particularly common in Ashkenazi Jews, among whom the heterozygote frequency is 8%. The current research in factor XI deficiency, pregnancy, and menstrual problems has been specifically reviewed [40].

References

1 Rizza CR, Rhymes IL, Austen DEG, et al. Detection of carriers of haemophilia: a 'blind' study. Br J Haematol 1975; 30: 447–56.
2 Lyon MF. Sex chromatin and gene action in the mammalian X-chromosome. Am J Hum Genet 1962; 14: 135–48.
3 Hallberg L, Hogdahl AM, Nilsson L, Rybo G. Menstrual blood loss and iron deficiency. Acta Med Scand 1966; 180: 639–50.
4 Higham JM, O'Brien PM, Shaw RW. Assessment of menstrual blood loss using a pictorial chart. Br J Obstet Gynaecol 1990; 97: 734–9.
5 Kadir RA, Economides DL, Sabin CA, et al. Assessment of menstrual blood loss and gynaecological problems in patients with inherited bleeding disorders. Haemophilia 1999; 5: 40–8.
6 Mauser Bunschoten MEP, van Houwelingen JC, Sjamsoedin Visser EJM, et al. Bleeding symptoms in carriers of Hemophilia A and B. Thromb Haemost 1988; 59: 349–52.

7 Kadir RA, Sabin CA, Pollard D, *et al.* Quality of life during menstruation in patients with inherited bleeding disorders. *Haemophilia* 1998; 4: 836–41.

8 Kouides P, Phatak P, Burkhart P, *et al.* Gynaecological and obstetrical morbidity in women with Type 1 von Willebrand disease: results of a patient survey. *Haemophilia* 2000; 6: 643–8.

9 Rozeik Ch, Scharrer I. Gynecological disorders and psychological problems in 184 women with von Willebrand disease. *Haemophilia* 1998; 4: 293 (abstract).

10 Kingman CE, Kadir RA, Lee CA, Economides DL. The use of levonorgestrel-releasing system for the treatment of menorrhagia in women with inherited bleeding disorders. *Br J Obstet Gynaecol* 2004; 111: 1–4.

11 Stewart A, Cummins C, Gold L, Jordan R, Phillips W. The effectiveness of the levonorgestrel-releasing intrauterine system in menorrhagia: a systematic review. *Br J Obstet Gynaecol* 2001; 108: 74–86.

12 Greer IA, Lowe GDO, Walker JJ, Forbes CD. Haemorrhagic problems in obstetrics and gynaecology in patients with congenital coagulopathies. *Br J Obstet Gynaecol* 1991; 98: 909–18.

13 Miller R. Genetic Counselling for Haemophilia. WFH Treatment of Haemophilia monograph 2002; No 25.

14 Ljund R, Petrini P, Nilsson IM. Diagnostic symptoms of severe and moderate haemophilia A and B — a survey of 140 cases. *Acta Paediatr Scand* 1990; 79: 196–200.

15 Antonarakis SE, Rossiter IP, Young M, *et al.* Factor VIII gene inversions in severe haemophilia A: Results of an international consortium study. *Blood* 1995; 86: 2206–12.

16 Giannelli F, Green PM, Sommer S. Haemophilia B (sixth edition); a database of point mutations and short additions and deletions. *Nucleic Acids Res* 1996; 24: 103–18.

17 Tedgard VI. Carrier testing and prenatal diagnosis of haemophilia — utilisation and psychological consequences. *Haemophilia* 1998; 4: 365–9.

18 Varekamp I, Suurmeijer TP, Brocker-Vriends AH, *et al.* Carrier testing and prenatal diagnosis for hemophilia: experiences and attitudes of 549 potential and obligate carriers. *Am J Med Genet* 1990; 37: 147–54.

19 Ranta S, Lehesjoki AE, Peippo M, Kaariainen H. Haemophilia A: experiences and attitudes of mothers, sisters, and daughters. *Pediatr Hematol Oncol* 1994; 11: 387–97.

20 Rhoads GG, Jackson LG, Schlesselman SE, *et al.* The safety and efficacy of chorionic villus sampling for early prenatal diagnosis of cytogenetic abnormalities. *N Engl J Med* 1989; 320: 609–917.

21 Firth HV, Boyd PA, Chamberlin PF, *et al.* Analysis of limb reduction defects in babies exposed to chorionic villus sampling. *Lancet* 1994; 343: 1067–71.

22 Froster UG, Jackson L. Limb defects and chorionic villus sampling: results from an international registry, 1992–1994. *Lancet* 1996; 347: 489–94.

23 Wilson RD, Farquharson DF, Wittmann BK, Shaw D. Cordocentesis: overall pregnancy loss rate as important as procedure loss rate. *Fetal DiagnTher* 1994; 9: 142–8.

24 Plattner G, Renner W, Went J, Beaudette L, Vain G. Fetal sex determination by ultrasound scan in the second and third trimesters. *Obstet Gynecol* 1983; 61: 454–8.

25 Bronshtein M, Rottem S, Yoffe N, Blumenfeld Z, Brandes JM. Early determination of fetal sex using transvaginal sonography: technique and pitfalls. *J Clin Ultrasound* 1990; 18: 302–6.

26 Witlow BJ, Lazanakis MS, Economides DL. The sonographic identification of fetal gender from 11 to 14 weeks gestation. *Ultrasound Obstet Gynaecol* 1999; 13: 301–4.

27 Hromadnikova I, Houbova B, Hridelova D, *et al.* Replicate real-time testing of DNA in maternal plasma increases the sensitivity of non-invasive fetal sex determination. *Prenat Diagn* 2003; 23: 235–8.

28 Kadir RA, Economides DL, Braithwaite J, *et al.* The obstetric experience of carriers of haemophilia. *Br J Obstet Gynaecol* 1997; 104: 803–10.

29 Ray JG. DDAVP use in pregnancy: an analysis of its safety for mother and child [review]. *Obstet Gynecol Surv* 1998; 53: 450–5.

30 Santagostino E, Mannucci PM, Gringeri A, *et al.* Eliminating parvovirus B19 from blood products [Letter]. *Lancet* 1994; 343: 798.

31 Goldsmith JC, Kletzel M. Risk of birth related intracranial hemorrhage in hemophilic newborns: results of a North American survey (abstract). *Blood* 1990; 76: 421a.

32 Kulkarni R, Lusher JM, Henry RC, Kallen DJ. Current practices regarding newborn intracranial haemorrhage and obstetric care and mode of deliveryof pregnant haemophilia carriers: a survey of obstetricians, neonatologists and haematologists in the United States, on behalf of National Haemophilia Foundation's Medical and Scientific Advisory Council. *Haemophilia* 1999; 5: 410–15.

33 Ljung R, Lindgren AC, Petrini P, Tengborn L. Normal vaginal delivery is to be recommended for haemophilia carrier gravidae. *Acta Paediatr* 1994; 83: 609–11.

34 Kletzel M, Miller C H, Becton DL, *et al.* Postdelivery head bleeding in hemophilic neonates. *Am J Dis Child* 1989; 143: 1107–10.

35 Cunningham FG, MacDonald PC, Gant NF. Abnormalities of the third stage of labor. In: Cunningham FG, MacDonald PC, Gant NF. *Williams Obstetrics,* 18th edn. London: Prentice-Hall, 1989: 415–24.

36 Lee CY, Madrazo B, Drukker BH. Ultrasonic evaluation of postpartum uterus in the management of postpartum bleeding. *Obstet Gynecol* 1981; 58: 227–32.

37 Walker ID, Walker JJ, Colvin BT, *et al.* Investigation and management of haemorrhagic disorders in pregnancy. *J Clin Pathol* 1994; 47: 100–8.

38 Kulkarni R. Perinatal management of newborn with haemophilia. *Br J Haematol* 2001; 112: 264–74.

39 Peyvandi F, Duga S, Akhavan S, Mannucci PM. Rare coagulation deficiencies. *Haemophilia* 2002; 8: 308–21.

40 Kadir RA, Economides DL, Lee CA. FXI deficiency in women. *Am J Med* 1999; 60: 48–54.

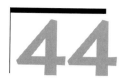

von Willebrand disease: molecular aspects

Ulrich Budde and Reinhard Schneppenheim

The von Willebrand factor gene and gene product

The protein is encoded by a gene that is located on chromosome 12p and is approximately 180 kilobases in size and composed of 52 exons. A nonprocessed pseudogene is located on chromosome 22. It duplicates the region spanning exons 23–34 with 97% homology. The gene product is synthesized by endothelial cells and megakaryocytes. The primary translation product undergoes a complex series of processing steps leading to the assembly of large von Willebrand factor (VWF) multimers, which are stored in specialized intracellular organelles (Weibel–Palade bodies, α-granules), while smaller multimers leave the cell constitutively [1]. Circulating VWF undergoes proteolytic cleavage under physiologic conditions. This proteolytic cleavage is responsible for the complex banding pattern of the individual oligomers and is apparently essential for the regulation of the size of the multimeric protein.

The mature VWF contains 2050 amino acids. Cysteines are abundant and cluster in two domains located at the amino and carboxy termini. In these regions, intermolecular disulfide bonds lead to dimerization (cysteine knot-like domain) and multimerization (cysteine-rich D3 domain). Because no free sulfhydryl groups are detectable, all cysteine residues that are not used for intermolecular bonds form intramolecular bonds that end in a complex tertiary structure of the VWF molecule. Of particular interest are two large loops in the A1 and A3 domains. The estimated carbohydrate content is approximately 18% of the total mass. Some of the carbohydrates express ABO antigens, which are responsible for a considerable part of the physiologic heterogeneity of the VWF level.

Because of the limited space of this chapter, not all known mutations can be addressed. The VWF mutation database is updated frequently and contains most of the hitherto known mutations [2].

von Willebrand disease with quantitative defects

Virtually complete absence of VWF (type 3)

The inheritance of von Willebrand disease (VWD) type 3 is autosomal recessive and the parents are often consanguineous.

Linkage analysis

Several studies have shown a linkage between VWD type 3 and the VWF gene by using the known restriction fragment length polymorphisms and the variable number of tandem repeats (VNTRs). Thus, in large enough families, carrier detection is easy by these methods in most cases.

Molecular defects

Because of the quantitative deficiency in type 3, restriction to functional domains of the molecule, which is successful in many families with qualitative (type 2) defects, will not be successful in a large number of type 3 patients. Most of the defects will be gene deletions, mRNA defects, stop codons, frameshift mutations, or splice-site mutations. Therefore, the identification of these defects, which are scattered over the whole gene (see Plate 4, opposite p. 00), is time-consuming and expensive [3]. The defects responsible for type 3 VWD are listed in Table 44.1.

Gene deletions

These defects, which were first detected in type 3 patients, are responsible for the disease in only a minority of patients [4,5]. On the other hand, the knowledge about large deletions in a given patient is clinically important, because most of them will develop alloantibodies after treatment with VWF-containing concentrates [6].

mRNA defects

Comparing the genomic DNA with platelet-derived cDNA will identify silent alleles, because heterozygous relatives of type 3 patients will be homozygous at the cDNA level, when one allele is not expressed. Using this method, which omits screening of the entire coding region, defects at the level of mRNA expression were detected in three families [7].

Stop codons

At least 18 different stop codons have been detected in patients with VWD type 3. One of these is recurrent and was found in Swedish, Italian, Dutch, Turkish, and German families [7]. A founder effect could be established for some, but not all, families.

Table 44.1 Molecular defects in von Willebrand disease type 3 (from ref. 3).

Type of defect	Nucleotide change	Amino acid change	Exon location
Gene deletions	Complete VWF gene deletion	Gene deletion	1–52
	Large partial VWF gene deletion	Gene deletion	17–18
	Large partial VWF gene deletion	Gene deletion	22–43
	Large partial VWF gene deletion	Gene deletion	23–52
	Large partial VWF gene deletion	Gene deletion	33–38
	Large partial VWF gene deletion	Gene deletion	42
	Large partial VWF gene deletion	Gene deletion	Unspecified
	8241del9	HYC2784del	51
mRNA expression defect	No VWF mRNA detectable	Not applicable	Not applicable
Stop codons	$171C \rightarrow A$	C57X	3
	$652C \rightarrow T$	Q218X	6
	$916G \rightarrow A$	W222X	7
	$970C \rightarrow T$	R324X	8
	$1093C \rightarrow T$	R365X	9
	$1117C \rightarrow T$	R373X	10
	$1858G \rightarrow T$	E620X	15
	$1930G \rightarrow T$	E644X	15
	$2116C \rightarrow T$	Q706X	16
	$3931C \rightarrow T$	Q1311X	28
	$4013C \rightarrow G$	S1338X	28
	$4036C \rightarrow T$	Q1346X	28
	$4626C \rightarrow G$	Y1542X	28
	$4975C \rightarrow T$	R1659X	28
	$5557C \rightarrow T$	R1853X	32
	$6635G \rightarrow T$	E2129X	37
	Not reported	Y2392X	42
	$7603C \rightarrow T$	R2535X	45
Frameshift insertions	1657insT	Frameshift	14
	2734insT	Frameshift	21
	4415insG	Frameshift	28
	4971insC	Frameshift	28
	7125insC	Frameshift	42
	7449insA	Frameshift	44
	7671insC	Frameshift	45
Frameshift deletions	187delG	Frameshift	3
	1930del20	Frameshift	15
	2430delC	Frameshift	18
	2641delC	Frameshift	20
	3385delAG	Frameshift	26
	4449delG	Frameshift	28
	4635delG	Frameshift	28
	6181delT	Frameshift	36
Splice-site mutations	$1110 - 1G \rightarrow A$	Not applicable	10
	$1534 - 3C \rightarrow A$	Not applicable	14
	$2443 - 1G \rightarrow C$	Not applicable	19
	$5053 + 1G \rightarrow T$	Not applicable	28
	$5170 + 10C \rightarrow T$	Not applicable	29
	$6977 - 1G \rightarrow C$	Not applicable	41
	$7437G \rightarrow A$	Not applicable	43
	$8155 + 3G \rightarrow T$	Not applicable	50

Continued

Table 44.1 *Continued*

Type of defect	Nucleotide change	Amino acid change	Exon location
Missense mutations	100C → G	R34G	3
	449T → A	L150Q	5
	817C → T	R273W	7
	823T → A	C275S	7
	1131G → T	W377C	10
	Gene conversion		28
	3943C → T	R1315C	28
	6187C → T	P2063S	36
	6520T → G	C2174G	37
	7085G → T	C2362F	42
Missense mutations, dimerization region	8012G → A	C2671Y	49
	8216G → A	C2739Y	51
	8262T → G	C2754W	52
	8411G → A	C2804Y	52
	8416T → C	C2806R	52

Table 44.2 Localization of molecular defects in von Willebrand disease (VWD) variants.

Localization of molecular defects	VWD variants
D1 domain	2A (IIC and IIC Miami)
D2 domain	2A (IIC)
D′ domain	2N
D3 domain	2M (Vicenza)
	2A (IIE and IIC Miami)
A1 domain	2B
	2M
	2 unclassified
	2A (IB)
	2A (smeary structure)
A2 domain	2A (IIA)
A3 domain	2M collagen-binding defect
Cysteine knot domain	2 (IID)

Frameshift mutations

Because only a few frameshift mutations are inframe and produce a gene product, most of these mutations will terminate the translational process prematurely and are functional stop codons. One single cytosine deletion in exon 18 (2430delC) has a very high prevalence in Poland, Sweden, and Germany but is rare or nonexistent in other countries ("Baltic mutation" [8]). This deletion was found to be causative in the original Åland families [9].

Splice-site mutations

Splice-site mutations result in exon skipping and terminate the transcription when the reading frame is changed. A number of these mutations have been reported in type 3 patients, and some have been shown to be causative for the type 3 phenotype [10].

Missense mutations

All the above listed mutations result in null alleles and the quantitative defect is thus plausible. The quantitative defect resulting from missense mutations is less obvious. For a few mutations, e.g., the propeptide mutation R723W, the expressed recombinant molecule was retained intracellularly [11]. Those mutations located in the cysteine knot result in a loss of cysteine residues. Expression studies showed a complete loss of dimerization in the homozygous state [12]. In some patients with homozygous mutations in exon 52, residual VWF can be shown in platelets. Thus, these patients may be homozygous type 2 or type 3 patients.

Classification issues

No cut-off level of VWF:Ag for the distinction between severe type 1, homozygous type 2, and type 3 has ever been defined. Thus, classification is clearly not unambiguous. The absence or presence of platelet VWF may distinguish between these patients. Expression of all candidate mutations and determination of intracellular and secreted VWF will help to resolve the remaining classification issues in the near future.

Partial deficiency of VWF (type 1)

Molecular defects

The inheritance of VWD type 1 is autosomal dominant with variable expressivity and penetrance [13]. Owing to the quantitative nature of the defect, most of the defects should be gene deletions, mRNA defects, stop codons, frameshift mutations, or splice-site mutations. Up to now, in rare cases mutations have been characterized as frameshifts, nonsense mutations, or deletions, which overlap with those in type 3.

Because the genetic mechanism remains elusive in most cases, two large studies were initiated in Europe and Canada. In July 2003, a first update of the European study was given during the International Society on Thrombosis and Hemostasis (ISTH) conference in Birmingham. At that time, 100 candidate mutations had been detected in 83 individuals. In contrast to the expected mutations that would result in null alleles, 71% were missense mutations, while a minority of families showed splicing errors, small insertions and deletions, nonsense mutations, and 5′ untranslated repeat (UTR) changes. As in type 3 patients, the quantitative defect resulting from missense mutations is not immediately obvious. For one mutation (C1149R), a dominant negative mechanism could be demonstrated by Eikenboom and colleagues [14,15]. The expressed recombinant molecule was secreted as wild-type homodimers only, and mutant wild-type heterodimers were retained in the endoplasmic reticulum.

Classification issues

Although type 1 VWD is defined as a quantitative defect without any detectable qualitative abnormalities, there is to date no consensus as to whether or not minor qualitative abnormalities, such as a small loss of the largest multimers or aberrant structural patterns, can be neglected.

Thus, during the European type 1 study, in roughly one-third of the families the diagnosis of type 1 was not compatible with phenotypic and genotypic data gained during the study. Because all participating laboratories had the best expertise in diagnosis of VWD, this indicated that, more than 75 years after the first description of VWD, diagnostic issues still exist. Many patients with presumed VWD type 1 and bleeding symptoms have VWD type 2 instead. The diagnosis of VWD type 2 subtypes depends on a standardized multimer analysis as the critical method. Molecular diagnosis can and should confirm the diagnosis in difficult cases.

von Willebrand disease with qualitative defects (see Plates 4 and 5, facing p. 212)

von Willebrand disease type 2A

The reduction in high-molecular-weight multimers (HMWMs) in subtype IIA (Table 44.3) is due either to their impaired intracellular transport (group 1 mutations) or to their enhanced proteolysis by the VWF-specific protease (group 2 mutations [16]). Most mutations causing this subtype are located in the A2 domain of VWF, although some (mostly mutations that affect cysteine residues) have been described in the A1 domain. They are listed in the VWF mutation database [2] and are reviewed in Meyer et al. [17].

Another cause of the deficiency of HMWM is defective posttranslational processing, which includes defects of dimerization at the VWF carboxy terminus (Table 44.4) in the subtype IID

Table 44.3 Localization of molecular defects in the A1 domain that cause a 2A (IIA) phenotype (modified from ref. 17). The number of families is that found by our group in German patients; the numbers for French families are given in ref. 17.

Exon	Defective amino acid(s)	Families (*n*)
28	G1505E*	
28	G1505R*	
28	S1506L*	2
28	F1514C*	
28	K1518E*	
28	L1540P*	
28	S1543F*	
28	Q1556R*	
28	L1562P*	
28	R1597G*	
28	R1597Q*	
28	R1597W*	2
28	V1604F*	
28	V1607D*	
28	G1609R*	4
28	P1627H	
28	I1628T*	4
28	G1629R*	
28	V1630E*	
28	E1638K*	
28	L1639P*	
28	P1648S*	
28	L1657I*	
28	V1665E*	
28	G1672R*	

*The reference is given in ref. 17.

Table 44.4 Localization of molecular defects in the cysteine knot. The number of families is that found by our group in German patients.

Exon	Defective amino acid(s)	Families (*n*)	Phenotype
52	C2754W	1	3
52	C2771R	1	2A (IID)
52	C2773R	1	2A (IID)
52	S2775C	1	2A (IID)
52	C2771Y	1	2A (IID)
52	dC8566	1	2A (IIE)

(58–60). Patients with this variant show odd-numbered oligomers [18] (see Plate 6, facing p. 212).

Defects of further polymerization of VWF dimers to multimers at their amino termini can be due to mutations in the D1 and D2 domain (Table 44.5) of the VWF propeptide, which are necessary to catalyze intermolecular disulfide bonding at the D3 domain of the mature VWF in the subtype IIC [19,20].

Mutations in the D3 domain (Tables 44.5 and 44.6) itself are described in subtypes IIE [21] and in the subtype IIC Miami [22,23]. In addition to a decrease in or absence of HMWMs, the multimer patterns of the subtypes IIE show an aberrant triplet structure. Surprisingly, the IIE phenotype is rather common and accounts for about one-third of patients with VWD type 2A. In such patients, we have identified a cluster of mutations in the VWF D3 domain that mainly affect cysteine residues that are potentially participating in intermolecular disulfide bonding at

the amino terminus of the mature VWF subunit as the essential domain of VWF multimerization. Interestingly, in families with the IIC Miami subtype of VWD 2A, the associated mutations also cluster in the D3 domain, suggesting a similar mechanism [24,25].

The IB (Table 44.7) phenotype with a relative loss of the largest multimers is represented by about 12% of our 2A patients. Some of the causative mutations have been allocated into the region of exon 28, where type 2M mutations have been described [26,27].

About 16% of our patients with subtypes of type 2A show a relative loss of the large multimers, with sometimes faint supranormal multimers and a triplet structure that is overlaid with amorphous material, giving the electrophoresis lane a smeary appearance. Gene defects have been located in exon 28 within the A1 domain [28] and in cases of VWD 2N in the D′ domain. In all cases, the mutations affected cysteine residues. Cysteine mutations may induce an unstable molecule [29], resulting in the observed smeary pattern of the electrophoretic lanes.

Most subtypes of VWD 2A are inherited in a dominant fashion, except subtype IIC and, in one case, subtype IID, both of which are inherited recessively.

von Willebrand disease type 2B

An important reason for the lack of HMWM is the enhanced affinity of VWF to platelet GPIb in patients with VWD type 2B (Table 44.8). In some of these patients, however, the enhanced affinity of VWF to GPIb is not correlated with loss of HMWMs, e.g., in VWD 2B New York/Malmö [30]. The inheritance is autosomal dominant. This subtype is well defined by the results of

Table 44.5 Localization of molecular defects in the prosequence (modified from ref. 17). The number of families is that found by our group in German patients, the numbers for French families are given in ref. 17.

Exon	Defective amino acid(s)	Families (n)	Phenotype
3	S58P	1	2A (IIC Miami)
6	L193P	1	2A (IIC Miami)
11	F404insNP		2A (IIC)*
	R436del6		2A (IIC)*
12	T441N	1	2A (IIC Miami)
12	R442H	1	2A (IIC Miami)
14	C524Y	1	2A (IIC)
14	N528S		2A (IIC)*
14	L536P	1	2A (IIC)
14	G550R	1	2A (IIC)
15	C623W		2A (IIC)*
15	A625insG		2A (IIC)*

*The reference is given in ref. 17.

Table 44.6 Localization of molecular defects in the D3 domain. The number of families is that found by our group in German patients.

Exon	Defective amino acid(s)	Families (n)	Phenotype
22	R976C	1	2A (IIE)
24	M1051T	1	2A (IIC Miami)
24	C1071F	1	2A (IIE)
25	C1091R	1	2A (IIE)
25	C1099Y	1	2A (IIC Miami)
25	C1109R	1	2A (IIE)
25	R1121M	1	2A (IIE)
26	C1126F	1	2A (IIE)
26	C1130Y	1	2A (IIE)
26	Y1146C	2	2A (IIE)
26	C1149Y	1	2A (IIE)
26	C1153Y	1	2A (IIE)
26	C1173F	1	2A (IIE)
26	C1173R	1	2A (IIE)
26	C1190R	1	2A (IIE)
27	D1195Y	1	2A (IIE)
27	R1205H	10*	2M (Vicenza)
28	L1278R	1	2A (IIE)
23	delExon 23	1	2A (IIE)
26	delExon 26	1	2A (IIE)

*Eight from Italian families.

Table 44.7 Localization of molecular defects in the A1-domain that do not cause a 2B phenotype (modified from ref. 17). The number of families is that found by our group in German patients, the numbers for French families are given in ref. 17.

Exon	Defective amino acid(s)	Families (n)	Phenotype
28	L1276P		2A/2M/unclassified*
28	R1315C	3	2A (IB)
28	G1324S		2M*
28	G1324A		2M*
28	R1343V	2	2M
28	E1359K		2M*
28	F1369I		2M*
28	R1374C		2A/2M/unclassified*
28	R1374H		2A/2M/unclassified*
28	R1374L		2A/2M/unclassified*
28	I1425F		2M*
28	Q1191del11		2M*
28	K1048delK		2M*
28	C1458Y	1	2A/2M/unclassified*

*The reference is given in ref. 17.

Table 44.8 Localization of molecular defects in the A1 domain that cause a 2B phenotype (modified from ref. 17). The number of families is that found by our group in German patients; the numbers for French families are given in ref. 17.

Exon	Defective amino acid(s)	Families (n)
28	P1266L*	3
28	H1268D*	
28	C1272G*	
28	C1272R*	1
28	M1304insM*	
28	R1306Q*	1
28	R1306M*	1
28	R1306W*	2
28	R1308C*	1
28	R1308P*	1
28	I1309V*	1
28	S1310F*	
28	W1313C*	
28	V1314F*	
28	V1314L*	
28	V1316M*	1
28	P1337L*	
28	R1341L*	
28	R1341Q*	2
28	R1341W*	
28	L1460V*	
28	A1461V*	

*The reference is given in ref. 17.

the ristocetin-induced platelet agglutination test (RIPA) and by the location of the mutations in a restricted region of the A1 domain. These mutations are listed in the VWF mutation database [2] and are reviewed in Meyer *et al.* [17].

von Willebrand disease type 2M

This type, which is inherited in a dominant fashion (Tables 44.8 and 44.9), includes patients with decreased VWF platelet-dependent functional parameters in the presence of HMWMs, disregarding further issues of differentiation such as an aberrant structure of individual multimers or the presence of ultralarge HMWM (supranormal multimers), as seen in the subtype VWD type 2M Vicenza. Subtype VWD 2M Vicenza is associated in several families with a mutation in the D3 domain of VWF [31]. The Vicenza type seems to be much more abundant than previously thought [32]. The problem in diagnosing VWD 2M is similar to the situation in VWD 1, as the quality of the multimer analysis leaves some range of interpretation. A careful re-evaluation of patients with VWD type 2M and patients with VWD type 1 who present with a discrepancy between VWF:Ag and either VWF:RCo or VWF:CB seems necessary.

Most of our type 2M (88%) patients have a triplet structure that is overlaid with amorphous material, giving the electrophoresis lane a smeary appearance.

Table 44.9 Localization of molecular defects in the A3 domain.

Exon	Defective amino acid(s)	Families (n)	
30	S1731T	1	2 M (CB)*
30	Q1734H	1	2 M (CB)
30	I1741T	1	2 M (CB)
30	Q1762R	1	2 M (CB)

*The reference is given in ref. 17.

Table 44.10 Localization of molecular defects in type 2N von Willebrand disease variants (modified from ref. 17). The number of families is that found by our group in German patients; the numbers for French families are given in ref. 17.

Exon	Defective amino acid(s)	Families (n)	Phenotype
18	R728W		2N*
18	G785E		2N*
18	E787K	1	2N
18	C788R		2N*
18	C788Y		2N*
18	T791M	1	2N
18	Y795C	1	2N; structure
18	M800V		2N*
19	R816W		2N*
19	R816Q		2N*
19	H817Q		2N*
20	R854Q	15	2N
20	R854W		2N*
20	C858F		2N*
20	D879N		2N*
24	Q1053H		2N*
24	C1060R		2 N; structure*
27	C1225G		2 N; structure*

*The reference is given in ref. 17.

Very recently, a mutation in the A3 domain (S1731T), which interfered with binding to collagens type I and type III, has been described and the causative role of this mutation was confirmed by expression studies [33]. We have detected three different heterozygous mutations (Q1734H, I1741T, Q1762R) in the same region of unrelated patients with defective VWF:CB. The causative role of these mutations could be confirmed by expression in 293 EBNA cells and subsequent analysis of VWF:Ag, VWF:CB, and VWF:RCo, and evaluation of the VWF multimers [34]. All four previously described mutations are in close proximity to three mutations that interfere with binding to collagen type III *in vitro* [35].

von Willebrand disease type 2N

This type (Table 44.10) comprises patients with defects in the FVIII-binding region of VWF [36–40]. Patients may be either homozygous or compound heterozygous for the FVIII-binding defect, or compound heterozygous for the FVIII-binding defect and a null allele. Accordingly, the phenotype may either mimic hemophilia A exactly or be combined with decreased VWF:AG [37,38]. As patients with an additional aberrant multimeric pattern are not uncommon, analysis of the multimeric structure should be included [29,39]. The inheritance is recessive. This type is well defined by the FVIII-binding defect and by the underlying mutations, which are located in the VWF:FVIII-binding domain (D' domain) or in its close neighborhood.

References

1 de Wit TR, van Mourik JA. Biosynthesis, processing and secretion of von Willebrand factor: biological implications. *Baillière's Clin Hematol* 2001; **14**: 241–55.

2 Von Willebrand factor (vWF) mutation data base: (http://www.shef.ac.uk/vwf/mutations.html).

3 Eikenboom JCJ. Congenital von Willebrand disease type 3: clinical manifestations, pathophysiology and molecular biology. *Baillière's Clin Hematol* 2001; **14**: 365–79.

4 Ngo KY, Glotz VT, Koziol JA, *et al.* Homozygous and heterozygous deletions of the von Willebrand factor gene in patients and carriers of severe von Willebrand disease. *Proc Natl Acad Sci USA* 1988; **85**: 2753–7

5 Schneppenheim R, Krey S, Bergmann F, *et al.* Genetic heterogeneity of severe von Willebrand disease type III in the German population. *Hum Genetics* 1994; **94**: 640–52.

6 Mannucci PM, Bloom AL, Larrieu MJ, Nilsson IM. Atherosclerosis and von Willebrand factor I: prevalence of severe von Willebrand's disease in western Europe and Israel. *Br J Haematol* 1984; **57**: 163–9.

7 Eikenboom JCJ, Ploos van Amstel HK, Reitsma PH, Briët E. Mutations in severe, type III von Willebrand's disease in the Dutch population: candidate missense and nonsense mutations associated with reduced levels of von Willebrand factor messenger RNA. *Thromb Haemost* 1992; **68**: 448–54.

8 Gazda H, Budde U, Krey S, *et al.* Delta C in exon 18 of the von Willebrand factor gene is the most common mutation in patients with severe von Willebrand disease type 3 in Poland. *Blood* 1997; **90**: 566a (Abstract).

9 Zhang ZP, Blombäck M, Nyman D, Anvred M. Mutations of von Willebrand factor gene in families with von Willebrand disease in the Aaland islands. *Proc Natl Acad Sci USA* 1993; **90**: 7937–40.

10 Eikenboom JCJ, Castaman G, Vos HL, *et al.* Characterization of genetic defects in recessive type 1 and type 3 von Willebrand disease patients of Italian origin. *Thromb Haemost* 1998; **79**: 709–17.

11 Schneppenheim R, Budde U, Obser T, *et al.* Expression and characterization of von Willebrand dimerization defects in different types of von Willebrand disease. *Blood* 2001; **97**: 2059–66.

12 Allen S, Abuzenadah AM, Hinks J, *et al.* A novel von Willebrand disease causing mutation (Arg273TRP) in the von Willebrand factor propeptide that results in defective multimerization and secretion. *Blood* 2000; **96**: 560–8.

13 Rodeghiero F, Castaman G. Congenital von Willebrand disease type 1: definition, phenotypes, clinical and laboratory assessment. *Baillière's Clin Haematol* 2001; **14**: 321–5.

14 Eikenboom JCJ, Matsushita T, Reitsma PH, *et al.* Dominant type 1 von Willebrand disease caused by mutated cysteine residues in the D3 domain of von Willebrand factor. *Blood* 1996; **88**: 2433–41.

15 Castaman G, Eikenboom JCJ, Missiaglia E, Rodeghiero F. Autoso-mal dominant type 1 von Willebrand disease due to G3639T mutation (C1130F) in exon 26 of the von Willebrand factor gene: description of five Italian families and evidence for a founder effect. *Br J Haematol* 2000; **108**: 876–9.

16 Lyons SE, Bruck ME, Bowie EJ, Ginsburg D. Impaired intracellular transport produced by a subset of type IIA von Willebrand disease mutations. *J Biol Chem* 1992; **267**: 4424–30.

17 Meyer D, Fressinaud E, Hilbert L, *et al.* Type 2 von Willebrand disease causing defective von Willebrand factor-dependent platelet function. *Baillière's Clin Hematol* 2001; **14**: 349–64.

18 Schneppenheim R, Brassard J, Krey S, *et al.* Defective dimerization of von Willebrand factor subunits due to a Cys Arg mutation in IID von Willebrand disease. *Proc Natl Acad Sci USA* 1996; **93**: 3581–6.

19 Gaucher C, Dieval J, Mazurier C. Characterization of von Willebrand factor gene defects in two unrelated patients with type IIC von Willebrand disease. *Blood* 1994; **84**: 1024–30.

20 Schneppenheim R, Thomas KB, Krey S, *et al.* Identification of a missense mutation in a family with von Willebrand disease type IIC. *Hum Genet* 1995; **95**: 681–6.

21 Schneppenheim R, Obser T, Schneppenheim S, *et al.* Von Willebrand disease type 2A with aberrant structure of individual oligomers is caused by mutations clustering in the von Willebrand factor D3 domain. *Blood* 2000; **96**: 566a (Abstract).

22 Schneppenheim R, Budde U, Ruggeri ZM. A molecular approach to the classification of von Willebrand disease. *Baillière's Clin Hematol* 2001; **14**: 281–98.

23 Budde U, Schneppenheim R. Von Willebrand factor and von Willebrand disease. *Rev Clin Exp Hematol* 2001; **5**: 335–63.

24 Ledford MR, Rabinowtz I, Sadler JE, *et al.* New variant of von Willebrand disease type II with markedly increased levels of von Willebrand factor antigen and dominant mode of inheritance: von Willebrand disease type IIC Miami. *Blood* 1993; **82**: 169–75.

25 Schneppenheim R, Obser T, Drewke E, *et al.* The first mutations in von Willebrand disease type IIC Miami. *J Thromb Haemost* 2001; Suppl. July: P1805.

26 Hilbert L, Jenkins PV, Gaucher C, *et al.* Type 2M vWD resulting from a lysine deletion within a four lysine residue repeat in the A1 loop of von Willebrand factor. *Thromb Haemost* 2000; **84**: 188–94.

27 Nitu-Whalley IC, Ridell A, Lee CA, *et al.* Identification of type 2 von Willebrand disease in previously diagnosed type 1 patients: a reappraisal using phenotypes, genotypes and molecular modelling. *Thromb Haemost* 2000; **84**: 998–1004.

28 Casonato A, Pontara E, Sartorello F, *et al.* Type 2M von Willebrand disease variant characterized by abnormal von Willebrand factor multimerization. *J Lab Clin Med* 2001; **137**: 70–6.

29 Jorieux S, Fressinaud E, Goudemand J, *et al.* Conformational changes in the D' domain of von Willebrand factor induced by CYS25 and CYS95 mutations lead to factor VIII binding defect and multimeric impairment. *Blood* 2000; **95**: 3139–45.

30 Weiss HJ, Sussman II. A new von Willebrand variant (type I, New York): increased ristocetin-induced palatelet aggregation and plasma von Willebrand factor containing the full range of multimers. *Blood* 1986; **68**: 149–56.

31 Schneppenheim R, Federici AB, Budde U, *et al.* Von Willebrand disease type 2M "Vicenza" in Italian and German patients: identification of the first candidate mutation (G3864R; R1205H) in 8 families. *Thromb Haemost* 2000; **83**: 136–40.

32 Zieger B, Budde U, Jessat U, *et al.* New families with von Willebrand disease type 2M (Vicenza). *Thromb Res* 1997; **87**: 57–64.

33 Ribba AS, Loisel I, Lavergne JM, *et al.* Ser968Tyr mutation within the A3 domain of von Willebrand factor (vWF) in two related patients leads to defective binding of vWF to collagen. *Thromb Haemost* 2001; **86**: 848–54.

34 Schneppenheim R, Obser T, Drewke R, *et al.* Isolated molecular defects of von Willebrand factor binding to collagen do not correlate with bleeding symptoms. *Blood* 2001; **98**: 41a (Abstract).

35 Romijn RA, Bouma B, Wuyster W, *et al.* Identification of the collagen-binding site of the von Willebrand factor A3-domain. *J Biol Chem* 2001; **30**: 9985–91.

36 Mazurier C, Goudemand J, Hilbert L, *et al.* Type 2N von Willebrand disease: clinical manifestations, pathophysiology, laboratory diagnosis and molecular biology. *Baillière's Clin Hematol* 2001; **14**: 337–47.

37 Nishino M, Girma JP, Rothschild C, *et al.* New variant of von Willebrand disease with defective binding to factor VIII. *Blood* 1989; **74**: 1591–9.

38 Mazurier C. Von Willebrand disease masquerading as haemophilia A. *Thromb Haemost* 1992; **67**: 391–6.

39 Allen S, Abuzenadah AM, Blagg JL, *et al.* A novel type 2N von Willebrand disease-causing mutation that results in defective factor VIII binding, multimerization, and secretion of von Willebrand factor. *Blood* 2000; **95**: 2000–7.

40 Schneppenheim R, Budde U, Krey S, *et al.* Results of a screening for von Willebrand disease type 2N patients with suspected haemophilia A or von Willebrand disease type 1. *Thromb Haemost* 1996; **76**: 598–602.

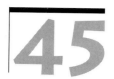

von Willebrand disease: epidemiology

Francesco Rodeghiero and Giancarlo Castaman

When Erik von Willebrand, in 1926, first investigated a family with a new bleeding disorder, subsequently universally known as von Willebrand disease (VWD) in recognition of his pioneering discovery [1], he was probably unaware that he was studying what would be recognized 60 years later as the most frequent inherited hemorrhagic disorder. Nowadays, there is a general consensus that VWD is often encountered in patients with mild bleeding symptoms or even in apparently normal subjects, and a prevalence up to 1% was estimated in a large epidemiologic investigation conducted by our group in 1987 [2]. However, a definite diagnosis of VWD remains often difficult or elusive, owing to the wide spectrum of clinical and laboratory manifestations and to the lack of strong penetrance and expressivity in its inheritance.

For these reasons, the actual prevalence of clinically significant cases of VWD is uncertain despite the ever-increasing number of diagnostic laboratory tools. Prevalence estimates are in fact critically influenced both by the clinical criteria used to select subjects and by the laboratory criteria used to confirm the diagnosis. Moreover, the assessment of the bleeding history is often more difficult in the epidemiologic than in the clinical setting. Physicians must rely on the patient's bleeding history, which is prone to personal feelings (recall bias), unless subjects have suffered from severe hemorrhages, possibly leading to hospitalization. No clinical methods are available to objectively quantify mild or intermediate bleeding symptoms, apart, possibly, from surgical bleeding and menorrhagia [3]. To further compound the problem, even normal subjects often refer with mild bleeding symptoms [4]. As a consequence, bleeding history taken at a referral center has not been shown to be predictive of subsequently diagnosed specific bleeding disorders [5]. Thus, it is important to understand the potential pitfalls that arise in prevalence estimation of VWD in relation to its clinical presentation. The use of different methods for prevalence estimation may indeed produce diverging results, with far lower prevalence figures obtained in hospital-based in comparison with population-based investigations, since different categories of subjects are considered (Figure 45.1).

Ascertainment and validity of epidemiologic data on von Willebrand disease

von Willebrand disease is usually classified in three subtypes on the basis of clinical and laboratory phenotypes. Type 1, ac-

counting for the large majority of cases, is represented by partial quantitative defects, type 2 by qualitative defects, and type 3 by virtual absence of VWF in plasma [6]. In practice, qualitative defects are suspected by measuring a significantly reduced VWF ristocetin cofactor activity to antigen ratio and confirmed by assessing the distribution of high/intermediate/low-molecular weight (MW) VWF multimers or more subtle abnormalities. This allows subclassification of type 2 into 2A (lack of high- and intermediate-MW multimers), 2B (lack of high-MW multimers), 2M (all species of multimers or even higher-MW multimers, as in the Vicenza type), or rarer variants [7]. However, from the point of view of clinical presentation and diagnostic approach, three distinct groups of VWD patients may be considered (Table 45.1).

In the first group (group A), patients present with a lifelong history of severe to moderate bleeding symptoms, often requiring hospitalization for transfusion, replacement therapy, surgical intervention (e.g., nose packing for epistaxis, dilation and curettage in women for menorrhagia). Iron deficiency anemia is also common, especially in women. Laboratory investigations show VWF activity levels below or around 10 IU/dL. Linkage with a mutant VWF gene is usually complete [8]. This group of patients comprises all subjects with recessive type 3 VWD, some with dominant type 1 with full penetrance and expressivity, and most type 2A and 2B VWD and type 2M Vicenza. Prevalence estimates for these patients may be reliably obtained from hospital-based cohorts, as it is highly unlikely that these patients have never been referred to specialized secondary centers, at least in Western countries.

The second group of patients (group B) comprises subjects with a milder but still definite bleeding diathesis. These patients have frequent spontaneous bleeding (such as mucocutaneous bleeding) and may be referred with bleeding after trauma or minor surgery, especially when mucous membranes are involved. Laboratory investigations show VWF activity levels around 30 IU/dL. Linkage analysis with mutations in the VWF gene is consistent with an autosomal dominant disease with variable penetrance in most cases [9]. This group of patients comprises most subjects with type 1 and some with type 2 VWD. Prevalence estimates for these patients are partly underestimated from hospital-based cohorts, because some patients may never seek hospital advice and hence give a falsely low prevalence. Very large, cross-sectional (population-based) investigations should be used.

The third group of patients (group C) comprises patients with

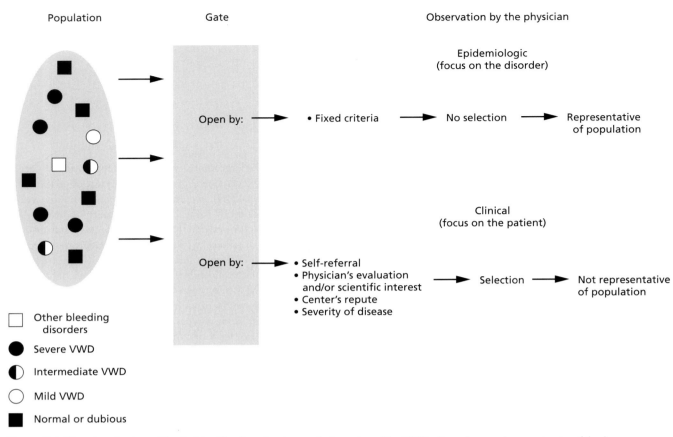

Figure 45.1 How the criteria used for the identification of patients to be investigated for VWD affects the prevalence estimates of the disease.

Table 45.1 Classification of von Willebrand disease according to clinical presentation and diagnostic approach.

	Severe VWD (group A)	Intermediate VWD (group B)	Mild VWD (group C)
Symptoms	Manifest bleeding	Intermediate	Mild or very mild
Cosegregation (linkage) of symptoms with low VWF/haplotype	Invariable	Variable	Inconsistent
VWF levels	About 10 IU/dL or less	About 30 IU/dL	40–50 IU/dL
Diagnosis	Easy	Repeated testing needed	Not always possible
Epidemiologic ascertainment	Referral-based: appropriate	Referral-based: underestimates	Cross-sectional: overestimates

a mild hemorrhagic diathesis. Bleeding symptoms are occasional, sometimes absent, even after trauma or minor surgery. Laboratory investigation shows VWF activity levels around 40–50 IU/dL, often requiring repeated measurements and adjustment for ABO group to achieve a correct diagnosis. Linkage analysis fails to detect association with VWF haplotype in up to 50% of the families, indicating a possibly spurious association [10]. Only cross-sectional, population-based studies could be used in this case and great care should be exercised to avoid falsely positive subjects possibly being identified as VWD just by chance.

For instance, based on the reported prevalence of hemorrhagic symptoms in normal and affected adults and children [2,4,5], and on an autosomal dominant pattern of disease transmission, one could estimate the probability of finding one or more subjects with a history of hemorrhage in a nuclear family with five subjects (two parents and three children, see Figure 45.2a) [11]. In the case of a healthy family, the probability of finding at least two family members with at least one hemorrhagic symptom is about 13%, compared with 70% in a VWD family (see Figure 45.2b for technical details). While this means that finding two or more subjects with a hemorrhagic history in such a family gives

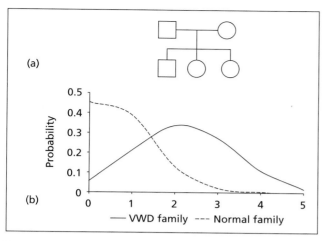

Figure 45.2 (a) Structure of the nuclear family considered for the simulation study. (b) Probability of finding exactly the number of hemorrhagic subjects reported in the abscissa for the family in (a), under the assumption of VWD being present in the family (solid line) or not (dashed line). To calculate the cumulative probability of having two or more subjects affected within a family, the probabilities reported for two, three, four, and five affected should be summed. For calculation, we assumed the prevalence of hemorrhagic symptoms in normal and VWD subjects reported by Rodeghiero [4] and Srámek *et al.* [5] and an autosomal dominant transmission of disease with a prevalence of 0.5%. The prevalence of hemorrhagic symptoms was decreased by about one-third in siblings to account for the age effect. The probability of finding one or more affected in the family was computed according to Weiss [11] in a computer-based simulation of 100 000 families.

a high likelihood of facing with a family with a hemostatic defect, it also means that about 13% of normal subjects could belong to a "hemorrhagic family" just by chance. Considering that (by definition) about 2.5% of normal subjects have a VWF activity level below the reference range, the probability of diagnosing an otherwise healthy subject as having VWD could be as high as 13% × 2.5%, or 1 in every 307 in the normal population. A similar simulation was recently reported by Sadler [12] to justify a proposal to use VWF level simply as a risk factor for bleeding in less severe cases. Noteworthy, in our large epidemiologic investigation [2], more conservative criteria in defining VWD were used and no more than 5% of the investigated population was classified as belonging to a bleeding family. Consequently, the misclassification rate of "probable" VWD (i.e., subjects belonging to a hemorrhagic family with reduced VWF activity) was one subject in every 800 investigated (5% × 2.5%). Furthermore, by considering the diagnosis as "definite" only in those with low VWF levels in at least another family member, the misclassification rate was as low as 5% × 2.5% × 2.5%, that is one subject in every 32 000 investigated.

Prevalence of severe VWD (group A VWD)

Most cases of clinically moderate to severe VWD are represented by type 3 and some cases of type 1, type 2A, and 2B VWD.

The prevalence of type 3 VWD is very low, ranging from 0.1 to 5.3 per million of the population. In 1982, Weiss *et al.* [13] reported a prevalence of severe VWD of 1.53 and 1.38 per million in Europe and North America respectively, based on the report from 195 referral centers worldwide. A subsequent re-evaluation of these subjects through measurement of VWF:Ag with a highly sensitive method (immunoradiometric assay) showed a prevalence of severe VWD (defined by an antigen level below 1 IU/dL) of 0.45 per million [14]. Significant differences in the prevalence of severe VWD were present in different countries, notably with a higher prevalence in Scandinavian countries (2.4–3.12 per million) [14]. The highest prevalence of type 3 VWD was, however, observed by Berliner *et al.* [15] in Arabs, in whom consanguinity is rather frequent, with an estimated prevalence of 5.3 per million.

Prevalence of intermediate VWD (group B VWD)

As for severe VWD, prevalence estimates for intermediate VWD are available only from hospital-based cohorts, as the number of patients registered at a single specialized center divided by the total population served by the center. The first data published with this methodology date back to 1984, when Nilsson estimated that there were about 530 known cases (230 families) of VWD in Sweden, corresponding to a prevalence of seven VWD patients per 100 000 inhabitants, the same figure as for hemophilia in that country [16]. This study, however, also includes patients with type 3. More recently, Bloom and Giddins [17] carried out an international survey on the prevalence of AIDS in VWD in 1991, trying to indirectly estimate the prevalence of VWD. A questionnaire was dispatched to the hemophilia center directors of 59 countries, soliciting information on the number of patients with VWD attending each center and the proportion of those treated with blood derivatives. Information was retrieved from 63% of the centers belonging to 37 countries concerning 16 664 identified patients, of whom 7534 were treated. The prevalence estimate was consequently very heterogeneous in the various countries, ranging from 3.7 to 239 cases per million inhabitants (Table 45.2). Surprisingly, the estimated prevalence for Scandinavia was about twice that reported by Nilsson [16] in the previously mentioned study. Whatever the limitations of this approach, the prevalence of patients with intermediate VWD requiring specific treatment has been estimated to range from 40 to 100 cases per million [16–19], a figure often quoted as a reliable estimation [20].

Prevalence of mild VWD

Four population-based studies are available. (Table 45.3) Rodeghiero *et al.* [2,21] evaluated 1218 schoolchildren aged 11–14 years in a well-defined territory of northern Italy. Diagnosis of VWD was considered "probable" in children with low

Table 45.2 Prevalence of referred VWD in ref. 17.

Area	Population (millions)	Patients reported	Percent of replies	Raw prevalence per million	Corrected prevalence per million
Scandinavia	21.5	4749	92	221	239
Rest of Europe	441	6514	65	14.8	23
Australasia	16	599	88	37	42
North America	237	2263	43	9.5	22
Israel	3.5	106	50	30.2	60.4
Far East	286	1673	71	5.8	8.1
South America	133	600	60	2.2	3.7
South Africa	24	80	44	3.3	7.4

VWF levels (VWF:RCo below an ABO-adjusted reference range) belonging to a family with more than two members, including or not the subject under investigation, with a bleeding history with two or more symptoms. A definite diagnosis was assigned if in addition to these criteria at least one other family member on the hemorrhagic side had a low VWF level. Ten children (four with probable and six with definite VWD) were classified as affected (0.82%). This figure could range from seven (0.57%) to 14 (1.15%) taking into account the 90% confidence interval for the lower limit of the normal range. It turned out that all these children had at least a bleeding symptom. This translates into a prevalence of 0.57–1.15%, or 5700–11 500 per million. Interestingly, in about half of the diagnosed families from this investigation, linkage was not subsequently confirmed [10].

In 1993, Werner *et al.* [22] published the results of a similar investigation carried out in 600 American schoolchildren aged 12–18 years undergoing well-child or school physical examinations at the pediatric ambulatory clinics of the hospitals located in Virginia, Ohio, and Mississippi. The criteria were seemingly less restrictive and included all three of at least one bleeding symptom, a family member with at least one bleeding symptom, and low VWF. The overall prevalence was estimated at 1.3%, with no racial difference (1.15% among Caucasians and 1.8% among blacks). These data have been confirmed in two additional studies, not reported as full papers. Miller *et al.* [23] in 1987 found a prevalence of VWD of 1.6% in adult blood donors from New York; however, the prevalence of symptomatic subjects with low VWF:RCo was 0.2%. In an additional study, Meriane *et al.* [24] studied the prevalence in Arabic-Turkish adult subjects. The figure was 1.23%, again with no racial differences. As a general comment, the prevalence of VWD appears to be similar in different ethnic groups. In all these studies, the same functional test (VWF:RCo) and separate normal ranges according to blood groups were used, thus giving uniformity to the results. Even though these figures appear high, it should be emphasized that the prevalence could probably be even higher since the sensitivity of the functional test is about 50%. This assumption stems from the demonstration by Miller *et al.* [25] that, among the obligatory carriers for type 1 disease, only 42% had abnormal VWF activity on their initial test. Only extensive haplotype or mutation detection studies could definitely clarify if these cases are really linked to VWF gene defects or caused by a complex interaction of different genetic and environmental influences producing a VWD-like phenotype. In a murine model, a phenotype mimicking VWD was produced by a mutation in the glycosyltransferase gene (*GALgt2*) [26] and the occurrence of similar mutations in human "VWD" cannot presently be ruled out.

Frequency of VWD subtypes

The relative frequencies of subtypes of VWD have been estimated only from the series of single institutions, and are obviously biased since they are based on severe and intermediate VWD patients (group A and B patients) only. On epidemiologic grounds, the prevalence of mild VWD (group C), which is almost invariably due to type 1 VWD, appears to be 100–1000 times higher than that of the group A and B. Consequently, type 1 VWD in the population should be at least 100-fold more common than the other subtypes. Nevertheless, in referred patients there is a rather homogeneous distribution of VWD subtypes (Table 45.4) [15,16,27–30]. Overall, the data could be summarized for a relative percentage frequency of 70, 17, and 13 for types 1, 2, and 3 VWD in the 592 patients considered in these studies. These data are quite in accordance with an extensive, recent survey carried out by Federici *et al.* [31] among Italian hemophilia centers, which reported a relative frequency of 73%, 21%, and 6% for types 1, 2, and 3 VWD respectively.

Prevalence of VWD in developing countries

Limited investigations have been carried out in developing countries, based on voluntary reporting in mail questionnaire-based survey through national or regional hemophilia centers [20]. In general, major under-reporting is evident compared with the expected prevalence. In a more recent unpublished survey, the ratio between severe hemophilia A (taken as a normalizing prevalence) and that of VWD in the same region was

Table 45.3 Estimates of prevalence of von Willebrand disease in ravious studies.

VWD severity	Study	Methodology	Population	Prevalence
Severe	Weiss et al. [13]	Mail survey to 354 hematology departments	USA, Canada, 17 European countries, Iran, Israel	1.38–1.51 per million
	Mannucci et al. [14]	Patients identified through a questionnaire; plasma VWF assay and recruitment of patients with VWF:Ag < 1% by IRMA*	Western European countries plus Israel	0.1–3.12 per million
	Berliner et al. [15]	Investigation of patients followed at a single center	Cases followed in Israel	5.3 per million among Arabs
Intermediate	Nilsson [16]	Cases registered at specialized centers in Sweden	230 Swedish families (530 patients) with VWD already known	70 cases per million inhabitants (about 15% severe type 3)
Mild	Rodeghiero et al. [2]	Anamnesis + VWF:RCo Family study	Caucasian children	0.82% (8200 per million)
	Rodeghiero et al. [21]	As above + VWF:Ag instead of VWF:RCo	As above	0.7%
	Miller et al. [23]	VWF:RCo	Adult blood donors	1.6% (0.2% bleeder)
	Meriane et al. [24]	Anamnesis + VWF:RCo Family study	Arabic-Turkish adult students	1.23%
	Werner et al. [22]	Anamnesis + VWF:RCo Family study	Caucasian and black children	1.3% (1.15% Caucasian; 1.81% black)

IRMA, immunoradiometric assay.

investigated, showing an under-reporting of more than 60% of cases of VWD. Surprisingly, the distribution of severity in reported cases is apparently not much different from that reported in developed countries, indicating the lack of a regional or national strategy for the detection of more severe cases (A. Srivastava and F. Rodeghiero, unpublished data). Sadly, deaths secondary to hemorrhage in VWD patients are still reported from these countries, despite cryoprecipitate and VWF/factor VIII concentrates being generally available, whereas similar cases are no longer described in economically more developed countries.

Practical implications

Severe VWD is a rare disorder, with a prevalence similar to that of other severe, homozygous coagulopathies, whereas the prevalence of intermediate VWD is probably similar to the cumulative prevalence of hemophilia A and B. The prevalence of mild VWD is still uncertain, but a reasonable estimate is possibly one case between every 1000–10 000 subjects. About 1% of the normal population could satisfy quite conservative epidemiologic criteria sufficient to diagnose VWD in *ad hoc* cross-sectional investigations. This rather high prevalence figure must be interpreted with caution, as many of these subjects will experience only minor or trivial bleedings during their lifetime and will probably never be referred for medical assistance. It is there-

fore of paramount importance to distinguish between a diagnosis satisfying only minimal criteria and a clinically meaningful diagnosis. While the first type of diagnosis is relevant for the epidemiologist but could be dangerous to the patient and his/her family in terms of generated anxiety and social burden, the second one is certainly more useful for the patient and the physician alike [4,32]. We will discuss here two instances aiming at clarifying this issue using an epidemiologic approach.

The case of presurgical screening

A prevalence of 1 per 500 subjects of a hemorrhagic disease may certainly be alarming for a surgeon facing an elective mucous surgery (e.g., tonsillectomy) and keen to avoid any hemorrhagic risk. However, despite such a high prevalence in the population, a presurgical screening is probably not cost-effective for two reasons. First, all available phenotypic laboratory tests have their specificity based on the "reference limit" concept, which means that the specificity is usually set at 97.5%. Even assuming a sensitivity of 100% for a laboratory test (a very optimistic estimate indeed), for every 1000 subjects screened, the test would identify 25 subjects as affected, of whom 23 would be false positives and only two would have mild VWD. Second, the chance of patients with mild VWD bleeding significantly after surgery may be less than 50%, which means that we need to screen more than 1000 subjects to avoid a surgical bleeding related to mild VWD, at the cost of excluding all the false positives.

Table 45.4 Frequency of von Willebrand disease subtypes in different sevies of patients.

Authors	Number of patients	Type 1 (%)	Type 2 (%)	Type 3 (%)
Tuddenham *et al.* [27]	134	75	19	6
Lenk *et al.* [28]	111	76	12	12
Nilsson [16]	106 families	70	10	20
Hoyer *et al.* [29]	116	71	23	6
Awidi [30]	65	59	29.5	11.5
Berliner *et al.* [15]	60	62	9	29
Overall	592	70	17	13

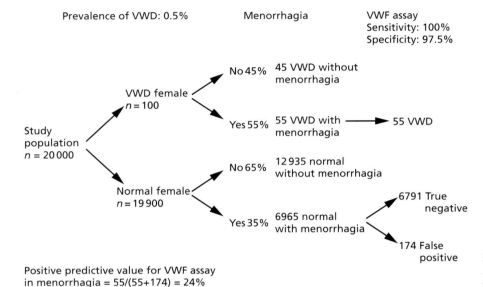

Figure 45.3 Positive predictive value for VWF assay in women referring menorrhagia. See text for assumptions.

The case of a diagnosis based on mild bleeding symptoms

Similarly, pursuing the diagnosis of mild VWD in a subject without a convincing personal or familial bleeding history poses the problems mentioned for presurgical screening and for cross-sectional epidemiologic surveys. As an example, we could examine the case of a woman investigated for VWD because of menorrhagia. Menorrhagia is found in 29–44% of otherwise healthy women [5,33] compared with 50–60% of VWD females [34]. Is screening for VWD advisable for all patients suffering menorrhagia? Let us consider a town with a population of 20 000 fertile women (Figure 45.3). Based on a prevalence of VWD of 0.5%, and on the above-mentioned figures, the ratio of VWD/normal in women with menorrhagia is 55/6965. By using the same laboratory test with a sensitivity of 100% and a specificity of 97.5% in all women complaining of menorrhagia, we would identify all the 55 VWD women but also 174 false positives, with a positive predictive value of only 24%. Thus, while it is recognized that menorrhagia could be the sole presenting symptom of a hemorrhagic disorder [34] and that, among women with menorrhagia, there is a high prevalence of VWD [35], generalized screening is not advisable. This is even truer if one considers that only a limited benefit is expected from a specific diagnosis in most women.

A clinically useful diagnosis

The two above-mentioned instances share a common feature: a laboratory diagnosis is made on the basis of a personal history with few symptoms (e.g., menorrhagia) or no symptoms at all (screening). In a recent multicenter survey, we demonstrated that the pretest probability (likelihood ratio) of VWD is significantly increased only when a clinically relevant history of hemorrhage is present (at least two hemorrhagic symptoms in the proband) [36]. Moreover, Figure 45.1 also highlights that at least two (but preferably three) family members should be present in a family to reasonably suspect VWD. Thus, every laboratory assessment should be undertaken only in subjects presenting with at least two separate hemorrhagic symptoms or having two first-degree relatives with hemorrhagic symptoms. It is also worth noting that the subjects and families identified by these criteria are also those that are more likely to benefit from an appropriate therapy (e.g., desmopressin treatment or prophylaxis).

Waiting for more specific clinical and laboratory tools that may allow us to better separate the wheat from the chaff in VWD, the epidemiologic data further reaffirm the concept that physicians should always base their diagnoses on sound clinical criteria that will translate their specific diagnosis into a beneficial way to treat or prevent the consequences of this still intriguing disorder [4].

Acknowledgment

We wish to thank Dr Alberto Tosetto for his helpful suggestions and for his invaluable contribution to the development of the epidemiologic simulations.

References

1 Von Willebrand EA. Hereditär pseudohemofili. *Finska Läkarsällskapets Handl* 1926; **67**: 7–112.
2 Rodeghiero F, Castaman G, Dini E. Epidemiological investigation of the prevalence of von Willebrand's disease. *Blood* 1987; **69**: 454–9.
3 Higham JM, O'Brien PM, Shaw RW. Assessment of menstrual blood loss using a pictorial chart. *Br J Obstet Gynaecol* 1990; **97**: 734–9.
4 Rodeghiero F. von Willebrand disease: still an intriguing disorder in the era of molecular medicine. *Haemophilia* 2002; **8**: 292–300.
5 Sramek A, Eikenboom JC, Briet E, *et al.* Usefulness of patient interview in bleeding disorders. *Arch Intern Med* 1995; **155**: 1409–15.
6 Sadler JE. A revised classification of von Willebrand disease. *Thromb Haemost* 1994; **71**: 520–3.
7 Castaman G, Federici AB, Rodeghiero F, Mannucci PM. Von Willebrand's disease in the year 2003: towards the complete identification of gene defects for correct diagnosis and treatment. *Haematologica* 2003; **88**: 94–108.
8 Keeney S, Cumming AM. The molecular biology of von Willebrand disease. *Clin Lab Haem* 2001; **23**: 209–30.
9 Casana P, Martinez F, Haya S, *et al.* Significant linkage and non-linkage of type 1 von Willebrand disease to the von Willebrand factor gene. *Br J Haematol* 2001; **115**: 692–700.
10 Castaman G, Eikenboom JCJ, Bertina R, Rodeghiero F. Inconsistency of association between type 1 von Willebrand disease phenotype and genotype in families identified in an epidemiologic investigation. *Thromb Haemost* 1999; **82**: 1065–70.
11 Weiss KM. *Genetic Variation and Human Disease.* Cambridge: Cambridge University Press, 1993.
12 Sadler JE. Von Willebrand disease type 1: a diagnosis in search of a disease. *Blood* 2003; **101**: 2089–93.
13 Weiss HJ, Ball AP, Mannucci PM. Incidence of severe von Willebrand's disease. *N Engl J Med* 1982; **307**: 127.
14 Mannucci PM, Bloom AL, Larrieu MJ, *et al.* Atherosclerosis and von Willebrand factor. I. Prevalence of severe von Willebrand's disease in Western Europe and Israel. *Br J Haematol* 1984; **57**: 163–9.
15 Berliner SA, Seligsohn U, Zivelin A, *et al.* A relatively high frequency of severe (type III) von Willebrand's disease in Israel. *Br J Haematol* 1986; **62**: 535–43.
16 Nilsson IM. Von Willebrand disease from 1926 to 1983. *Scand J Haematol* 1984; **33** (Suppl. 40): 21–43.
17 Bloom AL, Giddins JC. HIV infection and AIDS in von Willebrand's disease. An international survey including data on the prevalence of clinical von Willebrand's disease. In: Lusher JM, Kessler CM, eds. *Hemophilia and von Willebrand's Disease in 1990s.* Amsterdam: Elsevier Science Publishers, 1991: 405–11.
18 Bloom AL. The von Willebrand syndrome. *Semin Hematol* 1980; **17**: 215–27.
19 Bachman F. Diagnostic approach to mild bleeding disorders. *Semin Hematol* 1980; **17**: 292–312.
20 Sadler JE, Mannucci PM, Berntorp E, *et al.* Impact, diagnosis and treatment of von Willebrand disease. *Thromb Haemost* 2000; **84**: 160–74.
21 Rodeghiero F, Castaman G, Tosetto A. von Willebrand factor antigen is less sensitive than ristocetin cofactor for the diagnosis of type I von Willebrand disease — results based on an epidemiological investigation. *Thromb Haemost* 1990; **64**: 349–52.
22 Werner EJ, Broxson EH, Tucker EL, *et al.* Prevalence of von Willebrand disease in children: A multiethnic study. *J Pediatr* 1993; **123**: 893–8.
23 Miller CH, Lenzi R, Breen C. Prevalence of von Willebrand's disease among US adults. *Blood* 1987; **70** (Suppl. 1): 377 (Abstract).
24 Meriane F, Sultan Y, Arabi H, *et al.* Incidence of a low von Willebrand factor activity in a population of Algerian students. *Blood* 1991; **78**: 484 (Abstract).
25 Miller CH, Graham JB, Goldin LR, Elston RC. Genetics of classic von Willebrand's disease. I. Phenotypic variation within families. *Blood* 1979; **54**: 117–136.
26 Nichols WC, Cooney KA, Mohlke KL, *et al.* von Willebrand disease in the RIIIS/J inbred mouse strain as a model for von Willebrand disease. *Blood* 1994; **83**: 3225–8.
27 Tuddenham EGD. von Willebrand factor and its disorders: an overview of recent molecular studies. *Blood Rev* 1989; **3**: 251–62.
28 Lenk H, Nilsson IM, Holmberg L, Weissbach G. Frequency of different types of von Willebrand's disease. *Acta Med Scand* 1988; **224**: 275–80.
29 Hoyer LW, Rizza CR, Tuddenham EGD, *et al.* von Willebrand factor multimer patterns in von Willebrand's disease. *Br J Haematol* 1983; **55**: 493–507.
30 Awidi AS. A study of von Willebrand's disease in Jordan. *Ann Hematol* 1992; **64**: 299–302.
31 Federici AB, Castaman G, Mannucci PM. Guidelines for the diagnosis and treatment of von Willebrand disease in Italy. Italian Association of Hemophilia Centers (AICE). *Haemophilia* 2002; **8**: 607–21.
32 Rodeghiero F, Castaman G. Congenital von Willebrand disease type 1: definition, phenotypes, clinical and laboratory assessment. *Clin Haematol* 2001; **14**: 321.
33 Kadir RA, Economides DL, Sabin CA, *et al.* Assessment of menstrual blood loss and gynaecological problems in patients with inherited bleeding disorders. *Haemophilia* 1999; **5**: 40–8.
34 Edlund M, Blomback M, von Schoultz B, Andersson O. On the value of menorrhagia as a predictor for coagulation disorders. *Am J Hematol* 1996; **53**: 234–8.
35 Kadir RA, Economides DL, Sabin CA, *et al.* Frequency of inherited bleeding disorders in women with menorrhagia. *Lancet* 1998; **351**: 485–9.
36 Castaman G, Tosetto A, Cappelletti A, *et al.* Clinical presentation of type 1 von Willebrand disease (vWD) in obligatory carriers: final results from a collaborative, international, multicenter study. *J Thromb Haemost* 2003 (Suppl.): abs OC078.

46

von Willebrand disease: biological diagnosis

Edith Fressinaud and Dominique Meyer

Introduction

Von Willebrand factor (VWF) (Table 46.1) is a multimeric plasma protein that mediates platelet adhesion as well as platelet aggregation at sites of vascular injury; moreover, VWF acts as a chaperone protein for coagulation factor VIII (FVIII). Congenital deficiency of VWF causes von Willebrand disease (VWD), a bleeding disorder of variable severity that is divided into three categories [1]. Type 3 is easy to diagnose, with virtually complete deficiency of VWF. Type 2 is relatively easy to diagnose except in some forms, with various qualitative defects of VWF: three subtypes of type 2 are caused by an abnormal binding of VWF to platelets (2A, 2B, and 2M) and one is due to a defective binding of VWF to FVIII (2N), which mimics mild hemophilia A. In type 3 and type 2, molecular defects of the VWF gene are identified. VWD type 1, however, which is described as the common form of VWD and refers to partial, quantitative VWF deficiency, is difficult to diagnose and is probably widely overestimated [2]; moreover, the molecular basis of VWD type 1 is still unclarified.

Laboratory testing

Laboratory investigation should be performed after a careful study of personal and/or familial history of bleeding symptoms. It involves several levels of testing (Table 46.2): (i) screening tests; (ii) specific tests; (iii) discriminating tests.

Screening tests

Bleeding time

The bleeding time (BT) is usually performed using disposable apparatus with the modified Ivy method. The procedure is neither specific nor sensitive. A prolonged BT does not predict VWD; a normal BT does not necessarily exclude VWD [3].

Closure time

Evaluation of the closure time (CT) is done with an automated platelet function analyzer, called the PFA-100. Whole blood is aspirated through a capillary device to mimic the high shear stress conditions that occur *in vivo*. Thus, the PFA-100 is very sensitive to quantitative and qualitative abnormalities of VWF (except type 2N), and has consistently been found to be more sensitive than the BT [4]. Averaging reported data suggests that the sensitivity of the PFA-100 for VWD is around 90% [5], and it is now probably the case that diagnosis of VWD (except that of type 2N) may be excluded when the CT is normal. The PFA-100, however, is not specific for VWD; an abnormal CT requires VWF assays and, if the latter are normal, investigation of platelet function.

Platelet count

The platelet count is in the normal range in patients with all types of VWD, except those with type 2B, who often present with a mild thrombocytopenia.

Activated partial thromboplastin time

The activated partial thromboplastin time (aPTT) is sensitive to deficiencies in FVIII activity (FVIII:C). Since the FVIII:C levels may be low in VWD patients, the aPTT has some value as a screening test; it is consistently prolonged in VWD type 3 and in the type 2N variant. However, patients with mild VWD type 1 and other type 2 variants may have normal FVIII:C levels and thus a normal aPTT cannot exclude VWD.

Specific tests

The diagnosis of VWD relies on specific tests, i.e., VWF assays (antigen, ristocetin cofactor activity, collagen-binding activity, multimer distribution) and levels of FVIII protein bound to VWF in circulating blood. The study of the ratio of functional assays to VWF antigen, coupled to VWF multimer analysis, allows the identification of the type of VWD.

Blood levels of VWF have a broad normal range, extending from 40% to 240% of the mean [6]. VWF levels are influenced by ABO blood group, Lewis blood type, race, and age. ABO blood group accounts for approximatively 30% of the genetic variance of VWF [7]; in type O subjects, the VWF levels are 25–35% below those of persons with non-O blood type [6], which explains the over-representation of group O among VWD patients. VWF levels rise with increasing age and appear to be 15% higher in African-American blacks than in whites. Circumstantial factors transiently increase VWF levels, for example stress, exercise, trauma, surgery, and pregnancy (beginning in the second trimester). Several chronic conditions cause elevation of VWF levels: renal failure, diabetes, liver disease, athero-

Table 46.1 Recommended abbreviations for von Willebrand factor and its activities.

Mature protein	VWF
Antigen	VWF:Ag
Ristocetin cofactor activity	VWF:RCo
Collagen binding capacity	VWF:CB
Factor VIII binding capacity	VWF:FVIIIB

According to the von Willebrand Factor Subcommittee of the International Society on Thrombosis and Hemostasis (C. Mazurier and F. Rodeghiero, *Thromb Haemost* 2001; 86: 712).

Table 46.2 Tests for the laboratory diagnosis of von Willebrand disease.

Screening tests
Bleeding time
Closure time (PFA-100)
Platelet count
Activated partial thromboplastin time

Specific tests
VWF antigen
VWF ristocetin cofactor activity
VWF collagen-binding capacity
VWF multimer analysis
Factor VIII assay
VWF factor VIII-binding capacity

Discriminating tests
Ristocetin-induced platelet aggregation
Platelet VWF
Plasma VWF binding to platelets
VWF proteolysis
Propeptide assay
Antibodies to VWF
DNA analysis

sclerosis, inflammatory states, cancer, and hyperthyroidism. These level variations complicate the diagnosis of VWD. Thus, a clinical evaluation should be carefully performed at the time of the laboratory testing with the knowledge of drug intake. It is recommended that the evaluation be repeated once or even twice. It is also advisable to use ABO-matched reference ranges. Unfortunately, it is not yet possible to clearly define a cut-off VWF level between normal and abnormal.

von Willebrand factor antigen

The von Willebrand factor antigen (VWF:Ag) assay quantifies the total level of VWF protein. The old Laurell gel procedure (electro-immunodiffusion) has now been practically abandoned because of its lack of sensitivity in type 2 variants. The reference method is an enzyme-linked immunosorbent assay (ELISA) procedure [8]. Newer technologies are routinely used: a fast semi-automated ELISA available with the BioMerieux VIDAS system

[9] and a latex immunoassay (Diagnostica Stago) [10]. However, the sensitivity of both methods is lower than that of the conventional ELISA, and the latex immunoassay has the drawback of potential interference of rheumatoid factor, with the resulting possibility of false exclusion of VWD [10]. VWF:Ag assays may not detect patients with qualitative abnormalities of VWF; thus, the use of this assay alone is not recommended.

von Willebrand ristocetin cofactor activity

The von Willebrand ristocetin cofactor activity (VWF:RCo) is an indirect measurement of the affinity of VWF for platelet glycoprotein Ib (GPIb), thus testing the ability of VWF to bind to platelets in the presence of a compound called ristocetin, which preferentially recognizes high-molecular-weight (HMW) forms of VWF. This assay is typically performed using a platelet agglutination procedure monitored by aggregometry [11], by visual inspection [12], or, recently, by an automated method [13]. Ristocetin (1 mg/mL final concentration) is added to a suspension of normal washed platelets (fresh or commercial formalin- or paraformaldehyde-fixed and lyophilized) and to control or patient plasma at different dilutions. This assay is somewhat complex and poorly reproducible. An ELISA has also been described [14,15] using a monoclonal antibody against the GPIb binding site of VWF; it may thus differentially recognize samples with qualitative VWF defects. This promising assay exhibits a higher sensitivity and a lower intra-assay variability. VWF:RCo measurements are still considered as the most sensitive assays, allowing detection of all types of VWD (except type 2N).

The ratio of VWF:RCo to VWF:Ag provides good information on the type of VWD. In variants with an abnormal platelet-dependent function, this ratio is markedly decreased in type 2A and type 2M, and variable in type 2B. In contrast, type 1 and type 2N are characterized by a normal ratio. A threshold of 0.7 has been proposed: a ratio >0.7 is in favor of type 1 whereas a ratio <0.7 tends to define patients with type 2 (except 2N) [16].

von Willebrand factor collagen-binding activity

The capacity of VWF to bind to collagen (VWF:CB) is measured by an ELISA [17]. This assay is extremely sensitive to the lack of the HMW forms (the most functional) of VWF. Thus, the VWF:CB levels are very low in patients lacking those multimers, i.e., type 2A and most type 2B. Some investigators have proposed VWF:CB as a substitute for VWF:RCo since this assay appears to be more reproducible and easier to perform. This method, however, suffers from some drawbacks. The appropriate collagen type is still not entirely elucidated [18] and the value of this assay in detecting patients with type 1 is not accurately established; moreover, most patients with type 2M disease (with no abnormality of VWF multimers) are not identified using this assay. Thus, at present, the VWF:CB measurement cannot replace the VWF:RCo assay, which reflects the main function of VWF, i.e., interacting with platelets; the combined use of both assays tends to be recommended.

The ratio of VWF:CB to VWF:Ag allows the distinction between patients lacking HMW forms and those with no abnormality of VWF multimers. Thus, this ratio is decreased (<0.7) in type 2A and type 2B and normal in type 1 and type 2M.

von Willebrand factor multimer analysis

VWF multimer analysis by sodium dodecyl sulfate electrophoresis in agarose gels is a useful method for typing and subtyping of VWD [19]. This procedure, however, cannot be performed by all laboratories as it is technically complex, time-consuming, and difficult to standardize. The previous standard method of autoradiography using radiolabeled anti-VWF antibodies has been substituted in many laboratories by immunoblotting techniques combined with the colorimetric [20] or luminescent [21] detection of multimer bands. The analysis is performed using both low- and high-resolution gels. Low-resolution gels show three distinct profiles: (i) normal distribution (type 1 and type 2M); (ii) absence of HMW multimers (type 2A and most type 2B); and (iii) presence of supranormal multimers (Vicenza variant). High-resolution gels show distinct abnormalities in the various type 2 patients, such as the predominance of the protomer and a modification in the intensity or position of the satellite sub-bands of each multimeric unit.

Factor VIII assays

Factor VIII activity (FVIII:C) is measured by one-stage or two-stage clot-based assays, or chromogenic assays. FVIII antigen levels (FVIII:Ag) are measured by ELISA and results of activity and antigen are similar in VWD. Factor VIII levels usually parallel those of VWF:Ag, except in type 2N, in which the factor VIII levels are significantly lower, with a FVIII:C to VWF:Ag ratio lower than 0.5 [22].

Factor VIII-binding capacity of plasma VWF

The FVIII-binding capacity of VWF (VWF:FVIIIB) measures the affinity of VWF for FVIII. VWF:FVIIIB is determined by isolating patient VWF by immunoadsorption, followed by the binding of exogenous purified factor VIII; the bound factor VIII is measured either by a chromogenic assay [23] or by an ELISA method [22]. VWF:FVIIIB should be systematically performed when the FVIII:C to VWF:Ag ratio is decreased (<0.5), to distinguish VWD type 2N from mild to moderate hemophilia A. Today, this assay is performed only in some specialized laboratories.

Discriminating tests

Ristocetin-induced platelet agglutination (RIPA)

Ristocetin-induced platelet agglutination (RIPA) depends on both the concentration of VWF and the affinity of VWF for GPIb. Several concentrations of ristocetin (from 0.2 to 1.5 mg/mL) are added to patient platelet-rich plasma (PRP) in an aggregometer. RIPA is undetectable in VWD type 3 but is somewhat insensitive to mild quantitative deficiencies. Patients with type 2A and type 2M tend to show no or little aggregation at 1.3–1.5 mg/mL ristocetin. The major use of this assay is to detect type 2B where platelet aggregation occurs at low concentrations of ristocetin (<0.6 mg/mL) that have no effect on normal PRP, indicating the increased affinity of VWF for GPIb.

Platelet VWF content

Measurement of VWF:Ag and VWF:RCo, as well as multimeric analysis of VWF, may also be performed in platelet lysates [24]. In the past, a subclassification of type 1 has been proposed on the basis of the platelet VWF levels ("platelet-low" or "platelet-normal") [25], some patients with a slight decrease in larger multimers ("platelet-discordant") being now currently included among type 2A [1].

Plasma VWF binding to platelets

In vitro, VWF binding to platelets may be induced in the presence of the antibiotic ristocetin or a snake (*Bothrops jararaca*) venom component, botrocetin. These binding assays are GPIb dependent and thus useful for discriminating among VWD variants those with a decreased VWF affinity for GPIb (type 2A and type 2M) from those with an increased affinity (type 2B). Such assays may differentiate type 2B (increased affinity of patient plasma VWF for normal platelets) from pseudo-VWD (increased affinity of patient platelet GPIb for normal VWF). Since ristocetin and botrocetin involve distinct domains of VWF for binding to GPIb, a discrepancy between ristocetin- and botrocetin-induced VWF binding to platelets appears to characterize patients with typical type 2M [26].

Study of proteolysis of VWF

The susceptibility of VWF to proteolysis by the ADAMTS13 metalloprotease, which regulates its multimer size, may be interesting to investigate following incubation of VWF with the protease [27]. VWF of blood group O appears to be more sensitive to proteolysis [28]. Other genetic factors may influence proteolysis.

Propeptide immunoassay

The propeptide (previously called VWAgII), measured by ELISA, reflects the rate of synthesis of VWF [29]. Unlike plasma VWF, propeptide levels are not influenced by blood group. Levels are decreased in all inherited forms of VWD, contrasting with normal levels in acquired VWD.

Antibodies to VWF

Only patients with VWD type 3 may develop alloantibodies directed against VWF after replacement therapy, with a prevalence estimated between 7% and 10% [30]. These antibodies have polyclonal characteristics, and the majority have an inhibitory action against the GPIb binding site of VWF and thus inhibit RIPA and/or VWF:RCo [30].

Autoantibodies directed against VWF may be detected in acquired von Willebrand syndrome [31]. They are usually noninhibitory but promote a rapid clearance of the resulting immune complexes, which are difficult to detect *in vitro*.

DNA analysis

The genetic basis for VWD type 3 [32] and VWD type 2 [26] has been well documented in recent years, leading to better understanding of VWF structure–function relationship and to more precise defining of variants. In contrast, the molecular abnormalities in VWD type 1 are still poorly documented; two large studies in the European Union and Canada are in progress to investigate whether molecular biology can support the diagnosis of VWD type 1.

Databases for VWD mutations and polymorphisms have been established and can be accessed on the Internet at: http://mmg2.im.med.umich.edu/VWF and http://www.sheffield.ac.uk/vwf.

Strategy of diagnosis

The approach undertaken depends to some extent on the initial clinical presentation, the time available for testing and the laboratory methods locally available. We propose the strategy illustrated in Figure 46.1. Among screening tests, the only one appearing to have sufficient sensitivity to exclude VWD (except 2N) if normal is the CT measured with the PFA-100, provided that it is performed at an appropriate time: no pregnancy, no inflammatory state. Whatever the results of the BT, if there is a clinical reason to suspect VWD, VWF assays plus FVIII:C assay should be performed.

When VWF:RCo and VWF:Ag levels are undetectable, the diagnosis of *type 3* is rapidly made (Table 46.3). When they are decreased, the VWF:RCo to VWF:Ag ratio is critical to discriminate between a quantitative (type 1) or qualitative (type 2) defect of VWF; the VWF:CB to VWF:Ag ratio may be performed as an additional test.

Concordant levels of all VWF assays plus FVIII:C are in favor of a quantitative defect and multimer analysis is not essential (Table 46.3). Sadler [2] proposes to restrict the diagnosis of VWD *type 1* to patients with significant bleeding associated to clearly dominant inheritance and very low VWF levels (less than 15%?), other subjects being defined as having "low VWF level"; However, the boundary between both types is not clearly defined and awaits the results of ongoing studies (European and Canadian studies).

When the VWF:RCo to VWF:Ag ratio is low (<0.7), the VWF:CB assay is a useful additional test to discriminate between qualitative defects related to a loss of HMW VWF multimers (type 2A and type 2B) and those not associated with a loss of these multimers (type 2M). Patients with *type 2A* display a markedly decreased ratio of VWF:RCo or VWF:CB to VWF:Ag, and a decreased RIPA and ristocetin- or botrocetin-induced plasma VWF binding to GPIb (Table 46.3); the multimeric distribution of platelet VWF shows either a loss of HMW multimers or the presence of all molecular forms. Patients with *type 2M* may be misclassified as type 1 (or type 2A as a few mutations may lead to some decrease of the HMW multimers); the ratio of VWF:RCo to VWF:Ag is decreased, in contrast to the ratio of VWF:CB to VWF:Ag, which is normal (or less decreased) (Table 46.3); binding of plasma VWF to platelet GPIb is consistently decreased in the presence of ristocetin; it is either normal or abnormal (the latter when multimer distribution exhibits some abnormalities) in the presence of botrocetin (Table 46.3). The "Vicenza" variant, which is not so rare as described and is classified as type 2M, is characterized by very low levels of plasma VWF with no clear-cut abnormalities of the ratio of VWF:RCo to VWF:Ag and the presence of larger than normal plasma VWF multimers (Table 46.3).

RIPA is systematically indicated at low ristocetin concentrations to detect VWD *type 2B*; patients have a decreased ratio of VWF:RCo to VWF:Ag (but often less than in types 2A or 2M) and of VWF:CB to VWF:Ag. The key characteristics are enhanced RIPA and binding of plasma VWF to GPIb in the presence of low ristocetin concentrations (Table 46.3), or sometimes a spontaneous platelet aggregation, due to the adsorption of VWF multimers onto platelets; a large majority of patients exhibit intermittent thrombocytopenia, more pronounced during pregnancy or other circumstances of increased VWF levels, including administration of desmopressin. Thus, the multimeric structure of platelet VWF is normal while plasma VWF multimers are absent; in the mildest forms (formerly described as "type I New York" or "Malmö"), plasma VWF multimer distribution may be normal. It may be difficult to distinguish VWD type 2B and patients with pseudo-VWD, characterized by increased affinity of the platelet GPIb for normal VWF. Most laboratory features are similar, including enhanced RIPA and absence of plasma HMW multimers. A way to distinguish these two distinct disorders is to perform ristocetin-induced binding assay of patient plasma VWF to control platelet GPIb: the test is normal in case of pseudo-VWD; a simpler test consists in adding normal purified VWF to patient PRP in an aggregometer: platelet aggregation is induced in case of pseudo-VWD and not in case of VWD type 2B; however, a clear-cut distinction is only obtained by DNA analysis.

The observation of a decreased FVIII:C to VWF:Ag ratio (<0.5) leads to consider two diagnoses: mild hemophilia A or VWD type 2N. The distinction is done by the VWF:FVIIIB

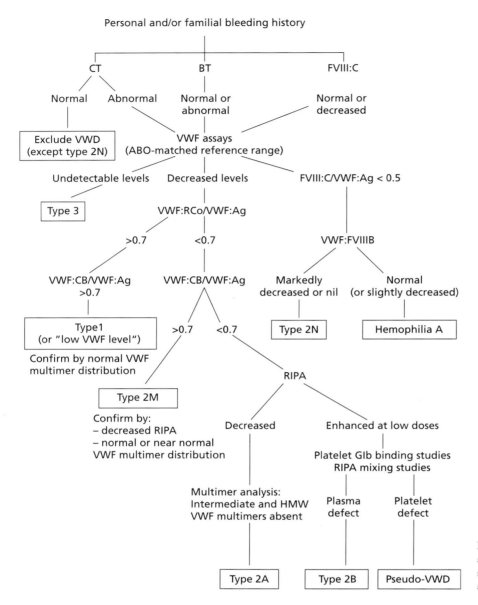

Figure 46.1 Flow chart for the laboratory diagnosis of VWD. This recommended approach should be considered as a general guide. For abbreviations, see text.

assay, which should be systematically considered. In all cases of VWD *type 2N*, the VWF:FVIIIB is markedly decreased or nil.

In difficult cases, DNA analysis, which is performed by only some research laboratories, improves VWD classification. However, in practice, the most important is to consider a test trial with desmopressin to make the appropriate choice of treatment in case of necessity. It is also necessary to deliver good information to patients, taking into account an adapted risk of bleeding.

In some patients, the diagnosis of acquired von Willebrand syndrome (AVWS) may be considered. AVWS presents with laboratory findings (prolonged BT, low FVIII:C and VWF levels) similar to those of congenital forms, commonly with a type 2A

phenotype, but patients, often elderly, are devoid of family history of VWD, have bleeding symptoms of recent onset, and appear with various underlying diseases. The latter are mainly lymphoproliferative disorders, immunologic diseases, and neoplasia. VWF is usually synthesized normally, but it is rapidly removed from plasma through different pathogenic mechanisms such as specific autoantibodies to VWF, nonspecific antibodies forming circulating immune complexes with rapid clearance, adsorption of VWF onto malignant cells, and increased proteolytic degradation [33,34]. Among autoantibodies to VWF, an inhibitor to VWF:RCo is rarely demonstrated. Propeptide levels are normal (unlike in inherited VWD).

Table 46.3 Phenotypic characterization of the different types of von Willebrand disease.

Type and subtype	1	2A	2M	2M "Vicenza"	2B*	2N	3
VWF:RCo/VWF:Ag ratio	Normal	Decreased	Decreased	Normal or slightly decreased	Decreased or nearly normal	Normal	Undetectable levels
VWF:CB/VWF:Ag ratio	Normal	Decreased	Normal	Normal	Decreased	Normal	Undetectable levels
VWF:FVIIIB	Normal	Normal	Normal	Normal	Normal	Decreased	–
Plasma multimers	Normal	Loss of large and intermediate	Normal (or slight decrease of large)	Presence of ultralarge	Loss of large or normal	Normal (or rarely decrease of large)	Undetectable
Platelet multimers	Normal	Normal or loss of large and intermediate	Normal	Normal	Normal	Normal	Undetectable
RIPA	Normal (or decreased)	Decreased (or nil)	Decreased (or nil)	Normal	Enhanced sensitivity at low doses	Normal	Nil
Ristocetin-induced VWF binding to platelets	Normal	Decreased	Decreased	Normal	Enhanced sensitivity at low doses	Normal	Not feasible
Botrocetin-induced VWF binding to platelets	Normal	Decreased	Normal or decreased	Normal	Enhanced sensitivity at low doses	Normal	Not feasible

*Patients exhibit intermittent or chronic thrombocytopenia.
RIPA, ristocetin-induced platelet agglutination.

References

1 Sadler JE. A revised classification of von Willebrand disease. *Thromb Haemost* 1994; **71**: 520–5.

2 Sadler JE. Von Willebrand disease type 1: a diagnosis in search of a disease. *Blood* 2003; **101**: 2089–93.

3 Rodgers RP, Levin J. A critical reappraisal of the bleeding time. *Semin Thromb Haemost* 1990; **16**: 1–20.

4 Fressinaud E, Veyradier A, Truchaud F, *et al.* Screening for von Willebrand disease with a new analyzer using high shear stress: a study of 60 cases. *Blood* 1998; **91**: 1325–31.

5 Favaloro EJ. Utility of the PFA-100 for assessing bleeding disorders and monitoring therapy: a review of analytical variables, benefits and limitations. *Haemophilia* 2001; **7**: 170–9.

6 Gill JC, Endres-Brooks J, Bauer PJ, *et al.* The effect of ABO blood group on the diagnosis of von Willebrand disease. *Blood* 1987; **69**: 1691–5.

7 Ørstavik KH, Kornstad L, Reisner H, Berg K. Possible effect of Secretor locus on plasma concentration of factor VIII and von Willebrand factor. *Blood* 1989; **73**: 990–3.

8 Ingerslev J. A sensitive ELISA for von Willebrand Factor (vWF:Ag). *Scand J Clin Lab Invest* 1987; **47**: 143–9.

9 Pittet JL, Barbalat V, Sanvert M, *et al.* Evaluation of a new automated ELISA test for von Willebrand factor using two monoclonal antibodies. *Blood Coagul Fibrinol* 1997; **8**: 209–15.

10 Veyradier A, Fressinaud E, Sigaud M, *et al.* A new automated method for von Willebrand factor antigen measurement using latex particles. *Thromb Haemost* 1999; **81**: 320–1.

11 MacFarlane DE, Stibbe J, Kirby EP, *et al.* A method for assaying von Willebrand factor (ristocetin cofactor). *Thromb Diath Haemorrh* 1975; **34**: 306–8.

12 Wright RD, Krauss JS. A comparison of two macroscopic platelet agglutination assays for von Willebrand factor. *Ann Clin Lab Sci* 1990; **20**: 73–8.

13 Miller CH, Platt SJ, Daniele C, Kaczor D. Evaluation of two automated methods for measurement of the ristocetin cofactor activity of von Willebrand factor. *Thromb Haemost* 2002; **88**: 56–9.

14 Murdock PJ, Woodhams BJ, Mathews KB, *et al.* Von Willebrand factor activity detected in a monoclonal antibody-based ELISA: an alternative to the ristocetin cofactor platelet agglutination assay for diagnostic use. *Thromb Haemost* 1997; **78**: 1272–7.

15 Vanhoorelbeke K, Cauwenberghs N, Vauterin S, *et al.* reliable and reproducible ELISA method to measure ristocetin cofactor activity of von Willebrand factor. *Thromb Haemost* 2000; **83**: 107–13.

16 Federici AB. Diagnosis of von Willebrand disease. *Haemophilia* 1998; **4**: 654–60.

17 Favaloro EJ, Grispo L, Exner T, Koutts J. Development of a simple collagen based ELISA assay aids in the diagnosis of, and permits sensitive discrimination between type I and type II von Willebrand's disease. *Blood Coagul Fibrinol* 1991; **2**: 285–91.

18 Neugebauer BM, Goy C, Seitz R. A collagen binding assay: an additional method for von Willebrand factor activity in therapeutic concentrates. *Thromb Haemost* 2002; **88**: 871–2.

19 Meyer D, Obert B, Pietu G, Lavergne JM, Zimmerman TS. Multimeric structure of factor VIII/von Willebrand factor in von Willebrand's disease. *J Lab Clin Med* 1980; **95**: 590–602.

20 Miller MA, Palascak JE, Thompson MR, Martolo OJ. A modified SDS agarose gel method for determining factor VIII/von Willebrand factor multimers using commercially available reagents. *Thromb Res* 1985; **39**: 777–80.

21 Schneppenheim R, Plendl H, Budde U. Luminography—an alternative assay for detection of von Willebrand factor multimers. *Thromb Haemost* 1988; **60**: 133–6.

22 Mazurier C, Goudemand J, Hilbert L, *et al.* Type 2N von Willebrand disease: clinical manifestations, pathophysiology, laboratory diagnosis and molecular biology. *Best Pract Res Clin Haematol* 2001; **14**: 337–47.

23 Nishino M, Girma JP, Rothschild C, *et al.* New variant of von Willebrand disease with defective binding to factor VIII. *Blood* 1989; **74**: 1591–9.

24 Rodeghiero F, Castaman G, Tosetto A, *et al.* Platelet von Willebrand factor assay: results using two methods for platelet lysis. *Thromb Res* 1990; **59**: 259–67.

25 Mannucci PM, Lombardi R, Bader R, *et al.* Heterogeneity of type I von Willebrand disease. Evidence for a subgroup with an abnormal von Willebrand factor. *Blood* 1985; **66**: 796–802.

26 Meyer D, Fressinaud E, Hilbert L, *et al.* Type 2 von Willebrand disease causing defective von Willebrand factor-dependent platelet function. *Best Pract Res Clin Haematol* 2001; **14**: 349–64.

27 Obert B, Tout H, Veyradier A, *et al.* Estimation of the von Willebrand factor-cleaving protease in plasma using monoclonal antibodies to vWF. *Thromb Haemost* 1999; **82**: 1382–5.

28 Bowen DJ. An influence of ABO blood group on the rate of proteolysis of von Willebrand factor by ADAMTS13. *J Thromb Haemost* 2003; **1**: 33–40.

29 McCaroll DR, Ruggeri ZM, Montgomery RR. Correlation between circulating levels of von Willebrand's antigen II and von Willebrand factor: discrimination between type I and type II von Willebrand disease. *J Lab Clin Med* 1984; **103**: 704–11.

30 Mannucci PM, Cattaneo M. Alloantibodies in congenital von Willebrand's disease. *Res Clin Lab* 1991; **21**: 119–25.

31 Mohri H, Motomura S, Kanamori H, *et al.* Clinical significance of inhibitors in acquired von Willebrand syndrome. *Blood* 1998; **91**: 3623.

32 Baronciani L, Cozzi G, Canciani MT, *et al.* Molecular characterization of a multiethnic group of 21 patients with type 3 von Willebrand disease. *Thromb Haemost* 2000; **84**: 536–40.

33 Mannucci PM, Lombardi R, Bader LR, *et al.* Studies of the pathophysiology of acquired von Willebrand's disease in seven patients with lymphoproliferative disorders or benign monoclonal gammopathies. *Blood* 1984; **64**: 614–21.

34 Michiels JJ, Budde U, van der Planken M, *et al.* Acquired von Willebrand syndromes: clinical features, aetiology, pathophysiology, classification and management. *Best Pract Res Clin Haematol* 2001; **14**: 401–36.

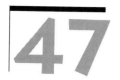

Classification and clinical aspects of von Willebrand disease

Augusto B. Federici

von Willebrand disease (VWD) is the most frequent inherited bleeding disorder and is due to a deficiency and/or abnormality of von Willebrand factor (VWF), the high-molecular-weight glycoprotein that plays a major role in early phases of hemostasis [1]. VWD is inherited in an autosomal dominant or recessive pattern, but women with milder VWD forms are apparently more symptomatic. VWD is also a very heterogeneous disorder, and therefore patients with mild VWD forms are sometimes under- and misdiagnosed because of physiologic changes in VWF within the same individual and the relative high variability of diagnostic tests [2–5].

Classification of VWD

The revised classification of VWD identifies two major categories, characterized by quantitative (types 1 and 3) or qualitative (type 2) VWF defects [6]. A partial quantitative deficiency of VWF identifies type 1 VWD, whereas type 3 VWD is marked by the total absence or only trace amounts of VWF in plasma and platelets. Type 1 is easily distinguished from type 3 by the moderate–mild VWF deficiency (usually in the range of 10–40 U/dL), the autosomal dominant inheritance pattern, and the presence of milder bleeding symptoms [2–6].

Four type 2 VWD subtypes have been identified, reflecting different pathophysiologic mechanisms. Type 2A and 2B VWD are marked by the absence of high-molecular-weight VWF multimers in plasma; in type 2B, there is increased affinity for platelet glycoprotein Ib–IX–V complex (GPIbα). The identification of qualitatively abnormal variants with decreased platelet-dependent function and the presence of normal multimers on gel electrophoresis has led to the addition of a new subtype, called 2M. If this definition is followed and more stringent criteria are applied to VWD diagnosis, many cases previously identified as type 1 should now be classified as type 2M because they are caused by single missense mutations affecting VWF function but not its multimeric structure and assembly [4]. Furthermore, type 2N (Normandy) also shows a full array of multimers since the defect lies in the N-terminal region of the VWF, where the binding domain for factor VIII (FVIII) resides. The subtype is phenotypically identified only by the FVIII/VWF binding test [2–4]. The current classification of VWD [6], summarized in Table 47.1, was proposed by Sadler in 1994 on behalf of the subcommittee on VWF of the Scientific Standardization Committees of the International Society of Thrombosis and Hemostasis (ISTH-

SSC). In a recent meeting of this subcommittee on VWF, several problems regarding the classification of type 1 versus type 2M VWD were raised and a working party was organized with the aims to prepare an updated version of VWD classification that will take into consideration the new developments in molecular and clinical markers of different VWD forms. This working party, chaired by Dr. Sadler and composed of the best experts in the field, has the duty to prepare updated guidelines for diagnosis and classification of VWD by 2005.

Clinical definition of severe versus mild forms of VWD

Type 3 is always severe, by definition, because it is characterized by unmeasurable VWF levels in both plasma and platelets and by low amounts of FVIII:C (<20 U/dL). Conversely, types 1 and 2 VWD are very heterogeneous and their clinical presentation is strictly related to the circulating levels of a functional VWF, measured as ristocetin cofactor activity (VWF:RCo).

In the last 5 years an international prospective study on the use of desmopressin in "severe forms of VWD" has been carried out by five European Hemophilia Centers in the framework of the 5th Project, sponsored by the European Community, and the results are now available [7].

For the first time, the Steering Committee of that study made an attempt to define patients with "severe VWD forms," using levels of FVIII/VWF activities as an index of severity, following the same criteria used for hemophiliacs. Patients with "severe VWD" were defined as those patients who were characterized by a lifelong history of bleeding (including at least two episodes of blood loss severe enough to require replacement therapy) and by the presence of at least one of the following laboratory abnormalities: bleeding time (BT) >15 min, VWF:RCo <10 IU/dL, FVIII:C <20 IU/dL. Therefore, in the group of "severe VWD forms" not only type 3 but also type 1, 2A, 2M, and 2N VWD, with low VWF:RCo and/or FVIII:C levels, were included [7]. Similar criteria have been used by the Steering Committee of the Italian National Registry on VWD to evaluate retrospective data on 1234 VWD patients, collected from 16 hemophilia centers on behalf of the Italian Association of Hemophilia Centers [3].

Following such a definition of "disease severity," based on the levels of defective VWF:RCo and/or FVIII:C, three different groups of VWD can be identified: a first group of "severe VWD forms" with VWF:RCo <10 U/dL and/or FVIII:C <20 U/dL [7];

Table 47.1 Classification of von Willebrand disease.

Quantitative deficiency of VWF

Type 1   Partial quantitative deficiency of VWF
Type 3   Virtually complete deficiency of VWF

Qualitative deficiency of VWF

Type 2   Qualitative deficiency of VWF
  2A   Qualitative variants with decreased platelet-dependent function associated with the absence of high-molecular-weight VWF multimers
  2B   Qualitative variants with increased affinity for platelet GPIb
  2M   Qualitative variants with decreased platelet-dependent function not caused by the absence of high-molecular-weight VWF multimers
  2N   Qualitative variants with markedly decreased affinity for factor VIII

Modified from ref. 8.

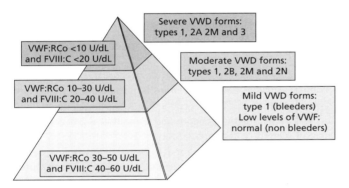

Figure 47.1 Pictorial representation of the three different degrees of VWD severity according to levels of FVIII/VWF activities: severe, moderate, and mild VWD forms. In the upper part of the pyramid, the most "severe VWD forms" (Types 3, 2A, 2M, 1) are included with levels of VWF:RCo <10 U/dL and/or FVIII:C <20 U/dL. The "moderate VWD forms" (Types 1, 2B, 2M, 2N) with levels of VWF:RCo 10–30 U/dL and/or FVIII:C 20–40 U/dL, and the "mild VWF forms" (VWF:RCo 30–50 U/dL and/or FVIII:C 40–60 U/dL) are described in the middle portion and in the base of the pyramid. Due to the physiologic changes of VWF and of the variability of the assays, a very "mild VWD form" with values of VWF:RCo and/or FVIII:C >40 U/dl can be diagnosed only when these low-borderline levels of FVIII/VWF activities are associated with personal and family bleeding history. Therefore, the lower the levels of VWF:RCo or FVIII:C the higher is the probability of a current VWD diagnosis: in this sense, the "severe VWD forms" might represent the "tip of the iceberg" of a large number of moderate and mild VWF defects.

a second group of "moderate VWD forms" with VWF:RCo 10–30 U/dL and/or FVIII:C 20–40 U/dL; and a third group of "mild VWD forms" with VWF:RCo 30–50 U/dL and/or FVIII:C 40–60 U/dL. A pictorial pyramidal representation of the three different degrees of VWD severity according to levels of both VWF:RCo and FVIII:C activities is shown in Figure 47.1

[5]. The "severe VWD forms" might represent the "tip of the iceberg" of a large number of underdiagnosed VWF with mild VWF defects. While no diagnostic problems occur in moderate–mild VWD with levels of VWF:RCo <40 U/dL, a definite diagnosis of VWD can be argued in case of patients with very mild VWD forms and VWF:RCo levels >40 U/dL. Moreover, it is well known that physiologic changes in VWF levels and the variability of the VWF:RCo assays can mask any mild defects of VWF. In very mild VWD forms, the limit between "disease" and "reduced levels of VWF in a normal individual" can be difficult in the absence of bleeding history in other members of the family, as recently reported [8]. On the other hand, many mild VWF defects remain undiagnosed in the absence of well-documented personal and family bleeding history and only the patients characterized by low VWF:RCo levels can be easily recognized and followed by the hemophilia centers (tip of the iceberg, in Figure 47.1). Of course, the clinical definition reported here is merely speculative, needs validation in a large number of patients, and must be discussed and approved within the working party of VWD classification still ongoing.

History and examination in the clinical diagnosis of VWD

Bleeding history is recognized by experts as the most critical issue in the triad of diagnostic criteria of VWD: bleeding symptoms, inheritance pattern, and low levels of VWF activity, measured as ristocetin cofactor activity (VWF:RCo).

Bleeding symptoms typical of VWD are easy bruising, epistaxes, oral cavity bleeding, and, in women, menorrhagia. It is particularly important to ascertain the response to hemostatic challenges such as surgeries or invasive procedures, trauma, and dental extractions. Women should be asked about postpartum bleeding, although symptoms of VWD may improve during pregnancy of women with moderate or mild forms of VWD. It is always important to establish whether bleeding has been lifelong or whether it is of recent onset, indicating an acquired abnormality: in this case, all the conditions associated with acquired von Willebrand syndrome (AVWS) should be excluded [9]. A detailed drug history should be taken since aspirin and NSAIDs are the commonest cause of platelet dysfunction [2–5].

Medical examination assesses the type of bleeding (bruising, ecchymoses, hematomas) if any is present at the time of consultation, but often the main purpose is to exclude an underlying disorder. Scars from previous trauma or surgery should be also examined to exclude other defects of primary hemostasis.

Criteria for evaluation of the bleeding history: a bleeding score

Bleeding histories are subjective and there is overlap between symptoms suffered by patients with VWD and normal individuals. In one study of children undergoing tonsillectomy, a history of easy bruising was present in 24% of those who did not bleed excessively at operation and in 67% of those who did [10]. More stringent criteria to define a positive mucocutaneous bleeding history have been proposed, but these criteria have been reported to be difficult to apply, and other, less stringent, criteria have been suggested, which appear to result in fewer indeterminate results [11]. It has also been shown that the discriminatory power of bleeding history is greater in a screening situation than when patients have already been referred for investigation [12].

Several attempts have been made recently by some clinicians, experts in VWD, to evaluate the sensitivity and specificity of bleeding symptoms, which are important especially in the mild cases of type 1 VWD, with VWF:RCo levels >40 U/dL. In a multicenter study of the clinical presentation of type 1 VWD in obligatory carriers of such a VWF defect, it has been shown that menorrhagia and epistaxis are not good predictors of type 1 VWD, while cutaneous bleeding and bleeding after dental extractions should be considered the most sensitive symptoms [13]. Based on these analyses, it has been proposed that laboratory screening for VWD should be performed in subjects with at least three minor bleeding symptoms or with at least two major symptoms if they include cutaneous bleeding or bleeding after dental extractions [13]. These recent findings have encouraged the use of a specific bleeding score to quantify the bleeding tendencies in different types of VWD. An example of a proposed bleeding score, based on the progressive severity of individual symptoms and used as a pilot template in some clinical studies on VWD patients, is reported in Table 47.2.

Family history and inheritance pattern

A positive family history compatible with the dominant forms of VWD requires that a first-degree relative or two second-degree relatives have a personal history of significant mucocutaneous bleeding and laboratory tests compatible with VWD. A complete dominant pattern is often not seen owing to incomplete penetrance. When available, the identity of VWF mutations or genetic markers linked to the VWF locus may permit linkage of the phenotype to more distant relatives.

The inheritance pattern of VWD type 3 is autosomal recessive. Before the era of molecular genetics, the autosomal recessive mode of transmission had already been described based on the phenotypes of severely affected patients and their symptomless relatives. Recent phenotypic and molecular genetic investigation of still living members of the family, originally described by Erik von Willebrand, confirmed the diagnosis of VWD and its autosomal recessive inheritance [14]. Recent studies of gene defects in an increased number of patients of different ethnic origins have shown that VWF mutations are located within the entire VWF gene, without any founder effect [15].

In type 2 VWD patients, the pattern of inheritance is mainly autosomal dominant, even though rare cases with recessive pattern have been reported [16]. Most type 2A cases are due to missense mutations in the A2 domain, with R1597W or Q or Y and

S1506L accounting for about 60%. Expression experiments have shown two possible mechanisms [17]. Group I mutations show impaired secretion of high-molecular-weight multimers, due to secondary defective intracellular transport. Group II mutations show normal synthesis and secretion of a VWF that is probably more susceptible to *in vivo* proteolysis. The majority of type 2B cases are due to missense mutations in the A1 domain, about 90% being caused by R1306W, R1308C, V1316M, and R1341Q mutations [16]. A few heterogeneous mutations are responsible for type 2M cases and are also located within the A1 domain. Therefore, most mutations are expressed, and the mutated recombinant VWFs have been compared with others found within the same domain. A recurrent mutation in type 2M Vicenza has been recently reported in families from Europe (R1205H), associated with a second nucleotide change (M740I) exclusively identified in some families from the Vicenza area [18,19].

Missense mutations in the FVIII-binding domain at the amino-terminal portion of VWF are responsible for type 2N [21]. The R854Q mutation is the most frequent and has been found in about 2% of the Dutch population. This mutation may cause symptoms only in homozygous or compound heterozygous states. Identification of the type 2N mutation, which is suspected in case of a marked reduction of FVIII in comparison to VWF and is confirmed by the FVIII/VWF binding test, is important for genetic counseling to exclude the state of carrier for hemophilia A [20].

Inheritance of the mild type 1 VWD is usually autosomal dominant, with variable phenotype and penetrance. Despite its high prevalence, the precise genetic cause of type 1 VWD is still elusive in most cases, especially those with a mild phenotype. Many type 1 VWD cases might be compound heterozygous, producing an apparent dominant transmission or, alternatively, the mutated allele is negatively influenced by the effects of gene(s) outside the VWF gene and by other nongenetic factors contributing to the expression of a bleeding phenotype [21]. In a few cases with high penetrance, missense mutations have been described, e.g., of a cysteine in the D3 domain, resulting in a dominant negative mechanism [22–24]. However, in most cases with variable penetrance the genetic molecular background has not yet been investigated. In some of these families, linkage studies failed to establish a relation between the phenotype and a given VWF allele [25].

In type 1 VWD, a number of genetic and nongenetic factors are likely to contribute to the wide variability of the clinical and laboratory phenotype. About 60% of the variation in VWF plasma is due to genetic factors, with ABO group accounting for only about 30%. In type O subjects, the VWF level is 25–35% lower than in non-O individuals. Thus, other unknown genetic factors may greatly influence VWF levels and, taken together with ABO blood groups and environmental effects, help explain the wide variety and incomplete penetrance of type 1 VWD. Furthermore, at least one subset of type 1 may have a combination of genetic modifier mutations outside the VWF gene, thus accounting for the failure of linkage studies. A possible example has been

Table 47.2 Criteria for calculating the bleeding score in patients with VWD (0–3)

Types of bleeding	Score			
	0	1	2	3
Epistaxis	Absent	<10 episodes/year No therapy	>10 episodes/year No or local therapy	DDAVP or FVIII/VWF concentrates
Cutaneous bleeding	Absent	<10 episodes/year No therapy	>10 episodes/year No or local therapy	DDAVP or FVIII/VWF concentrates
Bleeding from minor wounds	Absent	<10 episodes/year No therapy	>10 episodes/year No or local therapy	DDAVP or FVIII/VWF concentrates
Oral cavity bleeding	Absent	After minimal trauma only No therapy	Spontaneous No or local therapy	DDAVP or FVIII/VWF concentrates
Gastrointestinal bleeding	Absent	One episode No therapy	>1 bleeding episode No or local therapy	DDAVP or FVIII/VWF concentrates
Bleeding tooth extractions	Absent	Sometimes No or local therapy	Always Local therapy	DDAVP or FVIII/VWF concentrates
Bleeding after surgery	Absent	Minor bleeding No or local therapy	Major bleeding Local therapy	DDAVP or FVIII/VWF concentrates
Postpartum hemorrhage	Absent	Minor bleeding No or local therapy	Major bleeding Local therapy	DDAVP or FVIII/VWF concentrates
Muscle hematomas	Absent	After major trauma No or local therapy	After minor trauma No or local therapy	DDAVP or FVIII/VWF concentrates
Hamartomatosis	Absent	After major trauma No therapy	After minor trauma Local therapy	DDAVP or FVIII/VWF concentrates
Menorrhagia	Absent	No or local therapy	Birth control pills	DDAVP or FVIII/VWF concentrates
Total score				

From ref. 28.

provided by a murine model of VWD, the RIIIS/J inbred mouse strain [26]. Using a positional cloning approach, the authors succeeded in identifying MVWF as the unique allele for a previously known glycosyltransferase gene *Galgt2*. The *Galgt2* product is expressed primarily in the gut epithelium. Although its function in this tissue is unknown, gut-specific expression is conserved in humans, suggesting an important role for the corresponding post-translational modification. Other factors outside the VWF gene, such as platelet polymorphisms, have been proposed to modify the bleeding tendency of type 1 VWD, as reported [28]. Since many aspects of type 1 VWD abnormalities are still not understood, a specific project entitled Molecular and Clinical Markers for Diagnosis and Management of type 1 VWD has been carried out by 12 European Hemophilia Centers in the framework of the 5th Project sponsored by the European Community, and final results will be available in 2005.

Clinical features and bleeding symptoms in different VWD types

As reported above, the clinical expression of VWD is usually mild in most type 1 cases, increasing in severity in types 2 and 3. However, in some families the severity of bleeding manifestations varies, underlining the different molecular bases of the di-

verse phenotypes of this disorder, and its variable penetrance. In general, the severity of bleeding correlates with the degree of the reduction of VWF:RCo and FVIII:C activities, as reported in Figure 47.1, but not with the magnitude of BT prolongation or with the patient's ABO blood type. Mucocutaneous bleeding (epistaxis, menorrhagia) is a typical manifestation of the disease and may even affect the quality of life. VWD may be highly prevalent in patients with isolated menorrhagia [2–5]. Women with VWD may require treatment with antifibrinolytics, iron supplementation or an estroprogestinic pill to control heavy menses. Bleeding after dental extraction is the most frequent postoperative bleeding manifestation. Since FVIII:C is usually only slightly reduced, manifestations of a severe coagulation defect (hemarthrosis, deep muscle hematoma) are rare in type 1 VWD and are mainly post-traumatic. In type 1 VWD, bleeding after delivery is rare since FVIII/VWF levels tend to become normal at the end of pregnancy. Postoperative bleeding may not occur even in more severely affected type 1 VWD patients, but in those with type 3 VWD prophylaxis is always required [2–5].

To date, only a few detailed descriptions of symptoms in VWD patients have been provided [3,4,29,30] but only one study took into account the differentiation according to the VWD types [3,4]. Table 47.3 shows the relative frequency of bleeding symptoms in three large series of patients with VWD diagnosed at specialized centers. In the Scandinavian experi-

Table 47.3 Incidence (%) of bleeding symptoms in patients with VWD and in normal subjects

Symptoms	Iranian VWD Type 3 (*n* = 348)	Italian VWD (*n* = 1234) Type 1 (*n* = 609)	Type 2 (*n* = 550)	Type 3 (*n* = 66)	Scandinavian VWD (*n*= 264)	Normal (*n* = 500)
Epistaxis	77	61	63	66	62	5
Menorrhagia	69	32	32	56	60	25
Postextraction bleeding	70	31	39	53	51	5
Hematomas	NR	13	14	33	49	12
Bleeding from minor wounds	NR	36	40	50	36	0.2
Gum bleeding	NR	31	35	56	35	7
Postsurgical bleeding	41	20	23	41	28	1
Postpartum bleeding	15	17	18	26	23	19
Gastrointestinal bleeding	20	5	8	20	14	1
Joint bleeding	37	3	4	45	8	0
Hematuria	1	2	5	12	7	1
Cerebral bleeding	NR	1	2	9	NR	0

NR, not reported.

Bleeding symptoms in Italian patients have been recently recalculated according to the updated results of the Italian Registry of VWD [3,4].
For Scandinavian and Iranian studies see refs. 29 and 30.

ence, postpartum bleeding overlaps the percentage observed in normal females [29]. It is striking that the distribution of different types of bleeding (apart from joint bleeding) is similar for the different subtypes. However, the severity of bleeding manifestations (e.g., menorrhagia or gastrointestinal bleeding) is more marked in type 3 VWD, often requiring substitutive treatment.

Conclusions and future perspectives

VWD is the most frequent inherited bleeding disorder, but, mainly due to the large heterogeneity of VWF defects, clinical diagnosis can still be difficult for the general hematologist who may encounter these patients. Clinical diagnosis based on the appropriate phenotypic laboratory investigations is still the most common considering the difficulties and high costs of molecular diagnosis. However, molecular diagnosis can be useful to confirm specific VWF defects in VWD families.

It is still not clear whether most mild type 1 VWD patients really have a mutation in the VWF locus. The results of a large European study entitled Molecular and Clinical Markers for Diagnosis and Management of type 1 VWD, involving 154 VWD families, will be available in 2005 and will provide novel insights into these issues.

The members of the subcommittee on VWF of the SSC of the ISTH are working on the minimal requirements for a correct clinical and laboratory diagnosis of VWD leading to an updated classification of VWD. Such a classification should be clinically oriented for the current use of the general hematologists who usually follow these patients in their clinical practice. Ideally, each VWD type must be characterized by specific and standardized assays reflecting the basic and molecular mechanisms of the VWF defects.

Acknowledgments

A few data on diagnosis and management of VWD are derived from the Italian Registry of VWD sponsored by a grant from the Italian Ministry of Health. We wish to thank all the members of the Italian Association of Hemophilia Centers who participated in this Registry. The full manuscript containing all the data of the retrospective and prospective studies on 1234 Italian patients is now in preparation.

References

1 Ruggeri ZM. Structure of von Willebrand factor and its function in platelet adhesion and thrombus formation. *Best Pract Res Clin Haematol* 2001; **14**: 257–79.

2 Sadler JE, Mannucci PM, Berntorp E, *et al.* Impact, diagnosis and treatment of von Willebrand disease. *Thromb Haemost* 2000; **84**: 160–74.

3 Federici AB, Castaman G, Mannucci PM. Guidelines for diagnosis and treatment of von Willebrand disease in Italy. *Haemophilia* 2002; **5**: 607–21.

4 Castaman G, Federici AB, Rodeghiero F, Mannucci PM. von Willebrand's disease in the year 2003: toward the complete identification of gene defects for correct diagnosis and treatment. *Haematologica* 2003; **88**: 94–108.

5 Federici AB. Mild forms of von Willebrand disease: diagnosis and management. *Curr Hematol Rep* 2003; **2**: 373–80.

6 Sadler JE. A revised classification of von Willebrand disease. *Thromb Haemost* 1994; **71**: 520–3.

7 Federici AB, Mazurier C, Bertorp E, *et al*. Response to Desmopressin in patients with severe types 1 and 2 von Willebrand Disease: results of a multicenter prospective European study. *Blood* 2004; **103**: 2032–8.

8 Sadler JE. Von Willebrand disease type 1: a diagnosis in search of a disease. *Blood* 2003; **101**: 2089–93.

9 Federici AB, Rand JH, Bucciarelli P, *et al*. Acquired von Willebrand Syndrome: data from an International Registry. Thromb Haemost 2000; **84**: 345–9.

10 Nosek Cenkowska B, Cheang MS, Pizzi NJ, *et al*. Bleeding/bruising symptomatology in children with or without bleeding disorders. *Thromb Haemost* 1991; **65**: 237–41.

11 Dean JA, Blanchette VS, Carcao MD, *et al*. Von Willebrand disease in a pediatric-based population: comparison of type 1 diagnostic criteria and use of the PFA-100 and von Willebrand factor: collagen binding assays. *Thromb Haemost* 2000; **84**: 401–9.

12 Shramek A, Eikenboom JC, Briet E, *et al*. Usefulness of patient interview of bleeding disorders. *Arch Int Med* 1995; **155**: 1409–15.

13 Castaman G, Tosetto A, Cappelletti A, *et al*. Clinical presentation of type 1 von Willebrand disease in obligatory carriers: final results from a collaborative, international, multicentre study. *J Thromb Haemost* 2003; Suppl. 1: Abstract OC078.

14 Eikemboom JC. Congenital von Willebrand disease type 3: clinical manifestations, pathophysiology and molecular biology. *Best Pract Res Clin Haematol* 2001; **14**: 365–79.

15 Baronciani L, Cozzi G, Canciani MT, *et al*. Molecular defects in type 3 von Willebrand disease: updated results from 40 multiethnic patients. *Blood Cells, Mol Dis* 2003; **30**: 264–70.

16 Meyer D, Fressinaud E, Hilbert L, *et al*. Type 2 von Willebrand disease causing defective von Willebrand factor-dependent platelet function. *Best Prac Res Clin Haematol* 2001; **14**: 349–64.

17 Lyons SE, Bruck ME, Bowie EJW, *et al*. Impaired cellular transport produced by a subset of type IIA von Willebrand disease mutations. *J Biol Chem* 1992; **267**: 4424–30.

18 Schneppenheim R, Federici AB, Budde U, et al. Von Willebrand disease type 2 M "Vicenza" in Italian and German patients: identification of the first candidate mutation (G3864A; R1205H) in 8 families. *Thromb Haemost* 2000; **83**: 136–40.

19 Castaman G, Missiaglia E, Federici AB, et al. An additional candidate mutation (G2470A; M740I) in the original families with von Willebrand disease type 2 M Vicenza and the G3864A (R1205H) mutation. *Thromb Haemost* 2000; **84**: 350–1.

20 Mazurier C, Goudemand J, Hilbert L, *et al*. Type 2N von Willebrand disease: clinical manifestations, pathophysiology, laboratory diagnosis and molecular biology. *Best Prac Res Clin Haematol* 2001; **14**: 337–47.

21 Rodeghiero F, Castaman G. Congenital von Willebrand disease type 1: definition, phenotypes, clinical and laboratory assessment. *Best Prac Res Clinical Haematol* 2001; **14**: 321–35.

22 Eikenboom JCJ, Matsushita T, Reitsma PH , *et al*. Dominant type 1 von Willebrand disease caused by mutated cysteine residues in the D3 domain of von Willebrand factor. *Blood* 1996; **88**: 2433–41.

23 Castaman G, Eikenboom JCJ, Missiaglia E, Rodeghiero F. Autosomal dominant type 1 von Willebrand disease due to G3639T mutation (C1130F) in exon 26 of von Willebrand factor gene: description of five Italian families and evidence for a founder effect. *Br J Haematol* 2000; **108**: 876–9.

24 Eikenboom JCJ, Castaman G, Vos H, *et al*. Characterization of the genetic defects in recessive type 1 and type 3 von Willebrand disease patients of Italian origin. *Thromb Haemost* 1998; **79**: 709–17.

25 Castaman G, Eikenboom JCJ, Bertina R, Rodeghiero F. Inconsistency of association between type 1 von Willebrand disease phenotype and genotype in families identified in an epidemiologic investigation. *Thromb Haemost* 1999; **82**: 1065–70.

26 Mohlke KL, Purkayastha AA, Westrick RJ, *et al*. Mvwf, a dominant modifier of murine von Willebrand factor, results from altered lineage-specific expression of a glycosyltransferase. *Cell* 1999; **96**: 111–20.

27 Di Paola J, Federici AB, Mannucci PM, *et al*. Low platelet α2β1 levels in type 1 von Willebrand Disease correlate with impaired platelet function in a high shear stress system. *Blood* 1999; **93**: 3578–82.

28 Kunicki TJ, Federici AB, Solomon DR, *et al*. An association of candidate gene haplotypes and bleeding severity in von Willebrand disease (VWD) Type 1 pedigrees. *Blood* 2004; DO1 10.1182/blood 2004–01-0349.

29 Silwer J. von Willebrand's disease in Sweden. *Acta Paediat Scand* 1973; **238**: 1–159.

30 Lak M, Peyvandi F, Mannucci PM. Clinical manifestations and complications of childbirth and replacement therapy in 348 Iranian patients with type 3 von Willebrand disease. *Br J Haematol* 2000; **111**: 1223–9.

48 Treatment of von Willebrand disease: desmopressin

Pier M. Mannucci

Introduction

In von Willebrand disease (VWD), the principle of treatment or prevention of bleeding is the transient correction of the dual plasma deficiency of von Willebrand factor (VWF) and factor VIII (FVIII). The latter deficiency is secondary to that of VWF, its carrier and stabilizer in plasma [1]. Correction of both deficiencies can be achieved by administering the synthetic peptide desmopressin (DDAVP) or, in patients unresponsive to this agent, plasma or plasma fractions.

Desmopressin (DDAVP)

This peptide is an analog of the antidiuretic hormone vasopressin devoid of V1 agonist effects. Accordingly, its administration is not accompanied by such adverse effects as vasoconstriction, hypertension, uterus contraction, and colicky abdominal pain. Being a V2 agonist, the drug retains the antidiuretic activity of vasopressin. Desmopressin raises VWF by secreting this moiety into plasma from its natural site of synthesis and storage, the vascular endothelial cell [2]. It is not known how desmopressin raises FVIII in parallel with VWF.

Factor VIII and VWF increase three- to fivefold above baseline values when desmopressin is infused intravenously [3,4] (the most frequently used route of administration), subcutaneously [5], or intranasally [4] (the last two routes used mainly for self-treatment at home). The recommended dosages are 0.3 µg/kg by slow intravenous infusion or subcutaneous injection, and fixed doses of 300 µg in adults and 150 µg in children by intranasal spray. Lower and higher doses are less effective and no more effective respectively. The factor-raising effect of desmopressin is present in normal individuals as well as in patients with mild hemophilia and von Willebrand disease, except for those with undetectable levels of the factors (patients with severe hemophilia and with type 3 von Willebrand disease) [4].

Clinical use

These properties of desmopressin have been exploited therapeutically to treat patients with von Willebrand disease (and mild hemophilia) at the time of bleeding or before invasive surgical procedures [6–8]. The likelihood of an efficacious hemostatic response should be assessed with a test dose given to candidates for treatment either at the time of diagnosis or when an elective

treatment is planned [9]. Table 48.1 shows the schedule of desmopressin administration and blood sampling recommended to evaluate the degree of laboratory response to a test dose. On the basis of the results obtained in this manner, caregivers can evaluate whether or not the attained factor levels and the duration of their persistence in plasma are of such a degree that the successful management of any given clinical situation can be predicted (Table 48.2). In practical terms, patients with FVIII and VWF levels of 10–20% or more are the most likely to benefit from the therapeutic use of desmopressin. For instance, a patient with baseline levels of 5% should reach peak postinfusion levels of 15–20% (which may be sufficient to stop a posttraumatic hemarthrosis but not to handle dental extractions). On the other hand, a patient with baseline levels of 20–25% may reach levels as high as 50–70%, adequate to provide hemostasis during dental extractions. Major surgical procedures can be successfully carried out in patients with levels of 30–40%, because postdesmopressin levels in excess of 100% are usually reached.

Responses to desmopressin can also be predicted from knowledge of the different phenotypes of von Willebrand disease. Type 1, the most frequent phenotype, accounting for 60–80% of cases and due to the quantitative deficiency of VWF and of FVIII, is the most responsive to desmopressin [7–10]. Type 2, accounting for 20–30% of cases and due to a dysfunctional VWF protein synthesized in normal amounts, is generally poorly responsive to desmopressin, because the compound triggers the secretion into plasma of a dysfunctional moiety [7,8,11]. Exceptions to this general rule are some patients with the subtypes 2N, in whom FVIII increases markedly [8,12]. Type 3 von Willebrand disease, the most severe form, accounting for 2–5% of cases, is almost invariably unresponsive to desmopressin, because affected patients lack secretable VWF.

A limitation of DDAVP is a progressive decrease in the degree of factor rise observed in patients with von Willebrand disease (and mild hemophilia) treated repeatedly [13]. The only way to ascertain whether and when tachyphylaxis develops is to measure FVIII and VWF levels in plasma after each desmopressin infusion. Depending on the peak factor levels attained post infusion and on trough levels, the caregiver can decide whether treatment can be safely stopped because rebleeding is unlikely to occur, or whether it is necessary to revert to the infusion of plasma fractions.

The obvious advantages of desmopressin are the absent risk of transmission of blood-borne infections and its relatively low

Table 48.1 Schedule for the test dose of desmopressin to assess responsiveness in patients with von Willebrand disease (and mild hemophilia).

Step 1	Infuse over 30 min 0.3 µg/kg of desmopressin in 100 mL saline in newly diagnosed patients or in those who must undergo an elective treatment
Step 2	Obtain citrated blood samples 60 min after starting desmopressin (postinfusion peak) and at 4 h (to assess the rate of factor clearance)
Step 3	Measure FVIII coagulant activity and ristocetin cofactor or collagen-binding activity

If the subcutaneous or intranasal routes are preferred for desmopressin administration, the same schedule should be followed.

Table 48.2 Target levels of factor VIII and von Willebrand factor recommended in clinical situations for patients with von Willebrand disease.

Clinical situation	Target
Major surgery	Peak FVIII levels* of 100% and trough daily levels of at least 50% until healing is complete (usually 5–10 days)
Minor surgery	Peak FVIII levels of 60% and trough daily levels of at least 30% until healing is complete (usually 2–4 days)
Dental extractions	Peak FVIII levels of 60% (single dose)
Spontaneous bleeding episodes	Peak FVIII levels higher than 50% until bleeding stops (usually 2–4 days)
Delivery and puerperium*	Peak FVIII levels higher than 80% and trough levels of at least 30%, usually for 3–4 days

*For those who prefer to monitor and measure von Willebrand factor, the same target levels of ristocetin cofactor or collagen binding activity are recommended.

cost. For this reason, desmopressin is the treatment of choice in responsive patients with von Willebrand disease (and mild hemophilia). Desmopressin is listed by the World Health Organization (WHO) among essential drugs. However, not all countries have implemented WHO recommendations, and in many of them desmopressin is not available or is licensed only for the other main clinical indications of the compound, i.e., diabetes insipidus and nocturnal enuresis.

Monitoring treatment

The purpose of monitoring desmopressin treatment with laboratory testing is to establish whether or not the degree of correction over time of the FVIII and VWF defects is adequate to control bleeding, spontaneous or postoperative (Table 48.2). For minor bleeding episodes and invasive procedures such as dental extractions, monitoring is usually not necessary, because the hemostatic response is quite predictable if the dosages recommended above are used. For more severe bleeding episodes and major surgery, monitoring is usually necessary to establish whether or not the occurrence of tachyphylaxis has rendered the patient unresponsive.

FVIII assays are the tests of choice for monitoring treatment in patients with von Willebrand disease. VWF measurements such as ristocetin cofactor and collagen binding assays can also be used, but they are more technically demanding and less standardized than FVIII assays, more costly, and difficult to set up. Moreover, there is much less experience than for FVIII on peak and trough VWF levels needed to reach and maintain hemostasis (Table 48.2). If one chooses to monitor patients with VWF or assays, the same peak and trough levels recommended for FVIII are tentatively recommended (Table 48.2).

It is not usually necessary to monitor the skin bleeding time, not only because this test is difficult to standardize and has poor reproducibility, but mainly because it is a poor predictor of hemostasis during soft-tissue and postoperative bleeding. There is evidence, for instance, that surgical hemostasis is reached and maintained by desmopressin as well as by plasma fractions, even if the bleeding time is prolonged, provided sufficient levels of plasma FVIII are reached. It is also unnecessary to evaluate the post-treatment multimeric pattern of VWF, whereas knowledge of this pattern is necessary to establish the phenotype of von Willebrand disease and to decide the optimal treatment with desmopressin or plasma fractions.

Side-effects

Transient headache, facial flushing, and mild tachycardia are relatively frequent side-effects, usually well tolerated by patients. The antidiuretic effect is not perceived clinically in patients with a normal capacity to excrete water, if the drug is given at the recommended time intervals (every 12–24 h) and fluid intake is not excessive. Laboratory monitoring of osmolality and electrolytes is not necessary, but body weighing is a recommended simple and inexpensive precautionary measure. Severe symptoms due to water intoxication, such as cerebral edema and seizures, are rarely reported, more often in infants and young children [14] but sometimes also in adults. There are occasional reports of arterial thrombosis during treatment [15,16], so that the drug should be avoided in patients with overt cardiovascular disease. DDAVP can be safely used in pregnant women, because it is devoid of oxytocic properties.

Adjuvant treatments

Treatment with desmopressin is usually given in association with antifibrinolytic amino acids. Epsilon-aminocaproic acid and tranexamic acid are synthetic compounds that inhibit fibrinolysis by saturating the binding sites on plasminogen, thereby impeding plasmin formation. Epsilon-aminocaproic acid can be administered orally, intravenously, or topically at doses of 60 mg/kg every 6 h, tranexamic acid by the same routes at doses of 15 mg/kg every 8 h. In general, the effectiveness of these compounds in the treatment of bleeding disorders is explained by the role of local hyperfibrinolysis in the onset and maintenance of bleeding in such mucosal tracts as the nasopharynx and the gastrointestinal and genitourinary tracts. Sometimes in these situations, antifibrinolytic drugs are sufficient to stop bleeding without the need to revert to desmopressin or plasma products. More often, they are given as adjuvants, because they help to reduce the total amount of factors by stabilizing the formed fibrin clots. A typical example is dental surgery, in which these drugs can also be used locally, as mouthwashes. We recommend the use of antifibrinolytic amino acids together with desmopressin for the previously mentioned reasons. Even though desmopressin induces a brisk, short-term increase of tissue plasminogen activation, there is no evidence that this effect affects hemostasis in treated patients.

Concluding remarks

The therapeutic use of desmopressin in von Willebrand disease (and mild hemophilia) has now withstood the experience of nearly a quarter of a century. There is no doubt that the use of this compound at a time when plasma concentrates were not virus inactivated spared many patients with mild hemophilia and von Willebrand disease from blood-borne infections and the related ominous consequences [17], which were felt to be particularly dramatic in patients with mild bleeding disorders, who need treatment much less frequently than those with severe disease. The advent of virus-inactivated plasma concentrates and the availability of recombinant factors in hemophilia have currently rendered less crucial the safety afforded by a synthetic drug such as desmopressin. Hence its main appeal is its relatively low cost, particularly for developing countries. It is baffling that, despite its early inclusion in the WHO-recommended list of essential drugs, desmopressin is not licensed or available in many developing countries. For instance, it was hardly used until recently in the Islamic Republic of Iran, a country with good levels of hemophilia care delivery.

In terms of new nontransfusional treatments of hemophilia and von Willebrand diseases, it has been shown that the cytokine interleukin 11 leads to a gradual and sustained increase in FVIII and VWF in mice and dogs, different from the short-lasting effect elicited by desmopressin [18,19]. Should these early studies in animals be confirmed in humans, one might envision the use of desmopressin when a short-term increase in FVIII and VWF is needed (treatment of acute bleeding) and of interleukin 11 when a longer duration of the hemostatic effect is needed (management of major surgery).

References

1 Sadler JE. Biochemistry and genetics of von Willebrand factor. *Annu Rev Biochem* 1998; **67**: 395–424.

2 Kaufmann JE, Oksche A, Wollheim CB, *et al.* Vasopressin induced von Willebrand factor secretion from endothelial cells involves V2 receptors and cAMP. *J Clin Invest* 2000; **106**: 107–16.

3 Mannucci PM, Aberg M, Nilsson IM, Robertson B. Mechanism of plasminogen activator and factor VIII increase after vasoactive drugs. *Br J Haematol* 1975; **30**: 81–93.

4 Mannucci PM, Canciani MT, Rota L, Donovan BS. Response of factor VIII/von Willebrand factor to DDAVP in healthy subjects and patients with haemophilia A and von Willebrand disease. *Br J Haematol* 1981; **47**: 283–93.

5 Rodeghiero F, Castaman G, Mannucci PM. Prospective multicenter study on subcutaneous concentrated desmopressin for home treatment of patients with von Willebrand disease and mild or moderate hemophilia A. *Thromb Haemost* 1996; **76**: 692–6.

6 Mannucci PM, Ruggeri ZM, Pareti FI, Capitanio AM. Deamino–8-D-arginine vasopressin: a new pharmacological approach to the management of haemophilia and von Willebrand disease. *Lancet* 1977; **1**: 869–72.

7 Revel-Vilk S, Schmugge M, Carcao MD, *et al.* Desmopressin (DDAVP) responsiveness in children with von Willebrand disease. *J Pediatr Hematol Oncol* 2003; **25**: 874–9.

8 Federici AB, Mazurier C, Berntorp E, *et al.* Biological response to desmopressin in patients with severe type 1 and type 2 von Willebrand disease. Results of a Multicenter European Study. *Blood* 2004; **103**: 2032–8.

9 Rodeghiero F, Castaman G, Di Bona E, Ruggeri M. Consistency of responses to repeated DDAVP infusions in patients with von Willebrand's disease and hemophilia A. *Blood* 1989; **74**: 1997–2000.

10 Mannucci PM, Lombardi R, Bader R, *et al.* Heterogeneity of type I von Willebrand disease: evidence for a subgroup with an abnormal von Willebrand factor. *Blood* 1985; **66**: 796–802.

11 Ruggeri ZM, Mannucci PM, Lombardi R, *et al.* Multimeric composition of factor VIII/von Willebrand factor following administration of DDAVP: implications for pathophysiology and therapy of von Willebrand's disease subtypes. *Blood* 1982; **59**: 1272–8.

12 Mazurier C, Gaucher C, Jorieux S, Goudemand M, and the Collaborative Group. Biological effect of desmopressin in eight patients with type 2 N ("Normandy") von Willebrand disease. *Br J Haematol* 1994; **88**: 849–54.

13 Mannucci PM, Bettega D, Cattaneo M. Patterns of development of tachyphylaxis in patients with hemophilia and von Willebrand disease after repeated doses of desmopressin (DDAVP). *Br J Haematol* 1992; **82**: 87–93.

14 Smith TJ, Gill JC, Ambroso DR, Hathaway WE. Hyponatremia and seizures in young children given DDAVP. *Am J Hematol* 1989; **31**: 199–202.

15 Bond L, Bevin D. Myocardial infarction in a patient with hemophilia A treated with DDAVP. *N Engl J Med* 1988; **318**: 121 (letter).

16 Byrnes JJ, Larcada A, Moake JL. Thrombosis following desmopressin for uremic bleeding. *Am J Hematol* 1988; **28**: 63–5.

17 Mannucci PM, Ghirardini A. Desmopressin: twenty years after. *Thromb Haemost* 1997; **78**: 958.

18 Denis CV, Kwack K, Saffaripour S, *et al.* Interleukin 11 significantly increases plasma von Willebrand factor and factor VIII in wild type and von Willebrand disease mouse models. *Blood* 2001; **97**: 465–72.

19 Olsen EH, McCain AS, Merricks EP, *et al.* Comparative response of plasma vWF in dogs to upregulation of vWF mRNA by interleukin-11 versus Weibel-Palade body release by desmopressin (DDAVP). *Blood* 2003; **102**: 436–41

Treatment of von Willebrand disease: therapeutic concentrates

Peter Collins

Therapeutic concentrates

The treatment or prevention of bleeding in patients with von Willebrand disease (VWD) requires correction of the platelet–vessel wall defect and the secondary hemostatic defect caused by a deficiency of factor VIII (FVIII). These defects vary between patients and subtypes of VWD. The two hemostatic defects are important in different clinical situations; the platelet–vessel wall interaction is more important in microvascular bleeding, particularly from muscosal surfaces, whereas FVIII is more important for the control of deep tissue bleeding and promoting wound healing. The role of antifibrinolytic drugs is important in clinical situations in which mucosal bleeding or increased fibrinolytic activity is likely.

The optimal hemostatic treatment of VWD is with DDAVP (1-deamino-8-arginine vasopressin) [1] because pooled plasma-derived von Willebrand factor (VWF)-containing concentrates are associated with the potential risk of transmission of infectious agents. Not all patients with VWD are suitable for treatment with DDAVP, however, and VWF-containing concentrates are indicated. Patients who may need to be treated with pooled blood products should be vaccinated against hepatitis A and B [2]. This chapter will focus on the management of patients who need VWF-containing concentrates.

The use of VWF-containing concentrates is complicated by a lack of data relating the properties of these concentrates in *in vitro* tests and hemostatic effects *in vivo* [3]. Furthermore, correction of VWF levels in the plasma may not reproduce the physiologic action of VWF at the vessel wall under high shear. When making therapeutic decisions, most weight should be given to studies that demonstrate clinical hemostatic efficacy.

Indications for the use of VWF-containing concentrates

VWF-containing concentrates are indicated for VWD patients unresponsive or unsuitable for DDAVP. Many clinicians are cautious about treating young children with DDAVP because of the risk of hyponatremic seizures [4]. This must be balanced against the risk of exposing a young child to a pooled blood product. Atherosclerosis is a contraindication to DDAVP owing to the risk of arterial thrombosis [5,6]. Venous thromboembolism (VTE) has also been noted [7]. Some clinicians recommend an upper age limit for DDAVP use although there is no

clear consensus. The VWD subtype affects the decision on whether to use DDAVP or a VWF-containing concentrate (Table 49.1).

Type 3 von Willebrand disease

Patients with type 3 VWD must be treated with a VWF-containing concentrate because they will not respond to DDAVP.

Type 2B von Willebrand disease

Many clinicians suggest that DDAVP is contraindicated in type 2B VWD owing to the risk of thrombocytopenia [8]. There are a few reports, however, of DDAVP being used safely [9,10].

Type 2A and type 2M von Willebrand disease

The DDAVP response of patients with type 2A or 2M VWD is unpredictable, and a therapeutic trial should assess the response of VWF ristocetin cofactor (VWF:RCo) and FVIII [11,12]. Patients shown not to achieve adequate levels need a VWF-containing concentrate. This is likely for major operative procedures, when therapeutic levels of VWF and FVIII must be maintained for a prolonged period.

Type 2N VWD

DDAVP increases FVIII to normal in most patients but the half-life is significantly reduced [13]. Minor bleeds and procedures can often be treated with DDAVP. Major bleeds or procedures that require a prolonged correction of FVIII are likely to need a VWF-containing concentrate that normalizes the half-life and plasma level of endogenous FVIII [14].

Type 1 VWD

Most patients with type 1 VWD respond to DDAVP [1,12]. Some patients do not respond adequately, particularly if they lack platelet VWF [15]. Some patients have very good initial responses to DDAVP but the half-life of the released VWF and FVIII is short [16]. A DDAVP trial should include a 3–4 h time point to assess this. For major operations, it may not be possible to sustain adequate VWF and FVIII levels with DDAVP and patients may need a VWF-containing concentrate.

Table 49.1 Indications for the use of a VWF-containing concentrate to treat VWD.

Definite	Relative
Type 3 VWD	Age less than 2 years
Type 2B VWD*	Older age†
Inadequate response to DDAVP	Type 2A and 2M VWD‡
Atherosclerotic disease	Heart failure and patients on diuretics
	Type 2N VWD‡
	Acquired VWD

*There are reports of DDAVP being used safely in patients with type 2B VWD.
†There is a lack of consensus on an upper age limit and many clinicians do not regard age alone as a contraindication to DDAVP.
‡Some patients may respond to DDAVP for minor procedures and bleeding episodes.

Table 49.2. Important considerations when choosing a VWF-containing concentrate.

Hemostatic efficacy demonstrated in clinical trials
Viral inactivation steps
Plasma source
Side-effects
Availability

General properties required of a VWF-containing concentrate

Concentrates available for the treatment of VWD may contain FVIII and VWF or are very high-purity VWF (VHP-VWF) with minimal amounts of FVIII. The important considerations when choosing a concentrate are summarized in Table 49.2. The *in vitro* and *in vivo* characteristics of VWF-containing concentrates have been comprehensively reviewed [3].

It is often stated that the presence of high-molecular-weight multimers (HMWMs) is essential for the *in vivo* correction of the primary hemostatic defect. The degree of retention of HMWMs that is required remains controversial [3]. There are no data that compare multimer composition or other laboratory parameters of VWF-containing concentrates with hemostatic efficacy. However, an *in vivo* crossover study investigated the ability of four concentrates to correct laboratory parameters. Hemate-P, Factor 8Y, Alpha VIII, and VHP-VWF had similar VWF:RCo recoveries of 2.1–2.4 IU/mL per IU/kg infused. There was a more consistent normalization of bleeding time with Hemate-P, but the bleeding time did not correlate with VWF:RCo. No concentrate normalized VWF multimers *in vivo* [17]. Cryoprecipitate, with a full complement of HMWMs, does not consistently correct the bleeding time [18]. In practice,

however, many VWF-containing concentrates have established clinical efficacy [14,19–23].

VWF-containing concentrates

The availability of VWF-containing concentrates varies between countries, but commonly used products are shown in Table 49.3. In a survey of 25 large hemophilia centers in Europe and Japan, the concentrates perceived to be most useful for treating VWD were Hemate-P, Alphanate, VHP-VWF, and BPL 8Y [24]. Representative concentrates are described in more detail below.

Hemate-P

A number of reports support the use of Hemate-P in VWD. A retrospective report of 97 patients with all types of VWD who were treated for 73 surgical operations, 344 bleeding events, and 93 other events (invasive procedures and test doses) has been published [25]. The efficacy was excellent or good in 99% of surgical operations (including in 21 patients with type 3 and 19 with type 2 VWD), 97% for bleeding events and 86% of other events. Administration of 1 IU/kg FVIII can be expected to lead to a rise in circulating VWF:RCo of approximately 3.5–4 IU/dL. There have been other smaller reports of good hemostatic efficacy with Hemate-P in both adults [26] and children [27]. The practice of dosing based on VWF:RCo has been shown to be successful [28].

Hemate-P has been used as a continuous infusion to cover surgical procedures, deliveries, and bleeding episodes with good clinical efficacy and a reported reduction in concentrate use [29]. Data have been presented demonstrating that Hemate-P has a multimer structure with decreased HMWMs compared with normal plasma but better preservation of these multimers compared with other concentrates [17]. The clinical significance of this is unclear.

Alphanate

Alphanate has been the subject of a prospective study of treatment and prophylaxis using pre-established dosage regimens based on VWF:RCo [22]. Eighty-one patients with VWD were treated with Alphanate SD/HT (solvent/detergent and heat treated), and its predecessor Alphanate S/D (solvent/detergent treated). The two products have similar pharmacokinetic parameters in patients with type 3 VWD. Fifty-three patients were given one of these preparations to treat 87 bleeding episodes. Use for surgery was reported in 39 patients (six with type 1, 17 with type 2A, two with type 2B, and 14 with type 3 VWD) undergoing 71 surgical or invasive procedures. In all cases, adequate hemostasis was achieved, and none of the patients required the use of alternative blood products. Musculoskeletal and genitourinary bleeding required more treatments per bleeding episode and higher doses. It was demonstrated that surgery could be safely undertaken even when Alphanate did not correct the bleeding time [22]. The concentrate lacks HMWMs compared with plasma.

Fanhdi

Fanhdi has been reported to be efficacious in the management of VWD in a retrospective clinical study. In 22 patients, 12 bleeding episodes and 14 invasive procedures were treated with Fanhdi. There was 92% excellent or good efficacy and no adverse events [23].

VHP-VWF

This high-purity VWF concentrate contains only small amounts of FVIII and so does not normalize FVIII immediately. The amount of VWF in VWF:RCo is given on the vial. The multimer structure of the concentrate is well preserved but not normal [14,30].

Infused VWF stabilizes endogenously produced FVIII and, over 6–12 h, the FVIII will rise to normal levels [31]. This has implications for treatment regimens (see below).

Clinical efficacy has been demonstrated in a review of 75 patients (including four with type 3 and 22 with type 2 VWD) [14]. Adequate hemostasis was reported after one infusion for epistaxis and minor bleeding. Gastrointestinal bleeding required infusions once or twice daily for a more prolonged period. Successful treatment of 31 minor and 23 major surgical procedures was reported (see below) [14]. VHP-VWF concentrate has been used as a continuous infusion [32].

Factor 8Y

This is an intermediate-purity factor VIII with good clinical efficacy and correction of laboratory parameters [19,20]. Factor 8Y has been used as a continuous infusion [33]. The label states the amount of VWF:Ag per vial, as measured by ELISA. The product data sheet states that 1 IU of VWF:Ag is associated with 0.8 IU VWF:RCo and 0.4 IU FVIII. Pharmacokinetic analysis showed a lower clearance and recovery in patients with type 3 and 2A VWD compared with type 1 VWD (Table 49.3) [33]. The concentrate lacks HMWMs compared with normal plasma.

Venous thrombosis

Venous thrombosis has been associated with intermediate-purity VWF-containing concentrates [34,35]. Patients usually have other factors that contribute to venous thromboembolism (VTE) and high FVIII may add to the risk. It is advised that clinicians monitor FVIII daily and avoid high levels; venous thromboprophylaxis should be considered [35].

Dosing

The amount of VWF-containing concentrate required to correct the hemostatic defect in VWD is dependent on the type of bleed or surgery, the patient's baseline VWF:RCo and FVIII levels, and the subtype of VWD. Different types of surgery necessitate different target VWF:RCo and FVIII levels (Table 49.4) [36]. Many clinicians adjust the initial dose of VWF-containing concentrates dependent on the individual patient's baseline levels, and subsequent doses are calculated from measured recovery and fall-off levels [36]. Infusion of a VWF-containing concentrate increases FVIII as a result of the FVIII in the concentrate and by stabilizing endogenous FVIII [3].

It is becoming common practice to dose patients with regard to the VWF:RCo content of a VWF-containing concentrate. This has been shown to be effective in a prospective study [22] and a retrospective study involving both children and adults [28]. The VWF:RCo and FVIII levels required for hemostasis have not been established by clinical trials but a general consensus is that, at the time of a major procedure or to treat a significant bleed, the VWF:RCo and FVIII should be raised to above 80 IU/dL and maintained above 50 IU/dL until hemostasis is secured. The FVIII level is maintained above 50 IU/dL until wound healing is complete. Minor surgery may be performed successfully with a VWF:RCo and FVIII of about 50 IU/dL [36,37].

Some clinicians recommend fixed initial doses of VWF-containing concentrate irrespective of the patient's baseline levels. In a prospective study using Alphanate, bleeding episodes were treated with 40 IU/kg VWF:RCo (50 IU/kg for children) and surgery covered by 60 IU/kg VWF:RCo (75 IU/kg in children) [22]. Italian guidelines suggest an initial dose of 50 IU/kg for major surgery, 30 IU/kg for minor surgery, and 20 IU/kg for dental surgery [38].

Dosing of VHP-VWF concentrate differs from other concentrates because the deficiency of FVIII is corrected over 6–12 h by stabilization of endogenous FVIII [31]. VHP-VWF can be started 12–24 h before a planned procedure or FVIII can be infused in an emergency. Surgery is covered with an infusion of VHP-VWF 1 h preoperatively in patients with FVIII greater than 20 IU/dL (30 IU/dL for major surgery). A total of 31 minor and 23 major procedures have been reported [14]. The mean VWF:RCo in patients postinfusion was 100 IU/dL and the FVIII was above 50 IU/dL in almost all patients.

Patients with FVIII below 20–30 IU/dL received either one infusion of VHP-VWF concentrate given 12–24 h preoperatively, with a second infusion 1 h preoperatively, or one infusion of VHP-VWF concentrate and an infusion of FVIII 1 h preoperatively. The VWF:RCo was raised to greater than 100 IU/dL for major surgery and the FVIII was greater than 60 IU/dL in all patients. VWF:RCo was maintained at about 100 IU/dL for 1–16 days depending on the procedure. No further factor VIII was required and all patients had adequate hemostasis [14].

Monitoring therapy

A survey of experienced clinicians in Europe reported that, for surgery, 22 of 24 responders measured FVIII daily and 18 of 24 measured VWF:RCo daily. Only 5 of 24 monitored the bleeding

Table 49.3 Characteristics of some commonly used VWF-containing concentrates.

Product (manufacturer)	Plasma source	Manufacturing process	Viral inactivation	VWF:RCo/ FVIII ratio	In vivo recovery FVIII (IU/dL per IU/kg)	In vivo recovery VWF:RCo (IU/dL per IU/kg)	Reference
Hemate-P (ZLB Berhing)	Germany, Austria, USA	Glycine/sodium chloride treatment of cryoprecipitate	Pasteurized (60°C/10 h)	2.5:1	2.7 (1.9–3.7) (median (range))	2.1 (1.1–2.7) (median (range))	25
Alphanate (Alpha)	USA	Heparin ligand chromatography	S/D and dry heat (80°C/72 h)	1.6:1	2.1 ± 0.4 (mean ± SD)	2.9 ± 1.3 (mean ± SD)	22
Fandhi (Grifols)	USA	Heparin ligand chromatography	S/D and dry heat (80°C/72 h)	1.6:1	No data	No data	23
Factor 8Y (Bio Products Laboratory)	USA	Glycine/sodium chloride treatment of cryoprecipitate	Dry heat (80°C/72 h)	2:1	Type 3: 2.4 ± 1.1 (mean ± SD) / Type 1: 5.0 ± 4.5 (mean ± SD)	Type 3: 1.4 ± 0.05 (mean ± SD) / Type 2A: 2.0 ± 0.06 (mean ± SD) / Type 1: 2.3 ± 0.5 (mean ± SD)	33
VHP-VWF (LFB)	France	Ion and affinity-exchange chromatography	S/D	10:1	22.5 ± 24.3* (mean ± SD)	1.79 ± 0.24 (mean ± SD)	31
Immunate (Baxter)	USA, Austria, Sweden, Germany, Czech Republic	Ion-exchange chromatography	S/D and vapor heat (60°C/10 h)		1.9 (0.8–3.5) (mean (range))	1.8 (0.4–3.6) (mean (range))	21

*High recovery of FVIII at one hour is due to the low amount of infused FVIII and the stabilization of endogenous FVIII.
S/D, solvent/detergent treated.

Table 49.4 Target laboratory parameters for invasive procedures.

	Target VWF:RCo	Target FVIII
Major		
At the time of procedure	80–100 IU/dL	100 IU/dL complete
Subsequently	Maintain trough above 50 IU/dL until hemostasis secure	Maintain trough above 50 IU/dL until wound healing
Minor		
At the time of procedure	30–50 IU/dL	50 IU/dL
Subsequently	Unlikely to be important	Maintain trough of 50 IU/dL until wound healing complete

time, and two of these only on the first postoperative day [24]. A survey of 194 USA clinicians reported that for major surgery they aimed for a FVIII and VWF:RCo greater than 80%, with levels greater than 50% considered adequate for minor surgery [37].

Factor VIII

It is standard practice to monitor the FVIII level. FVIII is, however, only a surrogate marker of VWF function and does not necessarily reflect the VWF:RCo, particularly in patients with types 2 and 3 VWD. In these situations, the VWF:RCo may be considerably lower than the FVIII and mislead the clinician.

VWF:RCo

It has been recommended that VWF:RCo should be monitored aiming for target levels appropriate for the clinical situation (Table 49.4) [36], and this is common practice [24].

Bleeding time

A retrospective study of 76 patients unresponsive to DDAVP undergoing surgical procedures showed no correlation between correction of the bleeding time and surgical hemostasis. Furthermore, clinicians did not alter their management dependent on the bleeding time [39]. Adequate hemostasis has been achieved with concentrates that do not reproducibly correct the bleeding time [17,22]. The bleeding time may be useful if patients are bleeding abnormally in spite of replacement therapy. Some patients whose bleeding time is not corrected with infused VWF may respond to platelet infusions [40].

PFA-100

PFA-100 has been used to monitor replacement therapy in patients with VWD. Although convenient to use, the reliability of this method of monitoring hemostasis following the use of VWF-containing concentrates is not yet established and results should be interpreted with caution.

Management of surgery and other invasive procedures in VWD patients unresponsive to DDAVP

General considerations

Regular clinical assessment of hemostasis is crucial and it is important to recognize that abnormal bleeding may be the result of surgical bleeding rather than inadequate hemostasis. In patients who bleed in spite of apparently adequate treatment a full blood count, coagulation screen, and measurement of FVIII and VWF:RCo levels should be carried out urgently. A bleeding time may be useful. In patients with type 3 VWD, the development of an inhibitor to VWF needs to be considered and tested for [36].

Minor procedures

In general, a VWF:RCo and FVIII of 50 IU/dL should be adequate for a minor procedure and often only one infusion is required.

Dental treatment

For dental extraction or inferior dental nerve block, in patients unsuitable for DDAVP, treatment with a VWF-containing concentrate is indicated. Many clinicians aim to increase the VWF:RCo and FVIII to about 50 IU/dL with a single infusion of a VWF-containing concentrate. An antifibrinolytic should be given for 7–10 days following a dental extraction.

Major procedures

VWF:RCo should be raised to 80–100 IU/dL at the time of surgery and maintained above 50 IU/dL until hemostasis is secure [36,37]. The FVIII should be raised to about 100 IU/dL perioperatively and maintained above 50 IU/dL until wound healing is complete. This requires regular monitoring of VWF:RCo and FVIII. Dosing regimens for VHP-VWD differ and are described above. Continuous infusion of a VWF/FVIII or VHP-VWF concentrate has also been successfully used to cover major surgery [29,32,33].

The risk of VTE should be assessed in patients undergoing major surgery who receive VWF-containing concentrates. High levels of FVIII should be avoided and venous thrombophylaxis considered [34,35].

The use of VWF-containing concentrates in managing surgery depends, in part, on the subtypes of VWD.

Type 1 VWD

VWF-containing concentrates are more likely to be needed for larger operations or where prolonged correction of the hemostatic defect is required. In type 1 VWD, the VWF and FVIII levels often increase temporarily postoperatively owing to an acute-phase response.

Type 2A or type 2M VWD

Minor procedures can be performed under DDAVP cover in some patients but major procedures are likely to require a VWF-containing concentrate. Correcting the VWF:RCo level may lead to high FVIII levels, increasing the risk of VTE.

Type 2B VWD

Most clinicians recommend VWF-containing concentrates to cover invasive procedures in type 2B VWD.

Type 2N VWD

Minor procedures may be done with DDAVP. A VWF-containing concentrate normalizes the half-life of endogenous FVIII. Raising FVIII to about 100 IU/dL perioperatively and maintaining it above 50 IU/dL until wound healing provides adequate cover. Infusion of a VHP-VWF concentrate will also lead to normalization of the FVIII level over 6–12 h [13,14]. The improved half-life of factor VIII means that once-daily treatment is usually sufficient.

Type 3 VWD

Patients with type 3 VWD who are undergoing invasive procedures must be treated with a VWF-containing concentrate.

Patients who have alloantibodies to VWF are at risk of anaphylactic reactions with the use of VWF-containing concentrates [41]. Experience in managing these patients is limited; however, good hemostasis has been reported with the use of high doses or infusions of recombinant FVIII [38]. Recombinant FVIIa has also been used [42].

Acquired VWD

Some patients with acquired VWD who have failed to respond to DDAVP have responded to VWF-containing concentrates [43].

Treatment failure

Patients who have an inadequate clinical response to VWF-containing concentrates, despite correction of laboratory parameters, may respond to platelets or cryoprecipitate. Surgical bleeding, inhibitory activity, and other causes of hemostatic defects should be considered.

Platelets

The bleeding time may be shortened by platelet infusion [40]. If mucosal bleeding persists and the bleeding time remains prolonged after adequate replacement therapy with a VWF-containing concentrate, platelet infusions should be considered.

Cryoprecipitate

Cryoprecipitate is not virally inactivated and should not be used for the management of VWD unless other treatment modalities have failed or are unavailable [24,36]. Some patients who have not responded to a VWF-containing concentrate may respond to cryoprecipitate.

Conclusion

VWF-containing concentrates play a valuable role in the management of patients with VWD who are unsuitable for DDAVP. Further clinical trials that focus on hemostatic endpoints are required to investigate how to improve the use and monitoring of these products. The potential use of recombinant VWF concentrate is under investigation, but as yet a product suitable for clinical trials is not available [44].

References

1 Mannucci PM. Desmopressin (DDAVP) in the treatment of bleeding disorders: the first 20 years. *Blood* 1997; **90**: 2515–21.
2 Makris M, Conlon CP, Watson HG. Immunisation of patients with bleeding disorders. *Haemophilia* 2003; **9**: 541–6.
3 Menache D, Aronson DL. New treatments of von Willebrand disease: plasma derived von Willebrand factor concentrates. *Thromb Haemost* 1997; **78**: 566–70.
4 Smith TJ, Gill JC, Ambruso DR, Hathaway WE. Hyponatremia and seizures in young children given DDAVP. *Am J Hematol* 1989; **31**: 199–202.
5 Bond L, Bevan D. Myocardial infarction in a patient with hemophilia treated with DDAVP. *N Engl J Med* 1988; **318**: 121.
6 Grunwald Z, Sather SD. Intraoperative cerebral infarction after desmopressin administration in infant with end-stage renal disease. *Lancet* 1995; **345**: 1364–5.
7 Byrnes JJ, Larcada A, Moake JL. Thrombosis following desmopressin for uremic bleeding. *Am J Hematol* 1988; **28**: 63–5.
8 Holmberg L, Nilsson IM, Borge L, *et al.* Platelet aggregation induced by 1-desamino-8-D-arginine vasopressin (DDAVP) in Type IIB von Willebrand's disease. *N Engl J Med* 1983; **309**: 816–21.

9 Casonato A, Pontara E, Dannhaeuser D, *et al*. Re-evaluation of the therapeutic efficacy of DDAVP in type IIB von Willebrand's disease. *Blood Coagul Fibrinol* 1994; 5: 959–64.

10 Fowler WE, Berkowitz LR, Roberts HR. DDAVP for type IIB von Willebrand disease. *Blood* 1989; 74: 1859–60.

11 Gralnick HR, Williams SB, McKeown LP, *et al*. DDAVP in type IIa von Willebrand's disease. *Blood* 1986; 67: 465–8.

12 Michiels JJ, van de Velde A, van Vliet HH, *et al*. Response of von Willebrand factor parameters to desmopressin in patients with type 1 and type 2 congenital von Willebrand disease: diagnostic and therapeutic implications. *Semin Thromb Haemost* 2002; 28: 111–32.

13 Mazurier C, Gaucher C, Jorieux S, Goudemand M. Biological effect of desmopressin in eight patients with type 2N ("Normandy") von Willebrand disease. Collaborative Group. *Br J Haematol* 1994; 88: 849–54.

14 Goudemand J, Negrier C, Ounnoughene N, Sultan Y. Clinical management of patients with von Willebrand's disease with a VHP vWF concentrate: the French experience. *Haemophilia* 1998; 4 (Suppl. 3): 48–52.

15 Mannucci PM, Lombardi R, Bader R, *et al*. Heterogeneity of type I von Willebrand disease: evidence for a subgroup with an abnormal von Willebrand factor. *Blood* 1985; 66: 796–802.

16 Brown SA, Eldridge A, Collins PW, Bowen DJ. Increased clearance of von Willebrand factor post-DDAVP in type 1 von Willebrand disease: is it a potential pathogenic process? *J Thromb Haemost* 2003; 1: 1714–7.

17 Mannucci PM, Tenconi PM, Castaman G, Rodeghiero F. Comparison of four virus-inactivated plasma concentrates for treatment of severe von Willebrand disease: a cross-over randomized trial. *Blood* 1992; 79: 3130–7.

18 Mannucci PM, Moia M, Rebulla P, *et al*. Correction of the bleeding time in treated patients with severe von Willebrand disease is not solely dependent on the normal multimeric structure of plasma von Willebrand factor. *Am J Hematol* 1987; 25: 55–65.

19 Cumming AM, Fildes S, Cumming IR, *et al*. Clinical and laboratory evaluation of National Health Service factor VIII concentrate (8Y) for the treatment of von Willebrand's disease. *Br J Haematol* 1990; 75: 234–9.

20 Pasi KJ, Williams MD, Enayat MS, Hill FG. Clinical and laboratory evaluation of the treatment of von Willebrand's disease patients with heat-treated factor VIII concentrate (BPL 8Y). *Br J Haematol* 1990; 75: 228–33.

21 Auerswald G, Eberspacher B, Engl W, *et al*. Successful treatment of patients with von Willebrand disease using a high-purity double-virus inactivated factor VIII/von Willebrand factor concentrate (Immunate). *Semin Thromb Haemost* 2002; 28: 203–14.

22 Mannucci PM, Chediak J, Hanna W, *et al*. Treatment of von Willebrand disease with a high-purity factor VIII/von Willebrand factor concentrate: a prospective, multicenter study. *Blood* 2002; 99: 450–6.

23 Federici AB, Baudo F, Caracciolo C, *et al*. Clinical efficacy of highly purified, doubly virus-inactivated factor VIII/von Willebrand factor concentrate (Fanhdi) in the treatment of von Willebrand disease: a retrospective clinical study. *Haemophilia* 2002; 8: 761–7.

24 Lusher JM. Clinical guidelines for treating von Willebrand disease patients who are not candidates for DDAVP — a survey of European physicians. *Haemophilia* 1998; 4 (Suppl. 3): 11–4.

25 Dobrkovska A, Krzensk U, Chediak JR. Pharmacokinetics, efficacy and safety of Humate-P in von Willebrand disease. *Haemophilia* 1998; 4 (Suppl. 3): 33–9.

26 Berntorp E, Nilsson IM. Use of a high-purity factor VIII concentrate (Hemate P) in von Willebrand's disease. *Vox Sang* 1989; 56: 212–7.

27 Kreuz W, Mentzer D, Becker S, *et al*. Haemate P in children with von Willebrand's disease. *Hemostasis* 1994; 24: 304–10.

28 Lillicrap D, Poon MC, Walker I, *et al*. Association of Hemophilia Clinic Directors of Canada. Efficacy and safety of the factor VIII/von Willebrand factor concentrate, Haemate-P/Humate-P: ristocetin cofactor unit dosing in patients with von Willebrand disease. *Thromb Haemost* 2002; 87: 224–30.

29 Lubetsky A, Schulman S, Varon D, *et al*. Safety and efficacy of continuous infusion of a combined factor VIII-von Willebrand factor (vWF) concentrate (Haemate-PTM) in patients with von Willebrand disease. *Thromb Haemost* 1999; 81: 229–33.

30 Mazurier C, De Romeuf C, Parquet-Gernez A, Goudemand M. *In vitro* and *in vivo* characterization of a high-purity, solvent/detergent-treated factor VIII concentrate: evidence for its therapeutic efficacy in von Willebrand's disease. *Eur J Haematol* 1989; 43: 7–14.

31 Goudemand J, Mazurier C, Marey A, *et al*. Clinical and biological evaluation in von Willebrand's disease of a von Willebrand factor concentrate with low factor VIII activity. *Br J Haematol* 1992; 80: 214–21.

32 Smith MP, Rice KM, Bromidge ES, *et al*. Continuous infusion therapy with very high purity von Willebrand factor concentrate in patients with severe von Willebrand disease. *Blood Coagul Fibrinol* 1997; 8: 6–12.

33 Lubetsky A, Martinowitz U, Luboshitz J, *et al*. Efficacy and safety of a factor VIII-von Willebrand factor concentrate 8Y: stability, bacteriological safety, pharmacokinetic analysis and clinical experience. *Haemophilia* 2002; 8: 622–8.

34 Makris M, Colvin B, Gupta V, *et al*. Venous thrombosis following the use of intermediate purity FVIII concentrate to treat patients with von Willebrand's disease. *Thromb Haemost* 2002; 88: 387–8.

35 Mannucci PM. Venous thromboembolism in von Willebrand disease. *Thromb Haemost* 2002; 88: 378–9.

36 Pasi KJ, Collins PW, Keeling DM, *et al*. Management of von Willebrand disease. A guideline from the UK Haemophilia Centre Doctors' Organisation. *Haemophilia* 2004; 10: 218–31.

37 Cohen AJ, Kessler CM, Ewenstein BM. The Hemophilia Research Society of North America. Management of von Willebrand disease: a survey on current clinical practice from the haemophilia centres of North America. *Haemophilia* 2001; 7: 235–41.

38 Federici AB, Castaman G, Mannucci PM. Italian Association of Hemophilia Centers (AICE). Guidelines for the diagnosis and management of von Willebrand disease in Italy. *Haemophilia* 2002; 8: 607–21.

39 Foster PA. A perspective on the use of FVIII concentrates and cryoprecipitate prophylactically in surgery or therapeutically in severe bleeds in patients with von Willebrand disease unresponsive to DDAVP: results of an international survey. On behalf of the Subcommittee on von Willebrand Factor of the Scientific and Standardization Committee of the ISTH. *Thromb Haemost* 1995; 74: 1370–8.

40 Castillo R, Monteagudo J, Escolar G, *et al*. Hemostatic effect of normal platelet transfusion in severe von Willebrand disease patients. *Blood* 1991; 77: 1901–5.

41 Mannucci PM, Tamaro G, Narchi G, *et al*. Life-threatening reaction to FVIII concentrate in a patient with severe vWD and alloantibodies to von Willebrand factor. *Eur J Haematol* 1987; 39: 467–70.

42 Ciavarella N, Schiavoni M, *et al*. Use of recombinant factor VIIa (NovoSeven) in the treatment of two patients with type III von Willebrand's disease and an inhibitor against von Willebrand factor. *Hemostasis* 1996; 26: 150–4.

43 Kumar S, Pruthi RK, Nichols WL. Acquired von Willebrand's syndrome: a single institution experience. *Am J Hematol* 2003; 72: 243–347.

44 Schwarz HP, Turecek PL, Pichler L, *et al*. Recombinant von Willebrand factor. *Thromb Haemost* 1997; 78: 571–6.

50 Women and von Willebrand disease

Peter A. Kouides

Introduction

Since the first description of von Willebrand disease (VWD), the phenotypic expression of the disease in females has become more pronounced. Seventy-nine years ago, the index case in the kindred studied by von Willebrand was a girl who had multiple mucocutaneous symptoms and actually bled to death at the time of the fourth menstrual cycle after menarche. Furthermore, 16 of the 23 affected members of this kindred were females. Despite this thorough documentation, approximately 70 years elapsed until it was definitively reported in the literature that, because of the monthly challenge of menstruation and of intermittent childbirth, typical type 1 VWD carried a greater import in females than in males [1–6]. These studies have clearly documented a definite degree of obstetric and gynecologic morbidity in females with VWD. This chapter will highlight relevant epidemiology, clinical characteristics, and therapeutic issues in the patient with menorrhagia and/or postpartum hemorrhage related to VWD.

Epidemiology of von Willebrand disease in females

In the past 5 years, there has been a concerted effort internationally to determine the prevalence of VWD in women presenting with menorrhagia. These studies have included a total of approximately 350 women. Although there have been more differences than similarities in terms of study design, overall the general prevalence of VWD in women presenting for menorrhagia and subsequently referred for hemostasis testing is in the 7–20% range [7–10]. However, "mass" testing of all women is not feasible. In general, the probability of VWD in a female with menorrhagia would be highest if there are multiple mucocutaneous bleeding symptoms and menorrhagia since menarche, [7] and if the menstrual bleeding is ovulatory (regular periods).

Diagnostic aspects

In general, the fact that VWF levels fluctuate is well established; less well established is the degree and significance, if any, of the fluctuation in relation to the menstrual cycle and oral contraceptive (OC) use.

Regarding the potential fluctuation of VWF levels in relation to the menstrual cycle, a longitudinal study of 39 normal-menstruating volunteers conducted by Kadir *et al.* [11] found a statistically significant decrease in VWF during the first 3 days of menses. However, cross-sectional analysis revealed no difference. In addition, Onundarson *et al.* [12] found no difference in VWF levels in a cross-sectional analysis of 93 patients sampled at days 4–7, 11–15, and 21–28. However, a more recent cross-sectional study found that the VWF level was lowest during the first 4 days of menses and that the highest levels actually occurred on days 9–10 [13]. It is possible that in this study the groups were more finely divided than in other studies [13]. Given these conflicting results, it is most logical to advise the clinician that, when randomly measured VWF levels are normal or borderline low in a female with menorrhagia, independent of the day of menses, the test should be repeated during the first 3 days of the menstrual cycle. The intent would be to "capture" the "lowest" VWF level in that patient. Furthermore, this would be a practical approach as it is during those initial 3 days that the patient would be a candidate for intranasal or subcutaneous desmopressin (DDAVP) to raise the VWF levels [14].

Regarding OC use, based on an initial report over 20 years ago, which found increased VWF levels in three women with VWD taking prescribed OCs or conjugated estrogen (which is more than 10 times the dose in present-day OC) [15], hematologists are generally reluctant to test for VWD in women on OCs. It is assumed that hormonal therapy might "mask" the diagnosis. Interestingly, in a recent study by Kadir *et al.* [11], a low-dose monophasic estrogen (< 30 μg) OC actually led to a decrease in the VWF level, though this finding was not statistically significant. Again, as in the case of testing in relation to the menstrual cycle, a practical approach would be to still test women when on OC, particularly if they are indeed still experiencing menorrhagia or other mucocutaneous bleeding symptoms. This is because, intuitively, if the subnormal VWF levels are contributing to the bleeding, at that point in time, then the OC should not be raising the VWF levels.

A discussion of diagnostic aspects of VWD in women is not complete if mention is not made of the "false" diagnosis of VWD in the setting of hypothyroidism-related menorrhagia. Hypothyroidism can present with menorrhagia [16]. In turn, one mechanism may be through reduced VWF synthesis in the hypothyroid state. This is because correction of the hypothyroidism will result in normalization of the VWF levels and subsequent resolution of the menorrhagia [16].

Menorrhagia: clinical characteristics

A female with VWD certainly has a very high relative risk of menorrhagia compared with the general population, with the prevalence of menorrhagia by subjective report being 78–97% among women with known, primarily type 1, VWD. Using the more objective pictorial blood assessment chart (PBAC), the Royal Free London group reported that 74% of their patients with VWD (primarily type 1) had pictorial chart evidence for menorrhagia (score >100) [1]. Alternatively, the relative risk of menorrhagia in a woman with a low VWF level has been estimated at fourfold [17].

Not surprisingly, surrogate clinical characteristics of menorrhagia are pronounced in women with VWD: they use more tampons and pads than non-VWD menstruating women, have higher prevalence of anemia (28–66% [2,4,5]) and report more frequent staining of underwear [4]. In addition, again not surprisingly, these women also have a much higher frequency of other mucocutaneous bleeding symptoms. Table 50.1 summarizes the prevalence of these bleeding symptoms in comparison with a control group of non-VWD women from recent studies. These bleeding symptoms may ultimately prove useful in combination as a screening tool in predicting VWD in women presenting with menorrhagia.

Type 2 and type 3 VWD patients have not been as extensively studied as type 1 patients, but a study by Foster *et al.* on behalf of the International Society of Thrombosis and Hemostasis (ISTH) von Willebrand Factor Subcommittee reported a high prevalence of menorrhagia. They also noted that a quarter of the patients required hysterectomy [18]. Subsequent studies have focused on the more common type 1 patient and, even in this population, with the milder depression of the VWF level, there is a relatively high rate of hysterectomy for control of menorrhagia

(~8–18%) [1,2,4,5,19]. In two studies, underlying uterine pathology was noted in the hysterectomy specimen, and it can be postulated that mild VWD may "unmask" a uterine fibroid [1,4].

In type 1 VWD patients, menstrual bleeding will not be as dramatic as Erik von Willebrand's index case, who exsanguinated at the time of her fourth cycle (by genotyping her family, this patient has since been proved to have had type 3 disease [20]). Nonetheless, the morbidity of menorrhagia in type 1 patients is significant, both for the reasons noted above and also in terms of the cumulative impairment of quality of life resulting from heavy monthly menstruation. Four relatively large studies (involving nearly 400 patients) comparing women with VWD with non-VWD women have shown unequivocally that quality of life is indeed impaired in these women [2,4,6,19]. Approximately 40% of VWD women reported having to take time off work or school in the last year. Dysmenorrhea was also reported in approximately half the patients [2,4]. Remarkably, in a Canadian study using a standardized quality-of-life tool, women with VWD assessed their own health status as being compromised to an extent similar to that reported by HIV-positive patients with severe hemophilia and even greater than that experienced by adult survivors of brain tumors [21]. Furthermore, VWD was also reported to have a negative impact on cognition. The authors hypothesize that this may be a result of chronic iron deficiency anemia related to menorrhagia. However, the sample size was small ($n = 12$) so further study is needed to confirm these provocative findings.

A high rate of mid-cycle pain, termed mittelschmerz, has also been noted in VWD women [4]. Besides mid-cycle pain, these patients can develop an acute surgical abdomen from hemoperitoneum, presumably from bleeding into the corpus luteum with subsequent rupture [22]. There have been reports of this involv-

Table 50.1 Significant primarily nonmenstrual bleeding symptoms in women with vWD.

	Study population	Symptoms more common in vWD patients than in non-VWD patients
Royal Free London 1998 [7]	From a cohort of 150 women presenting with menorrhagia subsequently diagnosed with VWD ($n = 26$, presumed all type 1); comparison with the 124 non-VWD-related menorrhagia patients	Bruising Dentistry-related bleeding Surgery-related bleeding Postpartum hemorrhage Menorrhagia since menarche Multiple bleeding symptoms
Upstate NY Hemophilia Treatment Center Consortium study 2000 [4]	81 menstruating women registered at HTCs, all with type 1 VWD, compared with a cohort of 150 menstruating volunteers	Age (the younger the age, the higher the probability of VWD) History of dental-related bleeding Past or present history of anemia A diminished quality of life during menses in relation to family activities
Centers for Disease Control — Atlanta 2002 [6]	102 women with VWD (type not specified) registered at HTCs compared with 88 control subjects	Surgery-related bleeding Excessive gum bleeding Bleeding after minor injuries

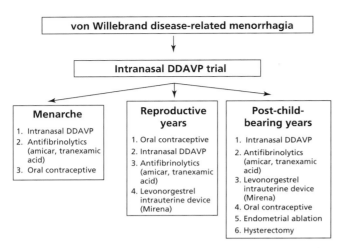

Figure 50.1 Age and preference-based algorithm for management of von Willebrand disease-related menorrhagia.

ing bleeding into the broad ligament, with the patient presenting with a positive iliopsoas sign [23]. Another consequence, conceivably, of prolonged impairment of quality of life could be the emergence of psychiatric disorders in terms of emotional impairment [21] and anxiety. Rozeik *et al.* [19], in Germany, reported that the prevalence of anxiety was significantly higher in their population of VWD women than the general baseline German population.

Menorrhagia: management

The management of menorrhagia related to VWD involves consideration of the patient's age, childbearing status, and preference, as depicted in Figure 50.1. Table 50.2 also summarizes the relative efficacy of various treatments in terms of the level of evidence. In the adolescent, surgical intervention is not an option, whereas an older patient beyond her childbearing years may personally choose a hysterectomy as definitive treatment in lieu of continued medical therapy with intranasal/subcutaneous DDAVP, or oral antifibrinolytic agents, or oral contraceptive therapy. Regardless of the patient's choice, it is reasonable to advise a laboratory trial for response to intranasal or subcuta-

neous DDAVP since not all type 1 patients will respond [5] and since knowledge of the degree of response is helpful for future reference if the patient ever has to undergo a procedure wherein DDAVP prophylaxis would be considered.

Desmopressin

If the recently diagnosed VWD patient being evaluated for menorrhagia is going to undergo a DDAVP trial as noted above, it is obvious to consider DDAVP as a frontline option after demonstrating that the VWF level has at least doubled. This certainly can be considered to be a frontline option in the adolescent. Until recently, available evidence has been only at level C (case series), with the subcutaneous form of DDAVP being rated effective 86% of the time and rated only no effect 14% of the time [24]. In another similar cohort study using the intranasal form of DDAVP and involving 721 daily uses in 90 women, 64% rated the treatment as excellent, 28% as good, and 8% reported no response [14]. In both cases, it should be emphasized that assessment was by patient report and not by the PBAC or the spectrophotometric method.

More recently, however, Kadir *et al.* [25] have measured the efficacy of intranasal DDAVP using the PBAC. Women were studied during two menstrual periods with one spray in each nostril (either placebo or 300 μg of DDAVP, respectively, on days 2 and 3 of the period). Thirty-nine women were recruited, of whom 30 had VWD and nine had other non-VWD bleeding disorders. Twenty-nine received trial medication and completed the PBAC during at least one period. Regardless of whether the first treatment period involved the placebo or the intranasal DDAVP, there was a reduction in the PBAC score that was statistically significant ($P = 0.0001$ with both placebo and DDAVP when compared with the baseline PBAC). There was a trend toward a lower score if intranasal DDAVP was administered. However, this was not statistically significant and there was no significant difference in quality of life in terms of absence from work or school or avoidance of social activities or use of other medications.

Similar results were noted in a related study of 20 women with menorrhagia and an underlying platelet disorder comparing 300 μg of intranasal DDAVP with placebo. There was no statistically significant decrease in blood loss from 230 cm^3 baseline

Table 50.2 Summary of levels of evidence of menorrhagia treatments.

Intervention	Efficacy in non-VWD menorrhagia	Level of evidence in non-VWD menorrhagia	Efficacy in VWD menorrhagia	Level of evidence in VWD menorrhagia
Tranexamic acid	Yes	A	Yes	C
Intranasal DDAVP	Not studied	–	±	C, B
Oral contraceptive	No	B	No	C
Mirena	Yes	B	Yes	C
Mefenamic acid	Yes	B	Not studied	–

A, randomized control trial; B, robust observational; C, case series.
Additional treatments studied for menorrhagia in general: Danazol, gonadotropin-releasing hormone, nonsteroidal anti-inflammatory drugs.

(measured spectrophotometrically) to 192 cm³ with DDAVP, compared with 213 cm³ with the placebo. However, there was a statistically significant decrease to 155 cm³ if the DDAVP was combined with tranexamic acid [26]. Perhaps the concurrent use of tranexamic acid offsets the rise of tissue plasminogen activator after DDAVP infusion, although Edlund *et al.* did not report increased fibrinolytic activity in menstrual fluid post-DDAVP [27].

Regarding side-effects of intranasal DDAVP, in both studies fluid intake was restricted to "1.5 L/day. Nonetheless, Kadir *et al.* [25] reported weight gain in 12%, compared with none with placebo. Interestingly, the prevalence of headache (23%) was no different from 24% of the placebo group.

In summary, more objective measurements of efficacy have not shown as great a benefit of intranasal DDAVP for VWD-related menorrhagia as prior studies using subjective assessment as the endpoint of efficacy. The question remains whether the efficacy of DDAVP can be improved without an increase in the adverse event rate in terms of altering the schedule from the standard use of one puff to each nostril on days 2 and 3 of menses to twice-daily dosing on the first 2 days or daily for 3 days. Also, further study of the efficacy and safety of combined therapy of intranasal DDAVP and antifibrinolytic therapy is warranted, as are studies exploring alternative hemostatic interventions.

Antifibrinolytic therapy

The rationale for antifibrinolytic therapy is well founded, as several studies have demonstrated increased fibrinolysis in uterine fluid in women with menorrhagia [27]. The seminal study by Bonnar *et al.* was a three-arm randomized comparison of oral tranexamic acid (1 g orally four times a day) and ethamsylate, a general hemostatic agent, and mefenamic acid, a prostaglandin synthetase inhibitor [28]. There were approximately 25 patients per arm, each with prior documented heavy menstrual blood flow as determined by the spectrophotometric method. There was a statistically significant 54% decrease in menstrual flow against baseline in the tranexamic acid arm, compared with no statistically significant decrease with the other agents. Further supportive evidence for tranexamic acid in menorrhagia has come from the evidence-based database of the Cochrane Review, which concluded that it is an efficacious agent in general for menorrhagia [29]. The actual effective dose and frequency, however, remains unclear at this time with a total of four VWD women reported in literature who received only daily dosing of 4 g in a single dose daily for 3 consecutive days [30]. However, one concern would be gastrointestinal distress at this dose.

Hormonal therapy

In the Cochrane database of systemic reviews, oral contraceptive therapy is not proven to be effective for the therapy of menorrhagia. Supporting this, in type 1 VWD patients, in one study of 41 patients with VWD-related menorrhagia, standard dose

OC was only 24% effective [4]. However, in a survey carried out through the ISTH of 40 women with type 2 or type 3 VWD, it was 80% effective [18]. At this point, for the VWD-related menorrhagia patient focused primarily on family planning, a trial of oral contraceptive is warranted in that it may also decrease menstrual flow. But on average, its efficacy appears to be lower compared with the hemostatic agents discussed above. Hormonal therapy delivered through an intrauterine device, however, may prove to be very efficacious for VWD-related menorrhagia, given a robust body of literature in Europe showing its efficacy for menorrhagia in general. Several studies have shown 74–97% efficacy [31]. Recently, Kadir and Lee [32] studied the intrauterine device, Mirena, which releases the second-generation progesterone levonorgestrel, over a 5-year period. In 15 women (12 with VWD, one with FIX deficiency, and two with FXI deficiency), after 9 months of use, 9/15 became amenorrheic, while, in the remaining six patients the maximum PBAC score was only 64 compared with a mean score of 216 before treatment!

Another less invasive alternative to hysterectomy would be endometrial ablation, but its long-term efficacy in VWD-related menorrhagia is not well established at this time. In a small series of patients with VWD-related menorrhagia, only two had long-term control beyond 4 years [33].

Obstetric aspects of von Willebrand disease

It has been well established that part of the "physiologic response" in pregnancy is a progressive elevation of the FVIII and VWF levels [34]. However, it should be stressed that there appears to be a proportionately lower elevation in the levels than in the normal pregnant patient. Consequently, not surprisingly, a higher rate of postpartum hemorrhage (PPH) than in the general population has been reported, with a rate of 16–29% PPH in the first 24 h [this is defined as primary PPH (PPPH)] [3,23,35]. The rate of PPPH in the general population is 3–5% [35]. Also, there appears to be a higher rate in type 2 and 3 patients than in type 1 patients [3,23,35]. The increased rate of PPPH may result in the need for red cell transfusions, as reported in 7% [3] to 17%[4] of type 1 patients.

The rise in the FVIII and VWF levels occurs in the second and third trimester, so clinicians should not assume that there will not be excessive bleeding during amniocentesis or a first-trimester abortion, as levels may not yet have increased at that time point [36]. The presentation of VWD as transfusion-dependent bleeding at miscarriage has been reported [3]. Excessive bleeding beyond a week post partum up to 5 weeks post partum has also been reported [4,37]. Consequently, it should be common practice to remind new mothers of this possibility in the weeks after delivery.

Management of VWD during pregnancy

As noted above, gestational palliation does occur during pregnancy so that, if such a pregnant woman needs a dental extraction or another invasive procedure, DDAVP is not necessary if the VWF levels are normalized. However, if the VWF levels are still subnormal, the following are, theoretically, of concern when administering DDAVP ante partum:

- vasoconstrictive effect leading to decreased placental flow;
- risk of premature labor given the potential oxytocic effect of desmopressin;
- risk of maternal and neonatal hyponatremia.

Maternal hyponatremia has been reported [38], but this is uncommon. There seems to be a sense among practitioners that DDAVP use ante partum is safe and that a dose during labor does not first require clamping of the umbilical cord. Mannucci [39] found no adverse events associated with DDAVP given in the second trimester in 31 women with VWD who underwent chorionic villus sampling.

The importance of obtaining VWF levels in the third trimester cannot be overemphasized. Documentation of normal levels at that point is very important information at the time of delivery for the anesthesiologist intuitively reluctant to give epidural analgesia, and for the obstetrician planning a cesarean section. Again, documentation of normal levels at that time would not necessitate DDAVP. But, certainly, measuring VWF levels 24 and 48 h post partum is not unreasonable if the plan is to administer DDAVP should the VWF levels decrease.

In the case of patients with type 2 or type 3 VWD, there is evidence that an expectant approach, as one would carry out in a type 1 patient in terms of observation alone at the time of delivery if the VWF levels are normal, is sufficient, provided that the FVIII level has increased above 50%. In turn, this is based on the premise that the FVIII level predicts deep-tissue hemostasis as opposed to the VWF level. However, this is based on a cohort of only five women [40]. As such, most clinicians would be more comfortable infusing a plasma-derived VWF containing FVIII concentrate such as Humate P or Alphanate SD. Theoretically, there could be a risk of postpartum thrombosis; although reports of thrombosis with VWF concentrates have so far come only from orthopedic settings, pregnancy can be considered to be a prothrombotic state of similar magnitude. There has been one report of thrombosis in a type 2B patient post partum (associated with the use of cryoprecipitate [41]). Dosing at delivery has typically been 40–80 U/kg of a plasma-derived VWF-containing FVIII concentrate. Postpartum prophylaxis has usually been 20–40 U/kg for at least 1 week post partum then tapered over several weeks [37].

In the case of VWD Normandy and type 2B VWD, management has been problematic. The use of recombinant FVIII concentrate has been reported in a type 2N patient with a FVIII level <50% at the time of delivery [42]. In the case of type 2B, platelet transfusions were given at the time of delivery, when the platelet count fell as low as 20 000/μL [43]. The use of a plasma-derived VWF containing FVIII concentrate should also be considered prophylactically [41].

Finally, DDAVP does not appear to cross into breast milk and can be safely administered in breastfeeding women.

References

1 Kadir RA, Economides DL, Sabin CA, et al. Assessment of menstrual blood loss and gynaecological problems in patients with inherited bleeding disorders. Haemophilia 1999; 5: 40–8.
2 Kadir RA, Sabin CA, Pollard D, et al. Quality of life during menstruation in patients with inherited bleeding disorders. Haemophilia 1998; 4: 836–41.
3 Kadir RA, Lee CA, Sabin CA, et al. Pregnancy in women with von Willebrand's disease or Factor XI deficiency. Br J Obstet Gynaecol 1998; 105: 314–21.
4 Kouides PA, Burkhart P, Phatak P, et al. Gynecological and obstetrical morbidity in women with type I von Willebrand disease: results of a patient survey. Haemophilia 2000; 6: 643–8.
5 Ragni MV, Bontempo FA, Cortese Hassett A. von Willebrand disease and bleeding in women. Haemophilia 1999; 5: 313–17.
6 Kirtava A, Drews C, Lally C, et al. Medical, reproductive and psychosocial experiences of women diagnosed with von Willebrand's disease receiving care in haemophilia treatment centres: a case–control study. Haemophilia 2003; 9: 292–7.
7 Kadir RA, Economides DL, Sabin CA, et al. Frequency of inherited bleeding disorders in women with menorrhagia. Lancet 1998; 351: 485–9.
8 Woo YL, White B, Corbally R, et al. von Willebrand's disease: an important cause of dysfunctional uterine bleeding. Blood Coagul Fibrinol 2002; 13: 89–93.
9 Edlund M, Blomback M, von Schoultz B, Andersson O. On the value of menorrhagia as a predictor for coagulation disorders. Am J Hematol 1996; 53: 234–8.
10 Dilley A, Drews C, Miller C, et al. von Willebrand disease and other inherited bleeding disorders in women with diagnosed menorrhagia. Obstet Gynecol 2001; 97: 630–6.
11 Kadir RA, Economides DL, Sabin CA, et al. Variations in coagulation factors in women: effects of age, ethnicity, menstrual cycle and combined oral contraceptive. Thromb Haemost 1999; 82: 1456–61.
12 Onundarson PT, Gumundsdottir BR, Arnfinnsdottir AV, et al. von Willebrand factor does not vary during the normal menstrual cycle. Thromb Haemost 2001; 85: 183–4 [letter].
13 Miller CH, Dilley A, Drews C, et al. Changes in von Willebrand factor and Factor VIII levels during the menstrual cycle. Thromb Haemost 2002; 87: 1082–3.
14 Leissinger C, Becton D, Cornell C, Gill JC. High-dose DDAVP intranasal spray (Stimate) for the prevention and treatment of bleeding in patients with mild haemophilia A, mild or moderate type 1 von Willebrand disease and symptomatic carriers of haemophilia A. Haemophilia 2001; 7: 258–66.
15 Alperin JB. Estrogens and surgery in women with von Willebrand's disease. Am J Med 1982; 73: 367–71.
16 Michiels JJ, Schroyens W, Berneman Z, Van der PM. Acquired von Willebrand syndrome type 1 in hypothyroidism: reversal after treatment with thyroxine. Clin Appl Thromb Haemost 2001; 7: 113–15.
17 Sadler JE. von Willebrand disease type 1: a diagnosis in search of a disease. Blood 2003; 101: 2089–93.
18 Foster PA. The reproductive health of women with von Willebrand disease unresponsive to DDAVP: results of an international survey. On behalf of the Subcommittee on von Willebrand Factor of the Scientific and Standardization Committee of the ISTH. Thromb Haemost 1995; 74: 784–90.
19 Rozeik C, Scharrer I. Gynecological disorders and psychological problems in 184 women with von Willebrand disease. Haemophilia 1998; 4: 293 [abstract].

20 Zhang ZP, Blomback M, Nyman D, Anvret M. Mutations of von Willebrand factor gene in families with von Willebrand disease in the Aland Islands. *Proc Natl Acad Sci USA* 1993; **90**: 7937–40.

21 Barr RD, Sek J, Horsman J, *et al.* Health status and health-related quality of life associated with von Willebrand disease. *Am J Hematol* 2003; **73**: 108–14.

22 Jarvis RR, Olsen ME. Type I von Willebrand's disease presenting as recurrent corpus hemorrhagicum. *Obstet Gynecol* 2002; **99** (5:Pt 2): t–8.

23 Greer IA, Lowe GD, Walker JJ, Forbes CD. Haemorrhagic problems in obstetrics and gynaecology in patients with congenital coagulopathies. *Br J Obstet Gynaecol* 1991; **98**: 909–18.

24 Rodeghiero F, Castaman G, Mannucci PM. Prospective multicenter study on subcutaneous concentrated desmopressin for home treatment of patients with von Willebrand disease and mild or moderate hemophilia A. *Thromb Haemost* 1996; **76**: 692–6.

25 Kadir RA, Lee CA, Sabin CA, *et al.* DDAVP nasal spray for treatment of menorrhagia in women with inherited bleeding disorders: a randomized placebo-controlled crossover study. *Haemophilia* 2002; **8**: 787–93.

26 Edlund M, Blomback M, Fried G. Desmopressin in the treatment of menorrhagia in women with no common coagulation factor deficiency but with prolonged bleeding time. *Blood Coagul Fibrinol* 2002; **13**: 225–31.

27 Edlund M, Blomback M, He L. On the correlation between local fibrinolytic activity in menstrual fluid and total blood loss during menstruation and effects of desmopressin. *Blood Coagul Fibrinol* 2003; **14**: 593–8.

28 Bonnar J, Sheppard BL. Treatment of menorrhagia during menstruation: randomised controlled trial of ethamsylate, mefenamic acid, and tranexamic acid. *BMJ* 1996; **313**: 579–82.

29 Cooke I, Lethaby A, Farquhar C. Antifibrinolytics for heavy menstrual bleeding. *Cochrane Database of Systematic Reviews* (Issue 2), 2000.

30 Onundarson PT. Treatment of menorrhagia in von Willebrand's disease. *Haemophilia* 1999; **5**: 76 [letter].

31 Stewart A, Cummins C, Gold L, Jordan R, Phillips W. The effectiveness of the levonorgestrel-releasing intrauterine system in menorrhagia: a systematic review. *Br J Obstet Gynaecol* 2001; **108**: 74–86.

32 Kingman CEC, Kadir RA, Lee CA, Economides DL. The use of Levonorgestrel-releasing intrauterine system for the treatment of menorrhagia in women with inherited bleeding disorders. *Br J Obstet Gynaecol* 2004 (in press*).*

33 Rubin G, Howard F, Wortman M, Kouides PA. The efficacy and safety of endometrial ablation for von Willebrand disease-related menorrhagia. *Haemophilia* 2004 (in press).

34 Stirling Y, Woolf L, North WR, *et al.* Hemostasis in normal pregnancy. *Thromb Haemost* 1984; **52**: 176–82.

35 Ramsahoye BH, Davies SV, Dasani H, Pearson JF. Obstetric management in von Willebrand's disease: a report of 24 pregnancies and a review of the literature. *Haemophilia* 1995; **1**: 140–4.

36 Sorosky J, Klatsky A, Norbert GF, Burchill RC. von Willebrand's disease complicating second trimester abortion. *Obstet Gynecol* 1980; **55**: 253–4.

37 Caliezi C, Tsakiris DA, Behringer H, *et al.* Two consecutive pregnancies and deliveries in a patient with von Willebrand's disease type 3. *Haemophilia* 1998; **4**: 845–9.

38 Chediak JR, Alban GM, Maxey B. von Willebrand's disease and pregnancy: management during delivery and outcome of offspring. *Am J Obstet Gynecol* 1986; **155**: 618–24.

39 Mannucci PM. How I treat patients with von Willebrand disease. *Blood* 2001; **97**: 1915–19.

40 Conti M, Mari D, Conti E, *et al.* Pregnancy in women with different types of von Willebrand disease. *Obstet Gynaecol* 1986; **68**: 282–5.

41 Mathew P, Greist A, Maahs JA, *et al.* Type 2B vWD: the varied clinical manifestations in two kindreds. *Haemophilia* 2003; **9**: 137–44.

42 Dennis MW, Clough V, Toh CH. Unexpected presentation of type 2N von Willebrand disease in pregnancy. *Haemophilia* 2000; **6**: 696–7.

43 Rick ME, Williams SB, Sacher RA, McKeown LP. Thrombocytopenia associated with pregnancy in a patient with type IIB von Willebrand's disease. *Blood* 1987; **69**: 786–9.

51 Factor II

Jan Astermark

Factor II (prothrombin) deficiency is a rare bleeding disorder that in the homozygous severe form is associated with high mortality. Milder deficiencies, however, may actually be underdiagnosed, since routine laboratory screening tests are often only slightly affected and many patients do not experience bleeding symptoms requiring medical care. This chapter will provide an overview of the structure and function of prothrombin and some clinical perspectives on the various deficiency states.

Biosynthesis

Prothrombin is synthesized as a preproprotein in hepatocytes and encoded by a gene, on chromosome 11, of 21 kb containing 14 exons and 13 intervening sequences [1]. The prepeptide directs the synthesized protein to the endoplasmic reticulum and is then removed prior to the process of post-translational modification. The mature molecule is a plasma glycoprotein and zymogen of a serine protease requiring vitamin K for normal biosynthesis [2]. The common feature of all vitamin K-dependent proteases is an N-terminal noncatalytic module containing γ-carboxyglutamic acid (Gla) residues, but, unlike the procoagulant factor VII (FVII), FIX, and FX, prothrombin consists not of epidermal growth factor (EGF)-like modules but of two kringle domains separated from the Gla module by a disulfide loop. The propeptide serves as an anchor for the γ-carboxylase, and is cleaved off before secretion [3]. The catalytic serine protease part contains the active site and is located at the C-terminal end of the molecule.

Structure and function

The binding of calcium to the Gla module is fundamental for proper folding of the vitamin K-dependent enzymes and for the accumulation of the factors on a negatively charged phospholipid membrane at concentrations high enough to promote fibrin formation [4,5]. The Gla residues have also been associated with normal intracellular transportation. The function of the kringles, named after a pastry because of their pretzel-like form, is to some extent unclear, although the second kringle seems to be involved in the binding of FVa and thrombin. Thrombin is the active form of prothrombin. It is formed by the cleavage of two peptide bonds by the prothrombinase complex composed of FXa, FVa, and calcium on a phospholipid surface (Figure 51.1).

In contrast to the other activated vitamin K-dependent coagulation factors, thrombin contains none of the noncatalytic modules and has therefore no phospholipid-binding capacity, but dissociates from the prothrombinase complex by diffusion. Thrombin exerts several pro- and anticoagulant effects. It triggers platelet aggregation and promotes coagulation by activating regulatory pathways and generating fibrin monomers by cleavage of a peptide bond in each of the α- and β-subunits of fibrinogen [6].

Prothrombin deficiency

Congenital prothrombin deficiency was first described by Quick in 1947 and further explored in subsequent reports [7,8]. The condition is inherited as an autosomal recessive trait and has been extensively reviewed by Girolami and coworkers [9]. The prevalence of congenital prothrombin deficiency is low, reported in the range of 1:1 000 000–2 000 000 [10,11]. Based on the immunoreactive component in plasma and the functional activity, two different phenotypic deficiencies have been described. In type 1 deficiency, or hypoprothrombinemia, the levels of antigen and functional activity are decreased to a similar extent, whereas in type 2 deficiency, or dysprothrombinemia, the enzyme itself is synthesized and present in plasma at a more or less normal level, but the coagulant activity is low. From what is presently known, complete prothrombin deficiency appears to be incompatible with life [12]. Mutations found in patients with hypo- and dysprothrombinemia have been reviewed and are summarized in Figure 51.2 [9,11,13]. The mutations associated with dysprothrombinemia are missense mutations, most of which interfere with the FXa binding site and the active site in the serine protease domain. In patients with hypoprothrombinemia, nonsense and small deletions have also been found, but the mechanisms by which these defects affect function largely remain to be settled. Compound heterozygosity for dys- and hypoprothrombinemia has been described [14]. In addition to isolated prothrombin deficiency, combined defects with the other vitamin K-dependent coagulation factors VII, IX, X, protein C and S have been found with variable clinical manifestations and in some cases associated with skeletal abnormalities [15–20]. The molecular defects are thought to reside in the gene of the γ-glutamyl carboxylase [21,22].

Acquired prothrombin deficiency is usually associated with neutralizing anticoagulants, the lupus anticoagulant–hypopro-

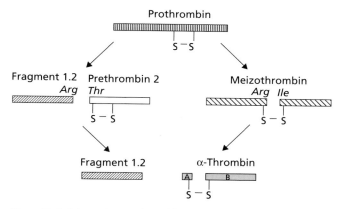

Figure 51.1 Schematic overview of the pathways for prothrombin activation. α-Thrombin is formed by the cleavage of two peptide bonds in prothrombin (Arg271 –|– Thr272) and (Arg320 –|– Ile321). Depending on which bond is cleaved first, fragment 1.2 and prethrombin 2 or meizothrombin is formed as an intermediate product. The activation by the prothrombinase complex is thought to mainly proceed through the formation of meizothrombin.

thrombinemia syndrome (LA-HPS), in patients with systemic lupus erythematosus (SLE), or following viral infections [23–26]. However, non-neutralizing antibodies accelerating the clearance of prothrombin have also been described [27,28].

Laboratory diagnosis

Specific tests are usually required to identify prothrombin deficiency. Screening tests such as prothrombin time (PT) and activated partial thromboplastin time (aPTT) are variably prolonged and in milder cases often more or less normal, suggesting that milder cases could be underdiagnosed [29]. Several specific diagnostic tools are available, some of which are based on viper venoms [9]. The most widely used test is a one-stage assay using thromboplastin as the activating agent. The test is reliable for screening purposes. In patients with homozygous type 1 prothrombin deficiency activity is usually less than 10% of normal, whereas subjects heterozygous for the same deficiency usually have values between 40% and 60%. Type 1 deficient patients generally have similar results regardless of the diagnostic method used, whereas the results for patients with type 2 deficiency may be inconsistent from method to method. Immunological methods are required to fully characterize the deficient state in terms of true hypo- or dysprothrombinemia.

Clinical manifestations

Clinically, heterozygotic patients with prothrombin deficiency are usually asymptomatic, but homozygote subjects with acti-

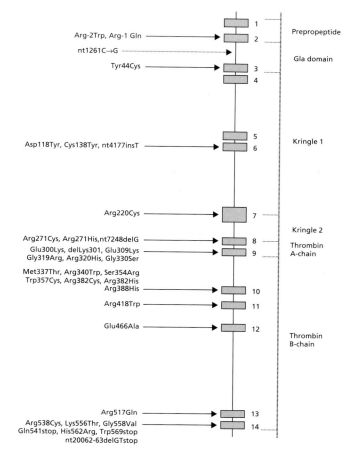

Figure 51.2 Mutations in the prothrombin gene associated with prothrombin deficiency projected on the corresponding exons and protein domains (modified from ref. 11).

vity levels less than 10% of normal may experience several different bleeding symptoms [9,30]. In a cohort of 14 patients with a plasma level of 4–10%, mucocutaneous bleeds from the nose, gums, and uterus were the most frequent bleeding symptoms. Joint and muscle bleeds were also relatively frequent and found in approximately one-third of the patients, some of whom developed arthropathy. Morbidity and mortality due to intracranial hemorrhage are high in patients with severe deficiency.

Therapeutic aspects

Patients with a coagulant activity above 30% usually do not require replacement therapy, but antifibrinolytics can be considered. In patients with more severe deficiency, replacement with the deficient factor must be given for surgery and in cases of trauma and more serious bleeding episodes. No pure prothrombin concentrate is available, but treatment can be given with either plasma and/or FIX complex concentrates [30]. The amount of plasma needed for transfusion is usually about 15–20 mL/kg body weight (BW), whereas FIX complex concentrates containing around 1 IU of prothrombin per U of FIX can be given in a dose of 20–30 IU/kg. Taking the long half-life of prothrombin into account (72 h), the infusion intervals must be adjusted to the clinical situation in order not to accumulate the enzyme and increase the risk of thrombotic events. In the current era of manufacturing processes, the risk of transmitting viruses is considered very low, although not negligible. Patients with acquired hypoprothrombinemia often require immunomodulating agents and usually respond to corticosteroids, cyclophosphamide, danazol, and/or intravenous gammaglobulins [31–35].

Concluding remarks

Prothrombin deficiency is rare, but important to recognize as patients with severe deficiency may experience life-threatening bleeding symptoms. Patients with milder deficiencies are probably underdiagnosed. An improved awareness of this condition may not only improve patient care, but also contribute to a better understanding of the hemostatic process.

References

1 Degen SJ, Davie EW. Nucleotide sequence of the gene for human prothrombin. *Biochemistry* 1987; **26**: 6165–77.

2 Furie B, Furie BC. The molecular basis of blood coagulation. *Cell* 1988; **53**: 505–18.

3 Furie B, Furie BC. Molecular basis of gamma-carboxylation. Role of the propeptide in the vitamin K-dependent proteins. *Ann NY Acad Sci* 1991; **614**: 1–10.

4 Swanson JC, Suttie JW. Prothrombin biosynthesis: characterization of processing events in rat liver microsomes. *Biochemistry* 1985; **24**: 3890–7.

5 Zhang L, Castellino FJ. Influence of specific gamma-carboxyglutamic acid residues on the integrity of the calcium-dependent conformation of human protein C. *J Biol Chem* 1992; **267**: 26078–84.

6 Hemker HC. Thrombin generation, an essential step in hemostasis and thrombosis. In: Bloom AL, Forbes CD, Thomas DP, Tuddenham EGD, eds. *Hemostasis and Thrombosis*, 3rd edn. Edinburgh: Churchill Livingstone, 1994: 477–90.

7 Quick AJ. Congenital hypoprothrombinemia and pseudo-hypoprothrombinemia. *Lancet* 1947; **ii**: 379–82.

8 Quick AJ, Hussey CV. Hereditary hypoprothrombinemias. *Lancet* 1962; **i**: 173–7.

9 Girolami A, Scarano L, Saggiorato G, *et al.* Congenital deficiencies and abnormalities of prothrombin. *Blood Coagul Fibrinol* 1998; **9**: 557–69.

10 Tuddenham EGD, Cooper DN. *The Molecular Genetics of Hemostasis and its Inherited Disorders.* Oxford: Oxford University Press, 1994.

11 Peyvandi F, Duga S, Akhavan S, Mannucci PM. Rare coagulation deficiencies. *Haemophilia* 2002; **8**: 308–21.

12 Sun WY, Witte DP, Degen JL, *et al.* Prothrombin deficiency results in embryonic and neonatal lethality in mice. *Proc Natl Acad Sci USA* 1998; **95**: 7597–602.

13 Akhavan S, Mannucci PM, Lak M, *et al.* Identification and three-dimensional structural analysis of nine novel mutations in patients with prothrombin deficiency. *Thromb Haemost* 2000; **84**: 989–97.

14 Akhavan S, Luciani M, Lavoretano S, Mannucci PM. Phenotypic and genetic analysis of a compound heterozygote for dys- and hypoprothrombinaemia. *Br J Haematol* 2003; **120**: 142–4.

15 Goldsmith GH Jr, Pence RE, Ratnoff OD, *et al.* Studies on a family with combined functional deficiencies of vitamin K-dependent coagulation factors. *J Clin Invest* 1982; **69**: 1253–60.

16 Vicente V, Maia R, Alberca I, *et al.* Congenital deficiency of vitamin K-dependent coagulation factors and protein C. *Thromb Haemost* 1984; **51**: 343–6.

17 Pauli RM, Lian JB, Mosher DF, Suttie JW. Association of congenital deficiency of multiple vitamin K-dependent coagulation factors and the phenotype of the warfarin embryopathy: clues to the mechanism of teratogenicity of coumarin derivatives. *Am J Hum Genet* 1987; **41**: 566–83.

18 Brenner B, Tavori S, Zivelin A, *et al.* Hereditary deficiency of all vitamin K-dependent procoagulants and anticoagulants. *Br J Haematol* 1990; **75**: 537–42.

19 Boneh A, Bar-Ziv J. Hereditary deficiency of vitamin K-dependent coagulation factors with skeletal abnormalities. *Am J Med Genet* 1996; **65**: 241–3.

20 McMahon MJ, James AH. Combined deficiency of factors II, VII, IX, and X (Borgschulte-Grigsby deficiency) in pregnancy. *Obstet Gynecol* 2001; **97**: 808–9.

21 Mutucumarana VP, Stafford DW, Stanley TB, *et al.* Expression and characterization of the naturally occurring mutation L394R in human γ-glutamyl carboxylase. *J Biol Chem* 2000; **275**: 32572–7.

22 Brenner B. Hereditary deficiency of vitamin K-dependent coagulation factors. *Thromb Haemost* 2000; **84**: 935–6.

23 Bernini JC, Buchanan GR, Ashcraft J. Hypoprothrombinemia and severe hemorrhage associated with a lupus anticoagulant. *J Pediatr* 1993; **123**: 937–9.

24 Galli M, Barbui T. Antiprothrombin antibodies: detection and clinical significance in the antiphospholipid syndrome. *Blood* 1999; **93**: 2149–57.

25 Schmugge M, Tolle S, Marbet GA, *et al.* Gingival bleeding, epistaxis and haematoma three days after gastroenteritis: the haemorrhagic lupus anticoagulant syndrome. *Eur J Pediatr* 2001; **160**: 43–6.

26 Baca V, Montiel G, Meillon L, *et al.* Diagnosis of lupus anticoagulant in the lupus anticoagulant-hypoprothrombinemia syndrome: report of two cases and review of the literature. *Am J Hematol* 2002; **71**: 200–7.

27 Bajaj SP, Rapaport SI, Barclay S, Herbst KD. Acquired hypoprothrombinemia due to non-neutralizing antibodies to prothrombin: mechanism and management. *Blood* 1985; **65**: 1538–43.

28 Lee ES, Hibsman BK, Liebman HA. Acquired bleeding disorder in a patient with malignant lymphoma: antibody-mediated prothrombin deficiency. *Cancer* 2001; **91**: 636–41.

29 Girolami A, De Marco L, Dal Bo Zanon R, *et al.* Rare quantitative and qualitative abnormalities of coagulation. *Clin Haematol* 1985; **14**: 385–441.

30 Peyvandi F, Mannucci PM. Rare coagulation disorders. *Thromb Haemost* 1999; **82**: 1207–14.

31 Simel DL, St Clair EW, Adams J, Greenberg CS. Correction of hypoprothrombinemia by immunosuppressive treatment of the lupus anticoagulant-hypoprothrombinemia syndrome. *Am J Med* 1987; **83**: 563–6.

32 Hift RJ, Bird AR, Sarembock BD. Acquired hypoprothrombinaemia

and lupus anticoagulant: response to steroid therapy. *Br J Rheumatol* 1991; **30**: 308–10.

33 Williams S, Linardic C, Wilson O, *et al.* Acquired hypoprothrombinemia: effects of danazol treatment. *Am J Hematol* 1996; **53**: 272–6.

34 Pernod G, Arvieux J, Carpentier PH, *et al.* B. Successful treatment of lupus anticoagulant-hypoprothrombinemia syndrome using intravenous immunoglobulins. *Thromb Haemost* 1997; **78**: 969–70.

35 Wong RS, Lau FY, Cheng G. Successful treatment of acquired hypoprothrombinemia without associated lupus anticoagulant using intravenous immunoglobulin. *Haematologica* 2001; **86**: 551.

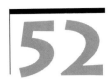# Factor V and combined factor V and VIII deficiencies

Flora Peyvandi and Marta Spreafico

Factor V deficiency

Within the coagulation cascade, factor V (FV) is one essential nonenzymatic cofactor of the prothrombinase complex, which catalyzes the conversion of prothrombin into thrombin [1,2]. FV shows high functional and structural homology with FVIII [3]. Both these proteins share the same A1–A2–B–A3–C1–C2 structure: the three A domains of FV and FVIII are approximately 30% amino acid identical to each other and to the triplicated A domain of ceruloplasmin, the major plasma copper transport protein [4]. The large B domain, having no homology with other proteins, is proteolytically removed during activation of FV and FVIII. Both C domains are tandem modules of approximately 150 amino acids and are part of the major subfamily of discoidin domains [5].

Factor V gene structure and protein

Human FV is synthesized by hepatocytes and megakaryocytes. Approximately 75% of FV is secreted, circulating in the blood as a precursor molecule, whereas the remaining 25% is stored in the platelet α-granules [6]. The FV that circulates in the blood is a single glycosylated polypeptide of 330 kDa that through proteolytic cleavages at three arginine residues (Arg709, Arg1018, Arg1545) [7,8], by thrombin and/or activated factor X (FXa), is converted into its active form (FVa), composed of two chains linked by a single Ca^{2+} ion: a 105-kDa heavy chain at the N-terminus and a 74- or 71-kDa light chain at the C-terminus. Cleavage by activated protein C (APC) at three arginine residues (Arg306, Arg506, Arg679) located in the FV heavy chain culminates in the inactivation of the procoagulant activity [9]. Thus, FV is indispensable for life, as was demonstrated in experimental knock-out mice lacking the FV gene that die either during mid-embryogenesis or immediately after birth from massive hemorrhagia [10]. The expression of a minimal FV activity due to the introduction of a liver-specific transgene, below the sensitivity threshold of the detection assay (<0.1%), leads mice to survive [11].

The human FV gene is more than 80 kb long and is located on chromosome 1q23 [12]. The genes for coagulation FV and FVIII are homologous in both structure and organization, suggesting their evolution from a common ancestral gene [13], but they differ in length, spanning ~80 kb and 186 kb respectively. The size difference is probably due to six introns in the FV gene that are much smaller than the corresponding introns in the FVIII gene

[12]. The FV gene coding sequence is divided into 25 exons ranging in size from 72 to 2820 basepairs (bp) and 24 introns varying between 0.4 kb and 11 kb. The sequence encoding the large B domain is contained within exon 13. FV cDNA is 6914 bp in length, corresponding to a coding region of 6674 bp, 91 bp of 5' untranslated region and 142 bp of 3' untranslated region. There are 83 bp encoding for the 28-amino acid hydrophobic signal peptide while in the protein of 2196 amino acids, 709 amino acids form the heavy-chain region, 836 amino acids form the connecting region and 651 amino acids form the light-chain region. The nucleotide sequence flanking the initiator ATG codon (AGCATGT) is very similar to the consensus Kozac translation initiator sequence. At the 3' end of the cDNA, the polyadenylation signal sequence (AATAAA) is located 12 nucleotides before the poly(A) tail [12].

Inherited FV deficiency

Human FV deficiency is an autosomal recessive bleeding disorder that has a prevalence of approximately 1 in 1 million and is characterized by low levels of FV associated with bleeding symptoms ranging from mild to severe [14]. In most of the affected individuals, phenotype is characterized by the concomitant deficiency of FV activity and antigen (type I deficiency); however, about 25% of the patients have normal antigen levels (type II deficiency), thus indicating that there is a dysfunctional protein [15].

Studies of the molecular basis of severe FV deficiency first took place in 1998 along with the identification of the first causative mutation [16]. However, presumably owing to the large size and complexity of the gene, relatively little information is still available. So far, a total of 26 distinct mutations that are associated with severe FV deficiency (Figure 52.1) [17,18] have been identified. Most of the mutations are located in the large exon 13, which encodes the entire B domain, whereas the remaining mutations are scattered throughout the gene. FV gene mutations encompass all types of lesions, ranging from missense mutations that are likely to impair the secretion or accelerate the degradation of factor V, to more frequent small deletions, frameshift (FS), nonsense, and splice-site mutations predicted to produce truncated proteins or no protein at all. Only a few mutations are present in more than one pedigree, which indicates that a founder effect is unlikely to explain most cases. So far, only one genetic defect associated with type II deficiency has been reported [19].

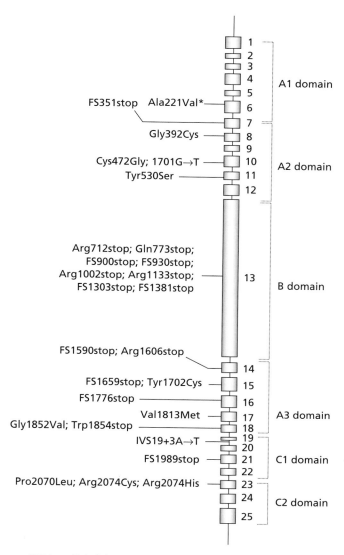

FS351stop Ala221Val*

Gly392Cys

Cys472Gly; 1701G→T

Tyr530Ser

A1 domain

A2 domain

Arg712stop; Gln773stop;
FS900stop; FS930stop;
Arg1002stop; Arg1133stop;
FS1303stop; FS1381stop

B domain

FS1590stop; Arg1606stop

FS1659stop; Tyr1702Cys

FS1776stop

Val1813Met

Gly1852Val; Trp1854stop

IVS19+3A→T

FS1989stop

Pro2070Leu; Arg2074Cys; Arg2074His

A3 domain

C1 domain

C2 domain

*FV type II deficiency-causing mutation

Figure 52.1 Mutations in the factor V gene, projected on the exons encoding the domains of the protein. Exons (rectangles) are drawn to scale while introns (lines) are not to scale.

Clinical manifestations in patients with FV deficiency

Generally, bleeding symptoms develop during the first 6 years of life, even bleeding from the umbilical stump was reported [20]. Frequent symptoms are epistaxis and menorrhagia, which occur in approximately 50% of patients and postoperative and oral cavity hemorrhages [14]. Other, less common, symptoms include hemarthroses and hematomas, which occur in about 25% of patients, whereas life-threatening bleeding episodes in the gastrointestinal tract and in the central nervous system are rare (6%) [20].

Discrepancy between the severe clinical phenotype that has been observed in the mouse knock-out model and the usually mild clinical phenotype of patients with FV deficiency is likely to be explained by the sensitivity of FV bioassay, much too low to detect the small amounts of FV that are probably sufficient to make the deficiency compatible with life and a mild clinical phenotype [11], but it must also be kept in mind that the absolute mass concentrations of coagulation factors can be quite different [21].

Combined deficiency of factor V and factor VIII

Combined FV and FVIII deficiency is an autosomal recessive bleeding disorder with an incidence of about 1 in 1 million, and it is a distinct clinical entity from FV deficiency and FVIII deficiency. The last are transmitted with different patterns of inheritance (autosomal recessive for FV, X-linked for FVIII) and involve proteins encoded by two different genes. The molecular mechanism of the association of the combined factor deficiency was not understood until 1998, when Nichols *et al.* [22] discovered that the cause of the deficiency was associated with mutations in the *LMAN1* gene (Lectin MANnose binding protein, previously referred to as *ERGIC-53*).

LMAN1 gene and protein

LMAN1 encodes a 53-kDa type 1 transmembrane protein with homology to leguminous lectin proteins. LMAN1 resides in the endoplasmic reticulum/Golgi intermediate compartment where, with a mannose-selective and calcium-dependent binding, it acts as a chaperone in the intracellular transport of both FV and FVIII [23].

LMAN1 is encoded by a gene of approximately 29 kb located on chromosome 18 and containing 13 exons (Figure 52.2). In the original study on the *LMAN1* gene, carried out by Nichols *et al.* [22], two distinct mutations were found in patients of Oriental Jewish ancestry, a splice-site mutation and a single-basepair insertion. In subsequent studies carried out in patients of various ethnic origins, 16 additional distinct mutations have been identified (splice site, insertions, deletion, nonsense codons) [24,25]. All the identified mutations are predicted to result in the synthesis of either a truncated protein product or no protein at all [23,24]. Mutations in *LMAN1* were found in approximately 70% of affected patients, but 30% of this population had no detectable mutation in *LMAN1*.

MCFD2 gene and protein

Recently, another locus correlated with the deficiency was identified in about 15% of affected families with no mutation in *LMAN1* [26]. The *MCFD2* (Multiple Coagulation Factor Deficiency 2) gene encodes a 16-kDa protein that forms a Ca^{2+}-dependent 1:1 stoichiometric complex with LMAN1 and acts as a cofactor for LMAN1, specifically recruiting correctly folded FV and FVIII in the endoplasmic reticulum [26]. MCFD2 is encoded by a gene of approximately 19 kb located on chromosome 2 and containing four exons (Figure 52.3).

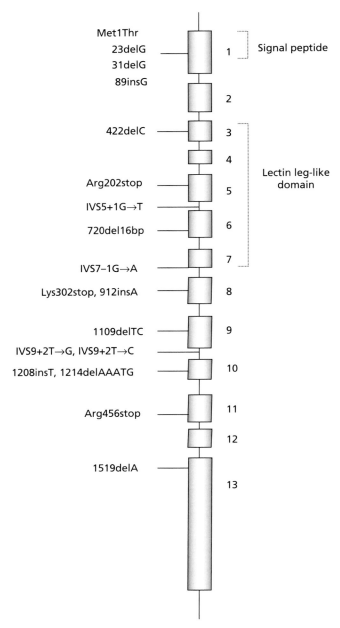

Figure 52.2 Mutation in the *LMAN1* gene, projected on the exons encoding the domains of the protein. Exons (rectangles) are drawn to scale while introns (lines) are not to scale.

Zhang *et al.* [26] identified seven distinct *MCFD2* mutations accounting for FV + FVIII deficiency in 9 of 12 families: three frameshift and two splice-site mutations, predicted to result in the complete loss of MCFD2 protein expression. They reported three frameshift and two splice-site mutations predicted to result in the complete loss of MCFD2 protein expression. Two missense mutations have also been identified. These two mutations are localized in a highly conserved region of the second EF-hand domain and eliminate the interaction with LMAN1 [26].

The presence of approximately 15% of affected patients in

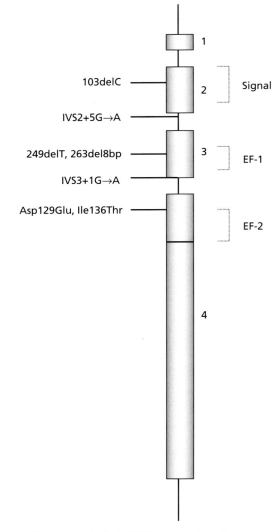

Figure 52.3 Mutation in the *MCFD2* gene, projected on the exons encoding the domains of the protein. Exons (rectangles) are drawn to scale while introns (lines) are not to scale.

whom the disorder is not linked to *LMAN1* or *MCFD2* mutations suggests the existence of a third locus associated with FV and FVIII deficiency. However, a misdiagnosis of FV deficiency associated to a mild hemophilia must be ruled out as a possible cause of combined deficiency. Therefore, all these cases need in-depth evaluation in a laboratory with standard techniques.

Inherited combined FV and FVIII deficiency

Combined FV and FVIII deficiency is characterized by concomitantly low levels (usually between 5% and 20%) of the two coagulation factors FV and FVIII, both as coagulant activity and antigen [27]. The phenotypes associated with mutations in *MCFD2* and *LMAN1* are indistinguishable and manifested only by deficiencies of the two proteins [26], although a selective delay in secretion of procathepsin C has been observed in

HeLa cells overexpressing a dominant-negative form of LMAN1 [28].

Clinical manifestations in patients with combined FV and FVIII deficiency

In the affected patients, FV and FVIII levels usually vary between 4% and 20%, and the deficiency usually manifests with mild symptoms. Frequent clinical manifestations of combined FV and FVIII deficiency are epistaxis and menorrhagia, which occur in 77% and 58% of patients respectively, and oral cavity hemorrhages, which occur in 51% of patients. Other symptoms include hemarthroses, which occur in about 25% of the patients, and cord bleeding (22%), whereas soft-tissue hematomas are unusual. Life-threatening bleeding episodes such as gastrointestinal and central nervous system bleeding are rare (4–7%) [14,29,30]. The concomitant presence of two coagulation defects does not enhance the hemorrhagic tendency that was observed in each defect separately (as for FV deficiency).

Treatment of factor V and combined factor V and VIII deficiencies

In patients with rare coagulation disorders, purified factor concentrates are not as widely available as they are for patients with hemophilia A and B. Dosages and frequency of treatment are based on minimal hemostatic levels of the deficient factor, plasma half-life, and type of bleeding episode [14]. The primary requisite in the choice of replacement material is the avoidance of transmission of blood-borne infectious agents. Solvent/detergent-treated plasma is an important and safe source of replacement recommended in the majority of these disorders. Also, virus-inactivated concentrates, when commercially available, are safe but expensive, especially for developing countries. Other important determinants in the choice of treatment are the healthcare facilities of the country where the patient is located and the cost of products.

There is now no FV concentrate available and FV is not present in cryoprecipitate or prothrombin complex concentrates [31]. Thus, replacement of FV is achieved through the use of fresh-frozen plasma (FFP), preferably with virus-inactivated plasma (15–20 mL/kg) [14]. The initial dose could be 15–20 mL/kg followed by 5 mL/kg every 12 h, with the dose adjusted based on FV levels and bleeding severity [32]. Studies of FV recovery recommend maintenance of a level of 20–25% of FV activity for surgery or in case of severe bleeding. For acute severe bleeding, the addition of platelet concentrates may aid in hemostasis by providing another source of FV that localizes at the site of bleeding [32]. The use of large amounts of plasma leads to a fluid overload and needs sometimes to be corrected by diuretic drugs.

In combined FV and FVIII deficiency to replace both FV and FVIII levels the treatment should be based on plasma and FVIII concentrates (see FV deficiency and hemophilia A treatment).

Prenatal diagnosis in rare coagulation disorders

Even though the cultural, religious, and economic roots of consanguineous marriages are deep in developing countries, this custom is becoming much less frequent in large cities and among younger generations.

Prevention of rare coagulation disorders, such as FV deficiency and combined FV and FVIII deficiency, through prenatal diagnosis of the underlying mutations is feasible in couples who have already had affected children. Gene mutations found in both parents need to be verified on DNA extracted from chorionic villus at 10–12 weeks' gestation.

Acknowledgment

We are grateful to Professor Pier M. Mannucci for his essential help in revising the text.

This study was supported by grants from the Fondazione Italo Monzino and Telethon, contract grant numbers: TS 044796 and GGP 030261.

References

1 Dahlback B. Blood coagulation. *Lancet* 2000; **355**: 1627–32.
2 Cripe LD, Moore KD, Kane WH. Structure of the gene for human coagulation factor V. *Biochemistry* 1992; **31**: 3777–85.
3 Kane WH, Davie EW. Blood coagulation factor V and VIII: structural and functional similarities and their relationship to hemorrhagic and thrombotic disorders. *Blood* 1988; **71**: 539–55.
4 Ortel TL, Takahashi N, Putnam FW. Structural model of human ceruloplasmin based on internal triplication, hydrophilic/hydrophobic character, and secondary structure of domains. *Proc Natl Acad Sci USA* 1984; **81**: 4761–5.
5 Baumgartner S, Hofmann K, Chiquet-Ehrismann R, Bucher P. The discoidin domain family revisited: new members from prokaryotes and a homology-based fold prediction. *Protein Sci* 1998; **7**: 1626–31.
6 Mann KG, Kalafatis M. Factor V: a combination of Dr Jekyll and Mr Hyde. *Blood* 2003; **101**: 23–30.
7 Foster WB, Nesheim ME, Mann KG. The factor Xa-catalyzed activation of factor V. *J Biol Chem* 1983; **258**: 13970–7.
8 Suzuki K, Dahlback B, Stenflo J. Thrombin-catalyzed activation of human coagulation factor V. *J Biol Chem* 1982; **257**: 6556–64.
9 Kalafatis M, Rand MD, Mann KG. The mechanism of inactivation of human factor V and human factor Va by activated protein C. *J Biol Chem* 1994; **269**: 31869–80.
10 Cui J, O'Shea KS, Purkayastha A, *et al.* Fatal hemorrhage and incomplete block of embryogenesis in mice lacking coagulation factor V. *Nature* 1996; **384**: 66–8.
11 Yang TL, Cui J, Taylor JM, *et al.* Rescue of fatal neonatal hemorrhage in factor V deficient mice by low transgene expression. *Thromb Haemost* 2000; **83**: 70–7.
12 Tuddenham EGD, Cooper DN. *The Molecular Genetics of Hemostasis and its Inherited Disorders.* Oxford: Oxford University Press, 1994.

13 Cripe LD, Moore KD, Kane WH. Structure of the gene for human coagulation factor V. *Biochemistry* 1992; **31**: 3777–85.

14 Peyvandi F, Duga S, Akhavan S, Mannucci PM. Rare coagulation deficiencies. *Haemophilia* 2002; **8**: 308–321.

15 Chiu HC, Whitaker E, Colman RW. Heterogeneity of human factor V deficiency. Evidence for the existence of an antigen-positive variant. *J Clin Invest* 1983; **72**: 493–503.

16 Guasch JF, Cannegieter S, Reitsma PH, *et al*. Severe coagulation factor V deficiency caused by a 4 bp deletion in the factor V gene. *Br J Haematol* 1998; **101**: 32–9.

17 Montefusco MC, Duga S, Asselta R, *et al*. Clinical and molecular characterization of six patients affected by severe deficiency of coagulation factor V: broadening of the mutational spectrum of FV gene and *in vitro* analysis of the newly identified missense mutations. *Blood* 2003; **102**: 3210–16.

18 Fu Q, Wu W, Ding Q, *et al*. Type I coagulation factor V deficiency caused by compound heterozygous mutation of F5 gene. *Haemophilia* 2003; **9**: 646–9.

19 Murray JM, Rand MD, Egan JO, *et al*. Factor V New Brunswick: Ala221-to-Val substitution results in reduced cofactor activity. *Blood* 1995; **86**: 1820–27.

20 Lak M, Sharifian R, Peyvandi F, Mannucci PM. Symptoms of inherited factor V deficiency in 25 Iranian patients. *Br J Haematol* 1998; **103**: 1067–69.

21 Mann KG. How much factor V is enough? *Thromb Haemost* 2000; **83**: 3–4.

22 Nichols WC, Seligsohn U, Zivelin A, *et al*. Mutations in the ER-Golgi intermediate compartment protein ERGIC-53 cause combined deficiency of coagulation factors V and VIII. *Cell* 1998; **93**: 61–70.

23 Itin C, Roche AC, Monsigny M, Hauri HP. ERGIC-53 is a functional mannose-selective and calcium-dependent human homologue of leguminous lectins. *J Cell Biol* 1996; **107**: 483–93.

24 Neerman-Arbez M, Johnson KM, Morris MA, *et al*. Molecular analysis of the ERGIC-53 gene in 35 families with combined factor V–factor VIII deficiency. *Blood* 1999; **93**: 2253–60.

25 Nichols WC, Valeri HT, Wheatley MA, *et al*. ERGIC-53 gene structure and mutation analysis in 19 combined factors V and VIII deficiency families. *Blood* 1999; **93**: 2261–66.

26 Zhang B, Cunningham MA, Nichols WC, *et al*. Bleeding due to disruption of a cargo-specific ER-to-Golgi transport complex. *Nat Genet* 2003; **34**: 220–5.

27 Giddings JC, Seligsohn U, Bloom AL. Immunological studies in combined factor V and factor VIII deficiency. *Br J Haematol* 1977; **37**: 257–64.

28 Vollenweider F, Kappeler F, Itin C, Hauri HP. Mistargeting of the lectin ERGIC-53 to the endoplasmic reticulum of HeLa cells impairs the secretion of a lysosomal enzyme. *J Cell Biol* 1998; **142**: 377–89.

29 Peyvandi F, Tuddenham EGD, Akhtari M, *et al*. Bleeding symptoms in 27 Iranian patients with factor V and VIII combined deficiency. *Br J Haematol* 1998; **100**: 773–6.

30 Seligsohn U, Zivelin A, Zwang E. Combined factor V and factor VIII deficiency among non-Ashkenazi Jews. *New Engl J Med* 1982; **307**: 1191–5.

31 Di Paola J, Nugent D, Young G. Current therapy for rare factor deficiency. *Haemophilia* 2001; **7**: 16–22.

32 Roberts HR, Lefkowitz JB. Inherited disorders of prothrombin conversion. In: Colman RW, Hirsh J, Marder VJ, Salzman EW, eds. *Hemostasis and Thrombosis,* 3rd edn. Philadelphia: J.B. Lippincott, 1994: 203–6.

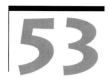# Congenital factor VII deficiency

Guglielmo Mariani and Alberto Dolce

Introduction

Factor VII (FVII) is the commonest deficiency amongst the rare, inherited coagulation disorders; a prevalence of 1 in 500 000 has been estimated, without racial or gender predilection for the defect [1,2]. Numerous mutations underlying this disorder (http://europium.csc.mrc.ac.uk) [3] have been described, which are predictive of considerable heterogeneity in genotype and phenotype (i.e. clotting activity) [4–10]. The clinical heterogeneity is a striking feature of this hemorrhagic disorder, which ranges in severity from lethal to mild, or even asymptomatic forms. The International FVII (IF7) deficiency Study Group has collected 515 cases with a FVII congenital deficiency and some data herein reported derive from this database [11]. In this chapter we will report on the most recent genetic and phenotypic aspects concerning this disorder and outline the issues related to its management.

Pathophysiology and genetics

The FVII gene is situated on chromosome 13, in proximity to the gene of FX. It is composed of eight exons and seven introns, with a gene organization that has many similarities with the other vitamin K-dependent proteins participating in the mechanisms of clotting.

Factor VII deficiency is not believed to be associated with complete absence of functional FVII, and this is in agreement with data from knock-out mice studies, which suggest that a complete absence of FVII is incompatible with life [12]. The minimal FVII level able to interact with tissue factor to prevent lethal bleeding in human subjects has not yet been defined [13,14]. At any rate, tissue factor (TF), the cofactor of activated FVII (FVIIa), is considered to be the true rate-limiting molecule of coagulation initiation [14]. As the FVIIa–TF complex is the initiator of blood coagulation, it appears logical that reduced levels of FVII clotting activity may cause a bleeding diathesis.

The number and type of FVII gene mutations in congenital FVII deficiency indicate the presence of a very heterogeneous genetic pattern: more than 100 different mutations have been described so far [3,11]. Missense mutations are the most frequent mutation type reported, occurring in about 80% of subjects, whereas splice-site, nonsense, and small deletion/frameshift mutations are rarer, with prevalences of about 12%, 5%, and 1–2% respectively. Most of the mutations have been described in exon 8, which contains a large part of the serine protease domain as well as sites of interaction with TF. For further details concerning the molecular genetics of FVII deficiency two web-based databases are available (http://193.60.222.13 and the aforementioned europium).

Factor VII deficiency is inherited in an autosomal recessive fashion. Homozygotes and compound heterozygotes are virtually indistinguishable as concerns both the bleeding (Figure 53.1) and the clotting phenotype: they exhibit the severest bleeding phenotypes, but a small number of homozygotes and double heterozygotes (about 15%) are asymptomatic [11]. In addition, the vast majority of the heterozygotes are asymptomatic.

Clinical picture and severity classification

Bleeding manifestations and the clinical presentation of FVII deficiency may vary widely; it is generally agreed that FVIIC levels do not predict the bleeding tendency in any individual patient. In the IF7 database [11], patients with FVIIC levels " 2% ($n = 123$) exhibited strikingly different bleeding phenotypes: 27 had mild disease, 34 moderate disease, and only 56 severe disease; a few even experienced thrombotic episodes [15]. This observation suggests that extragenic components are important in modulating the clinical phenotype.

The prevalence of the hemorrhagic manifestations, as found in the IF7 database, is shown in Table 53.1. Life-threatening bleedings [central nervous system (CNS) and gastrointestinal (GI)] are known to present first [16]. Those leading to handicap (hemarthrosis and muscle hematoma) manifest when children start to walk: although clinically indistinguishable from those occurring in hemophilic patients, they are not gender related and are less frequent than in hemophilia (Table 53.1).

Owing to the high prevalence of menorrhagia, this event requires particular attention in terms of prevention and treatment. It must be noted that this type of bleeding is frequently the cause of a severe, long-lasting, iron-deficiency anemia.

As there is a very poor correlation between FVII levels and the bleeding tendency, FVIIC levels cannot be used to distinguish classes of severity. We therefore propose a three-grade classification based on clinical findings. The severe form is characterized by life-threatening and potentially crippling hemorrhages (CNS, GI bleeding and hemarthrosis), prevalent in the first years of life. The other classes of severity (moderate and mild forms) differ only in quantitative terms concerning the symptoms (with

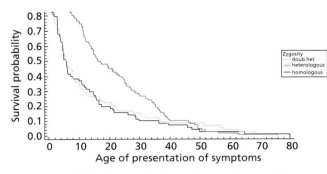

Figure 53.1 Bleeding-free survival curves by mutation zygosity.

Table 53.1 Prevalence of symptoms in congenital FVII deficiency.

Symptoms*	Patients (%)*
Epistaxis	60.9
Easy bruising	45.4
Gum bleeding	30.2
Hemarthrosis	18.4
GI bleeding	14.0
Hematuria	8.2
CNS bleeding	5.7
Bleeding after dental extraction	4.1
Thrombosis	3.5
Cephalohematoma	1.0
Rectal bleeding	1.0
Hemoptysis	0.6
Postpartum bleeding	0.6
Retroperitoneal bleeding	0.6
Umbilical bleeding	0.6
Wound bleeding	0.6
Compartment syndrome	0.3
Postoperative bleeding†	23.8
Menorrhagia‡	62.9

*Percentage of symptomatic subjects.

†Prevalence in surgical patients.

‡Frequency found in women aged >10.4 (age of the first episode recorded in the IF7 database).

CNS, central nervous system; GI, gastrointestinal.

the exclusion of those characterizing the severe cases), patients with moderate disease exhibiting three or more different bleeding symptoms and those with mild disease only one or two.

On the whole, FVII deficiency is associated, in the majority of patients, with a mild hemorrhagic disorder, characterized by hemorrhages of the mucous membranes and the skin (i.e., epistaxis, menorrhagia, gum bleeding, easy bruising) (Table 53.1). In fact, the mild and moderate forms account for about two-thirds of cases.

Diagnosis

Factor VII is currently measured by two methods: (i) factor VII coagulant activity (FVIIC) and (ii) factor VII protein (or antigen, FVIIAg).

There are true deficiencies [i.e. low or very low FVIIC levels associated with similar levels of FVIIAg: CRM (cross-reacting material) negative)]: these account for about half of the cases, while the dysfunctional forms (CRM-positive, i.e., low levels of FVIIC with normal levels of FVIIAg) account for about 10%. The remaining deficiencies are characterized by levels of FVIIAg higher than those of FVIIC but lower than normal (CRM-reduced).

The laboratory procedure to diagnose FVII deficiency is straightforward as it is the only clotting defect characterized by an isolated, prolonged prothrombin time (with normal aPTT); the diagnosis can be confirmed by the specific assay for FVIIC [17]. The results may vary widely depending on the thromboplastins used; to start with, it is advisable to perform the FVIIC assay using TF extracted from human tissues or produced by the recombinant technology mimicking the human TF (with an International Sensitivity Index close to 1). The FVIIAg assay is not needed for a formal diagnosis but is important for the identification of dysfunctional variants.

Isolated FVII deficiency can easily be differentiated from the so-called FMFD (familial multiple factor deficiency) type III because in the latter the aPTT is also prolonged, the levels of all the other vitamin K-dependent proteins (including protein C and S) are depressed, and, finally, because there is some response to vitamin K administration as well.

Inhibitors to FVII are very rare. This is partly explained by the mutational spectrum underlying the disorder, which could never lead to a complete absence of the protein. FVII deficiency has been found to be associated with hepatic congenital enzymic defects, such as the Dubin–Johnson and the Gilbert syndromes [18,19].

Management

Factor VII is a protein with a low concentration (350–450 ng/mL) and a very short half-life (3–4 h). It is important to keep this in mind when creating a treatment strategy. The low plasma concentration of the factor makes difficult the preparation of high-purity concentrates from plasma; it also makes fresh-frozen plasma (FFP) unsuitable for prolonged treatments. Treatment materials available are listed in Table 53.2. An activated, recombinant FVII preparation (rFVIIa, NovoSeven) has recently been licensed in Europe for use in congenital FVII deficiency.

In children and for prolonged administration (i.e., prophylaxis or surgery), rFVIIa should be used as first-line treatment (single dose of 15–30 µg/kg body weight) [20,21]. For the severe bleeds, multiple administration schedules (20–30 µg/kg) should be adopted, 4–6 h apart. For the mild bleeds a single, higher dose (30–40 µg/kg) would suffice.

Table 53.2 Treatment materials for congenital FVII deficiency.

Materials	Potency (IU/mL*)	Advantages	Disadvantages
Fresh-frozen plasma	1	Cost and easily available; limited effectiveness	Risk of viral transmission; circulatory overload; unsuitable for (major) surgery
Virus-attenuated fresh-frozen plasma	1	Virally attenuated (reduced risk of viral transmission); limited effectiveness	Circulatory overload; unsuitable for (major) surgery
Prothrombin complex concentrates (four factors)	5–10	Suitable for surgery; virally attenuated (reduced risk of viral transmission)	Other vitamin K-dependent factors present in concentrations higher than FVII, possibly activated; risk of thrombosis
Plasma-derived FVII concentrate†	20–30	Suitable for surgery; virally attenuated (reduced risk of viral transmission); effective	Other vitamin K-dependent factors/inhibitors present in high concentrations
rFVIIa‡	> 25 000	Very effective for any indication (at low doses); no risk of viral transmission	Cost

*Expressed in IU/mL, where 1 U corresponds to 100% of pooled normal plasma.
†Three brands available: (i) Facteur VII, LFB, Lille, France; (ii) Factor VII concentrate, BLP, UK; (iii) Provertin™, Baxter Immuno.
‡NovoSeven™, Novonordisk, Bagsværd, Denmark.

Table 53.3 Surgical interventions, replacement therapy and bleeding related to surgery.

	Bleeding without substitution therapy	Bleeding with substitution therapy	Odds ratio (α) = 0.05
Severe and moderate	12/23 (52.2%)	24/89 (26.9%)	3 (CI 1.2–7.6)
Mild	14/36 (38.9%)	12/44 (27.3%)	1.7 (CI 0.7–4.3)

The average dose capable of normalizing the prothrombin international normalized ratio (PT-INR) in severely affected patients has been found to be 20 µg/kg [20].

Also effective are pdFVII concentrates; they are safe as submitted to viral attenuation methods. For the spontaneous bleeding episodes a single dose of 20–40 IU/kg body weight would suffice if bleeding is mild, but for the severe bleeds it is advisable to repeat the administration two or three times.

It is important to note that the plasma recovery and half-life of FVIIa are similar to those of the native molecule [22].

Replacement therapy for surgery in FVII deficiency is an open issue: its need has been questioned, at least in asymptomatic subjects, whatever the FVII:C levels [23].

In our database [11] (Table 53.3), the risk of postsurgical bleeding in patients classified as having moderate or severe disease was high, and included a significant proportion of patients who bled despite replacement therapy. These data emphasize that management of this bleeding disorder, in terms of substitution therapy and therapy schedules, is not yet optimal.

At any rate, the minimal, protective FVII levels appear to be about 10–12%. To maintain these trough levels, repeated administrations (three to four/day) are needed, at least for the first postoperative days.

Thrombosis in FVII deficiency is not a very rare event — our group has observed 11 such events [15]; most such cases have been venous thromboembolism associated with surgical interventions and/or replacement therapy. Rare and frequent thrombophilias appear not to be an issue in this context; nor is the underlying FVII gene mutation or the bleeding phenotype. This situation is similar to that observed in hemophilia B and suggests that the risk of thrombosis in this hemorrhagic disorder should be considered in evaluating both the need for and the dose of substitution therapy, especially in the surgical setting.

Acknowledgments

The authors gratefully acknowledge the contribution of Francesco Bernardi and the cooperation of the members of the IF7 Steering Committee and of the Study Group at large.

References

1 Roberts HR, Escobar MA. Less common congenital disorders of hemostasis. In: Kitchens CS, Alving BM, Kessler CM, eds. *Consultative Hemostasis and Thrombosis*. Philadelphia: WB Saunders, 2002: 57.

2 Peyvandi F, Jenkins PV, Mannucci PM, *et al*. Molecular characterisation and three-dimensional structural analysis of mutations in 21 unrelated families with inherited factor VII deficiency. *Thromb Haemost* 2000; **84**: 250–7.

3 McVey JH, Boswell E, Mumford AD, Kemball-Cook, Tuddenham EGD. Factor VII deficiency and the FVII mutation database. *Hum Mutat* 2001; **17**: 3–17.

4 Triplett DA, Brandt JT, Batard MA, *et al*. Hereditary factor VII deficiency: heterogeneity defined by combined functional and immunochemical analysis. *Blood* 1985; **66**: 1284–7.

5 Perry DJ. Factor VII deficiency. *Br J Haematol* 2002; **118**: 689–700.

6 Bernardi F, Castaman G, Pinotti M, *et al*. Mutation pattern in clinically asymptomatic coagulation factor VII deficiency. *Hum Mutat* 1996; **8**: 108–15.

7 Millar DS, Kemball-Cook G, McVey JH, *et al*. Molecular analysis of the genotype-phenotype relationship in factor VII deficiency. *Hum Genet* 2000; **107**: 327–42.

8 Herrmann FH, Wulff K, Auberger K, *et al*. Molecular biology and clinical manifestation of hereditary factor VII deficiency. *Semin Thromb Hemost* 2000; **26**: 393–400.

9 Wulff K, Herrmann FH. Twenty-two novel mutations of the factor VII gene in factor VII deficiency. *Hum Mutat* 2000; **15**: 489–96.

10 Giansily-Blaizot M, Aguilar-Martinez P, Biron-Andreani C, *et al*. Study Group of Factor Seven Deficiency. Analysis of the genotypes and phenotypes of 37 unrelated patients with inherited factor VII deficiency. *Eur J Hum Genet* 2001; **9**: 105–12.

11 The IF7SG (International Factor VII Study Group) database: unpublished data.

12 Rosen E, Liang Z, Zollman A, Roahrig J, Castellino FJ. Examining the role of coagulation factor VII using FVII-insufficient mice [abstract]. *J Thromb Haemost* 2003; **1** (Suppl.): SY23.

13 Butenas S, van't Veer C, Mann KG. "Normal" thrombin generation. *Blood* 1999; **94**: 2169–78.

14 Rapaport SI, Rao LV. The tissue factor pathway: how it has become a "prima ballerina". *Thromb Haemost* 1995; **74**: 7–17.

15 Mariani G, Herrmann FH, Schulman S, *et al*. Thrombosis in inherited factor VII deficiency. *J Thromb Haemost* 2003; **1**: 2153–8.

16 Ragni MV, Lewis JH, Spero JA, Hasiba V. Factor VII deficiency. *Am J Hematol* 1981; **10**: 79.

17 Mariani G, Liberti G, D'Angelo T, LoCoco L. Factor VII activity and antigen. In: *Laboratory Techniques in Thrombosis. A Manual*. Jespersen J, Bertina RM, Haverkate F (eds). Kluwer Academic Publishers, Dordrecht, 1999: 99–106.

18 Levanon M, Rimon S, Shani M, *et al*. Active and inactive factor VII in Dubin-Johnson syndrome with factor VII deficiency, hereditary factor VII deficiency and coumarin administration. *Br J Haematol* 1972; **23**: 669.

19 Seligshon U, Shani M, Ramot B. Gilbert syndrome and factor VII deficiency. *Lancet* 1970; **i**: 1398.

20 Mariani G, Testa MG, Di Paolantonio T, *et al*. The use of recombinant, activated factor VII in the treatment of congenital factor VII deficiencies. *Vox Sang* 1999; **77**: 131–6.

21 Ingerslev J, Knudsen L, Hvid I, *et al*. Use of recombinant factor VIIa in surgery in factor VII deficient patients. *Hemophilia* 1997; **3**: 215–8.

22 Berrettini M, Mariani G, Schiavoni M, *et al*. Pharmacokinetic evaluation of recombinant, activated factor VII in patients with inherited factor VII deficiency. *Haematologica* 2001; **86**: 640–5.

23 Blaizot MG, Biron-Andreani C, Aguilar-Martinez P, *et al*. Inherited factor VII deficiency and surgery: clinical data are the best criteria to predict the risk of bleeding. *Br J Haematol* 2002; **117**: 172–5.

54 Factor X and factor X deficiency

David J. Perry

Introduction

Factor X (FX) (synonyms: autoprothrombin III, Stuart–Prower factor) is one of the vitamin K-dependent clotting factors and occupies a central position in the coagulation cascade at the point of convergence of the intrinsic and extrinsic pathways. FX was identified in the early 1950s by two groups, which independently reported a novel clotting factor deficiency in patients with a hemorrhagic tendency that closely resembled FVII deficiency [1,2]. The deficient clotting factor in these individuals was termed "Stuart–Prower" factor after the index patients. In 1954, Duckert and colleagues [3] reported a factor, deficient in patients receiving coumarin anticoagulants, that was distinct from FVII and FIX and which they called factor X before the official Roman numeral nomenclature was established in 1962.

Factor X gene

The gene for FX (*F10*) maps to the long arm of chromosome 13 at 13q34–ter approximately 28 kb downstream of the FVII gene. The gene consists of eight exons spread over ~27 kb of genomic sequence (Figure 54.1) and shares significant homology with the other vitamin K-dependent clotting factors in both organization and structure. Each of the exons of the FX gene encodes specific domains of the FX protein: exon I encodes the signal peptide; exon II encodes the propeptide and γ-carboxyglutamic acid (Gla)-rich domain; exon III encodes a short linking segment of aromatic amino acids termed the "aromatic stack"; exons IV and V encode regions homologous to epidermal growth factor (EGF); exon VI encodes the activation peptide at the amino terminus of the heavy chain, and exons VII and VIII encode the active serine protease domain containing the catalytic triad His236, Asp228, and Ser379.

The FX cDNA consists of 120 bp (basepairs) coding for the 40-amino-acid pre-pro-leader sequence, 1344 bp encoding the 488 amino acids of the mature protein and a 3′ untranslated region of 10 bp preceding the poly(A) tail (Figure 54.1).

Factor X protein structure and function

Factor X is synthesized by the liver and secreted into the plasma as an inactive zymogen, where it circulates as a two-chain molecule with a concentration of ~8–10 μg/mL. FX is synthesized with a 40-residue pre-pro sequence containing the hydrophobic signal sequence that targets the protein for secretion (residues −37 to −22) and which is cleaved prior to secretion of the mature protein into the plasma. Extensive post-translational modifications (glycosylation, γ-carboxylation, and β-hydroxylation) of FX occur before it is functionally active.

The first 39 residues of the light chain of FX contain 11 glutamic acid residues, which are modified by a vitamin K-dependent γ-carboxylation step to form Gla residues. Ten of these residues are encoded by exon II (the "Gla" domain) and the eleventh by exon III. Gla residues mediate conformational changes in FX that allow Ca^{2+}-dependent binding to negatively charged phospholipid membranes. In its two-chain form, mature FX consists of a light chain of 139 amino acids and a heavy chain of 346 residues. The two chains are connected by an Arg–Lys–Arg (RKR) tripeptide and by a disulfide bond between residues Cys89 and Cys124 (Figure 54.1). The heavy chain of FX contains the activation peptide (residues 143–195), which is cleaved when FX is activated. The heavy chain also contains the triad of amino acids — His236, Asp282, and Ser379 – which constitute the catalytic site.

A partial crystal structure of a large fragment of FXa that lacks only the N-terminal 45 residues has been solved and has been used to model a number of FX mutations [4].

The role of factor X

Physiologically, FX is activated by FIXa or by FVIIa, although *in vitro* FX can also be activated by Russell viper venom, a metalloproteinase isolated from the venom of the snake *Vipera russelli*. FX is converted to FXa by cleavage of the Arg194–Ile195 peptide bond located in the heavy chain. Cleavage releases a 52-residue peptide — the FX activation peptide — which can be assayed as a marker of FX activation.

Activation of the coagulation cascade occurs following exposure of tissue factor (TF) to plasma. The formation of a complex, comprising TF, FVIIa, and calcium ions, in the presence of an appropriate phospholipid membrane, activates FX to FXa and FIX to FIXa. A variety of cell types including endothelial cells, fibroblasts, monocytes, macrophages, and tumor cells appear to be capable of providing a suitable phospholipid surface for activation. The presence of all the constituents results in a 10-fold decrease in K_m for the reaction and a 1000-fold increase in k_{cat} accelerating the generation of FXa by at

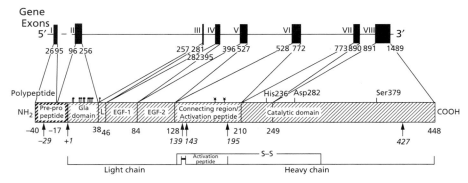

Figure 54.1 The human factor X gene (*F10*) and its encoded polypeptide. The upper part of the figure represents the *F10* gene, with the eight exons shown by filled boxes. The positions of the first and last nucleotides of each exon are shown (nucleotides are numbered according to Leytus *et al.* [25]). The lower part of the figure shows the polypeptide structure and the various functional domains encoded by specific exons. Darker hatching indicates the pre-propeptide and lighter hatching the mature protein. Codons initiating each exon are shown (residue +1 is the first amino acid of the mature protein). Residue −29 indicates the site of probable cleavage by the signal peptidase. The light chain is encoded by residues +1 to 139 and the heavy chain by residues 143 to 448. The connecting tripeptide (RKR) is located between residues 140 and 142 and the activation peptide resides within the heavy chain at residues 143 to 195. Activation of factor X occurs through cleavage at Arg194 –I– Ile195. Residue 427 shows the site of cleavage of factor X that generates factor Xaβ. His236, Asp282, and Ser379 are the residues that constitute the catalytic triad; (↑) indicates the position of the 11 Gla residues; (⸷) indicates the position of the two glycosylation sites.

least 10 000-fold relative to rates observed for factor VIIa and Ca^{2+} alone.

Activation of FX via the extrinsic pathway is dependent upon the interaction of FIXa, FVIIIa, Ca^{2+}, and a phospholipid surface — platelets and/or endothelial cells. FVIIIa serves as a cofactor in the activation of FX, accelerating the maximal velocity of the reaction approximately 200 000-fold, while phospholipid has been shown to significantly decrease the K_m of FIXa for FX by some 5000-fold.

FXa is the major physiologic activator of prothrombin, but its enzymatic activity is accelerated some 280 000-fold in the presence of FVa, Ca^{2+} ions, and a suitable negatively charged phospholipid membrane. The phospholipid membrane provides a surface that increases the local concentration of FVa, FXa, and prothrombin, although FVa also appears to increase the catalytic efficiency of FXa.

The principal regulators of FX activity are antithrombin and tissue factor pathway inhibitor (TFPI). FXa is inhibited by antithrombin to form a stable inactive complex that is rapidly removed from the circulation by the liver. The inhibitory activity of antithrombin is accelerated by various sulfated glycosaminoglycans. TFPI is the major inhibitor of the extrinsic pathway and rapidly forms a 1:1 complex with FXa, which then binds to the TF–FVIIa complex to form a quaternary complex [5]. The quaternary Xa/TFPI/TF–VIIa complex lacks any VIIa–TF catalytic activity.

Factor X deficiency

Diagnosis

The diagnosis of FX deficiency is suspected following the finding of a prolonged prothrombin time (PT) and activated partial thromboplastin time (aPTT), which corrects (unless an inhibitor is present) in a 50:50 mix with normal plasma. The diagnosis of FX deficiency is confirmed by measuring plasma FX levels. FX can be measured either immunologically or functionally. Numerous methods exist to measure FX antigen in plasma, including electroimmunoassay, antibody neutralization, immunodiffusion, radioimmunoassay, laser nephelometry, and enzyme-linked immunosorbent assay (ELISA). FX antigen is reduced in some cases of FX deficiency in which there is a total reduction in the levels of circulating FX, but it may be entirely normal in patients with a dysfunctional FX molecule. FX antigen levels are reduced to approximately 50% of normal in patients on coumarin therapy, although FX activity is lower. The reduction in FX antigenic levels in such patients may reflect an increased catabolism of the acarboxylated form or reduced secretion by the hepatocyte.

The most widely used functional FX assays employ human FX as a substrate to which dilutions of normal or test plasma are added and correction in clotting times is compared in assays based on either the PT or the activated partial thromboplastin time (aPTT). Russell viper venom (RVV) can also activate FX and, by using FX-deficient substrate plasma, an assay can be devised that is specific for FX. As with the PT- and aPTT-based assays for FX, some variants have been reported in which the RVV assay of FX is normal.

A chromogenic FX assay offers an accurate and reliable alternative to clotting assays, but there are concerns about such assays, and in particular the nonspecific nature of the substrate, which may give rise to spuriously high results in some patients with FX deficiency. The full spectrum of tests is required only for detailed protein characterization.

Factor X levels are low at birth and age/gestation-related ranges for FX are essential if a deficiency is suspected [6]. The diagnosis of mild FX deficiency may be especially difficult in premature or young neonates, when vitamin K deficiency may complicate assessment. Reassessment after vitamin K replacement may be necessary. It is important to exclude vitamin K deficiency or other acquired causes of a clotting disorder before the diagnosis of FX deficiency is made. In some cases, family studies may help in establishing the diagnosis of FX deficiency.

Clinical features

Factor X deficiency is inherited in an autosomal recessive manner. It is among the rarest of the inherited coagulation disorders, with an estimated prevalence in the UK of 1:500 000, but its heterozygous form is more common, with an estimated frequency of ~1:500, although such individuals are usually asymptomatic. Some heterozygotes can exhibit bleeding symptoms, and this may be due either to insufficient enzymatic activity by the normal FX or to an inhibition of a reaction step in the coagulation pathway by the mutant gene product. Because FXa is part of the prothrombinase complex, a dysfunctional FXa molecule may compete with the normal FXa for FVa binding sites. The net effect would be to decrease the formation of an active prothrombinase complex.

In contrast to hemophilia A and B, in which the risk of bleeding increases as the FVIII or FIX level falls, FX deficiency, in common with many of the other rare inherited bleeding disorders, shows a variable bleeding tendency with a poor correlation between absolute factor levels and bleeding (Figure 54.2). Although FX deficiency produces a variable bleeding tendency, patients with severe deficiency [FX activity (FX:C) <1 U/dL] tend to be the most seriously affected of patients with rare coagulation defects [7]. Less severely affected patients may bleed only after a challenge to the hemostatic system, e.g., trauma or surgery. Some cases are identified during routine screening or family studies.

Patients with FX deficiency may present at any age, and severely affected individuals (FX:C <1 U/dL) can present in the

neonatal period with umbilical stump bleeding. The most frequent symptom in FX deficiency is epistaxis, and this is seen with all severities of deficiency. Other mucosa-type bleeding is less frequent and occurs mainly in patients with severe deficiencies. Menorrhagia occurs in half of women of reproductive age. Hemarthroses, severe postoperative hemorrhage, and central nervous system hemorrhage have been reported. Recurrent hemarthroses may result in severe arthropathy. Moderately affected patients (FX:C 1–5 U/dL) may bleed only after hemostatic challenge, e.g., trauma or surgery. Mild FX deficiency (FX:C 6–10 U/dL) may be identified incidentally during routine screening or family studies. Patients who are only mildly affected may experience easy bruising or menorrhagia.

The thrombogram has been used to investigate the relation between FX levels, in an attempt to establish at what level of FX normal thrombin generation is achieved [8]. In FX deficiency, half-normal endogenous thrombin potential (EPT) was seen at an FX concentration of 5%. Ten individuals with FX deficiency (FX levels 1–50% of normal) were studied and when functional FX activity was below 10% the parameters of the thrombogram, lag time and peak height were markedly abnormal. The endogenous thrombin potential was similar irrespective of the method of activation of factor X (extrinsic pathway or intrinsic pathway). In patients with a FX activity between 10% and 50%, only the lag time of thrombogram and the peak height were abnormal but the EPT remained within normal limits. These patients had no bleeding even after trauma, and this work suggests that the threshold range of FX required to obtain normal thrombin generation is approximately 10% of normal.

Classification of factor X deficiency

The classification of FX deficiency is complex and based upon the results of various functional (PT, aPTT, and RVV time-based assays) and immunologic assays. Classical hereditary FX deficiency (CRM⁻) is characterized by a prolonged PT, prolonged aPTT, prolonged RVV time, and deficiencies in both FX activity and FX antigen. In contrast, CRM⁺ disease has been described and, in such cases, FX antigen is normal or near normal, but the PT, aPTT, RVV, and chromogenic FX assays show variable activity. A further group of patients exhibit variant FX molecules, which are present in reduced amounts (CRMʳ).

Molecular basis of factor X deficiency

Factor X mutations are thought to be rare because of the central role of FX in the coagulation cascade. The FX knock-out mouse has a lethal phenotype, with death occurring either *in utero* or within a few days of birth, and this is consistent with the hypothesis that a complete absence of FX is a lethal disorder [9]. A mutational website for FX mutants does not exist, but approximately 63 mutations within the *F10* gene have been reported [10,11].

The earliest reported molecular abnormality affecting the *F10* gene was reported by Scambler and Williamson, who described

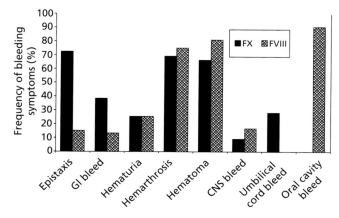

Figure 54.2 Prevalence of bleeding symptoms in 150 patients with haemophilia A (FVIII) matched for age and severity with patients with factor X deficiency.

a female monosomic for 13q34 and who was found to be deficient in FVII and FX [12]. Interestingly, her brother was trisomic for 13q34 and had elevated levels of these factors. A number of other gene deletions of varying size have also been reported and are summarized in refs 10 and 11.

The vast majority of the mutations described in FX deficiency are single point mutations resulting in amino acid substitutions (missense mutations) and affecting primarily exon 8, the largest exon in the *F10* gene and which encodes the catalytic domain.

Nonsense mutations occur when the nucleotide substitution produces a stop codon, or when a nucleotide deletion/insertion results in a frameshift and a stop codon further downstream. This may result in the synthesis of a truncated protein and a clinically significant deficiency. In the case of FX deficiency, no nonsense mutants have been reported. This, together with the observation that most patients with severe FX deficiency have low but measurable factor activity and the FX knock-out data, suggests that a complete absence of FX is incompatible with life.

Several cases of FX deficiency have been reported in which there is also a deficiency of the other vitamin K-dependent clotting factors. In such cases, a defect in the γ-carboxylation mechanism has been proposed as a causative mechanism either at the carboxylase step or at the level of the vitamin K reductase

Acquired factor X deficiency

An acquired rather than an inherited deficiency of FX is seen in a number of diverse disorders.
• Liver disease/oral anticoagulants/vitamin K deficiency: the differentiation of inherited FX deficiency from acquired deficiencies should include consideration of liver disease and vitamin K deficiency (malabsorption, warfarin, and other oral anticoagulants), although in such cases there are commonly deficiencies of the other vitamin K-dependent or hepatic-derived clotting factors.
• Amyloidosis: an association between amyloidosis and acquired FX deficiency was first reported by Korsan-Bengsten in 1962 [13] and subsequently by others. In general, there is only a modest reduction in FX antigen but a marked reduction in FX activity. Removal of endogenous FX from the plasma of these patients as well as exogenous FX appears to be mediated via the amyloid fibrils, which are deposited throughout the vasculature. FX has been shown to bind directly to amyloid fibrils. Treatment of the amyloidosis has limited benefit but may result in some improvement in FX levels. Splenectomy has been reported to be useful, probably because the spleen acts as a large reservoir of amyloid material. Exogenously administered FX is rapidly cleared from the circulation and is therefore of little if any benefit
• Miscellaneous: FX deficiency has been reported in association with a number of other disorders, including myeloma (without amyloidosis), following exposure to the fungicide methylbromide, and in association with various tumors including spindle cell tumors, acute myeloid leukemia treated with amsacrine, and

renal/adrenal carcinomas. Finally, two cases of acquired FX deficiency in patients with leprosy and a single case in association with a *Mycoplasma pneumoniae* chest infection have been documented.

Treatment of factor X deficiency

Inherited FX is a rare disorder, and there are no generally agreed guidelines for the management of this disorder. Current therapeutic options to manage patients with FX deficiency include fibrinolytic inhibitors, plasma, and intermediate-purity FIX concentrates (prothrombin complex concentrates). Recombinant VIIa (rVIIa) has been used successfully to treat acquired FX deficiency secondary to amyloidosis [14].

The need for replacement therapy is guided by the particular hemorrhagic episode. The biological half-life of FX is 20–40 h [15], so an adequate level can be achieved with repeated infusions. Factor levels of 10–20 IU/dL are generally sufficient for hemostasis, even in the immediate postoperative period [16], although some recent data suggest that levels of 5 IU/dL may be sufficient for adequate hemostasis [17].

Mucosal bleeding

Tranexamic acid

Tranexamic acid, a fibrinolytic inhibitor, may be of value in the management of patients with FX deficiency. In practice, 10 mL of a 5% solution of tranexamic acid is used as a mouthwash every 8 h. However, this is not commercially available and will need to be made up by the hospital pharmacy department. In women with menorrhagia, tranexamic acid 15 mg/kg 8-hourly (in practice, 1 g 6- to 8-hourly) may be effective when taken for the duration of the menstrual period.

Fibrin glue

Fibrin glue can be effective in facilitating local hemostasis. Currently, two products are licensed for use in the UK – Tisseel (Baxter) and Quixil (Omrix), although the latter is licensed only for use in liver surgery [18].

Fresh-frozen plasma (FFP)

FFP has been successfully used to manage patients with FX deficiency. A dose of 20 mL/kg followed by 3–6 mL/kg twice daily is recommended, aiming to keep FX:C trough levels above 10–20 IU/dL.

Prothrombin complex concentrates (PCCs)

In many centers, PCCs are used to manage patients with FX deficiency, particularly severe FX deficiency. The calculated required dosage for treatment is based on the empirical finding that 1 IU of FX per kg body weight raises the FX level by 1.5% of normal. Tranexamic acid should not be used concurrently with prothrombin complex concentrates because of the risk of thrombosis. The half-life of FX is 20–40 h and daily treatment is not usually required. However, in cases where replacement therapy is given, levels should be monitored on a daily basis. In children, the biologic half-life of FX may be shorter, and fall-off studies may be required to establish an appropriate dosing regimen [17].

Management of the acute bleed in patients with severe factor X deficiency

No specific factor X concentrates are available and prothrombin complex concentrates are probably the treatment of choice at present.

Fibrin glue

This may be effective in facilitating local hemostasis.

Fresh-frozen plasma

If prothrombin complex concentrates are not available or are contraindicated, FFP can be used and is usually given as a loading dose of 10–20 mL/kg, followed by 3–6 mL/kg twice daily [16], aiming to keep X:C trough levels above the 10–20 IU/dL needed for effective hemostasis. A virally inactivated plasma should be used.

Prothrombin complex concentrates

PCCs are the treatment of choice for patients with severe factor deficiency. However, PCCs should be used with caution, if at all, in patients with concomitant liver disease, large hematomas, or major trauma, in the neonate, or in those with antithrombin deficiency, because of the risk of precipitating a thrombosis [19]. PCCs have been used as regular prophylaxis in patients with severe FX deficiency [20]. Kouides *et al.* [20] reported the case of a patient who received 30 IU/kg of Profilnine twice weekly as part of a home treatment program. If breakthrough bleeding occurred, another dose was administered, but no more than two doses in 24 h or on more than three consecutive days. A trough level drawn 48 h post infusion showed an FX level of 30 IU/dL. Over a 12-month follow-up period, no bleeding episodes were reported. A recent paper reported four cases of FX deficiency in which primary prophylaxis was successfully undertaken using a PCC, commencing in the case of one child at the age of 1 month [17]. The four patients reported all had severe FX deficiency and presented within 24–72 h of birth with a severe bleeding diathesis. Unpublished data at the Royal Free Hospital (London) of a patient with severe FX deficiency (factor X:C < 1 IU/dL) have shown that 10 IU/kg of Defix (SNBTS) given every third day provides effective prophylaxis against hemarthroses.

Recombinant factor VIIa

Recombinant factor VIIa (rFVIIa) has been used to treat amyloid-associated FX deficiency [14] but data on its use in patients with inherited FX deficiency are limited. Adequate levels of FX appear to be important for the action of rFVIIa and therefore, in severe factor X deficiency, rFVIIa may be ineffective [21].

Management of surgery in patients with severe factor X deficiency

Surgery in individuals with severe FX deficiency (FX <1 IU/dL) has been successfully performed following infusion of either FFP or PCCs. In the case of FFP, a level of 35 IU/dL was achieved prior to surgery and FX levels were maintained above 20 IU/dL in the postoperative period, with no bleeding reported [22]. An FX level of 20 IU/dL appears to be sufficient for efficient hemostasis. However, a recent report has shown that a lower FX level, in the region of 0.05 IU/mL (5 IU/dL), achieves adequate hemostasis [17]. Similarly, data using the thrombogram suggest that FX levels of 10 IU/dL may be effective [8].

Management of severe factor X deficiency in pregnancy

Factor X levels increase during pregnancy [23], but women with severe FX deficiency and a history of adverse outcome in pregnancy may benefit from aggressive replacement therapy [24]. However, the potential for thrombosis associated with replacement therapy must be considered.

Management of the neonate with severe factor X deficiency

In families in which both parents are known to have FX deficiency, pregnancy and delivery should be managed in such a way as to minimize the potential risk of bleeding to both the mother and baby. This requires close liaison with the obstetric unit, including obstetric anesthesiologists, and a management plan should be prepared for the delivery and subsequent investigation of the neonate. An FX assay should be performed prior to delivery. At birth a cord blood sample should be taken for FX assay.

Cranial ultrasound scanning should be undertaken in severely affected neonates because of the increased risk of intracranial hemorrhage. Prophylaxis during the neonatal period may be necessary in severely affected neonates although, even with appropriate replacement therapy, hemorrhage may occur.

Management of moderate factor X deficiency (factor X:C >2 IU/dL)

Patients with FX levels greater than 10 IU/dL, or a lower level and no significant bleeding history (despite hemostatic challenges), require no replacement therapy. However, the nature of the surgery and any bleeding history in relation to previous hemostatic challenges must be considered.

References

1 Telfer TP, Denson KW, Wright DR. A new 'coagulation' defect. *Br J Haematol* 1956; **2**: 308–16.
2 Hougie C, Barrow HM, Graham JB. Stuart Clotting defect. Segregation of an hereditary hemorrhagic state from the heterozygous heretofore called 'stable factor' (SPCA, proconvertin, factor VII) deficiency. *J Clin Invest* 1957; **36**: 485–93.
3 Duckert F, Fluckiger P, Koller F. Le role de facteur X dans la formation de la thromboplastine sanguine. *Revue d'Hematologie* 1954; **9**: 489–92.
4 Uprichard J, Perkins SJ, Peyvandi F, Perry DJ. Molecular modelling of mutations in human factor X deficiency. *Blood Coagul Fibrinol* 2001; **12**: A10.
5 Jesty J, Lorenz A, Rodriguez J, Wun TC. Initiation of the tissue factor pathway of coagulation in the presence of heparin: control by antithrombin III and tissue factor pathway inhibitor. *Blood* 1996; **87**: 2301–7.
6 Williams MD, Chalmers EA, Gibson BE. The investigation and management of neonatal hemostasis and thrombosis. *Br J Haematol* 2002; **119**: 295–309.
7 Peyvandi F, Mannucci PM, Lak M, *et al.* Congenital factor X deficiency: spectrum of bleeding symptoms in 32 Iranian patients. *Br J Haematol* 1998; **102**: 626–8.
8 Al Dieri R, Peyvandi F, Santagostino E, *et al.* The thrombogram in rare inherited coagulation disorders: its relation to clinical bleeding. *Thromb Haemost* 2002; **88**: 576–82.
9 Dewerchin M, Liang Z, Moons L, *et al.* Blood coagulation factor X deficiency causes partial embryonic lethality and fatal neonatal bleeding in mice. *Thromb Haemost* 2000; **83**: 185–90.
10 Perry DJ. Factor X and its deficiency states. *Haemophilia* 1997; **3**: 159–72.
11 Uprichard J, Perry DJ. Factor X deficiency. *Blood Rev* 2002; **16**: 97–110.
12 Scambler PJ, Williamson R. The structural gene for human coagulation factor X is located on chromosome 13q34. *Cytogen Cell Genet* 1985; **39**: 231–3.
13 Korsan-Bengsten LHP, Ygge J. Acquired factor X deficiency in a patient with amyloidosis. *Thrombosis et Diathesis Haemorrhagica* 1962; **7**: 558–66.
14 Boggio L, Green D. Recombinant human factor VIIa in the management of amyloid-associated factor X deficiency. *Br J Haematol* 2001; **112**: 1074–5.
15 Roberts HR, Lechler E. Survival of transfused factor X in patients with Stuart disease. *Thrombosis et Diathesis Haemorrhagica* 1965; **13**: 305–13.
16 Knight RD, Barr CF, Alving BM. Replacement therapy for congenital Factor X deficiency. *Transfusion* 1985; **25**: 78–80.
17 McMahon C, Smith J, Goonan C, *et al.* The role of primary prophylactic factor replacement therapy in children with severe factor X deficiency. *Br J Haematol* 2002; **119**: 789–91.
18 UKHCDO. Guidelines on the selection and use of therapeutic products to treat haemophilia and other hereditary bleeding disorders. *Haemophilia* 2003; **9**: 1–23.
19 Kohler M. Thrombogenicity of prothrombin complex concentrates. *Thromb Res* 1999; **95** (4 Suppl. 1): S13–7.
20 Kouides PA, Kulzer L. Prophylactic treatment of severe factor X deficiency with prothrombin complex concentrate. *Haemophilia* 2001; **7**: 220–3.
21 Allen GA, Monroe DM III, Roberts HR, Hoffman M. The effect of factor X level on thrombin generation and the procoagulant effect of activated factor VII in a cell-based model of coagulation. *Blood Coagul Fibrinol* 2000; **11** (Suppl. 1): S3–7.
22 Knight RD, Barr CF, Alving BM. Replacement therapy for congenital Factor X deficiency. *Transfusion* 1985; **25**: 78–80.
23 Condie RG. A serial study of coagulation factors XII, XI and X in plasma in normal pregnancy and in pregnancy complicated by preeclampsia. *Br J Obstet Gynaecol* 1976; **83**: 636–9.
24 Kumar M, Mehta P. Congenital coagulopathies and pregnancy: report of four pregnancies in a factor X-deficient woman. *Am J Hematol* 1994; **46**: 241–4.
25 Leytus SP, Foster DC, Kurachi K, Davie EW. Gene for human factor X: a blood coagulation factor whose gene organization is essentially identical with that of factor IX and protein C. *Biochemistry* 1986; **25**: 5098–102.

Factor XI deficiency

Uri Seligsohn

History

Factor XI (FXI) deficiency was first described in 1953 by Rosenthal *et al.* [1] as a new type of hemophilia, later termed hemophilia C. Its presence in two sisters and their maternal aunt was interpreted as an indication that the mode of inheritance was autosomal dominant. However, a seminal study in 1961 clearly established that transmission of the disorder was autosomal recessive [2], and distinguished between patients with major FXI deficiency, with an activity of less than 20 U/dL, and patients with minor deficiency with an activity of 30–60 U/dL. This study, as well as a later study [3], also delineated that FXI deficiency was particularly common in Jews.

In the classical "waterfall" or "cascade" scheme of coagulation, designed in 1964, FXI was assigned with a role in the initial "contact phase" of the intrinsic system. It was shown that negatively charged surfaces trigger activation of factor XII (FXII), later found to occur in the presence of prekallikrein (PK) and high-molecular-weight kininogen (HK), and that FXIIa, in turn, activates FXI. FXIa then activates factor IX (FIX) in the presence of Ca^{2+}, which leads through additional reactions to the generation of thrombin. Yet this sequence of reactions was hard to reconcile with the clinical observations, which indicated that patients with severe deficiencies of FXII, PK, or HK had no bleeding tendency, whereas patients with FXI deficiency exhibited a significant bleeding tendency, particularly following trauma. This enigma was resolved in 1991 by two groups of researchers who showed that FXI was activated by thrombin, thereby bypassing the initial contact reactions [4,5]. These observations enabled design of a revised scheme of coagulation [4] in which FXII, PK, and HK play no role, while FXI is important for generating thrombin following its initial formation by the tissue factor–factor VII pathway (see Chapter 1).

Biochemical features and function of factor XI

Factor XI is a 160-kDa glycoprotein that consists of two identical polypeptide subunits of 80 kDa linked by a disulfide bond. Each subunit contains 607 amino acids organized in a heavy chain with four tandem repeats of 90 or 91 amino acids, designated "apple domains," and a light chain in which a serine protease domain is located. The first apple domain contains the binding sites for HK, with which FXI circulates as a complex,

and for prothrombin. Apple 3 contains the binding sites for platelets and FIX, and apple 4 harbors the binding site for FXII and is important for the dimerization of the subunits [6,7].

The gene encoding for FXI (GenBank M18295) consists of 15 exons and 14 introns and is located on chromosome 4q34–35 close to the gene that encodes for PK [8]. FXI is synthesized in the liver and circulates in the blood at a concentration of 3–7 µg/mL. The physiologic activator of FXI is thrombin, which converts zymogen FXI to a serine protease (FXIa) by cleavage of the Arg369–Ile370 bond, giving rise to a 47-kDa heavy chain and a 33-kDa light chain. Recent evidence suggests that this reaction is greatly accelerated when FXI is bound to activated platelets in the presence of prothrombin and Ca^{2+} ions or HK and Zn^{2+} ions [9]. Conceivably, one of the FXI subunits binds to the platelet membrane while the other subunit binds to FIX [6], thereby enabling efficient activation of FXI by thrombin and then activation of FIX by FXIa. FXIa initially cleaves FIX at the Arg146–Ala147 bond in the presence of Ca^{2+} ions and subsequently an Arg180–Val181 bond yielding fully activated factor IXaβ and an activation peptide. FIXa then activates FX in the presence of factor VIIIa, negatively charged phospholipids and Ca^{2+}, and FXa in turn converts prothrombin to thrombin in the presence of factor Va, negatively charged phospholipids, and Ca^{2+}.

Factor XI activated by thrombin is essential for sustained thrombin generation, which is particularly important after clot formation. It is at this stage that thrombin activates procarboxypeptidase B, also termed thrombin-activatable fibrinolysis inhibitor (TAFI). Activated TAFI removes terminal lysine residues, which are the sites of plasminogen binding, from fibrin, leading to impaired conversion of plasminogen to plasmin by tissue plasminogen activator and to diminished fibrinolysis [10]. Factor XI can thus be regarded as a procoagulant and an indirect inhibitor of fibrinolysis. This conclusion is supported by the clinical observation that patients with severe FXI deficiency are specifically prone to bleeding when trauma is inflicted at sites where there is enhanced fibrinolytic activity [11]. FXIa is inhibited by antithrombin in the presence of heparin, protease nexin II, C_1-inhibitor, and protein C inhibitor.

Inheritance and functional defect

Factor XI deficiency is inherited as an autosomal recessive disorder. Homozygotes or compound heterozygotes have a FXI

321

activity of less than 15 U/dL and heterozygotes have an activity range of 25–70 U/dL or are within normal limits. Vertical transmission of severe FXI deficiency or apparent dominance has been observed in Jewish families but stems from matings between homozygotes and heterozygotes in this population, in which the prevalence of mutant genes and affected individuals is high [3]. In the vast majority of patients with FXI deficiency, activity of FXI is concordant with antigenicity [12]. Only one patient has so far been shown to harbor unequivocally a dysfunctional FXI, with 100 U/dL antigenicity and less than 1 U/dL activity [13].

Mutations

Three mutations in the FXI gene, termed types I, II, and III, were first described in 1989 in six Ashkenazi Jews who had severe FXI deficiency [14]. Type I mutation is a G to A change at the splice junction of the last intron of the gene, type II mutation is a G to T change in exon 5 leading to Glu117ter, and type III mutation is a T to C change in exon 9, giving rise to Phe283Leu substitution. Homozygotes for type II mutation have a mean FXI activity of 1.2 U/dL, homozygotes for type III mutation have a mean FXI activity of 9.7 U/dL, and compound heterozygotes for types II and III mutations have a mean activity of 3.3 U/dL [11]. Types II and III mutations are the predominant mutations causing FXI deficiency in Ashkenazi Jews [11,15]. Table 55.1 demonstrates that in 295 Jewish patients of various ethnic origins with severe FXI deficiency, 52% of the alleles carried type II mutation, 46% type III mutation, 1% type I mutation, and 1% other mutations. At the time of this writing, 47 mutations have been published and 25 more were reported as abstracts at scientific meetings. Databases listing published mutations will be available (http://www.med.unc.edu/isth/; http://archive.uwcm.ac.uk/uwcm/mg/search/119891.html). Of the 47 published mutations, 26 are missense mutations, seven are nonsense mutations, six are deletions and/or insertions, and eight are splice-site mutations [14,16–31]. Interestingly, expression of eight missense mutations, five located in the fourth apple domain and the oth-

ers located in apple 1, revealed impaired secretion of FXI from transfected cells [16,17,28]. For one of these mutations, the type III mutation (Phe283Leu) in apple 4, the impaired secretion was related to defective dimerization [16]. Several polymorphisms have also been described and used for analysis of haplotypes in populations in which FXI deficiency is prevalent [28,32].

Prevalence and ethnic distribution

The highest prevalence of FXI deficiency has been observed in Ashkenazi Jews [3]. Among 531 individuals of Ashkenazi Jewish origin, the allele frequency of type II and type III mutations was 0.0217 and 0.0254 respectively [33]. Thus, 9.1% of subjects belonging to this ethnic group are predicted to be carriers of either mutation and 1 in 450 individuals (0.22%) is expected to be afflicted by severe FXI deficiency. Another ethnic group, the Iraqi Jews, who represent the ancient gene pool of Jews from Babylonian times 2500 years ago, have been found to harbor only the type II mutation. Among 507 subjects, an allele frequency of 0.0167 was found, predicting heterozygosity in 1/30 individuals and homozygosity in 1/3600 individuals in the general Iraqi Jewish community [33]. Among 947 subjects from other Jewish ethnic groups, an allele frequency of 0.0027 for the type II mutation was found and none was found to bear the type III mutation. Interestingly, among 382 Arabs, type II mutation was detected with an allele frequency of 0.0065. A study of intragenic polymorphisms in patients with severe FXI deficiency from all these ethnic groups enabled haplotype analysis, which disclosed distinct founder effects for the type II and type III mutations [32] (Figure 55.1). Based on the distribution of allelic variants at a microsatellite marker flanking the FXI gene, (D4S171), the type II mutation was estimated to have occurred more than 120 generations ago, while the type III mutation was of a more recent origin [34] (Figure 55.2). Another cluster of patients with FXI deficiency was observed in Basques residing in south-western France, and a recent study revealed that the predominant mutation in this population is Cys38Arg, with an allele frequency of 0.005 [28]. Another cluster of FXI-deficient patients among Caucasians living or originating in the UK has been described [35]. Preliminary data indicate that all affected patients harbor a C128X mutation and haplotype analysis is consistent with a founder effect .

Factor XI deficiency has also been reported sporadically in other patients of English, African-American, German, Indian, Italian, Korean, Japanese, Chinese, Portuguese, Swedish, Yugoslav, Arab, and Iranian origin [12,16–31,36].

Bleeding manifestations in patients with severe deficiency

Spontaneous bleeding manifestations are rare in patients with severe FXI deficiency. The common presentation is an injury-related bleeding tendency, particularly at sites where tissues con-

Table 55.1 Molecular analysis in 295 unrelated Jewish patients with severe factor XI deficiency.

Mutant allele	n	%
Type II: Glu117Ter	306	51.86
Type III: Phe283Leu	271	45.93
Type I: IVS 14 + 1 (GGT → GAT)	7	1.19
Type IV: 14 basepair deletion (IVS 14/exon 15)	2	0.34
Gly555Glu	2	0.34
Tyr427Cys	1	0.17
Glu323Lys	1	0.17
Total	590	100

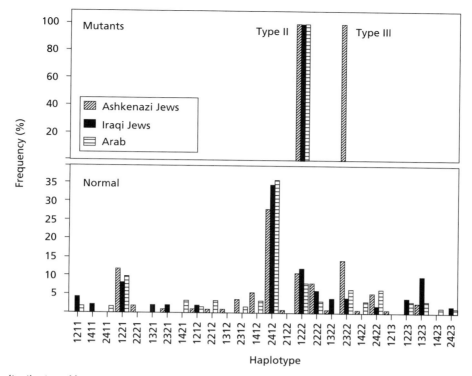

Figure 55.1 Frequency distribution of factor XI gene haplotypes observed in Ashkenazi Jews, Iraqi Jews, and Arabs. The numbers on the abscissa denote, from bottom to top, the allele numbers of polymorphisms in introns A, B, E, and M. For example, the haplotype designated 1-2-1-1 comprises allele 1 of intron A polymorphism, allele 2 of intron B polymorphism, allele 1 of intron E polymorphism, and allele 1 of intron M polymorphism. The lower and upper panels represent normal chromosomes and chromosomes bearing type II or type III mutations respectively. Note that all chromosomes carrying the type II mutation are characterized by the same 1-2-2-2 haplotype that is observed in 8–12% of normal chromosomes. The chromosomes bearing the type III mutation are confined to Ashkenazi Jews, all characterized by haplotype 2-3-2-2. From Peretz et al. [32].

tain activators of the fibrinolytic system, such as the oral cavity, nose, tonsils, and urinary tract [11]. At other sites of trauma, such as encountered during orthopedic surgery, appendicectomy, circumcision, or cuts in the skin, bleeding is less common. Postpartum hemorrhage occurs in only 20–30% of affected women [37]. Patients who are homozygotic for type II mutation, whose FXI activity is 1 U/dL or less, are more vulnerable to bleeds following injury than homozygotes for type III mutation, or compound heterozygotes for type II and type III mutations whose FXI levels are 2–15 U/dL [11,15]. Some patients with a very low level of FXI may not bleed at all following trauma [2], while in others the bleeding tendency varies in the same patient over time even when provoked by similar hemostatic challenges [11,37]. Bleeding can be brisk at the time of injury and persists unless treated, or can begin several hours following trauma.

Bleeding manifestations in heterozygotes

Whether or not heterozygotes with partial FXI deficiency exhibit a bleeding tendency is controversial. In one study, bleeding was observed in 9/94 (9.6%) of patients who underwent surgical procedures, including tooth extractions, tonsillectomy, and nasal operation [2]. In another study, no bleeding was observed following urologic surgery unless FXI activity was 25 U/dL or less [38]. In contrast, two studies from the UK and Iran [36,37,39] described injury-related bleeding in 48–60% of cases, as well as spontaneous bleeding manifestations, even including hemarthroses [36]. An assessment of the risk of bleeding in a large cohort of patients with severe and partial FXI deficiency yielded an odds ratio of 13 [confidence interval (CI) 3.8–45] for patients with severe FXI deficiency and an odds ratio of 2.6 (CI 0.8–9.0) for patients with partial deficiency [40]. In spite of these uncertainties, it can be concluded that patients with partial FXI deficiency may exhibit a bleeding tendency but that the risk is substantially lower than in patients with severe FXI deficiency. Whatever the cause of the discrepancy among the studies, patients with partial FXI deficiency who have a bleeding history should be carefully examined for additional inherited disorders of hemostasis such as platelet dysfunction or von Willebrand disease (VWD), and for acquired hemostatic defects.

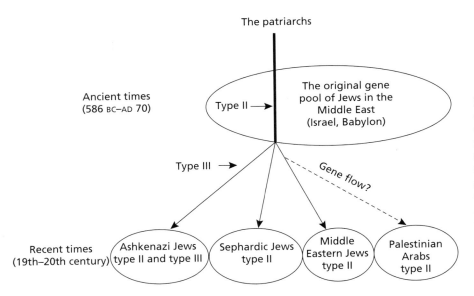

Figure 55.2 A simplified scheme showing the common origin of the three major segments of contemporary Jews and explaining the current distribution of the type II and type III mutations. The predicted time when type II and type III mutations occurred in the factor XI gene are indicated by horizontal arrows. We speculate that gene flow has been responsible for the transfer of type II mutation from Middle Eastern Jews to Palestinian Arabs after the settlement of Arabs in Israel in the seventh century AD. From Peretz *et al.* [32]. Copyright American Society of Hematology, used with permission.

Thrombosis

The effect of FXI in promoting coagulation and inhibiting fibrinolysis could hypothetically predict that, in patients with severe FXI deficiency, thrombosis would occur infrequently. However, unlike patients with severe hemophilia A or hemophilia B, in whom the incidence of acute myocardial infarction is significantly reduced, patients with severe FXI deficiency are not protected against such events. In a recent study of 96 adult patients with severe FXI deficiency, 16 (17%) have had an acute myocardial infarction, which occurred at median ages of 64.5 and 58 years in women and men respectively [41]. The observed incidence of acute myocardial infarction in this cohort was not statistically different from the expected incidence in the general population. As anticipated, one or more of the conventional atherosclerotic risk factors was detected in 13 of the 16 patients who had an acute myocardial infarction (81%), whereas, among patients with severe FXI deficiency who had not experienced an acute myocardial infarction, the presence of these risk factors was significantly lower. Venous thromboembolism was not observed in this study but anecdotal cases have been reported [42]. Conceivably, some protection against venous thromboembolism may be conferred by severe FXI deficiency because high levels of FXI constitute a risk factor for such venous thrombosis [43]. However, only a study of a very large number of patients with FXI deficiency would enable assessment of whether or not patients with severe FXI deficiency are protected against venous thromboembolism.

Association of factor XI deficiency with other disorders

Factor XI deficiency has been described in association with various other inherited bleeding disorders, e.g., VWD, platelet dys-

functions, and deficiencies of factors VII, VIII, and IX (for review see ref. 44). These associations are probably coincidental, although the probability of the common occurrence of combined deficiency of factors VII, IX, and XI, observed in five families, seems too remote to be coincidental. No mechanism for these exceptional families has been provided. Noonan syndrome and Gaucher disease have also been observed in patients with FXI deficiency. While the association between FXI deficiency and Noonan syndrome has not been explained, the association between Gaucher disease and FXI deficiency was shown to stem from the relatively high prevalence of the mutant genes of both disorders in Ashkenazi Jews, i.e., 1/19 for Gaucher disease and 1/11 for FXI deficiency. It was also demonstrated that the segregation of Gaucher disease and FXI deficiency in the same family was independent [45].

Development of inhibitors

Inhibitors to FXI have been described in patients with severe FXI deficiency. Fortunately, bleeding manifestations in such patients are not aggravated following inhibitor formation, but trauma or surgery presents a serious hemostatic challenge (see below under "Therapy"). In a recent study of 118 unrelated patients with severe FXI deficiency, seven were found to harbor an inhibitor [46]. All seven patients had received plasma replacement therapy prior to the development of the inhibitor and all were homozygous for the type II null allele, which is associated with extremely low levels of FXI. Of 84 patients with other genotypes, i.e., type III homozygotes or type II and type III compound heterozygotes (of whom 43 had received plasma), none was found to have an inhibitor to FXI. Patients with these genotypes have measurable levels of FXI in the range 2–15 U/dL. These observations suggest that only homozygotes or compound heterozygotes for two null alleles are prone to the development of an inhibitor following exposure to exogenous FXI. This study also revealed that the seven patients who developed an inhibitor were among 21 homozygotes for the type II mutation who had received plasma, which suggests that 33% of patients with almost no FXI have a predilection for development of an inhibitor. The antibodies isolated from patients with an inhibitor display various effects, i.e., impaired FXI activation by thrombin or by FXIIa, inhibition of binding of FXI to HK, and diminished activation of FIX by FXIa [46].

Diagnosis

Excessive bleeding following injury, such as tooth extraction, tonsillectomy, nose surgery, and urologic procedures, or an incidental finding of a prolonged activated partial thromboplastin time (aPTT) are the common modes of presentation of FXI deficiency. Spontaneous bleeding such as menorrhagia or postpartum bleeding, and injury involving tissues that do not contain increased amounts of activators of fibrinolysis, lead less commonly to the diagnosis of the disorder. All patients with severe FXI deficiency (activity of less than 15 U/dL) exhibit an aPTT value that is more than two standard deviations above the normal mean [47]. Heterozygotes may have a slightly prolonged aPTT but values are frequently within the normal range [47]. Similarly, FXI levels overlap with normal levels. [3,37,39]. Therefore, for diagnosis of partial FXI deficiency in suspected heterozygotes, only genotyping for the responsible mutation can be diagnostic. For the two common mutations prevalent in Jewish subjects (type II and III) as well as the common Basque mutation and others, simple polymerase chain reaction (PCR) and restriction analyses are available [28,33].

Because severe FXI deficiency can remain asymptomatic until injury is inflicted, it is desirable for all Ashkenazi Jews in need of surgery (particularly at sites of enhanced fibrinolysis) to undergo hemostatic screening tests including aPTT.

FXI activity is commonly measured by an aPTT-based assay, although the intra- and inter-laboratory coefficient of variation is significant. Other tests, e.g., radioimmunoassay, electroimmunoassay, and an amidolytic assay, have been described but are only performed in specialized laboratories.

Therapy

Spontaneous bleeding is rare in patients with severe FXI deficiency, and when it occurs it is usually mild and terminates without therapy. Sometimes, spontaneous bleeding follows the inadvertent use of antiplatelet agents and discontinuation of their use solves the problem. Deliveries are infrequently complicated by excessive bleeding in patients with severe FXI deficiency and thus on-demand, rather than preventive, blood product therapy can be advocated.

Surgery or trauma can be associated with excessive and prolonged bleeding unless treated properly. Consequently, careful

evaluation of patients with severe FXI deficiency prior to surgery is indispensable, as well as meticulous planning of the procedure and the postsurgical course. The following are some considerations and guidelines:

1 The surgical procedure should be absolutely indicated.
2 Previous bleeding episodes and their severity should be taken into account.
3 A test for an inhibitor to FXI should be performed and its presence ruled out.
4 The prothrombin time and platelet count should be normal.
5 The genotype of the patient should be determined because it has been shown to be associated with the risk of bleeding [11] and the development of inhibitors to FXI [46].
6 Use of antiplatelet drugs should be discontinued 1 week before surgery.
7 Both site and type of surgery are significantly related to the risk of bleeding and, hence, planning of surgery should be tailored accordingly. Examples include: (i) patients in need of tooth extraction can be treated only by tranexamic acid (see below); (ii) for prostatectomy and other lower urinary tract surgery, both blood component therapy and local flushing by saline containing tranexamic acid can be used; (iii) for nasal surgery and tonsillectomy, replacement therapy and parenteral tranexamic acid administration are advisable; (iv) for major surgery, plasma or FXI concentrate infusions should be targeted at trough FXI levels of 45 U/dL for at least 10 days; for minor surgery a trough level of 30 U/dL during 5 days is usually sufficient [38].
8 Assessment of the cardiovascular status of the patient is essential for two reasons: (i) when use of fresh-frozen plasma is planned, the patient's incapacity to tolerate volume overload can be a serious impediment; (ii) compromised cardiovascular function confers a risk of thrombosis when an FXI concentrate is used.
9 Replacement therapy should be started prior to surgery and carefully monitored thereafter by assays of FXI activity.
10 The surgeon should be guided to use ligation rather than cauterization because cauterized tissues are vulnerable sites for blood oozing that can occur after surgery.
11 Use of fibrin glue during surgery can significantly contribute to successful hemostasis.

Replacement therapy is usually by fresh-frozen plasma (FFP) [38]. The main disadvantages of this mode of therapy are potential transmission of infectious agents, allergic reactions, and—as mentioned—volume overload. Treatment of FFP by solvent/detergent or by pasteurization has increased its safety, with preservation of FXI activity [48].

Two concentrates of FXI have been produced, one in the UK and the other in France, and found to be safe with regard to transmission of infectious agents. However, approximately 10% of patients who were treated by these products developed arterial thrombosis or venous thromboembolism, which was fatal in several cases. Since almost all patients who developed these unfortunate complications were elderly and had pre-existing cardiovascular disease [48], these products should be avoided in such patients or used with extreme caution. Caution should also be exercised in patients with prothrombotic states such as pregnancy and malignant disorders. Notwithstanding these limitations, FXI concentrates have been successfully used in many patients. Studies have shown a 90% recovery of FXI after infusion of these concentrates and a half-life of 46–52 h. The relatively small volume that needs to be infused, the excellent *in vivo* recovery of FXI, and the extended half-life of FXI substantially facilitate therapy.

For several types of minor surgery, such as tooth extractions and skin biopsy, there is no need for replacement therapy. In 19 patients with severe FXI deficiency who have had a history of bleeding following tooth extractions or trauma, tooth extractions were uneventfully performed under treatment of only tranexamic acid started 12 h prior to surgery and continued until 7 days after surgery [49]. Fibrin glue can also be used in such cases and in patients undergoing resection of skin lesions.

The approach to patients with partial FXI deficiency who need surgery varies among centers. Excessive bleeding following surgery in some patients with FXI levels of approximately 50 U/dL is used to support the view that such patients need replacement therapy during surgery [39]. Other observations of patients who underwent uneventful prostatectomy with a level of 30 U/dL support the view that replacement therapy is unnecessary during most surgical procedures in patients with partial FXI deficiency [38]. Notwithstanding these inconsistencies, a reasonable practice in patients with partial FXI deficiency can be:

1 Obtain a detailed history of bleeding.
2 If a clear history of bleeding tendency is obtained, perform a thorough investigation of other potential inherited or acquired hemostatic disorders; abnormal results should be taken into account in the planning of surgery.
3 Use tranexamic acid and/or fibrin glue when there is a bleeding history or when high-risk surgery such as prostatectomy is planned.
4 Use replacement therapy in patients with an unequivocal bleeding tendency (after ruling out other hemostatic defects) aiming at a trough FXI level of 45 U/dL for 5 days after surgery.

Surgery in patients who have developed an inhibitor to FXI presents a great challenge. When the titer of the inhibitor is very low, use of an FXI concentrate can suffice, but an anamnestic reaction is to be expected. Recombinant factor VIIa (rFVIIa) has been successfully used in such a patient during cataract extraction [50]. *In vitro*, rFVIIa was shown to correct the abnormality in thrombin generation of plasma from such patients [45]. Clearly, more observations on the use of rFVIIa are needed before defining its role in treatment of patients with an inhibitor to FXI and perhaps in patients with severe FXI deficiency without an inhibitor.

References

1 Rosenthal R, Dreskin O, Rosenthal N. New hemophilia-like disease caused by deficiency of a third plasma thromboplastin factor. *Proc Soc Exp Biol Med* 1953; **82**: 171–4.

2 Rapaport SI, Proctor RR, Patch NJ, Yettra M. The role of inheritance of PTA deficiency: evidence for the existence of major PTA deficiency and minor PTA deficiency. *Blood* 1961; **18**: 149–65.

3 Seligsohn U. High gene frequency of factor XI (PTA) deficiency in Ashkenazi Jews. *Blood* 1978; **516**: 1223–8.

4 Gailani D, Broze GJ. Factor XI activation in a revised model of blood coagulation. *Science* 1991; **253**: 909–12.

5 Naito K, Fujikawa K. Activation of human blood coagulation factor XI independent of factor XII. Factor XI is activated by thrombin and factor XIa in the presence of negatively charged surfaces. *J Biol Chem* 1991; **266**: 7353–8.

6 Gailani D, Ho D, Sun MF, *et al.* Model for a factor IX activation complex on blood platelets: dimeric conformation of factor XIa is essential. *Blood* 2001; **97**: 3117–22.

7 Baglia FA, Walsh PN. Prothrombin is a cofactor for the binding of factor XI to the platelet surface and for platelet-mediated factor XI activation by thrombin. *Biochemistry* 1998; **37**: 2271–81.

8 Kato A, Asakai R, Davie EW, Aoki N. Factor XI gene (F11) is located on the distal end of the long arm of human chromosome 4. *Cytogenet Cell Genet* 1989; **52**: 77–8.

9 Baglia FA, Badellino KO, Li CQ, *et al.* Factor XI binding to the platelet glycoprotein Ib-IX-V complex promotes factor XI activation by thrombin. *J Biol Chem* 2002; **277**: 1662–8.

10 Bouma BN, Marx PF, Mosnier LO, Meijers JC. Thrombin-activatable fibrinolysis inhibitor (TAFI, plasma procarboxypeptidase B, procarboxypeptidase R, procarboxypeptidase U). *Thromb Res* 2001; **101**: 329–54.

11 Asakai R, Chung DW, Davie EW, Seligsohn U. Factor XI deficiency in Ashkenazi Jews in Israel. *N Engl J Med* 1991; **3253**: 153–8.

12 Saito H, Ratnoff OD, Bouma BN, Seligshon U. Failure to detect variant (CRM+) plasma thromboplastin antecedent (factor XI) molecules in hereditary plasma thromboplastin antecedent deficiency: a study of 125 patients in several ethnic backgrounds. *J Lab Clin Med* 1985; **106**: 718–22.

13 Zivelin A, Ogawa T, Bulvik S, et al. Severe factor XI deficiency caused by a Gly555 to Glu mutation (factor XI — Glu555): a cross-reactive material defective in factor XI activation. *J Thromb Haemost* 2004 (in press).

14 Asakai R, Chung DW, Ratnoff OD, Davie EW. Factor XI (plasma thromboplastin antecedent) deficiency in Ashkenazi Jews is a bleeding disorder that can result from three types of point mutations. *Proc Natl Acad Sci USA* 1989; **86**: 7667–71.

15 Hancock JF, Wieland K, Pugh RE, *et al.* A molecular genetic study of factor XI deficiency. *Blood* 1991; **77**: 1942–8.

16 Meijers JC, Mulvihill ER, Davie EW, Chung DW. Apple four in human blood coagulation factor XI mediates dimer formation. *Biochemistry* 1992; **31**: 4680–4.

17 Pugh RE, McVey JH, Truddenham EG, Hancock JF. Six point mutations that cause factor XI deficiency. *Blood* 1995; **85**: 1509–16.

18 Imanaka Y, Lal K, Nishimura T, *et al.* Identification of two novel mutations in non-Jewish factor XI deficiency. *Br J Haematol* 1995; **90**: 916–20.

19 Peretz H, Zivelin A, Usher S, Seligsohn U. A 14-bp deletion (codon 554 del AAGgtaacagagtg) at exon 14/intron N junction of the coagulation factor XI gene disrupts splicing and causes severe factor XI deficiency. *Hum Mutat* 1996; **8**: 77–8.

20 Wistinghausen B, Reischer A, Oddoux C, *et al.* Severe factor XI deficiency in an Arab family associated with a novel mutation in exon 11. *Br J Haematol* 1997; **99**: 575–7.

21 Martincic D, Zimmerman SA, Ware RE, *et al.* Identification of mutations and polymorphisms in the factor XI genes of an African American family by dideoxyfingerprinting. *Blood* 1998; **92**: 3309–17.

22 Alhaq A, Mitchell M, Sethi M, *et al.* Identification of a novel mutation in a non-Jewish factor XI deficient kindred. *Br J Haematol* 1999; **104**: 44–9.

23 Mitchell M, Cutler J, Thompson S, *et al.* Heterozygous factor XI deficiency associated with three novel mutations. *Br J Haematol* 1999; **107**: 763–5.

24 Sato E, Kawamata N, Kato A, Oshimi K. A novel mutation that leads to a congenital factor XI deficiency in a Japanese family. *Am J Hematol* 2000; **63**: 165–9.

25 Iijima K, Udagawa A, Kawasaki H, *et al.* A factor XI deficiency associated with a nonsense mutation (Trp501stop) in the catalytic domain. *Br J Haematol* 2000; **111**: 556–8.

26 Kawaguchi T, Koga S, Hongo H, *et al.* A novel type of factor XI deficiency showing compound genetic abnormalities: a nonsense mutation and an impaired transcription. *Int J Hematol* 2000; **71**: 84–9.

27 Dossenbach-Glaninger A, Krugluger W, Schrattbauer K, *et al.* Severe factor XI deficiency caused by compound heterozygosity for the type III mutation and a novel insertion in exon 9 (codons 324/325 +G). *Br J Haematol* 2001; **114**: 875–7.

28 Zivelin A, Bauduer F, Ducout L, *et al.* Factor XI deficiency in French Basques is caused predominantly by an ancestral Cys38Arg mutation in the factor XI gene. *Blood* 2002; **99**: 2448–54.

29 Tsukahara A, Yamada T, Takagi A, *et al.* Compound heterozygosity for two novel mutations in a severe factor XI deficiency. *Am J Hematol* 2003; **73**: 279–84.

30 Mitchel M, Harrington P, Cutler J, Rangarajan S. Eighteen unrelated patients with factor XI deficiency, four novel mutations and a 100% detection rate by denaturing high-performance liquid chromatography. *Br J Haematol* 2003; **121**: 500–2.

31 Wu WM, Wang HL, Wang XF, *et al.* Identification of two novel factor XI nonsense mutations Trp228stop and Trp383stop in a Chinese pedigree of congenital factor XI deficiency. *Zhonghua Xue Ye Xue Za Zhi* 2003; **24**: 126–8.

32 Peretz H, Mulai A, Usher S, *et al.* The two common mutations causing factor XI deficiency in Jews stem from distinct founders: one of ancient Middle Eastern origin and another of more recent European origin. *Blood* 1997; **90**: 2654–9.

33 Shpilberg O, Peretz H, Zivelin A, *et al.* One of the two common mutations causing factor XI deficiency in Ashkenazi Jews (type II) is also prevalent in Iraqi Jews, who represent the ancient gene pool of Jews. *Blood* 1995; **85**: 429–32.

34 Goldstein DB, Reich DE, Bradman N, *et al.* Age estimates of two common mutations causing factor XI deficiency: recent genetic drift is not necessary for elevated disease incidence among Ashkenazi Jews. *Am J Hum Genet* 1999; **64**: 1071–5.

35 Bolton-Maggs PHB, Peretz H, Butler R, *et al.* A common ancestral

mutation (C128X) occurring in 11 non-Jewish families from the UK with factor XI deficiency. *J Thromb Haemost* 2004; **2**: 918–24.

36 Peyvandi F, Lak M, Mannucci PM. Factor XI deficiency in Iranians: its clinical manifestations in comparison with those of classic hemophilia. *Haematologica* 2002; **87**: 512–4.

37 Bolton-Maggs PH, Patterson DA, Wensley RT, Tuddenham EG. Definition of the bleeding tendency in factor XI-deficient kindreds — a clinical and laboratory study. *Thromb Haemost* 1995; **73**: 194–202.

38 Sidi A, Seligsohn U, Jonas P, Many M. Factor XI deficiency: detection and management during urological surgery. *J Urol* 1978; **119**: 528–30.

39 Bolton-Maggs PH, Young Wan-Yin B, McCraw AH, *et al.* Inheritance and bleeding in factor XI deficiency. *Br J Haematol* 1988; **69**: 521–8.

40 Brenner B, Laor A, Lupo H, *et al.* Bleeding predictors in factor-XI-deficient patients. *Blood Coagul Fibrinol* 1997; **8**: 511–5.

41 Salomon O, Steinberg DM, Dardik R, *et al.* Inherited factor XI deficiency confers no protection against acute myocardial infarction. *J Thromb Haemost* 2003; **1**: 658–61.

42 Brodsky JB, Burgess GE. Pulmonary embolism with factor XI deficiency. *JAMA* 1975; **234**: 1156–7.

43 Meijers JC, Tekelenburg WL, Bouma BN, *et al.* High levels of coagulation factor XI as a risk factor for venous thrombosis. *N Engl J Med* 2000; **342**: 696–701.

44 Gailani D, Broze GJ. Factor XI and the contact system. In: Scriver CR, Beaudet AL, Sly WS, Valle D, eds. *The Metabolic and Molecular Basis of Inherited Diseases,* 8th edn. New York: McGraw-Hill, 2000: 4433–53.

45 Seligsohn U, Zitman D, Many A, Klibansky C. Coexistence of factor XI (plasma thromboplastin antecedent) deficiency and Gaucher's disease. *Isr J Med Sci* 1976; **12**: 1448–52.

46 Salomon O, Ziveiln A, Livnat T, *et al.* Prevalence, causes, and characterization of factor XI inhibitors in patients with inherited factor XI deficiency. *Blood* 2003; **101**: 4783–8.

47 Seligsohn U, Modan M. Definition of the population at risk of bleeding due to factor XI deficiency in Ashkenazic Jews and the value of activated partial thromboplastin time in its detection. *Isr J Med Sci* 1981; **17**: 413–5.

48 Bolton-Maggs PHB. Factor XI deficiency and its management. *Haemophilia* 2000; **6**: 100–9.

49 Berliner S, Horowitz I, Martinowitz U, *et al.* Dental surgery in patients with severe factor XI deficiency without plasma replacement. *Blood Coagul Fibrinol* 1992; **3**: 465–8.

50 Lawler P, White B, Pye S, *et al.* Successful use of recombinant factor VIIa in a patient with inhibitor secondary to severe factor XI deficiency. *Haemophilia* 2002; **8**: 145–8.

Factor XIII

Hans H. Brackmann and Vytautas Ivaskevicius

Background

Coagulation factor XIII (FXIII) belongs to a family of transglutaminases. It is the last enzyme to be activated in the blood coagulation pathway and functions to cross-link α- and γ-fibrin chains, resulting in a stronger clot with an increased resistance to fibrinolysis [1]. Congenital FXIII deficiency is a rare autosomal recessive disorder, affecting 1 in 1–3 million individuals. The prevalence of this disorder is higher in countries where consanguineous marriages are common. The phenotype is due to the deficiency or absence of FXIII. Patients suffering from this condition are characterized by lifelong bleeding diathesis and impaired wound healing, with the severity and frequency of symptoms correlating with the residual FXIII activity.

In plasma, FXIII proenzyme circulates in the form of a tetramer composed of two catalytic A subunits bound to two carrier B subunits (A_2B_2) [2]. Intracellularly, FXIII is found as a homodimer of the two A subunits (A_2) [3].

Each A subunit is composed of an activation peptide (residues 1–37) and four distinct domains: the beta sandwich (residues 38–183), central core (residues 184–515), beta barrel 1 (residues 516–627), and beta barrel 2 (residues 628–730) regions [4,5]. The central core domain contains a catalytic triad formed through hydrogen bond interactions between Cys314, His373, and Asp396 [6]. These three residues are absolutely conserved among all members of the transglutaminase family. The B subunit is composed of 10 tandem repeats or glycoprotein I (GP-I) structures designated Sushi domains [7]. The A subunit constitutes the catalytic moiety and the B subunit is thought to play a role in stabilization of the A subunit. On activation by thrombin and Ca^{2+}, the A and B subunits dissociate. The A subunit is then cleaved to produce the catalytically active form of the protein, FXIIIA* [8]. FXIIIA* catalyzes the Ca^{2+}-dependent formation of glutamyl–lysine bonds between fibrin monomers, alpha$_2$-plasmin inhibitor, and fibronectin. These reactions increase the mechanical strength of the fibrin clot and its resistance to proteolytic degradation, and enhance the assembly of the extracellular matrix.

FXIII A subunit protein is encoded by the F13A gene mapping to the short arm of chromosome 6 (p24–25) and spanning more than 160 kb of genomic DNA. It consists of 15 exons encoding a mature protein of 731 amino acids [9,10]. The F13B gene is located on the long arm of chromosome 1 (q32–32.1) and contains 12 exons encoding the mature B subunit protein of 641 amino acids [11,12].

Clinical manifestations

Factor XIII (fibrin-stabilizing factor) was discovered in 1944 by K.C. Robbins [13]. Sixteen years later, the first case of severe FXIII deficiency was described in a boy with bleeding diathesis in whom the only abnormality in the clotting tests was the solubility of his clots in 5M urea [14]. Since that original description, over 250 cases have been reported from all parts of the world.

Patients with FXIII deficiency have a bleeding tendency that is usually severe. In affected individuals, the most common manifestation is bleeding from the umbilical cord after birth. Intracranial hemorrhage appears in 25% of the patients and is the leading cause of death. Superficial bruising and hematomas in subcutaneous tissue and muscle are common, and bleeding at these sites may recur if not treated. Patients may bleed around the joint after trauma, but spontaneous hemarthrosis is much less frequent than in hemophiliacs [15]. The most frequent symptom of mucosal tract bleeding (Table 56.1) is bleeding in the oral cavity (lips, tongue, gums), followed by menorrhagia and epistaxis. Minor or major surgery without replacement therapy in 84% of patients leads to postsurgical bleeding. Intraperitoneal bleeding in women of reproductive age may occur in 20% of all cases at the time of ovulation [16]. Deficiency of FXIII results in "delayed bleeding" after trauma, while primary hemostasis in individuals with these traits is normal. The delayed bleeding is caused by premature lysis of hemostatic clots.

In addition to a lifelong bleeding tendency, abnormal wound healing in affected individuals and habitual spontaneous abortion in affected females are common [15]. Wound-healing complications are probably due to fibrinolytic abnormalities and altered vascular permeability [17], while repeated abortions in affected females are caused by severe hemorrhage in the placenta [18]. Nowadays, patients are diagnosed early and treated appropriately, so the severe bleeding complications associated with the deficiency are rarely seen [19]. A minority of homozygous or, rarely, heterozygous patients suffer a very mild bleeding syndrome that comes to light only when they present with a hemorrhagic complication, e.g., after surgery [2,20,21].

Classification

The Scientific and Standardization Commmittee (SSC) in 1999 approved a new classification of FXIII deficiency at the DNA level: XIIIA deficiency (former type II deficiency) and XIIIB defi-

Table 56.1 Prevalence of bleeding symptoms in 93 Iranian patients with FXIII deficiency according to Lak *et al.* [16].

Symptoms	Percent
Mucosal tract bleeding	
Mouth bleeding	48
Menorrhagia	35
Epistaxis	32
Hematuria	10
Gastrointestinal bleeding	10
Soft-tissue bleeding	
Umbilical cord bleeding	73
Hematoma	58
Hemarthrosis	55
CNS bleeding	25
Other symptoms	
Surgical bleeding	84
Miscarriages	50

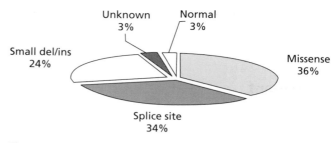

Figure 56.1 Mutation profile in 19 (38 alleles) patients with XIIIA deficiency. Eighteen patients had severe deficiency (homozygous or compound heterozygous), while one heterozygous patient (carrier) had developed mild deficiency (from ref. 26).

ciency (former type I deficiency), and a possible combined deficiency of XIIIA and XIIIB [15].

In inherited XIIIA deficiency (>95% of all cases) plasma levels of FXIIIA measured as functional activity or antigen are usually undetectable, whereas the FXIIIB subunit is reduced but detectable. No case of FXIIIA deficiency in which the plasma levels of FXIII antigen are normal but its functional activity is impaired has been described [19]

Diagnosis of FXIII deficiency

The standard laboratory clotting tests (PT, aPTT, fibrinogen level, platelet counts, bleeding time) are normal in FXIII deficiency. Laboratory diagnosis still relies on the standard clot solubility test. The stabilized clot is suspended in a solution of 1% monochloracetic acid or in a solution of 5M urea. Rapid dissolution should occur (within minutes to 1 h). Nevertheless clot solubility test is a qualitative test and is positive only if FXIII activity in the patient's plasma is zero, or very close to zero. If clot solubility in these reagents is found, it is important to perform some simple mixing experiments with normal plasma to make sure that the observed clot solubility is the result of FXIII deficiency and not due to the presence of a FXIII inhibitor [22].

The suggested diagnosis by solubility test should be confirmed by estimation of FXIII activity using one of the several quantitative assays, e.g., photometric assays (Berichrom FXIII, Dade Behring, Marburg, Germany) or incorporation assays (dansylcadaverine-casein assay). The plasma FXIII activity varies within the normal population, ranging between 53.2% and 221.3% (mean 105 ± 28.56% standard deviation) of the standard normal plasma value [23]. Notably, healthy newborns have reduced FXIII levels compared with adults. Low plasma levels, <5% of normal, are sufficient to control bleeding [24].

Quantitative assays are inaccurate at levels of FXIII activity between 0 and 10% of normal [22]. When investigating a patient with suspected inherited FXIII activity, it is useful to estimate activity in dilutions of normal plasma with both the deficient plasma and buffer [25]. The concentrations of the A and B subunits should then be determined by an immunologic technique [22]. Confirmation of the disease is the detection of causative mutation in the F13A or F13B genes.

Molecular defects

Nucleotide substitutions resulting in missense or nonsense mutations, small deletions/insertions, and splice defects do not appear to be clustered in specific regions but are scattered throughout the F13A gene. [22]. Nevertheless, the majority of missense mutations detected in the F13A gene are located in the catalytic core domain. One-third of missense mutations occur at CpG dinucleotides that are known as mutations hotspots. Splice-site mutation in intron E (IVS5–1 G → A) is the most common gene defect in European XIIIA severely deficient patients and is due to an ancient founder effect (see also Figure 56.1) [26].

To date, only five families with isolated B subunit deficiency have been described in the literature. The lack of XIIIB most likely causes instability of XIIIA and secondary XIIIA deficiency [15]. Severe XIIIB deficiency is not necessarily associated with severe phenotype [27].

The role of single nucleotide polymorphisms

The allelic variance of FXIIIA has been known for many years. Leu34 and Leu564 variants have higher FXIII specific activity, whereas the Phe204 variant results in lower FXIII specific activity [22]. Increased fibrinogen concentrations are associated with decreases in permeability, with tighter clot structures in the presence of FXIIIA Val34 alleles compared with those in the presence of Leu34 alleles [28]. A strong risk factor for myocardial infarction ($P = 0.002$) was found in carriers with combined status of prothrombin 20210A and FXIIIA Leu34 alleles [29]. The

Leu34 variant may also mitigate the severity of FXIII deficiency [22]. The Phe204 polymorphism may be associated with recurrent miscarriage [23].

Treatment

Whole blood, fresh-frozen plasma, stored plasma, and cryoprecipitate have all been used successfully in the treatment of FXIII deficiency and are adequate sources of FXIII. As quite low levels of FXIII in plasma are sufficient for control of bleeding, and the *in vivo* half-life of FXIII after infusion is long (11–14 days), prophylaxis is practicable [22].

No pharmacokinetics and tolerability differences have been observed between FXIII prepared from human plasma and that from placenta [30]. Nowadays, patients are mainly treated by plasma-derived pasteurized concentrates (Fibrogammin P, Aventis Behring). In case of mild to moderate bleeding, the recommended dosage is 20–30 IU/kg body weight monthly, while in severe bleeding (especially intracranial hemorrhages) the dosage must be increased to 50 IU/kg body weight. The half-life of FXIII is 11–14 days; thus, the bleeding risk may be increased 2–3 weeks after the last infusion. The best interval between substitutions is 14 days. Pregnant females should receive prophylactic treatment as soon as possible. In addition to prophylactic therapy, affected individuals who undergo surgery or trauma will require more intensive replacement therapy [22,31].

If FXIII concentrate is not available, fresh-frozen plasma is given prophylactically in doses of 2–3 mL/kg of body weight every 4–6 weeks. Cryoprecipitate can be administered in a dose of one bag per 10–20 kg body weight every 3–4 weeks [32].

FXIII inhibitors

In inherited FXIII deficiency, inhibitors such as antibodies to injected FXIII arise very rarely. Only two cases have been published, and no information on management of these cases is available [33,34]. Rarely, FXIII inhibitors arise *de novo*, in the course of other diseases, e.g. in systemic lupus erythematosus [35], and often in relation to chronic therapy with a variety of drugs, especially isoniazid, penicillin, and phenytoin. Bleedings in these cases may be severe and difficult to treat. Several patients have died of cerebral hemorrhage [2]. Most of the inhibitors described are antibodies (IgG immunoglobulins). Treatments attempted include immunosuppression with steroids and cyclophosphamide, administration of large doses of FXIII, and plasma immunoadsorption. Inhibitors may also appear in patients without any obvious chronic disease [36].

Acquired FXIII deficiency

This remains a doubtful entity. Low plasma levels of FXIII activity have been reported in a whole variety of conditions, predom-

Table 56.2 Diseases with acquired FXIII deficiency (from ref. 27).

Liver disorders
  Acute and chronic hepatitis
  Acute liver failure

Inflammatory bowel disorders
  Henoch–Schönlein syndrome
  Crohn's disease
  Ulcerative colitis
  Hemorrhagic gastritis

Hematologic disorders
  Leukemia
  Myeloproliferative and myelodysplastic syndrome

Disseminated intravascular coagulation (DIC)

Sepsis

Major surgical interventions

inantly leukemias, severe liver disease, and disseminated intravascular coagulation (Table 56.2). In these cases, plasma FXIII levels are usually in the range of 50–75%. Whether the low FXIII contributes to hemorrhagic complications in these diseases remains to be proven. Treatment with FXIII concentrate of patients bleeding from the small bowel in Henoch–Schönlein purpura and from the large bowel in ulcerative colitis has been reported to be effective in controlling the bleeding [37]. The benefits of such therapy in these circumstances cannot be recommended until more scientific evidence emerges in support of such an approach, and the possible mechanisms of FXIII action in these situations elucidated [22].

References

1 Tuddenham EGD, Cooper, DN. *The Molecular Genetics of Hemostasis and its Inherited Disorders.* Oxford: Oxford University Press, 1994.
2 Lorand L, Losowsky MS, Miloszewski KJ. Human factor XIII: fibrin-stabilizing factor. *Prog Hemost Thromb* 1980; 5: 245–90.
3 Schwartz ML, Pizzo SV, Hill RL, McKee PA. Human Factor XIII from plasma and platelets. Molecular weights, subunit structures, proteolytic activation, and cross-linking of fibrinogen and fibrin. *J Biol Chem* 1973; 248: 1395–407.
4 Yee VC, Pedersen LC, Le Trong I, *et al.* Three-dimensional structure of a transglutaminase: human blood coagulation factor XIII. *Proc Natl Acad Sci USA* 1994; 91: 7296–300.
5 Yee VC, Pedersen LC, Bishop PD, *et al.* Structural evidence that the activation peptide is not released upon thrombin cleavage of factor XIII. *Thromb Res* 1995; 78: 389–97.
6 Pedersen LC, Yee VC, Bishop PD, *et al.* Transglutaminase factor XIII uses proteinase-like catalytic triad to crosslink macromolecules. *Protein Sci* 1994; 3: 1131–5.
7 Ichinose A, McMullen BA, Fujikawa K, Davie EW. Amino acid sequence of the b subunit of human factor XIII, a protein composed of ten repetitive segments. *Biochemistry* 1986; 25: 4633–8.

8 Takagi T, Doolittle RF. Amino acid sequence studies on Factor XIII and the peptide released during its activation by thrombin. *Biochemistry* 1974; **13**: 750–6.

9 Board P, Coggan M, Miloszewski K. Identification of a point mutation in factor XIII A subunit deficiency. *Blood* 1992; **80**: 937–41.

10 Ichinose A, Davie EW. Primary structure of human coagulation factor XIII. *Adv Exp Med Biol* 1988; **231**: 15–27.

11 Webb GC, Coggan M, Ichinose A, Board PG. Localization of the coagulation factor XIII B subunit gene (F13B) to chromosome bands 1q31–32.1 and restriction fragment length polymorphism at the locus. *Hum Genet* 1989; **81**: 157–60.

12 Bottenus RE, Ichinose A, Davie EW. Nucleotide sequence of the gene for the b subunit of human factor XIII. *Biochemistry* 1990; **29**: 11195–209.

13 Robbins KC. A study of the conversion of the fibrinogen to fibrin. *Am J Physiol* 1944; **142**: 581–8.

14 Duckert F, Jung E, Shmerling DH. A hitherto undescribed congenital haemorrhagic diathesis probably due to fibrin stabilising factor deficiency. *Thromb Diath Haemorrh* 1960; **5**: 179–86.

15 Ichinose A. Physiopathology and regulation of factor XIII. *Thromb Haemost* 2001; **86**: 57–65.

16 Lak M, Peyvandi F, Ali Sharifian A, *et al.* Pattern of symptoms in 93 Iranian patients with severe factor XIII deficiency. *J Thromb Haemost* 2003; **1**: 1852–3.

17 Herouy Y, Hellstern MO, Vanscheidt W, *et al.* Factor XIII-mediated inhibition of fibrinolysis and venous leg ulcers. *Lancet* 2000; **355**: 1970–1.

18 Koseki-Kuno S, Yamakawa M, Dickneite G, Ichinose A. Factor XIII: A subunit-deficient mice developed severe uterine bleeding events and subsequent spontaneous miscarriages. *Blood* 2003; **102**: 4410–12.

19 Peyvandi F, Duga S, Akhavan S, Mannucci PM. Rare coagulation deficiencies. *Haemophilia*. 2002; **8**: 308–21.

20 Miloszewski KJA, Losowsky MS. Fibrin stabilisation and factor XIII deficiency. In: Francis L, ed. *Fibrinogen, Fibrin Stabilisation and Fibrinolysis*. Chichester: Ellis Horwood, 1988: 175–202.

21 Egbring R, Seitz R, Gürten GV. Bleeding complications in heterozygotes with congenital factor XIII deficiency. In: Mosseson MW, Amrani DL, Siebenlist KR, Diorio JP, eds. *Fibrinogen 3*. Amsterdam: Elsevier Science 1988: 341–446.

22 Anwar R, Miloszewski KJ. Factor XIII deficiency. *Br J Haematol* 1999; **107**: 468–84.

23 Anwar R, Gallivan L, Edmonds SD, Markham AF. Genotype/phenotype correlations for coagulation factor XIII: specific normal polymorphisms are associated with high or low factor XIII specific activity. *Blood* 1999; **93**: 897–905.

24 Walls WD, Losowsky MS. Plasma fibrin-stabilizing factor activity in acquired disease. *Br J Haematol* 1968; **15**: 327.

25 Miloszewski K, Walls WD, Losowsky MS. Absence of plasma transamidase activity in congenital deficiency of fibrin stabilizing factor (Factor 13). *Br J Haematol* 1969; **17**: 159–62.

26 Ivaskevicius V, Hilgenfeld R, Sicker T, *et al.* Mutation profiling in congenital FXIIIA deficiency: Detection of 6 novel mutations. *Transfusion Med Hemother* 2003; Suppl. 1: 29.

27 Saito M, Asakura H, Yoshida T, *et al.* A familial factor XIII subunit B deficiency. *Br J Haematol* 1990; **74**: 290–4.

28 Lim BC, Ariens RA, Carter AM, *et al.* Genetic regulation of fibrin structure and function: complex gene–environment interactions may modulate vascular risk. *Lancet* 2003; **361**: 1424–31.

29 Butt C, Zheng H, Randell E, *et al.* Combined carrier status of prothrombin 20210A and factor XIII-A Leu34 alleles as a strong risk factor for myocardial infarction: evidence of a gene–gene interaction. *Blood* 2003; **101**: 3037–41.

30 Brackmann HH, Egbring R, Ferster A, *et al.* Pharmacokinetics and tolerability of factor XIII concentrates prepared from human placenta or plasma: a crossover randomised study. *Thromb Haemost* 1995; **74**: 622–5.

31 Egbring R, Seitz R, Kroeniger A. Faktor-XIII-Erkrankungen: Klinik und Therapie. In: Mueller-Berghaus G, Poetzsch B, eds. *Hämostaseologie*, 1st edn. Berlin: Springer-Verlog, 1999: 299–302 [in German].

32 Roberts HR, Bingham MD. Other coagulation factor deficiences. In: Loscalzo J, Schafer AI, eds. *Thrombosis and Hemorrhage*, 3rd edn. Philadelphia: Lippincott Williams & Wilkins, 2003: 592–3.

33 Lorand L, Urayama T, De Kiewiet JW, Nossel HL. Diagnostic and genetic studies on fibrin-stabilizing factor with a new assay based on amine incorporation. *J Clin Invest* 1969; **48**: 1054–64.

34 Henriksson P, McDonagh J, Villa M. Type I autoimmune inhibitor of factor XIII in a patient with congenital factor XIII deficiency. *Thromb Haemost* 1983; **50**: 272.

35 Lorand L, Velasco PT, Hill JM, *et al.* Intracranial hemorrhage in systemic lupus erythematosus associated with an autoantibody against factor XIII. *Thromb Haemost* 2002; **88**: 919–23.

36 Tosetto A, Rodeghiero F, Gatto E, *et al.* An acquired hemorrhagic disorder of fibrin crosslinking due to IgG antibodies to FXIII, successfully treated with FXIII replacement and cyclophosphamide. *Am J Hematol* 1995; **48**: 34–9.

37 Lorenz R, Heimüller M, Classen M, Tornieporth N. Additional substitution of factor XIII concentrate in the treatment of ulcerative colitis.In: McDonagh J, Seitz R, Egbring R, eds. *FXIII: Second International Conference*. Marburg: FK Schattauer Verlagsgesellschaft mbH, 1993.

57 Fibrinogen

Michael Laffan

Introduction

Fibrinogen is a soluble 340-kDa dimeric plasma glycoprotein. Its principal role results from its conversion into the insoluble fibrin clot by the action of thrombin. However, it also has important interactions with platelets, endothelial cells, and cells involved in the inflammatory response.

Fibrinogen structure

Each half of the fibrinogen molecule is composed of three polypeptide chains designated Aα, Bβ, and γ. The properties of each chain are listed in Table 57.1.

The amino termini of the three pairs of polypeptide chains are held together by disulfide bridges (two γ–γ and one α–α) to form the globular E domain (see Plate 7, facing p. 212). All of the 58 cysteine residues in each six-chained molecule are incorporated into 29 disulfide bridges. From this central E domain, the two sets of three chains extend in an antiparallel fashion in a coiled coil to the D domain, which is composed of the somewhat separate globular carboxy termini of the γ and β-chains. From this domain, the alpha chain extends back in a structure called the Cα domain, with its carboxy terminus lying adjacent to the E domain.

A variant γ-chain, denoted γ', is produced by a variation in mRNA splicing that results in the replacement of amino acid residues 408–411 by a novel 20-amino-acid segment terminating at residue 427. In the process, a platelet-binding site is lost and high-affinity binding sites for factor XIII (FXIII) and thrombin gained. The γ' variant constitutes approximately 10% of plasma fibrinogen. A less common (<2%) α chain variant, "αE," is also produced by splice variation and has an additional 236 carboxy-terminal amino acids.

Genetics and regulation of synthesis

The sequences of the three fibrinogen (FG) chains exhibit a high degree of homology, suggesting that they have arisen by duplication events. This conclusion is supported by similarities in the intron–exon structure of the three genes *FGA*, *FGB*, and *FGG* and their genomic position in a contiguous cluster on chromosome 4q23–32, with Bβ in the opposite transcriptional orientation to Aα and γ. Expression of the three genes is highly coordinated,

but at the protein level production of the Bβ chain seems to be a limiting factor in humans. The liver appears to be the only major site of fibrinogen synthesis in humans, producing 1.7–5.0 g per day, sufficient to cope with a plasma half-life of 3–5 days. Synthesis of fibrinogen is up-regulated by interleukin 6 (IL-6) as part of the acute-phase reaction, but IL-1β and transforming growth factor beta (TGF-β) have the opposite effect. Several polymorphisms of the fibrinogen genes have been described, and most interest has focused on the −455G/A dimorphism in the *FGB* gene. This is estimated to account for 1–5% of the population variation in fibrinogen levels. The presence of the A allele is associated with a 0.15 g/L rise in fibrinogen level [1]. Other studies have detected this effect only in smokers or in those with coronary artery disease, suggesting a dynamic effect of the allele [2,3].

Plasma fibrinogen is a heterogeneous pool resulting from differential splicing of mRNA transcripts (Table 57.1) and from partial cleavage in plasma by thrombin and plasmin. Fibrinogen is also found in platelets, but the bulk of this is derived from glycoprotein IIb–IIIa-mediated endocytosis of plasma fibrinogen, which is then stored in alpha granules, rather than from synthesis by megakaryocytes. Thus, platelet fibrinogen is absent in severe forms of Glanzmann's thrombasthenia [4,5]

Fibrin clot formation

Conversion of fibrinogen into the insoluble fibrin clot can be considered to take place in three stages:
1 thrombin cleavage of fibrinopeptides A and B;
2 assembly of insoluble fibrin monomers into protofibrils and fibers;
3 cross-linking by FXIII.

The initiating event in fibrin formation is the cleavage of the Aα Arg14–Gly15 bond by thrombin, releasing fibrinopeptide A (FPA). This exposes an "A" site in the E domain, which can then bind to a pre-existing "a" site on the γ chain of another molecule's D domain. Thus begins a staggered assembly of half-overlapping fibrin monomers, which extends to form a double-stranded protofibril (Figure 57.1). At this stage, FXIII activation by thrombin has already occurred and cross-linking has begun (see below).

Cleavage of fibrinopeptide B (FPB) follows that of FPA. However, this sequential release of FPA and then FPB reflects the differing affinity of thrombin for these two substrates rather than a change in conformation after FPA release [6]. Fibrin polymer-

332

Table 57.1 Characteristics of the fibrinogen polypeptides and their variants.

Chain	Aα	Bβ	γ
Amino acid residues	610	461	411
Molecular weight	66 500	52 000	46 500
Variants (% total)	AαE +296aa (2%)		γ′ +408–427 (10%)
Thrombin cleavage	R16-17G	R14–15G	–
Cys residues	8	11	10
Factor XIII cross-link residues (Gln acceptor, Lys donor)	Gln: 221, 237, 328, 366 Lys: 208, 219, 224, 418, 427, 429, 446, 448, 508, 539, 556, 580, 583, 601, 606	None	Gln: 398, 399 Lys: 406
Glycosylation sites	AE 667	Bβ364	γ52
RGDF motif	95–98		
RGDS motif	572–575		
Dodecapeptide (platelet binding)			400–411

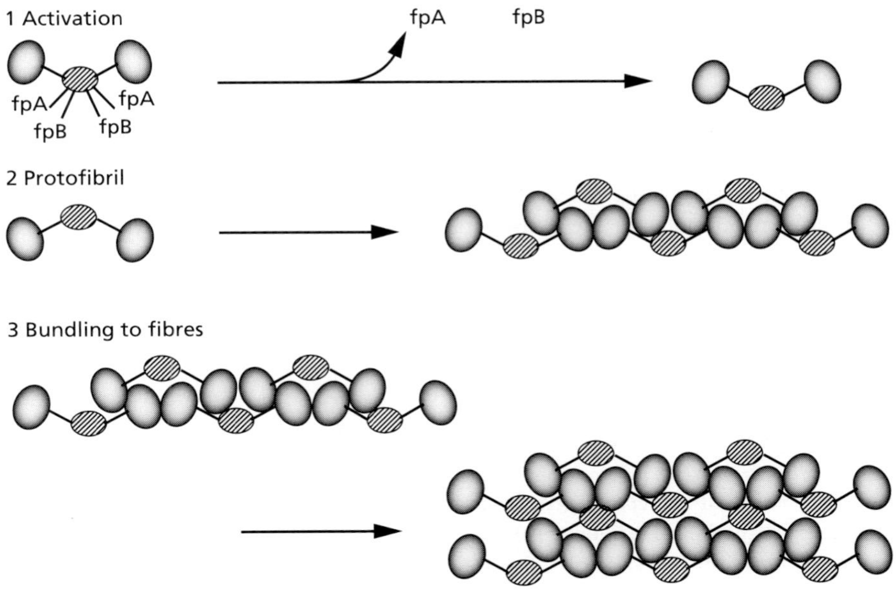

Figure 57.1 A schematic representation of the conversion of fibrinogen to a fibrin clot by thrombin. Thrombin cleavage of fibrinopeptide A (amino acids 1–16 of the Aα-chain) followed by cleavage of fibrinopeptide B (amino acids 1–14 of the Bβ-chain) leads to formation of fibrin monomers. Fibrin monomers then self-assemble in a half-staggered linear overlap to form protofibrils. Protofibril formation is governed by the interaction of the thrombin exposed 'a' site on the E domain with 'A' site on the D domain. The protofibrils are then bundled into fibrin fibres through interaction of the 'b' site on the E domain with the 'B' site located on the D domain (from Roberts: *Br J Haematol* 2001; **114**: 24–57).

ization facilitates FPB cleavage, but it remains incomplete, with only 33% of the potential FPB being released. FPB release exposes a "B" site in the E domain, which binds to a corresponding "b" site on the carboxy terminus of a β-chain in an adjacent molecule. This facilitates lateral assembly of thick fibers. FPB cleavage also releases the Cα domain from its noncovalent association with the E domain, freeing it to participate in lateral interactions with other Cα domains [7]. Nonetheless, FPA release appears to be sufficient for the entire process of clot formation, although it is enhanced by FPB removal and mutations of the FPB cleavage site result in prolonged clotting times and reduced

functional fibrinogen assay results. FPB cleavage alone (e.g., by Venzyme [8]) is not sufficient to induce fibrin clot formation under normal conditions.

Lateral association of fibrils leads to formation of thick fiber bundles. Convergence of two or three double-stranded fibrils results in tetra- and trimolecular branch points, effectively joining the nascent fibers and producing a complex three-dimensional network [9].

Formation of fibrin also accelerates the formation of activated FXIII. In plasma, fibrinogen functions as a carrier protein for The a_2b_2 FXIII tetramer, which appears to bind specifically to the γ′ chains. Fibrin polymer formation accelerates FXIII cleavage, but the a subunit is not active until the activation peptide has been released and it has dissociated from the b subunit. One or both of these dissociation events are facilitated by binding of activated FXIII to the γ′ region of fibrin. The active a subunit released then binds to fibrin in the Aα 242–424 region. Thus, fibrin formed from γ′ containing fibrinogen is more extensively cross-linked and γ′ levels are a risk factor for coronary heart disease [10]. Platelet FXIII comprises the a units only and is not dependent on fibrin for activation.

FXIII-mediated cross-linking begins by joining D domains in an end-to-end or longitudinal fashion via reciprocal γGln398–γLys406 links [11]. Side-to-side links between γ-chains then follow. Cross-linking between alpha chains occurs more slowly but at multiple sites (Table 57.1). "α" chain cross-linking is important in blocking plasmin access to the coiled coil regions linking D and E domains and thus preventing breakdown of the fibrin clot. Finally, some cross-linking between α- and γ-chains takes place [12].

At the same time, fibrin formation exposes binding sites for tissue plasminogen activator (tPA) and plasminogen. High-affinity sites for both tPA and plasminogen are exposed in the Aα392–610 segment (Cα) and lower-affinity sites on Aα 148–160 and γ312–324 (D domain). Adjacent binding of tPA and plasminogen greatly reduces the K_m and increases the V_{max} for the activation reaction [13]. The plasmin thus activated then cleaves fibrin, exposing further carboxy-terminal lysine residues of Cα, allowing more plasminogen and tPA to bind, accelerating and targeting the fibrinolytic system. This process is now known to be in competition with the activity of TAFI (thrombin-activatable fibrinolysis inhibitor), which selectively removes these lysine residues and thus limits fibrinolysis. FXIII also cross-links antiplasmin to Lys303 in the α-chain while retaining its antiplasmin activity.

Fibrinogen interaction with other cells

In addition to its self-associating properties, fibrin also has other important interactions. Fibrinogen has three potential integrin-binding motifs (Table 57.1), all of which appear to be important in different aspects of platelet binding. The γ-terminal sequence is involved in platelet adherence and aggregation whereas the two α-chain RGD sequences are important in promoting clot retraction [14]. Mice with fibrinogen lacking the terminal γ-chain sequence have a severe bleeding tendency [14]. Fibrinogen binding to endothelial cell integrins is mediated by the Aα RGD sequence at 572–574 [15]. However, fibrin-specific binding to endothelial cells is mediated by the β15–42 region exposed by thrombin cleavage. Fibrin or fibrin peptide interaction with endothelial cells results in numerous changes, including release of Weibel–Palade bodies, prostacyclin and tPA, and monolayer disruption [16–18]. Finally, fibrinogen is important in mediating adherence and migration of activated monocytes and neutrophils through endothelium [19].

Measuring fibrinogen

An international standard for fibrinogen assays has been prepared [20]. The normal plasma concentration of fibrinogen is approximately 1.7–4.0 g/L when measured by clotting assays and slightly higher (2.5–6.0 g/L) by immunoassay. Local normal ranges should be determined. The ability to detect abnormalities of fibrinogen depends critically on the assay methods used, and guidelines for fibrinogen assays have recently been published in the UK [21]. A deficiency or abnormality of fibrinogen may be first suspected from prolongation of clotting times. In afibrinogenemia, all the clotting times will be prolonged, but in less marked deficiency or the presence of a dysfibrinogenemia, it may be only the thrombin time that is prolonged.

Although the international reference method for fibrinogen measurement has traditionally been by the total clottable fibrinogen method, this is not practical for routine laboratory use. In routine hospital practice, fibrinogen is usually assayed by a functional (clotting) assay, either that of Clauss or as a measure derived from the optical changes occurring during the prothrombin time performed on an automated analyzer (derived fibrinogen: PT-Fg). In the Clauss assay [22], a high concentration of thrombin (approx 100 units) is used to clot a diluted aliquot of patient plasma. The clotting time is then compared with a standard curve prepared using dilutions of a reference plasma. When automated, the assay is quite reproducible (CV 3–9%) and the combination of dilution and high thrombin concentration makes it relatively insensitive to the effect of heparin. It is, however, sensitive to high concentrations of fibrin(ogen) degradation products and some kits contain agents to overcome these effects.

The PT-Fg assay generally results in a slightly higher estimation of fibrinogen than the Clauss assay. This is particularly so when coagulation is deranged for some reason or an abnormal fibrinogen is present. The PT-Fg is therefore not recommended [21], although it remains in widespread use as a result of its low cost and convenience. Fibrinogen can also be assayed using immunologic techniques, but this requires the use of monoclonal antibodies to avoid interference from degraded and partially degraded fibrinogen fragments. The performance of different fibrinogen assays has been reviewed [23].

When a low fibrinogen is determined by clotting assay then the presence of a dys- or hypofibrinogen can be resolved by performing a physicochemical or immunologic assay. In practice, a simple (gravimetric) clot weight determination is usually sufficient to demonstrate the discrepancy between function and protein characteristic of a dysfibrinogenemia [23].

Afibrinogenemia

The complete absence of fibrinogen, *afibrinogenemia*, is accompanied by a clinical syndrome that is surprisingly mild and generally less severe than hemophilia (Table 57.2) [24]. An early

Table 57.2 Relative frequency of bleeding symptoms in 55 patients with afibrinogenemia compared with 100 patients with severe hemophilia A (factor VIII 1%) (from ref. 24).

Symptom	In afibrinogenemia (%)	In hemophilia A (%)
Umbilical cord bleeding	45/55 (85)	0
Central nervous system bleeding	3/55 (10)	4/100 (4)
Hemarthrosis	30/55 (54)	86/100 (86)
Muscle hematoma	40/55 (72)	93/100 (93)
Gastrointestinal bleeding	0	10/100 (10)
Urinary tract bleeding	0	12/100 (12)
Epistaxis	40/55 (72)	50/100 (50)
Menorrhagia	14/20 (70)	Not applicable
Oral cavity bleeding	40/55 (72)	55/100 (55)
Postoperative bleeding	23/55 (40)	36/100 (36)
Thrombotic symptoms	2/55 (4)	0

and characteristic feature is umbilical cord bleeding. Thereafter, muscle bleeds and hemarthroses are relatively frequent but rarely result in disability. Unlike hemophilia, epistaxis is also common (72%) and spontaneous splenic rupture is reported. Bleeding is sometimes followed by poor wound healing [24]. In mice rendered afibrinogenemic by disruption of the FGA gene, all three chains are absent from plasma and a similar phenotype is seen: bleeding begins shortly after birth in approximately 30% but is not usually severe and the mice survive into maturity [25].

In affected women, menorrhagia is common and recurrent abortion is seen, presumed to reflect poor implantation, as is also observed in the fibrinogen-deficient mice. Afibrinogenemic mice are still capable of developing atheromatous plaques although murine plaques are not as complex as those in humans [26].

Remarkably, spontaneous thrombosis (venous and arterial) has been reported in patients with afibrinogenemia. A plausible explanation is that an increase in free thrombin results from the loss of the thrombin-binding capacity of fibrin and that this results in excessive platelet activation [27].

Genetics and molecular biology

Inheritance of afibrinogenemia is autosomal recessive and the disorder is thus more common in populations favoring consanguineous marriages. The estimated frequency in Europe is 1 in 10^6. Obligate heterozygotes have plasma fibrinogen levels of approximately half normal but are asymptomatic. The majority of cases appear to arise from mutations in the FGA gene, in particular a recurrent 11-kb deletion probably resulting from a nonhomologous recombination mediated by 7-bp (basepair) direct repeats. However, the most common recurrent mutation occurs at the donor splice site of FGA intron 4 [28]. A number of other truncating mutations in FGA, as well as FGB and FGG, are also described. Surprisingly, a small number of missense mutations also cause afibrinogenemia as a result of intracellular retention of the abnormal protein [29].

Therapy

The basis of therapy is replacement of fibrinogen. Historically, the principal source has been cryoprecipitate, which contains approximately 1.5 g fibrinogen per unit. Plasma-derived and virally inactivated concentrates are available and are the recommended choice but are not yet licensed. A level of 1 g/L is regarded as sufficiently hemostatic to arrest bleeding (20–40 mg/kg of fibrinogen concentrate). Bleeding problems may be sufficient to warrant prophylactic treatment and the long half-life of fibrinogen allows prophylactic infusions of fibrinogen concentrate or cryoprecipitate to be given weekly. In one report, a dose of 100 mg/kg/week was sufficient to maintain a trough level of 0.5 g/L, which prevented recurrence of hemorrhage [30]. However, in the context of primary prophylaxis, even lower levels may be effective in preventing bleeding and infusions every 2–4 weeks have been reported as successful [31]. Menorrhagia may be controlled by use of the combined oral contraceptive pill. Replacement therapy is not usually complicated by the development of antifibrinogen antibodies, but these have been reported [32].

Prophylactic therapy appears necessary for successful completion of pregnancy: fibrinogen replacement must be begun before 5 weeks' gestation to prevent abortion and maintained at >1.0 g/L throughout the pregnancy. Fibrinogen consumption increases markedly as gestation progresses and the amount and frequency of fibrinogen infusion must be increased accordingly. A level of >1.5 g/L is recommended for delivery [33].

Dysfibrinogenemia

Dysfibrinogens are usually inherited in an autosomal dominant fashion but a few cases are found as recessives with asymptomatic heterozygotes. Dysfibrinogen generally arises from missense mutations in any of the three FG genes, but small deletions or insertions may also be responsible and the clinical phenotype is correspondingly diverse. A database of mutations responsible is available at www.geht.org/databaseang/fibrinogen/. The diagnosis is suspected from prolonged coagulation times with low fibrinogen by functional assay. Determination of a discrepantly high fibrinogen protein concentration confirms the presence of a dysfibrinogen. Rare examples where the clotting times are shortened or where the functional and immunologic assays are concordant have been described.

The majority of dysfibrinogens are found incidentally and have no associated phenotype (55%), whereas 20% are associated with thrombosis and 25% with hemorrhage. A few cases have been reported with both hemorrhagic and thrombotic problems (e.g., Marburg, Bethesda III, and Baltimore I). Prophylactic anticoagulation or prophylactic replacement therapy is rarely required and is not warranted on the basis of the diagnosis alone. Studies of dysfibrinogens have been very informative in unraveling the structure–function relationships of fibrinogen [34]

Dysfibrinogens associated with thrombosis

Although usually detected as a result of a prolonged thrombin clotting time, a dysfibrinogen is reported in approximately 0.8% of patients with thrombosis: rarer than the anticoagulant deficiencies but, unlike them, associated with both venous and arterial events, although venous are more common. The rarity of each individual dysfibrinogen makes it difficult to be certain there is a causal relationship underlying the association, but a survey conducted by the ISTH in 1995 [35] concluded that it was genuine: an increased incidence of thrombosis was found in affected relatives of the dysfibrinogenemia proband but in none of 88 unaffected relatives. As with other thrombophilic traits, women affected with dysfibrinogenemia appear to suffer an increased rate of pregnancy complications [35]. It is postulated that dysfibrinogens may increase the risk of thrombosis either by producing clots that are more resistant to fibrinolysis or by failing to sequester normal amounts of thrombin, resulting in increased amounts of the free enzyme. Several mutations at or close to the thrombin cleavage sites have been reported in association with thrombosis (Marburg, Malmö, New York, and Naples), presumably via the latter mechanism [36]. The best-described association with thrombosis is of the fibrinogen Dusart Arg554Cys (also called Paris V and Chapel Hill III) as it has occurred several times [37]. The new Cys residue cross-links with albumin, resulting in formation of thin but plasmin-resistant fibrin fibers [38]. Similar phenomena have been reported in other dysfibrinogens with free thiol groups [39,40]. In one case, that of fibrinogen Oslo I [41], the dysfibrinogen was associated with thrombosis, shortened clotting times, and enhanced platelet activation.

Dysfibrinogens associated with bleeding

Some dysfibrinogens, particularly those with fibrinogen levels <1 g/L, are associated with an increased frequency of bleeding. The mechanisms are diverse, e.g., fibrinogen Bremen (Gly17Val) results in delayed polymerization and symptomatic bleeding as a result of impaired interaction of the "A" and "a" sites [42]. Many other examples can be found in the database. The symptoms are usually mild and may be associated with wound dehiscence. For those patients with a history of bleeding associated with a dysfibrinogen or hypofibrinogen, tranexamic acid or replacement therapy may be needed as for afibrinogenemia.

Dysfibrinogens associated with amyloidosis

Several mutations in the Aα chain gene have been found to cause hereditary renal amyloidosis (R554L, E526V, and 4904delG and 4897delT, both of which lead to premature termination at codon 548). The fibrinogen behaves normally from a coagulation point of view and cannot be detected by this means. The role of fibrinogen was originally revealed by sequence analysis of the amyloid deposits [43]. The only curative approach appears to be liver transplantation. [44]

Acquired dysfibrinogenemia

An acquired abnormality of fibrinogen typically arises in association with liver disease, especially hepatocellular carcinoma, owing to an increased number of sialic acid residues. The thrombin time is prolonged but the Clauss fibrinogen assay is normal or more frequently elevated. This is not associated with any bleeding tendency and can be ignored. A similar abnormality of fibrinogen is seen in neonates, reflecting hepatic immaturity. Occasionally, laboratory results simulating the presence of a dysfibrinogenemia may be produced by a paraprotein or auto-antibody interfering with fibrin polymerization. Although the fibrinogen may in fact be normal, this can nonetheless result in a hemorrhagic tendency.

References

1 Tybjaerg-Hansen A, Agerholm-Larsen B, Humphries SE, *et al*. A common mutation (G-455 → A) in the beta-fibrinogen promoter is an independent predictor of plasma fibrinogen, but not of ischemic heart disease. A study of 9127 individuals based on the Copenhagen City Heart Study. *J Clin Invest* 1997; **99**: 3034–9.

2 Laffan MA. Fibrinogen polymorphisms and disease. *Eur Heart J* 2001; **22**: 2224–6.

3 Humphries SE, Henry JA, Montgomery HE. Gene–environment interaction in the determination of levels of haemostatic variables involved in thrombosis and fibrinolysis. *Blood Coagul Fibrinol* 1999; **10**: S17–21.

4 Coller BS, Seligsohn U, West SM, *et al*. Platelet fibrinogen and vitronectin in Glanzmann thrombasthenia: evidence consistent with specific roles for glycoprotein IIb/IIIA and alpha v beta 3 integrins in platelet protein trafficking. *Blood* 1991; **78**: 2603–10.

5 Belloc F, Heilmann E, Combrie R, *et al*. Protein synthesis and storage in human platelets: a defective storage of fibrinogen in platelets in Glanzmann's thrombasthenia. *Biochim Biophys Acta* 1987; **925**: 218–25.

6 Mullin JL, Gorkun OV, Binnie CG, Lord ST. Recombinant fibrinogen studies reveal that thrombin specificity dictates order of fibrinopeptide release. *J Biol Chem* 2000; **275**: 25239–46.

7 Gorkun OV, Veklich YI, Medved LV, *et al*. Role of the alpha C domains of fibrin in clot formation. *Biochemistry* 1994; **33**: 6986–97.

8 Shainoff JR, Dardik BN. Fibrinopeptide B in fibrin assembly and

metabolism: physiologic significance in delayed release of the peptide. *Ann NY Acad Sciences* 1983; **408**: 254–68.

9 Mosesson MW. Fibrinogen and fibrin polymerization: appraisal of the binding events that accompany fibrin generation and fibrin clot assembly. *Blood Coagul Fibrinol* 1997; **8**: 257–67.

10 Lovely RS, Falls LA, Al-Mondhiry HA, *et al*. Association of gammaA/gamma' fibrinogen levels and coronary artery disease. *Thromb Haemost* 2002; **88**: 26–31.

11 Spraggon G, Everse SJ, Doolittle RF. Crystal structures of fragment D from human fibrinogen and its crosslinked counterpart from fibrin [erratum appears in *Nature* 1997; **390**: 315]. *Nature* 1997; **389**: 455–62.

12 Shainoff JR, Urbanic DA, DiBello PM. Immunoelectrophoretic characterizations of the cross-linking of fibrinogen and fibrin by factor XIIIa and tissue transglutaminase. Identification of a rapid mode of hybrid alpha-/gamma-chain cross-linking that is promoted by the gamma-chain cross-linking. *J Biol Chem* 1991; **266**: 6429–37.

13 Medved L, Nieuwenhuizen W. Molecular mechanisms of initiation of fibrinolysis by fibrin. *Thromb Haemost* 2003; **89**: 409–19.

14 Holmback K, Danton MJ, Suh TT, *et al*. Impaired platelet aggregation and sustained bleeding in mice lacking the fibrinogen motif bound by integrin alpha IIb beta 3. *EMBO J* 1996; **15**: 5760–71.

15 Suehiro K, Gailit J, Plow EF. Fibrinogen is a ligand for integrin alpha5beta1 on endothelial cells. *J Biol Chem* 1997; **272**: 5360–6.

16 Andersson RG, Saldeen K, Saldeen T. A fibrin(ogen) derived pentapeptide induces vasodilation, prostacyclin release and an increase in cyclic AMP. *Thromb Res* 1983; **30**: 213–18.

17 Gerdin B, Lindeberg G, Ragnarsson U, *et al*. Structural requirements for microvascular permeability-increasing ability of peptides. Studies on analogues of a fibrinogen pentapeptide fragment. *Biochim Biophys Acta* 1983; **757**: 366–70.

18 Fukao H, Matsumoto H, Ueshima S, *et al*. Effects of fibrin on the secretion of plasminogen activator inhibitor-1 from endothelial cells and on protein kinase C. *Life Sci* 1995; **57**: 1267–76.

19 Languino LR, Duperray A, Joganic KJ, *et al*. Regulation of leukocyte–endothelium interaction and leukocyte transendothelial migration by intercellular adhesion molecule 1-fibrinogen recognition. *Proc Natl Acad Sci USA* 1995; **92**: 1505–9.

20 Whitton CM, Sands D, Hubbard AR, Gaffney PJ. A collaborative study to establish the 2nd International Standard for Fibrinogen, Plasma. *Thromb Haemost* 2000; **84**: 258–62.

21 Mackie IJ, Kitchen S, Machin SJ, *et al*. Guidelines on fibrinogen assays. *Br J Haematol* 2003; **121**: 396–404.

22 de Maat MM, Lowe GDO, Haverkate F. Fibrinogen. In: Jespersen J, Bertina R, Haverkate F, eds. *Laboratory Techniques in Thrombosis. A Manual*. Dordrecht: Kluwer Academic Publishers; 1999: 79–88.

23 Mackie J, Lawrie AS, Kitchen S, *et al*. A performance evaluation of commercial fibrinogen reference preparations and assays for Clauss and PT-derived fibrinogen. *Thromb Haemost* 2002; **87**: 997–1005.

24 Lak M, Keihani M, Elahi F, *et al*. Bleeding and thrombosis in 55 patients with inherited afibrinogenaemia. *Br J Haematol* 1999; **107**: 204–6.

25 Suh TT, Holmback K, Jensen NJ, *et al*. Resolution of spontaneous bleeding events but failure of pregnancy in fibrinogen-deficient mice. *Genes Dev* 1995; **9**: 2020–33.

26 Xiao Q, Danton MJ, Witte DP, *et al*. Fibrinogen deficiency is compatible with the development of atherosclerosis in mice. *J Clin Invest* 1998; **101**: 1184–94.

27 Chafa O, Chellali T, Sternberg C, *et al*. Severe hypofibrinogenemia associated with bilateral ischemic necrosis of toes and fingers. *Blood Coagul Fibrinol* 1995; **6**: 549–52.

28 Neerman-Arbez M. The molecular basis of inherited afibrinogenaemia. *Thromb Haemost* 2001; **86**: 154–63.

29 Duga S, Asselta R, Santagostino E, *et al*. Missense mutations in the human beta fibrinogen gene cause congenital afibrinogenemia by impairing fibrinogen secretion. *Blood* 2000; **95**: 1336–41.

30 Parameswaran R, Dickinson JP, de Lord S, *et al*. Spontaneous intracranial bleeding in two patients with congenital afibrinogenaemia and the role of replacement therapy. *Haemophilia* 2000; **6**: 705–8.

31 Neerman-Arbez M, Honsberger A, Antonarakis SE, Morris MA. Deletion of the fibrinogen [correction of fibrogen] alpha-chain gene (FGA) causes congenital afibrogenemia [erratum appears in *J Clin Invest* 1999; **103**: 759]. *J Clin Invest* 1999; **103**: 215–18.

32 Ra'anani P, Levi Y, Varon D, *et al*. Congenital afibrinogenemia with bleeding, bone cysts and antibodies to fibrinogen. *Harefuah* 1991; **121**: 291–3.

33 Kobayashi T, Kanayama N, Tokunaga N, *et al*. Prenatal and peripartum management of congenital afibrinogenaemia. *Br J Haematol* 2000; **109**: 364–6.

34 Matsuda M, Sugo T, Yoshida N, *et al*. Structure and function of fibrinogen: insights from dysfibrinogens. *Thromb Haemost* 1999; **82**: 283–90.

35 Haverkate F, Samama M. Familial dysfibrinogenemia and thrombophilia. Report on a study of the SSC Subcommittee on Fibrinogen. *Thromb Haemost* 1995; **73**: 151–61.

36 Koopman J, Haverkate F, Lord ST, *et al*. Molecular basis of fibrinogen Naples associated with defective thrombin binding and thrombophilia. Homozygous substitution of B beta 68 Ala–Thr. *J Clin Invest* 1992; **90**: 238–44.

37 Wada Y, Lord ST. A correlation between thrombotic disease and a specific fibrinogen abnormality (A alpha 554 Arg → Cys) in two unrelated kindred, Dusart and Chapel Hill III. *Blood* 1994; **84**: 3709–14.

38 Koopman J, Haverkate F, Grimbergen J, *et al*. Molecular basis for fibrinogen Dusart (A alpha 554 Arg → Cys) and its association with abnormal fibrin polymerization and thrombophilia. *J Clin Invest* 1993; **91**: 1637–43.

39 Vakalopoulou S, Mille-Baker B, Mumford A, Manning R, Laffan M. Fibrinogen Bbeta14 Arg → Cys: further evidence for a role in thrombosis. *Blood Coagul Fibrinol* 1999; **10**: 403–8.

40 Koopman J, Haverkate F, Grimbergen J, *et al*. Abnormal fibrinogens Ijmuiden (B beta Arg → Cys) and Nijmegen (B beta Arg44 → Cys) form disulfide-linked fibrinogen-albumin complexes. *Proc Natl Acad USA* 1992; **89**: 3478–82.

41 Egeberg O. Inherited fibrinogen abnormality causing thrombophilia. *Thromb Diathesis Haemorrhagica* 1967; **17**: 176–87.

42 Wada Y, Niwa K, Maekawa H, *et al*. A new type of congenital dysfibrinogen, fibrinogen Bremen, with an A alpha Gly-17 to Val substitution associated with hemorrhagic diathesis and delayed wound healing. *Thromb Haemost* 1993; **70**: 397–403.

43 Hamidi Asl L, Liepnieks JJ, Uemichi T, *et al*. Renal amyloidosis with a frame shift mutation in fibrinogen aalpha-chain gene producing a novel amyloid protein. *Blood* 1997; **90**: 4799–805.

44 Gillmore JD, Booth DR, Rela M, *et al*. Curative hepatorenal transplantation in systemic amyloidosis caused by the Glu526Val fibrinogen alpha-chain variant in an English family. *Q J Med* 2000; **93**: 269–75.

58 Miscellaneous rare bleeding disorders

Amy Shapiro and Rekha Parameswaran

Congenital bleeding disorders encompass both quantitative and qualitative abnormalities of proteins regulating the procoagulant and fibrinolytic pathways, platelets, and blood vessels (Table 58.1). There is often a history of recurrent episodes of bleeding beginning in early childhood, which may include abnormal bruising, petechiae, epistaxis, menorrhagia, and prolonged bleeding after trauma, tooth extraction, and surgical procedures. Characteristic patterns of bleeding may point to the affected area of coagulation, e.g., rebleeding after achieving initial hemostasis may suggest defects in the fibrinolytic pathway (Table 58.2). The severity of the clinical phenotype will vary depending on the area of coagulation affected and the level of deficiency — both determined by the mutation, which often results from a compound heterozygous or homozygous defect. The true incidence of these rare bleeding disorders is not well established owing to lack of a centralized national/international reporting mechanism. This is confounded by the difficulty in establishing the diagnosis.

Deficiencies within the fibrinolytic system

Inhibition of fibrinolysis by specific protease inhibitors occurs at the level of plasminogen activators via plasminogen activator inhibitors, and at the level of plasmin via α_2-antiplasmin. Deficiencies of plasminogen activator inhibitor 1 (PAI-1) and α_2-antiplasmin are not associated with abnormalities of common screening coagulation tests (Table 58.3), yet can manifest significant hemorrhagic complications.

Plasminogen activator inhibitor-1 (PAI-1) deficiency

PAI-1 is the principal inhibitor of urokinase-type plasminogen activator (uPA) and tissue-type plasminogen activator (tPA), and plays an important role in the regulation of extracellular matrix remodeling and in the regulation of the fibrinolytic system. In blood, PAI-1 is bound to the adhesion protein vitronectin and is associated with vitronectin in fibrin clots [1]. Ginsberg et al. [2] assigned the PAI-1 gene to human chromosome 7 and by nucleotide sequence analysis found that the PAI-1 cDNA encodes a protein containing 402 amino acids with a predicted nonglycosylated molecular mass of 45 kDa. Klinger et al. [3] localized it to 7q21.3-q22 by *in situ* hybridization .

PAI-1 deficiency leads to excessive fibrinolytic activity with subsequent hemorrhagic manifestations. Congenital PAI-1 deficiency is an extremely rare autosomal recessive disorder. In a 9-year-old girl from an Old Order Amish community, Fay et al. [4] identified homozygosity for a frameshift mutation: a dinucleotide (TA) insertion in exon 4 resulting in the synthesis of a truncated, nonfunctional protein. The TA insertion represented a duplication of nucleotides 4975 and 4976. The mature PAI-1 protein has 379 amino acids. The mutation caused a shift in the reading frame after the codon for amino acid 210, resulting in a new stop codon (TGA) 45 codons into the aberrant reading frame. The predicted protein product lacked the 169 C-terminal amino acids of the wild-type protein, including the active center, Arg346–Met347. The patient had several episodes of major hemorrhage, all in response to trauma or surgery.

Fay et al. [5] have described more comprehensively the phenotype associated with PAI-1 deficiency by characterizing multiple individuals in this Old Order Amish kindred and by prospectively following affected individuals. Allele-specific oligonucleotide hybridization was used to genotype individuals, and serum PAI-1 antigen was measured by enzyme-linked immunosorbent assay. Nineteen individuals who were heterozygous for the null allele and seven homozygotes with complete deficiency were described. Abnormal bleeding was noted only in homozygous affected individuals. Fibrinolysis inhibitors, including epsilon-aminocaproic acid and tranexamic acid (Table 58.4), were effective in treating and preventing bleeding episodes. Other than abnormal bleeding, no significant developmental or other abnormalities were observed in homozygotes.

Clinical manifestations of PAI-1 deficiency are restricted to abnormal bleeding, which can be observed after injury or surgery in homozygous or compound heterozygous affected individuals. Heterozygous PAI-1 deficiency has not been associated with abnormal bleeding, even after trauma or surgery. Levels of PAI-1 in heterozygotes are approximately 50% of those in unaffected individuals.

Accurate diagnosis is important as this disorder is effectively managed with fibrinolytic inhibitors, thereby decreasing the use of blood product support and risk of uncontrolled hemorrhage. Unless the genetic defect leads to complete absence of the protein, as in the cases reported by Fay et al., the diagnosis of PAI-1 deficiency is difficult and at times is assumed rather than proven. If the defect results in a dysproteinemic state, PAI-1 antigen levels will be detected; however, the activity assay,

Table 58.1 Rare bleeding disorders.

Factor	PAI-1	α_2-Antiplasmin	Prekallikrein	High-molecular-weight kininogen
Synonyms			Fletcher factor	Fitzgerald factor Williams factor Flaujeac factor
Gene map locus	7q21.3–q22	17pter-p12	4q35	3q27
Molecular weight (daltons)	52 000	70 000	107 000	120 000
Normal plasma concentration (μg/mL)	0.01	60	50	70
Mode of inheritance	Autosomal recessive	Autosomal recessive	Autosomal recessive	Autosomal recessive
Biochemical features	Glycoprotein serpin synthesized in liver	Single-chain glycoprotein synthesized in liver	Single-chain serine protease	Single-chain cofactor
Clinical features	Bleeding in homozygotes; morphologic/developmental abnormalities absent	Bleeding in homozygotes	No clinical abnormalities	No clinical abnormalities
Prophylaxis and treatment	Antifibrinolytics Fresh-frozen plasma (FFP) as required	Antifibrinolytics FFP as required	None required	None required

Table 58.2 Bleeding patterns of rare deficiencies.

	Deficiency		
Age	PAI-1	α_2-Antiplasmin	Platelet function disorders
Neonates	Intracranial hemorrhage possible	Intracranial hemorrhage in full-term neonates Bleeding from umbilical cord stump	Bruising at birth; intracranial hemorrhage possible
Children	Bleeding with surgery, injury including hemarthroses	Spontaneous hemarthroses Bleeding with injury or surgery	Epistaxis Easy bruising Oropharyngeal and gastrointestinal bleeds Bleeding with injury or surgery
Adolescents	Menorrhagia Bleeding with surgery, injury including hemarthroses	Intramedullary hematomas of long bones Bleeding with injury or surgery	Oropharyngeal and gastrointestinal bleeds Bleeding with injury or surgery
Adults	Bleeding with surgery or trauma	Intramedullary hematomas of long bones	Oropharyngeal and gastrointestinal bleeds Bleeding with injury or surgery
All ages	Bleeding with surgery and injury	Surgical bleeding Soft-tissue and muscle bleeds Epistaxis Menorrhagia	Oropharyngeal and gastrointestinal bleeds Bleeding with surgery and injury

with normal ranges that are reported to start at zero, are nondiscriminatory for a deficiency. The true incidence of P AI-1 deficiency is therefore unknown and unable to be determined at this time due to the inadequate present state of laboratory testing for this deficiency. Therefore, both PAI-1 antigen and activity should be measured to screen individuals for possible PAI-1 deficiency, and a clinical trial of antifibrinolytic agents should be considered if there is a high index of suspicion and all other known bleeding disorders are excluded.

PAI-1 deficiency most often is characterized as a moderate bleeding disorder with bleeding episodes most commonly due to some precipitating event or injury. A spectrum of bleeding patterns has been observed, including intracranial and joint bleeding after mild trauma, delayed surgical bleeding, severe menstrual bleeding, and frequent bruising. Though bleeding occurs only secondary to injury and surgery, these episodes may be life-threatening and require prompt intervention for adequate resolution. Bleeding episodes may be effectively treated with a 5- to 7-day course of oral tranexamic acid or epsilon-aminocaproic acid, but the exact duration of treatment depends upon the episode experienced. Persistent excessive menorrhagia may be managed with hormonal suppression and long-term prophylactic antifibrinolytic therapy if

Table 58.3 Laboratory tests in rare disorders.

Test	PAI-1	α₂-Antiplasmin	Prekallikrein	High-molecular-weight kininogen	Platelet disorders	Vascular disorders	Disseminated intermittent coagulation
Platelet count	Normal	Normal	Normal	Normal	Normal	Normal	Decreased
Platelet function analyzer-100	Normal	Normal	Normal	Normal	Abnormal	Normal	Normal
Prothrombin time (PT)	Normal	Normal	Normal	Normal	Normal	Normal	Prolonged
Activated partial thromboplastin time (aPTT)	Normal	Normal	Markedly prolonged and corrects with mixing studies	Markedly prolonged and corrects with mixing studies	Normal	Normal	Prolonged
Euglobin clot lysis time (ELT)	Shortened	Shortened	Normal	Normal	Normal	Normal	Normal
Thrombin time	Prolonged	Prolonged	Normal	Normal	Normal	Normal	Prolonged
Fibrinogen–fibrin degradation products (FDP)	Normal	Normal	Normal	Normal	Normal	Normal	Increased

necessary. More severe bleeding events such as intracranial bleeding with evacuation of hematoma may be managed with intravenous fibrinolytic inhibitors and infusions of fresh-frozen plasma [6].

α₂-Antiplasmin

α₂-Antiplasmin (α₂-AP) is the most important plasma inhibitor of plasmin, the main enzyme responsible for fibrinolysis [7,8]. Welch et al. [9] assigned the α₂-AP locus to human chromosome 17. With a regional mapping panel, the assignment could be narrowed to region 17pter–p12. The gene contains 10 exons and nine introns distributed over about 16 kilobases (kb) of DNA. The reactive site and plasminogen binding site are encoded by the tenth exon. α₂-AP contains 464 amino acids. It has a carboxy-terminal extension of 51 amino acid residues, which contains a binding site that reacts with the lysine binding site of both plasminogen and plasmin.

Kluft et al. [10] have described a 15-year-old male, with homozygous defect for α₂-AP deficiency, with a hemorrhagic diathesis associated with injury from early childhood onward. He had a normal plasma concentration of α₂-AP antigen (83%) but a minimal α₂-AP level was recorded functionally. Kluft et al. [11] characterized the kindred and reported that a younger 5-year-old sister was likewise an apparent homozygote with 2% level recorded functionally and 92% antigen levels. The two identified homozygotes were found to have very low functional levels as determined by the immediate plasmin inhibition test. Eight heterozygotes were identified by half-normal activities and normal antigen concentrations.

Inherited in an autosomal recessive manner, homozygous deficiency is associated with a severe hemorrhagic diathesis, including spontaneous bleeds into joints which often present

early in life. The complete congenital absence of α₂-AP has been found to be associated with a distinct hemorrhagic diathesis. Intracranial hemorrhage (ICH) in a full-term newborn infant requires coagulation evaluation including α₂-AP as ICH has been reported to occur with this deficiency. Early identification of this disorder is critical to achieving optimal outcome as recurrent ICH may occur and lead to morbidity and mortality.

Intramedullary hematomas in the diaphyses of long bones is an unusual, distinctive pattern of bleeding that has been reported with α₂-AP deficiency [12,13].

A specific alpha α₂-AP assay should be performed when a patient presents with a bleeding diathesis indicative of this disorder in the face of normal screening coagulation testing [12]. α₂-AP levels are measured using a chromogenic substrate. Unlike PAI-1 deficiency, the activity assay normal range does discriminate between low normal and a deficient state. Based on the results of functional and immunologic assays, two types of biologic deficiencies can be recognized: type I (quantitative), defined by a similar deficiency of α₂-AP by both assays; and type II (qualitative) in which there is a discrepancy between the abnormal low activity level and a normal antigen level.

Some heterozygous individuals (40–60%) have been reported to experience a mild bleeding tendency. However, the real importance of bleeding in heterozygotes is controversial. The majority of heterozygous subjects identified in family studies of homozygous patients and isolated reported cases have not experienced clinical bleeding. The fact that the spectrum of severity exhibited by homozygous or compound heterozygous affected individuals varies from severe to moderate may relate to the type of genetic defects and their specific impact on enzymatic function and other as yet unidentified factors.

Table 58.4 Hemostatic agents.

	Drug		
	Aminocaproic acid	Tranexamic acid	Recombinant factor VIIa
Mechanism of action	Inhibitor of plasminogen activation	Competitive inhibitor of plasminogen activation; noncompetitive plasmin inhibition at higher concentrations	When complexed with tissue factor, NovoSeven® can activate FX to FXa, as well as FIX to FIXa. FXa, in complex with other factors, then converts prothrombin to thrombin, which leads to the formation of a hemostatic plug by converting fibrinogen to fibrin and thereby inducing local hemostasis
Dosage forms	500-mg tablets; 250 mg/mL syrup; 250 mg/mL injection in 20-cm^3 and 100-cm^3 vials	500-mg tablets (not available in the USA); 100 mg/mL injection	Intravenous form. Available as single-use vials of 1.2 mg, 2.4 mg, and 4.8 mg
Oral dosage	3 g every 4 h or 10 mg followed by 5 g every 6 h	25 mg/kg 3 or 4 times per day; absorption not affected by food	No oral dosage form available
Pediatric dosage	200 mg/kg orally followed by 100 mg/kg every 6 h Alternatively 50–100 mg/kg per dose	Limited data in children to date; dosing instructions for adults may be used	90–120 μg/kg bolus every 2–3 h
Dose modification		Reduce dose in renal impairment	No dose modifications for end-organ dysfunction
Monitoring parameters	Laboratory monitoring evaluation usually not performed	Laboratory monitoring evaluation usually not performed; higher concentrations may prolong thrombin time	Laboratory monitoring evaluation not performed
Contraindications	DIC (disseminated intravascular coagulation); upper urinary tract bleeding	Defective vision; subarachnoid hemorrhage	Known hypersensitivity to any component of the drug; known hypersensitivity to mouse, hamster, or bovine proteins
Adverse events	Urinary obstruction if used for upper genitourinary tract bleeding	Visual changes with prolonged treatment	Potential risk of thrombosis
Use in pregnancy	Category C	Category B	Category C
Drug interactions	Concomitant use with oral contraceptives or estrogens may lead to hypercoagulable state	Concomitant use with oral contraceptives or estrogens may lead to hypercoagulable state	None known

Treatment with antifibrinolytic therapy is utilized to treat patients who bleed, or to avoid hemorrhagic complications in those who are undergoing surgical interventions [12]. These agents prevent the binding of plasminogen to fibrin and thereby inhibit endogenous fibrinolysis and stabilize the hemostatic plug. These agents can be administered orally or intravenously.

Deficiencies within the contact system

The kallikrein–kinin system was first recognized as a plasma and tissue proteolytic system responsible for liberation of vasoactive, proinflammatory bradykinin. These plasma proteins were grouped together as the contact system as they required contact with artificial negatively charged surface for zymogen activation. Over the last 20 years, deficiencies of these proteins, including factor XII, high-molecular-weight kininogen, and prekallikrein, although resulting in prolongation of the screening tests reflecting the intrinsic pathway such as the activated partial thromboplastin time (aPTT), have not been demonstrated to lead to a hemorrhagic diathesis. [14]

Prekallikrein (Fletcher factor)

Prekallikrein (PK) is produced by a single gene that maps to chromosome 4 [15]. PK is estimated to have a circulating concentration in blood of 35–50 µg/mL [16]. The disorder is transmitted in an autosomal recessive manner.

Cases of PK deficiency are discovered incidentally by marked prolongation of the partial thromboplastin time (PTT), which corrects with extended incubation in the presence of a contact activator. Plasmas deficient in factors VIII, IX, XI, and XII correct the prolonged PTT on mixing studies. Prekallikrein assays reveal levels <2% of normal levels in patients with homozygous prekallikrein deficiency. In general, the remainder of the coagulation profile is normal. In liver disease, plasma PK is decreased [16]. Women on oral contraceptives have increased PK levels, but women in their second and third trimester of pregnancy do not [16,17]. Severe PK deficiency has no clinically significant effect on hemostasis.

High-molecular-weight kininogen (Williams, Fitzgerald, Flaujeac factor)

The pivotal protein for contact system assembly on cell membranes is high-molecular-weight kininogen (HMWK). Normal human plasma contains two molecular forms of kininogens: high-molecular and low-molecular weight. Each protein consists of three domains: an amino-terminal heavy chain, a bradykinin moiety, and a carboxy-terminal light chain. Hereditary HMWK deficiency is composed of cases of isolated deficiency of the high-molecular-weight form and other cases in which both the high- and low-molecular-weight forms are missing (total kininogen deficiency). The inheritance is autosomal recessive. A prolongation of aPTT is noted, which corrects with mixing studies. Levels of factor VIII, IX, XI, XII, and PK are all normal. HMWK level can be assessed by coagulation and immunologic methods. No bleeding tendency has been reported even in the face of complete absence of these proteins [18].

Platelet function disorders

With the congenital platelet function defects, mucocutaneous bleeding such as ecchymoses, epistaxis, gum bleeding, and menorrhagia are common clinical manifestations, whereas spontaneous deep-tissue hemorrhages such as muscle hematomas or hemarthroses seldom occur in affected patients [19]. Congenital platelet function defects are a heterogeneous group of disorders that cannot be distinguished from each other on clinical grounds alone, except that the most severe defects, such as Glanzmann's thrombasthenia, may often be recognized through early, recurrent clinical bleeding.

Glanzmann's thrombasthenia (GT)

Glanzmann's thrombasthenia (GT) is an autosomal recessive bleeding disorder characterized by a quantitative deficiency or a functional abnormality of the major platelet membrane integrin receptor: the glycoprotein (GP) IIb–IIIa complex. The

GPIIb–IIIa complex functions as a platelet receptor for fibrinogen, von Willebrand factor (VWF), fibronectin, and vitronectin. Thrombasthenic platelets fail to aggregate and form an adequate hemostatic plug at the site of vessel injury. A molecular defect affecting one of the two GP-coding genes is sufficient to result in a deficit of both GPIIb and GPIIIa, and, hence, the thrombasthenic phenotype. Large rearrangements within the GPIIb or GPIIIa coding genes appear to be unusual, whereas small modifications in the nucleotide sequence of the coding regions occur with higher frequency [20]. To date, 18 mutant alleles have been described and purported to cause GT.

This disorder is grouped into three types according to the amount of immunologically detectable GPIIb–IIIa. Genetic, biochemical, and immunologic studies are important to correlate genetic defects with protein and clinical phenotype. Essential diagnostic features are a normal platelet count and morphology, a prolonged bleeding time, and absence of platelet aggregation in response to ADP, collagen, epinephrine, thrombin, and all aggregating agents that ultimately depend on fibrinogen binding to platelets. However, ristocetin-induced platelet binding and agglutination will occur with GT platelets. Other laboratory testing may include flow cytometry for GP IIb–IIIa evaluation and GPIIb–IIIa platelet membrane surface receptor analysis using monoclonal antibodies. Although, by definition, all patients with GT have a virtually complete failure of platelet aggregation, a number of variant forms of GT have been described in which the glycoproteins are present in normal or near-normal amounts but are functionally defective. Heterozygotes express approximately one-half the number of normal GPIIb–IIIa complexes but do not exhibit a bleeding tendency. In homozygous or compound heterozygous affected individuals, the disorder is characterized by mild to severe mucocutaneous bleeding. Molecular biologic techniques have enabled us to detect heterozygote carriers who are clinically asymptomatic.

D-Amino-D-arginine vasopressin (DDAVP) is not useful in this disorder. The mainstay of therapy has consisted of platelet transfusions. However, platelet alloimmunization as a result of platelet transfusions is an important adverse consequence and platelet transfusions must be judiciously employed. Leukocyte-depleted blood products should be used to prevent alloimmunization. Platelets matched via human leukocyte antigen (HLA) may be used in a further attempt to prevent platelet alloimmunization. The successful use of NovoSeven® to attain hemostasis in this disorder has been reported and should be considered as first-line therapy, thus reserving platelet transfusions and their possible subsequent sequelae for episodes not responding to NovoSeven® [21].

Hermansky–Pudlak syndrome (HPS)

Hermansky–Pudlak syndrome (HPS) is a rare, often fatal, autosomal recessive disorder in which partial oculocutaneous albinism, bleeding, and lysosomal storage deficiency are associated with defects of diverse cytoplasmic organelles, including melanosomes, platelet dense granules, and lysosomes [22]. The prolonged bleeding time is due to the lack of storage organelles (dense bodies) in platelets [23]. A consistent finding in HPS is storage pool-deficient platelets. HPS can be diagnosed by lack of platelet dense bodies seen by electron microscopy [24]. Patients can develop restrictive lung disease, with the onset of pulmonary fibrosis noted most often in the third or fourth decade. Inflammatory bowel disease, secondary to accumulation of ceroid-like material in phagocytes, with onset of symptoms between 12 and 30 years of age, has been reported. Rivera et al. [25] have described the successful use of NovoSeven® for treatment of gastrointestinal bleed with adjunctive use of Amicar and platelet transfusions.

Vascular diseases

Osler–Weber–Rendu syndrome

Vascular diseases may mimic coagulopathies by presenting as a hemorrhagic state. The archetypal example of an inherited disorder resulting in hemorrhage from dilated vessels of the microvasculature (telangiectasia) is hereditary hemorrhagic telangiectasia (HHT, Osler–Weber–Rendu syndrome). Linkage analyses have indicated there are at least three HHT loci, including the genes for endoglin on chromosome 9 and activin-like receptor kinase (ALK1) on chromosome 12 [26]. This autosomal dominant disorder is characterized by hemorrhage from nasal, mucocutaneous, and gastrointestinal telangiectasias, in addition to vascular anomalies in other organs, particularly in the pulmonary, hepatic, and cerebral circulations. Associated brain and pulmonary lesions are sources of substantial morbidity and mortality [27]. Multiple treatments for epistaxis have been used, including cauterization, septal dermatoplasty, laser ablation, estrogen therapy, and transcatheter embolotherapy of arteries leading to the nasal mucosa. Antifibrinolytic therapy has been used for the treatment of bleeding in this disorder [28].

Chest radiography, arterial blood gas measurements, and finger oximetry remain important in screening persons with suspected pulmonary arteriovenous malformations. Pulmonary angiography is required in order to plan treatments by interventional radiology or surgery. Surgical management of pulmonary arteriovenous malformations has evolved from lobectomy to wedge resection to ligation of the arterial supply of the malformation. Transcatheter embolotherapy with detachable balloons or stainless-steel coils has also been used to close such malformations. Long-term follow-up of treated patients is important, because the interval growth of malformations may require further intervention. Those with a pulmonary arteriovenous malformation should receive antibacterial prophylaxis at the time of a dental or surgical procedure. Others who are affected or at risk and who have a family history of pulmonary arteriovenous malformations should use prophylaxis until the possibility that they may have such a malformation is ruled out. It is important that persons with HHT be aware of their diagnosis and its implications and that they inform healthcare providers that they are affected. Educational materials for patients and providers are available from the HHT Foundation International [29].

Role of fresh-frozen plasma in rare bleeding disorders

Bleeding episodes in the case of rare factor deficiencies such as PAI-1 and α_2-AP may at times require treatment with replacement therapy in the form of fresh-frozen plasma (FFP), especially given that specific factor replacement therapy is unavailable.

Prospective controlled clinical trials have not revealed any significant difference in clinical efficacy and tolerance between FFP and solvent/detergent-treated plasma. With the exception of emergency situations when timely clotting assay results are not available, the administration of plasma for a coagulopathy should be preceded by appropriate laboratory testing. Fresh-frozen plasma from one donation of whole blood usually consists of 175–250 mL and contains 1 IU/mL of clotting factors. Transfusion of 1 mL/kg of FFP can increase a clotting factor level by 1 IU/100 mL if the patient is in a steady state. However, increased turnover due to blood loss and/or consumption may reduce in vivo recovery to 0.5–1.0 IU/100mL or lower. Hence, the infusion of at least 10 mL plasma/kg is often required to increase the deficient plasma protein to a minimal hemostatic level [30]. Side-effects resulting from the administration of plasma are uncommon but must be considered, especially when long-term replacement therapy is contemplated. Acute volume overload is an issue of concern with the infusion of large volumes of FFP. Evidence of the clinical efficacy of plasma is mainly based on expert opinion, case reports, and controlled and uncontrolled observational studies.

Summary

Optimal management of rare bleeding disorders requires careful evaluation of the clinical situation for which therapy is required. Therapeutic interventions should be administered only after careful consideration of the risk–benefit ratio and not merely to treat an abnormal laboratory result. The safest yet most efficacious therapy should be provided. With the advent of advanced testing for viral blood-borne pathogens such as hepatitis A, B, and C, HIV, and cytomegalovirus (CMV), the risk of blood-borne viral infections has decreased; however, the transfusion of any blood product may be associated with potential side-effects and, without an inactivation procedure, pathogens for which no test is available or performed may potentially be transmitted. Therapeutic interventions are tailored to the specific deficiency. For example, antifibrinolytics are utilized as primary hemostatic agents to achieve hemostasis in PAI-1 and α_2-AP deficiency, whereas in GT they may be used as adjunctive agents for specific bleeding events such as oropharyngeal hemorrhage. New agents such as NovoSeven® offer an increased range of therapeutic options for these rare disorders in the absence of specific replacement products (Table 58.4). The off-label use of recombinant activated factor VIIa as a panhemostatic agent is being increasingly described, including the use in platelet function disorders.

The management of menorrhagia has until recently been the domain of the gynecologist. Hematologists are now addressing the issue of optimal management of menorrhagia in patients with bleeding disorders. The use of oral contraceptive agents, antifibrinolytics, intranasal DDAVP, and levonorgestrel-impregnated intrauterine devices all have been described [31].

Improved diagnostic tests are needed for some of these rare disorders, especially PAI-1 deficiency. National and international registries are required to better define the incidence, clinical manifestations, and outcome of treatment. A North American registry (www.hemophilia-forum.org/) maintains data pertaining to the use of NovoSeven® for treatment of bleeding episodes in Glanzmann's thrombasthenia. Systematic data collection on response to interventions, especially those using panhemostatic agents such as NovoSeven®, are required to assess long-term safety and efficacy.

References

1 Stefansson S, McMahon GA, Petitclerc E, Lawrence DA, et al. Plasminogen activator inhibitor-1 in tumor growth, angiogenesis and vascular remodeling. *Curr Pharm Des* 2003; **9**: 1545–64.

2 Ginsburg D, Zeheb R, Yang AY, et al. cDNA cloning of human plasminogen activator-inhibitor from endothelial cells. *J Clin Invest* 1986; **78**: 1673–80.

3 Klinger KW, Winqrist R, Andreasen PA, et al. Assignment of the human plasminogen activator inhibitor type 1 (PAI-1) gene to 7q21.3-q22 and genetic linkage to markers on chromosome 7 (Abstract). *Am J Hum Genet* 1987; **41**: A172.

4 Fay WP, Shapiro AD, Shih JL, et al. Complete deficiency of plasminogen-activator inhibitor type I due to a frameshift mutation. *N Engl J Med* 1992; **327**: 1729–33.

5 Fay WP, Parker AC, Condrey LR, Shapiro AD. Human plasminogen activator inhibitor-1 (PAI-1) deficiency: characterization of a large kindred with a null mutation in the PAI-1 gene. *Blood* 1997; **90**: 204–8.

6 Shapiro AD, Fay WP, Condrey LR, Kalsbeck JE. A report of severe intracranial bleeding in an infant with plasminogen activator inhibitor (PAI-1) deficiency: successful treatment with antifibrinolytic therapy and surgical evacuation. *Blood* 1996; **88**: Abstract 134.

7 Collen D. Identification and some properties of a new fast- reacting plasmin inhibitor in human plasma. *Eur J Biochem* 1976; **69**: 209–16.

8 Aoki N, Moroi M, Matsuda M, Tachiya K. The behaviour of alpha 2-antiplasmin inhibitor in fibrinolytic states. *J Clin Invest* **60**: 361–9.

9 Welch, SK, Francke U. Assignment of the human alpha(2)-plasmin inhibitor gene (PLI) on chromosome 17, region pter–p12, by PCR analysis of somatic cell hybrids. *Genomics* 1992; **13**: 213–14.

10 Kluft, C, Vellenga E, Brommer EJP. Homozygous alpha-2-antiplasmin deficiency [Letter]. *Lancet* 1979; **ii**: 206.

11 Kluft C, Nieuwenhuis HK, Rijken DC. Alpha-2-antiplasmin Enschede: dysfunctional alpha-2-antiplasmin molecule associated with an autosomal recessive hemorrhagic disorder. *J Clin Invest* 1987; **80**: 1391–400.

12 Takahashi Y, Tanaka T, Nakajima N, et al. Intramedullary multiple hematomas in siblings with congenital alpha-2-plasmin inhibitor deficiency: orthopedic surgery with protection by tranexamic acid. *Haemostasis* 1991; **21**: 321–7.

13 Devaussuzenet VMP, Doucou-le-Pointe H, Doco AM, et al. A case of intramedullary haematoma associated with congenital alpha-2-plasmin inhibitor deficiency. *Pediatr Radiol* 1998; **28**: 978–80.

14 Colman RW, Schmaier AH. Contact system: a vascular biology modulator with anticoagulant, profibrinolytic, antiadhesive, and proinflammatory attributes. *Blood* 1997; **90**: 3819–43.

15 Beaubien, G, Rosinski-Chupin I, Mattei M, et al. Gene structure and chromosomal localization of plasma kallikrein. *Biochemistry* 1991; **30**: 1628.

16 Fisher CA, Schmaier AH, Addonizio VP, Colman RW. Assay of prekallikrein in human plasma: comparison of amidolytic, esterolytic, coagulation, and immunochemical assays. *Blood* 1982; **59**: 963–70.

17 Chhibber G, Cohen A, Lane S, et al. Immunoblotting of plasma in a pregnant patient with hereditary angioedema. *J Lab Clin Med* 1990; **115**: 112.

18 Lefrere JJ, Horellou MH, Gozin D, et al. A new case of high-molecular-weight kininogen inherited deficiency. *Am J Hematol* 1986; **22**: 415–19.

19 Nair S, Ghosh K, Kulkarni B, et al. Glanzmann's thrombasthenia: updated. *Platelets* 2002; **13**: 387–93.

20 Perutelli P, Mori PG. Biochemical and molecular basis of Glanzmann's thrombasthenia. *Haematologica* 1992; **77**: 421–6.

21 Poon MC. Use of recombinant factor VII in hereditary bleeding disorders. *Curr Opin Hematol* 2001; **8**: 312–18.

22 Feng GH, et al. Mouse pale ear (ep) is homologous to human Hermansky-Pudlak syndrome and contains a rare 'AT-AC' intron. *Hum Mol Genetics* 1997; **6**: 793–7.

23 Berz F, Weiss M, Belohradsky BH. Albinism, thrombopathy, ceroid storage disease – Hermansky–Pudlak syndrome. Overview and description with immunodeficiency [Trans.]. *Klin Padiatr* 1996; **208**: 83–7.

24 Witkop CJ, Almadovar C, Nunez BPMB. Hermansky–Pudlak syndrome (HPS). An epidemiologic study. *Ophthalm Paediatr Genet* 1990; **11**: 245–50.

25 Rivera E, Santiago PJ, Cordova AI. Use of recombinant factor VII in Hermansky–Pudlak syndrome. *Blood* 2001; **98** (Suppl.).

26 Shovlin CL. Molecular defects in rare bleeding disorders: hereditary haemorrhagic telangiectasia. *Thromb Haemost* 1997; **78**:145–50.

27 Guttmacher AE, Marchuk DA, White RI. Hereditary hemorrhagic telangiectasia. *N Engl J Med* 1995; **333**: 918–24.

28 Saba HI, Morelli GA, Logrono LA. Treatment of bleeding in hereditary hemorrhagic telangiectasia with aminocaproic acid. *N Engl J Med* 1994; **330**: 1789–90.

29 Wimmer PJ, Howes DS, Rumoro DP, Carbone M. Fatal vascular catastrophe in Ehlers-Danlos syndrome: a case report and review. *J Emerg Med* 1996; **14**(1): 25–31.

30 Hellstern P, Muntean W, Schramm W, et al. Practical guidelines for the clinical use of plasma. *Thromb Res* 2002; **107** (Suppl. 1): S53–7.

31 Siegel JE, Kouides PA. Menorrhagia from a haematologist's point of view. Part II: management. *Haemophilia* 2002; **8**: 339–47.

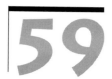

59

Quality of life in hemophilia

Sylvia v. Mackensen and Alessandro Gringeri

Introduction

Hemophilia is a congenital disorder characterized by spontaneous and post-traumatic bleeding events in joints, muscles, and other soft tissues. These manifestations, when not prevented, inexorably lead to severe pain, arthropathy, and disability, to the detriment of quality of life (QoL). The modern management of hemophilia has visibly influenced not only clinical symptoms, orthopedic outcome, and survival of patients, but also the perceived well-being [1].

Nevertheless, other concerns continue to challenge hemophilia management: the risk for plasma-derived and recombinant concentrates of contaminating viruses or prions and the risk of development of inhibitory antibodies, still involving about 25% of patients who are exposed for the first time to coagulation factors.

All these characteristics of hemophilia care require the absorption of a huge amount of human and economic resources, in a time of ever-increasing awareness of limited medical resources [2,3]. These staggering costs must be considered in the context not only of morbidity and mortality but also of QoL.

Improvement of patient's well-being and QoL has always been one of the goals of healthcare professionals and is indeed more and more regarded as one of the most relevant health outcomes in medicine [4]. Health outcome data are essential to optimize treatments and allocate resources in a cost-intensive chronic disease such as hemophilia, in which traditional outcome measures such as mortality are no longer influenced by diverse treatment options.

Quality of life

Several definitions ranging from operational to more philosophical approaches are available and well accepted in the international QoL field [5].

Definition of "quality of life"

A general definition of QoL was provided by the World Health Organization, which defined QoL as "individuals' perceptions of their position in life in the context of culture and value systems in which they live, and in relation to their goals, expectations, standards, and concerns" [6]. In medicine, the term QoL much more implies how the disease or the treatment is affecting the different aspects of life. Therefore, the term "health-related quality of life" was created: "Health-related quality of life (HR-QoL) is a multidimensional construct pertaining to the physical, emotional, mental, social and behavioral components of well-being and function as perceived by the patients and/or observers" [7]. HR-QoL is influenced not only by a disease and its treatment but also by personal characteristics such as coping or internal locus of control, as well as by living conditions and socioeconomic status.

Issues concerning quality of life

Quality of life assessment is considered an important outcome measure from an epidemiologic perspective, describing the well-being and function of patients, from a clinical perspective evaluating treatment intervention effects on well-being, and from a health economics perspective, which associates analyses of quality and cost of care.

Quality of life research is based on different theoretical models such as the concept of satisfaction, social comparison approaches, and expectation models, as well as on the so-called needs models. A widely used utility measure is the patient preference measure, assessing the importance attributed to different health status conditions.

One of the most important issues in QoL assessment is the direct perception of patients. It is well known that observers overestimate some aspects of QoL of patients, whereas psychologic aspects are often underestimated. Self-rated measures in which the patient is directly asked — so-called subjective measures — are recommended [8]. Other-rated measures, or "proxy" measures, are used in young children or patients unable to answer (e.g., mentally impaired patients). In this case, parents or other care-givers involved with the patient should be asked.

Instrument characteristics

In QoL assessment, it is important to distinguish between measures for adults and measures for children. Instruments for children should be especially developed considering age groups and developmental status. In small children, the parents' reports of children's well-being are necessary, while in grown-up children the comparison between children's and parent's perspectives turns out to be of interest by itself [9].

Development of QoL instruments

For the construction of a new instrument different steps must be considered: (i) development; (ii) translation (for international use); (iii) testing; and (iv) norming [10]. An instrument should be *developed* by specifying measurement goals and by generating items by focus groups (healthcare professionals and patients). Subsequently, items should be pretested and patients should be asked about how they understood each single item (cognitive debriefing). After item review and reduction, the questionnaire can be piloted in order to examine its feasibility. In international studies, the questionnaire must be *translated* into the relevant languages following internationally recommended translation rules [11], with forward and backward translations. The questionnaire must then be *psychometrically tested* with respect to reliability, validity, and responsiveness. *Reliability* is an indicator of reproducibility of an instrument and consistency of results. It can be examined with the internal consistency coefficient (Cronbach's alpha), which indicates the extent to which the items are interrelated, or with the test–retest reliability, which is based upon analysis of correlations between repeated measurements. *Validity* testing examines whether an instrument measures what it intends to measure. Construct validity gives information about the theoretical relationship of the items to each other and can be examined in terms of convergent validity (comparing new items with similar well-established questionnaires) and discriminant validity (differentiating clinical subgroups of patients). *Responsiveness* is the ability of a scale to detect changes over time and therefore is tested only in longitudinal studies. Finally, the questionnaire should be *normed* [12], through the application of a scale, to a representative sample of the national population in order to obtain information about age, sex, and other factors.

Measures of quality of life

Individual QoL measurements, such as interviews and psychometrically constructed questionnaires, have been developed in the past 30 years. They are represented by one-dimensional measures that assess just one dimension of QoL (index, summary) and multidimensional measures that assess several dimensions of QoL. Originally, only generic instruments were available, and these have been followed by disease-specific measures.

Generic instruments

Generic instruments can be used irrespectively of a specific disease in patients with different conditions or in the general population. The most frequently used generic questionnaires are briefly described:
• The Medical Outcomes Study 36-Item Health Survey (SF-36) [13] is the most widely used generic questionnaire, translated and validated in several languages. The SF-36 consists of 36 items covering eight dimensions of general health status, namely physical functioning, role–physical, bodily pain, general health, vitality, social functioning, role–emotional, and mental health.
• The Sickness Impact Profile (SIP) [14] is another measure assessing the perceived health status and consists of 136 items.
• With the Nottingham Health Profile (NHP) [15], emotional, social, and physical distress is assessed. The questionnaire consists of 38 items pertaining to the dimensions covering sleep, pain, emotional reactions, social isolation, physical morbidity, and energy level.
• The EuroQol (EQ-5D) [16], validated in many languages, asks five questions about mobility, self-care, usual activities, pain/discomfort, anxiety/depression, followed by a global question concerning the actual health status, the last providing a utility score frequently used in health economics.
• The World Health Organization Quality of Life Assessment Questionnaire (WHOQoL) [17] assesses a respondent's perception and subjective evaluation of various aspects of life. The WHOQoL consists of six domains (physical, psychologic, level of independence, social relationships, environment, and spirituality/religion/personal beliefs) with overall 100 items. A short-form version with 16 items has also been developed.
• For the evaluation of QoL in children, several instruments have been developed. Most of these measures have been validated only on a national level. One of the instruments validated in different languages is the Child Health Questionnaire (CHQ) [18], which assesses QoL in children from the parents' perspective. It consists of several subdimensions such as "general health perceptions," "physical functioning," and "mental health."
• Another psychometrically tested instrument translated in several languages is the KINDL questionnaire, originally developed for the assessment of QoL in the general pediatric population. The KINDL is available as a self-administered and as a proxy version for three age groups (4–7, 8–12, and 13–16 years of age) and consists of 24 items pertaining to six dimensions (physical function, psychologic well-being, self-esteem, family, friends, and school) and an additional chronic generic dimension [19].

Disease-specific instruments

Although generic instruments allow comparisons of the investigated patient population with other patient groups or with the general population, they are not able to provide a clear pattern of symptoms or impairments related to a specific disease and are not sensitive enough to treatment consequences. For this reason, disease-specific measures are especially developed for the assessment of QoL in patients with specific health diseases, such as cancer, respiratory, metabolic, or cardiovascular diseases, as well as neurologic, psychiatric, rheumatologic conditions, etc. [20].

The assessment of QoL in children with chronic diseases has increased, but it is still in need of development. QoL evaluation in children should involve the parents' perceptions of children's QoL as well as their own QoL rating, also including the opinions of siblings.

Only recently, the first hemophilia-specific questionnaire (*Hemo-QoL*) [21] was developed as a self-administered questionnaire for children, as well as a proxy version for their parents. Three age group versions are now available (4–7 years, 8–12 years, and 13–16 years). The Hemo-QoL has been validated in six European languages (German, French, Italian, Spanish, Dutch, and English). Another hemophilia-specific questionnaire for children is the *CHO-KLAT* [22], which was developed in Canada.

Some developmental work is ongoing for the assessment of QoL in adult patients and of treatment satisfaction.

Pharmacoeconomics and HR-QoL

HR-QoL assessment is increasingly used in pharmacoeconomics. In fact, the fundamental nature of pharmacoeconomics is an estimate of costs and outcomes of alternative health programs. The outcome of a medical intervention is represented by the health status perceived by the patient and includes symptoms, performance, compliance, care satisfaction, and QoL. HR-QoL is often essential for assessing cost-effectiveness. Cost–utility analysis is a type of cost-effectiveness analysis in which effectiveness is weighted for a factor that considers HR-QoL. Cost–benefit analyses are also based on patient preferences.

Choosing a measure

When choosing a measure we must keep in mind which kind of investigation we want to perform. In fact, generic instruments can measure general health status in different patient populations ("cross-illness comparison") and can allow comparison with the general population. Disease-specific measures can study specific problems of a selected cluster of patients and are more sensitive than generic measures: this allows the detection of small changes and makes these measures suitable for the assessment of a specific treatment intervention over time ("within-subject comparison"). The choice of a specific instrument relies upon its validation in the respective country, the reported sensitivity and even the number of items included. Moreover, the choice of a specific measure depends on the areas and dimensions mainly investigated by the instrument.

Quality-of-life research in hemophilia

For an adequate HR-QoL assessment of patients with hemophilia, validated instruments are necessary.

A literature research performed in 2003 detected 144 publications with the keywords "quality of life" and "hemophilia." In most of them, QoL was mentioned only as a condition of the patient that is considered important. In these studies, it was mainly stated that, for example, prophylactic treatment or home therapy is improving the QoL of patients, but without measuring QoL. In only a few studies were measurements of QoL used.

Results from generic instruments

One of the first studies was conducted in 935 Dutch hemophilia patients and showed that QoL did not differ from that of the general population [23]. In another study on clinical outcomes and resource utilization associated with hemophilia care in more than 1000 European patients, QoL, assessed by the SF-36, in patients on prophylaxis was better than in patients receiving on-demand treatment [24]. Miners *et al.* [1] found of their study, in which SF-36 and EQ-5D were administered to 249 British hemophiliacs, that patients with severe hemophilia had poorer levels of QoL. They suggested that early primary prophylaxis might increase their QoL. A French study of 116 patients with severe hemophilia showed that physical function and social relation were acceptable, whereas QoL scores in the pain dimension of the SF-36 were impaired [25]. Another study that administered the SF-36 to 150 Finnish patients with bleeding disorders showed that QoL levels were associated with the clinical severity [26]. In a Spanish study of 70 patients, using the SF-36, QoL was negatively affected by severe hemophilic arthropathy [27]. In a Canadian survey of patients with mild, moderate, and severe hemophilia, the Health Utility Index mark 2 (HUI-2) and mark 3 (HUI-3) were used. Hemophiliacs reported a greater burden of morbidity than the general population, being linearly correlated with the severity of hemophilia [28]. QoL is often assessed after a treatment, as was done by Schick *et al.* [29] in 11 hemophilia patients after knee arthroplasty, using the SF-12, WOMAC, and Knee Society Score. Even though several publications exist concerning psychologic issues in hemophilic patients with HIV, only a few assess QoL with appropriate instruments [30].

HR-QoL in children with severe hemophilia (*n* = 27) was investigated by Liesner *et al.* [31] in the UK in 1996. Prophylaxis significantly decreased the average number of bleeds compared with prior prophylaxis, and families reported an improved health perception. In a multicenter study concerning the effects of two prophylactic treatment regimes, 128 children with hemophilia from Sweden and the Netherlands were investigated, including QoL measures [32]. Clinical scores and QoL were similar in both prophylactic groups. High-dose prophylaxis significantly increased treatment costs; however, arthropathy could only be slightly reduced after a follow-up of 17 years. In a study of 140 American children with hemophilia, Shapiro *et al.* [33] found that those with fewer bleeding events had higher physical functioning scores as assessed by the Child Health Questionnaire (CHQ) and were similar to the general population.

Only recently, the relationship between health economics and QoL has been examined in hemophilia patients using, for example, the standard gamble technique [34] or the quality-adjusted life years (QALYs) approach [1]. Szucs *et al.* [35], in their study of the socioeconomic impact of hemophilia treatment involving 50 German hemophiliacs, found significant differences between patients and healthy men concerning limitations in physical activities, pain, and general health scores as assessed by the SF-36.

In a huge European study involving more than 1000 patients with hemophilia, it was shown that prophylaxis was associated with higher costs but better QoL scores as measured by the SF-36 [3]. In an Italian study of 56 hemophilic patients, combining QoL (SF-36) and utility assessment (EQ-5D), low scale values were found in the general health perceptions and higher scale values in social functioning [36]. Another Italian study involving 52 Italian hemophilic patients with inhibitors prospectively evaluated cost of care and QoL [2]. HR-QoL, measured by the SF-36 and the EQ-BD questionnaires, was similar to that of patients with severe hemophilia without inhibitors. In comparison with other diseases, physical functioning was similar to that of patients with diabetes and on dialysis, whereas mental well-being was similar to that in the general population. This study showed that management of hemophilia complicated by inhibitors required large amounts of resources, but it provided a satisfactory QoL. In a cost–utility analysis in six hemophilic children with inhibitors, Eckert *et al.* [37] included the Child-Health Questionnaire (CHQ) for the assessment of QoL and the EQ-5D for utility valuation. HR-QoL improvements were observed in several important areas as perceived by both patients and their families.

Results from disease-specific instruments

In a Dutch study, 31 patients with severe hemophilia were investigated using a generic QoL instrument (SIP) and a disease-specific instrument, the Arthritis Impact Scale (AIMS) [38]. This questionnaire is an arthritis-specific measure but not a specific QoL measure. Physical health components of the Dutch AIMS and the SIP were significantly correlated, but not the psychosocial components. Another arthritis-specific questionnaire (CHAQ, Children's Health Assessment Questionnaire) was used in another Dutch study, in which hemophilic children ($n = 39$) on prophylaxis were compared with their healthy peers. Although 90% of hemophilic children had no disabilities in activities of daily living (ADL), 79% reported that the disease impacted on their lives [39].

The first disease-specific QoL questionnaire for children and adolescents with hemophilia (Hemo-QoL) was recently field-tested in six European countries (Germany, Italy, France, Spain, the Netherlands, and the UK), involving 339 children from 20 centers [40]. The psychometric structure of the questionnaire showed acceptable psychometric properties for the three age group versions as well as the accompanying parent forms. HR-QoL was shown to be satisfactory: young children were bothered only in the dimension "family" and "treatment," whereas older children had higher impairments in the social dimensions, such as "perceived support" and "friends." Hemo-QoL also showed that the initial burden induced by prophylaxis in younger children is highly compensated by improvements in HR-QoL in older children, as indicated by impaired scores in the dimension "feeling" in smaller children and improved scores in the dimension "school & sport" in older children [41]. Using psychosocial determinants of QoL such as coping, locus of con-

trol, life satisfaction, and social support, it was apparent that QoL is dependent not only on clinical but also on psychosocial characteristics [42].

Hemophilia-specific questionnaires for adults are currently being developed by different international groups, e.g., in the USA, Spain, France, and Italy, but none of them has been published yet.

Conclusions

Quality of life has always been one of the main concerns of a physician, together with control of pain and prolongation of survival. In hemophilia, modern management has already been successful in improving the clinical health outcomes and, recently, has been aimed at improving the more comprehensive well-being of patients with hemophilia.

A literature search showed that QoL is considered one of the most relevant health outcome measures in clinical trials in hemophilia, even though it was only rarely appropriately assessed. Generally, the SF-36 was included for QoL assessment, followed by the EQ-5D [43], only rarely the SIP [38], or the WHO-QoL [29]. Additional questionnaires, such as the Satisfaction in Daily Life (SDL), the Activities of Daily Living (ADL), or the WOMAC questionnaire [29,39], were sometimes included. All of these questionnaires are generic questionnaires and do not fulfill the criteria of disease-specific instruments.

Since disease-specific questionnaires have become available only in the last few years, there are few studies using arthritis-specific instruments such as the AIMS-2 questionnaire [38] or the CHAQ [39]. In one study only, a hemophilia-specific QoL questionnaire (Hemo-QoL) for hemophilic children was used [40].

Generic and disease-specific questionnaires showed impairment in QoL in patients with severe hemophilia, compared with patients with mild and moderate disease and with the general population [1,26,28]. Poor orthopedic status as well as HIV coinfection were associated with a worse perception of QoL [27,30]. Studies in children demonstrated that QoL levels measured by a generic instrument were associated with the frequency of bleeding [32]. On the other hand, in other studies patients with inhibitors have reported levels of QoL similar to those of severe hemophiliacs without inhibitors [2], clearly indicating how a high quality of care, albeit expensive, can influence the burden of inhibitors in patients with hemophilia.

Health status measures have demonstrated QoL improvement in studies evaluating the impact of prophylaxis, both in adults [2,3] and in children [32,41], independent of the frequency of bleeding or the influence on the natural history of hemophilic arthropathy. In other words, these studies emphasized how prophylaxis could improve patients' well-being independent of its impact on bleeding tendency and its ability to influence the progression to severe arthropathy.

Further efforts should be made to develop and validate cross-cultural hemophilia-specific questionnaires all over the world, covering the most important dimensions of health-related QoL of patients with hemophilia (physical functioning, social functioning, emotional well-being, satisfaction of care, treatment preferences, impairments and healthcare needs, perceived utilities). QoL evaluation should be included in all clinical evaluations of treatment options, from product licensing studies to gene therapy trials, as one of the main outcomes. Finally, health-related QoL questionnaires should be part of the medical armamentarium for the global assessment and care of patients with hemophilia.

References

1 Miners AH, Sabin CA, Tolley KH, *et al.* Assessing health-related quality-of-life in individuals with haemophilia. *Haemophilia* 1999; 5: 378–85.

2 Gringeri A, Mantovani LG, Scalone L, Mannucci PM. Cost of care and quality of life in hemophilia complicated by inhibitors: the COCIS Study Group. *Blood* 2003; 102: 2358–63.

3 Schramm W, Royal S, Kroner B, *et al.*; for the European haemophilia economic study group. Clinical outcomes and resource utilization associated with haemophilia care in Europe. *Haemophilia* 2002; 8: 33–43.

4 Cella DF, Tulsky DS. Measuring quality of life today: methodological aspects. *Oncology* 1990; 4: 29–38.

5 Spilker B. *Quality of Life Assessment in Clinical Trials.* New York: Raven Press, 1996.

6 Orley J. and the WHOQOL-Group. The development of the WHO Quality of Life Assessment Instruments (the WHOQOL). In: Orley J, Kuyken W, eds. *Quality of Life Assessment. International Perspectives.* Berlin: Springer Verlag, 1994: 41–57.

7 Bullinger M. Quality of life – definition, conceptualization and implications – a methodologist's view. *Theor Surg* 1991; 6: 143–49.

8 Bowling A. *Measuring Health. A Review of Quality of Life Measurement Scales.* Milton Keynes: Open University Press, 1991.

9 Eiser C, Morse R. A review of measure of quality of life for children with chronic illness. *Arch Dis Child* 2001; 84: 205–11.

10 Juniper E, Guyatt GH, Jaeschke R. How to develop and validate a new health-related Quality of Life instrument. In: B. Spilker, ed. *Quality of Life and Pharmacoeconomics in Clinical Trials.* Philadelphia: Lippincott-Raven, 1996: 49–56.

11 Acquadro C, Jambon B, Ellis D, Marquis P. Language and translation issues. In: Spilker B, ed. *Quality of Life and Pharmacoeconomics in Clinical Trials.* Philadelphia: Lippincott-Raven, 1996: 575–85.

12 Guyatt GH, Feeny DH, Patrick DL. Measuring health-related quality of life. *Ann Intern Med* 1993; 118: 622–9.

13 Ware JE, Snow KK, Kosiniski M, Gandek B. *SF-36 Health Survey Manual and Interpretation Guide.* Boston, MA: New England Medical Centre, 1993.

14 Bergner M, Bobbit RA, Carter WB, Gilson BS. The Sickness Impact Profile: development and final revision of a health status measure. *Med Care* 1981; 19: 787–805.

15 Hunt SM, McKenna SP, McEwen J, *et al.* The Nottingham Health Profile: subjective health status and medical consultations. *Soc Sci Med* 1981; 15: 221–9.

16 Kind P. The EuroQol Instrument: an index of health-related quality of life. In: Spilker B, ed. *Quality of Life and Pharmacoeconomics in Clinical Trials.* Philadelphia: Lippincott-Raven, 1996: 191–201.

17 Power M, Harper A, Bullinger M. The World Health Organization WHOQOL-100: tests of the universality of Quality of Life in 15 different cultural groups worldwide. *Health Psychol* 1999; 18: 495–505.

18 Landgraf I, Abetz L, Ware JE. *Child Health Questionnaire (CHQ): a Users' Manual.* Boston: The Health Institute Press, 1997.

19 Ravens-Sieberer V, Bullinger M. Assessing the health related quality of life in chronically ill children with the German KINDL. First psychometric and content-analytic results. *QoL Res* 1999; 7: 399–408.

20 Bowling A. *Measuring Disease. A Review of Disease-specific Quality of Life Measurement Scales.* Milton Keynes: Open University Press, 2001.

21 Bullinger M, v. Mackensen S, Fischer K, *et al.* Pilot testing of the Haemo-QoL quality of life questionnaire for haemophiliac children in six European Countries. *Haemophilia* 2002; 8 (Suppl. 2): 47–54.

22 Young N, Bradley C, Blanchette V, *et al.* Development of a health-related quality of life measure for boys with haemophilia: The Canadian Haemophilia Outcomes-Kids Life Assessment Tool (CHO-KLAT). *Haemophilia* 2004; 10 (Suppl. 1): 34–43.

23 Rosendaal FR, Smit C, Varekamp I, *et al.* Modern haemophilia treatment: medical improvements and quality of life. *J Intern Med* 1990; 228: 663–40.

24 Royal S, Schramm W, Berntorp E, *et al.* Quality-of-life differences between prophylactic and on-demand factor replacement therapy in European haemophilia patients. *Haemophilia* 2002; 8: 44–50.

25 Molho P, Rolland N, Lebrun T, *et al.* Epidemiological survey of the orthopaedic status of severe haemophilia A and B patients in France. The French Study Group. *Haemophilia* 2000; 6: 23–32.

26 Soloviева S. Clinical severity of disease, functional disability and health-related quality of life. Three-year follow-up study of 150 Finnish patients with coagulation disorders. *Haemophilia* 2001; 7: 53–63.

27 Aznar J, Magall M, Querol F, *et al.* The orthopaedic status of severe haemophiliacs in Spain. *Haemophilia* 2000; 6: 170–6.

28 Barr RD, Saleh M, Furlong W, *et al.* Health Status and Health-Related Quality of Life Associated with Haemophilia. *Am J Hematol* 2002; 71: 152–60.

29 Schick M, Stucki G, Rodriguez M, *et al.* Haemophilic arthropathy: assessment of quality of life after total knee arthroplasty. *Clin Rheumatol* 1999, 18: 468–72.

30 Bussing R, Johnson S. Psychosocial issues in hemophilia before and after the HIV crisis: a review of current research. *Gen Hosp Psychiatry* 1992; 14: 387–403.

31 Liesner RJ, Khair K, Hann IM. The impact of prophylactic treatment on children with severe haemophilia. *Br J Haematol* 1996; 92: 973–8.

32 Fischer K, Astermark J, Van-Der-Bom J, *et al.* Prophylactic treatment for severe haemophilia: comparison of an intermediate-dose to a high dose regimen. *Haemophilia* 2002; 8: 753–60.

33 Shapiro A, Donfield S, Lynn H, *et al.* Defining the impact of hemophilia: the Academic Achievement in Children with Hemophilia Study. *Pediatrics* 2001; 108: E105.

34 Naraine V, Risebrough N, Oh P, *et al.* Health-related quality-of-life treatments for severe haemophilia: utility measurements using the Standard Gamble technique. *Haemophilia* 2002; 8: 112–20.

35 Szucs TD, Offner A, Schramm W. Socioeconomic impact of haemophilia care. Results of a pilot study. *Haemophilia* 1996; 2: 211–17.

36 Trippoli S, Vaiani M, Linari S, *et al.* Multivariate analysis of factors influencing quality of life and utility in patients with haemophilia. *Haematologica* 2001; 86: 722–8.

37 Ekert H, Brewin T, Boey W, *et al.* Cost-utility analysis of recombinant factor VIIa (NovoSeven) in six children with long-standing inhibitors to factor VIII or IX. *Haemophilia* 2001; 7: 279–85.

38 de-Joode E, van-Meeteren N, van-den-Berg H, *et al.* Validity of

health status measurement with the Dutch Arthritis Impact Measurement Scale 2 in individuals with severe haemophilia. *Haemophilia* 2001; 7: 190–7.

39 Schoenmakers M, Gulmans V, Helders P, van-der-Berg H. Motor performance and disability in Dutch children with haemophilia: a comparison with their healthy peers. *Haemophilia* 2001; 7: 293–8.

40 v. Mackensen S, Bullinger M, the Haemo-QoL Group. Development and testing of an instrument to assess the quality of life of children with haemophilia in Europe (Haemo-QoL). *Haemophilia* 2004; 10 (Suppl. 1): 17–25.

41 Gringeri A, v. Mackensen S, Auerswald G, *et al.*, for the Haemo-QoL Study Group. Health status and health-related quality of life of children with haemophilia from six west European countries. *Haemophilia* 2004; 10 (Suppl. 1): 26–33

42 Bullinger M, v. Mackensen S, the Haemo-QoL Group. Quality of life in children and families with bleeding disorders. *J Pediatr Haematol Oncol* 2003; 25: 64–67.

43 Fischer K, van der Bom JG, van den Berg HM. Health-related quality of life as outcome parameter in haemophilia treatment. *Haemophilia* 2003; 9 (Suppl. 1): 75–82.

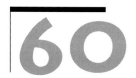

60 The economics of hemophilia treatments

Alec H. Miners

Introduction

All purchasers and providers of healthcare have a finite amount of resources on which they can draw. It follows that, although some healthcare technologies will be offered to patients, others will not because of insufficient funds. Difficult decisions must therefore be made to determine which technologies and services can and cannot be provided.

Economics, as a discipline, is concerned with the allocation of resources. "Health economics" is concerned with the allocation of health resources. More specifically, (healthcare) economic evaluations attempt to generate information on the costs and (health) benefits of a technology [1]. The general principle of this approach is that resources should be allocated toward those technologies that provide the most "benefit" for every pound, dollar, or euro spent — or the most "cost-effective"— and away from those that are considered to be relatively inefficient.

The basic objectives of an economic evaluation are to identify, measure, and value the costs and benefits of the technology at hand and to compare them with the costs and benefits of technology that it is ultimately seeking to replace. The statistic produced at the end of this process is called an "incremental cost-effectiveness ratio" (ICER). The ICER is defined as the difference in costs between two technologies divided into the difference in treatment benefits. Evaluations that do not consider the costs and benefits of more than one technology are likely to be partial rather than full economic evaluations, which are less useful for decision-making purposes, as they do not provide full information on the cost-effectiveness of the treatment at hand.

$$ICER = [cost_A - cost_B]/[benefit_A - benefit_B]$$

where $cost_A$ and $cost_B$ are the costs and $benefit_A$ and $benefit_B$ are the benefits associated with programs A and B respectively. For example, if programs A and B had incurred total costs of £2000 and £500 per year respectively and produced 8 and 2 years of patient survival respectively, the ICER would be £250 per life-year gained [(£2000 – £500)/(8 years – 2 years)]. In other words, here it would cost an additional £250 for every extra life-year produced if resources were allocated toward technology A instead of technology B.

The ICER is the statistic traditionally used to assess whether or not a technology is economically viable (or cost-effective). The lower the ICER, the more cost-effective the allocation in resources appears to be. Importantly, the ICER places emphasis on the return (in terms of benefit gain) that is generated per unit of currency spent rather than the total cost of treatment per se. Whether or not a technology is cost-effective, however, depends on the decision-maker's willingness to pay for an extra unit of health. In this instance, it would depend upon the decision-maker's willingness to pay £250 per additional life-year.

Arguably, one of the most important characteristics of the ICER is that it quantifies the amount of health that is generated for an estimated cost rather than the total cost of treatment per se. That is, economic evaluations produce estimates on cost-effectiveness, not on the budget required to treat people with the technology. The two are different concepts and should not be confused. This also means that a relatively costly technology (such as a hemophilia treatment) could be viewed as cost-effective compared with another technology as long as it also results in sufficiently large increases in health.

This aim of this chapter is to review the published evidence on the cost-effectiveness of healthcare technologies for people with hemophilia, although no attempt has been made to identify publications in a systematic manner. The chapter is divided into three main sections: strategies for treating/removing inhibitors, the different types of clotting factor, and prophylactic therapy.

The existing evidence base

Treatment strategies for inhibitors

A recent systematic review by researchers at Sheffield University, UK [2], identified three economic evaluations of treatment options for people with inhibitors to treatment [3–5]. The authors of the review also undertook a fourth evaluation.

All four evaluations assessed the cost-effectiveness of treatment options for people with hemophilia A, although one also included treatment options for inhibitors to factor IX (FIX) [5]. Three of the four evaluations were explicitly based on decision-analytic techniques [2–4], and all examined the costs and effects of treatment options for people with high-responding inhibitors (defined as >5–10 BU). Two of the four evaluations assessed the cost-effectiveness of removing inhibitors with immune tolerance therapy (ITT) [2,4]. The remaining two evaluations and one of the evaluations that had also examined the outcome of ITT, compared the cost-effectiveness of the various clotting factors given as a result of a bleed, most notably recombinant factor VIIa (rFVIIa). The key characteristics of these studies are described in Table 60.1.

Table 60.1 The key characteristics of existing economic evaluations of inhibitor treatments.

Author/Year/Country	Technology	Comparator	Results	Other key characteristics
Colowick et al., 2000; USA [4]	ITT followed by standard FVIII replacement Dose: FVIII 100 IU/kg/day for 420 days	No ITT and indefinite use of alternative clotting agents Minor/moderate bleeding episodes: APCC Major bleeding episodes: pFVIII	ITT was less costly and more effective compared with no ITT (ITT cost $1.9 million, year 65; no ITT cost $2.9 million, year 60)	• FVIII inhibitor • Treatment of a 5-year-old with high-responding inhibitor (25 BU) • Analysis based on a Markov model • Lifetime costs and patient survival assessed • 2.5-fold increase in annual mortality rate for people with inhibitors • Only included costs of clotting agents
Ekert et al., 2001; Australia [5]	rFVIIa 90 µg/kg per bleed repeated in 2 h	Usual care (no other details provided)	ICER of A$50 000 if rFVIIa is used instead of usual care	• Treatment of FVIII and FIX inhibitors • Treatment for high-responding inhibitors (12–240 BU at baseline) • Health outcomes measured in terms of QALYs • Wide range of healthcare costs included • 18-month costs and QALYs assessed • Included data on six people • Before and after study design
Odeyemi et al., 2002; UK [3]	First line treatment of a minor bleed with rFVIIa 2.3 doses (90 µg/kg over 24 h) assumed to stop 92% of bleeds	APCC	rFVIIa was less costly and reduced the time taken to stop a bleed compared with APCC (per bleed APCC cost £20 500; rFVIIa cost £11 800)	• Treatment for high-responding inhibitors (>10 BU) • Wide range of healthcare costs included • Modeled using a decision tree • Data estimated using expert opinion
Knight et al., 2003; UK [2]	Various: 1 ITT (using either the Bonn, Malmö or low-dose protocols) 2 APCC/rFVIIa/pFVIII used in a variety of orders and according to bleeding severity	The treatment regimens were compared with each other and with standard FVIIIs	Numerous ICERs presented; key messages: rFVIIa is cost-effective compared with APCC; The Malmö ITT strategy was the most cost-effective ITT option if the maximum willingness to pay for a QALY is £30 000; The Malmö ITT strategy was less costly and more effective than all methods and treating with APCC/rFVIIa/pFVIII	• Treatment for high-responding FVIII inhibitors (≥ 10 BU) • Health outcomes measured in terms of QALYs • Lifetime costs and QALYs assessed • Many different treatment strategies evaluated • Analysis based on a Markov model • Performed in conjunction with a systematic review of the clinical literature • Wide range of healthcare costs included

ITT, immune tolerance therapy; APCCs, activated prothrombin complex concentrates; pFVIII, porcine FVIII; rFVIIa, recombinant factor VIIa; QALY, quality-adjusted life-year.

Both evaluations of ITT concluded that it was more cost-effective than routine therapy with clotting agents such as activated prothrombin complex concentrates (APCC), porcine factor VIII (pFVIII), or recombinant factor VIIa (rFVIIa) following a bleed (or no ITT). Indeed, the results from both evaluations suggest that ITT is less costly and more effective than these alternatives. The evaluation by Knight et al. [2] went a step further and attempted to identify the most cost-effective of three ITT protocols: The "Malmö" regimen, "Bonn (high-dose)," and "low-dose" protocols. The results from this analysis showed that the Bonn protocol was the most costly (£3.4 million per person) and the most effective [33 quality-adjusted life-years (QALYs) per person] ITT regimen. The next most costly (£2.5 million per person) and effective (29 QALYs per person) regimen was the low-dose protocol followed by the Malmö protocol, with mean per person costs and effects of £2.1 million and 28 QALYs respectively. Although the Malmö protocol was associated with lowest number of QALYs, the authors considered it to be the most cost-effective treatment option. This was because the use of either the low-dose or Bonn regimen instead of the Malmö protocol was associated with incremental QALYs of approximately £60 000 and £148 000.

Odeyemi et al. [3] assessed the cost-effectiveness of treating minor bleeds in patients with high-responding inhibitors (>10 BU) with rFVIIa instead of APCCs. The evaluation was performed using a decision model, although a number of variables were estimated using expert opinion and were not based on the results from primary studies as such. The results from the evaluation suggested that treating with rFVIIa was not only less costly (by approximately £10 000 per bleed) compared with using APCCs, it also reduced the time taken to stop a bleed. In a similar evaluation, Ekert et al. [5] assessed the cost-effectiveness of using rFVIIa to treat a bleed instead of treatment with "usual care." However, as "usual care" was not well defined and the evaluation included only six people, the results of the study are difficult to interpret and are unlikely to be robust.

Increasing purity of clotting factor

To the best of knowledge, and excluding a number of costing studies, only one economic evaluation of the different types of clotting factors exists [6]. At first glance, this is somewhat surprising given that clinical opinion clearly favors the use of the highest purity (i.e., recombinant) agents and that different purities of clotting factor vary considerably in terms of acquisition cost, particularly if added up over a lifetime of use.

The evaluation by Hay et al. [6] was a cost–utility analysis (health benefits were expressed as QALYs) of treatment options for people with hemophilia A. The analysis was based on a decision-analytic model that synthesized the results from a number of separate studies. The time horizon for the evaluation ranged between 2 and 20 years. The aim of the study was to determine the largest increase per unit of clotting factor that could be paid for a move from using intermediate/very-high-purity clotting factor to ultra-pure/recombinant products, meaning

that it did not assess the cost-effectiveness of ultra-pure/recombinant products per se.

Three scenarios were modeled to reflect different treatment populations: people with HIV (human immunodeficiency virus) infection but no HCV (hepatitis C virus), people with HCV infection but no HIV, and people who were HIV and HCV seronegative. In the first scenario, the presumed benefits of increased clotting factor purity were a decrease in the rate of HIV progression and a decrease in the likelihood of parvovirus B19 seroconversion. In the second scenario, the main benefit was assumed to be a reduction in the probability of liver failure. In the final scenario, it was assumed that the main benefit of switching to a higher purity clotting factor reduced the probability of hepatitis A (HAV) and B (HBV) seroconversion. In none of the scenarios was the transmission of other viruses considered. Only the costs of providing the clotting factors and the treatment costs for the relevant viruses were included in the analysis. Clotting factor consumption was assumed to be 40 000 IU per person per annum. Both costs and QALYs were discounted at 3% per annum.

The results from the analysis that used a 20-year time horizon (which is arguably the most appropriate given that treatment is lifelong) suggested that the most decision-makers should be willing to pay on top of the cost of providing intermediate/very-high-purity clotting factor to instead provide ultra-pure/recombinant products was US$0.30 and US$0.46 per unit of clotting factor for scenarios 1 and 2 respectively. No numerical results were presented for the third scenario because, the authors claim, the costs and benefits of preventing HAV and HBV infection were negligible. Or, in other words, the ultra-pure/recombinant products were not considered to be cost-effective in this scenario.

It is interesting to note than none of the scenarios considered the possibility of transmitting either HIV or HCV. This is probably because the marginal risk of transmission with increasing clotting factor purity is so small that on their own these possibilities are likely to result in an extremely high ICER per QALY. Thus, they have been excluded from the analysis. It is also interesting to note that arguably one of the main (theoretical) benefits of the higher-purity clotting factors is that they are less likely to result in transmissions of as yet unknown viruses. It is difficult, if not impossible, to include such theoretical benefits in any formal consideration of cost-effectiveness, because by definition they are unknown, which is an important limitation of the analysis. Another limitation of the analysis is that very few sensitivity analyses were performed, chiefly around the improvements in QoL that were assumed to be gained as a result of switching agents. Thus, it is difficult to assess the robustness of the results.

Prophylaxis with clotting factor

Five full economic evaluations of prophylaxis with clotting factor have been published [7–11] (Table 60.2). These include the analysis by Bohn et al. [7], although strictly speaking it is a cost analysis rather than an economic evaluation as it does not

Table 60.2 The key characteristics of existing economic evaluations of routine prophylaxis with clotting factor compared with treatment on demand.

Author/Year/Country	Results	Key characteristics
Szucs *et al.*, 1996; Germany [11]	Healthcare costs accounted for on demand 94% and prophylaxis 99% of TCs TC on demand: DM17 200 TC prophylaxis: DM28 200 ICER: DM2500 per joint bleed averted	Cost-effectiveness analysis Six-month study involving 50 individuals Secondary prophylaxis Cost and effect data from a single source Not all individuals had severe hemophilia Healthcare and indirect costs included No modeling undertaken No sensitivity analysis performed
Smith *et al.*, 1996; USA [10]	Clotting factor use accounted for >90% of TCs 1 TC on demand: US$870 000 for ages 3–50 2 TC prophylaxis: US$1 267 000 for age 3–20 years followed by treatment on demand 20 to 50 years 3 TC prophylaxis: US$1 655 000 for age 3–50 years Prophylaxis significantly more costly than on demand (*P* < 0.05) ICER (1) vs.(2): US$1100 per bleed averted ICER (1) vs. (3): US$1380 per bleed averted Sensitivity analysis showed that the TC of 3 would equal the TC of 1 if the cost of clotting factor was 4 cents per unit	Cost-effectiveness analysis Two-year study involving 97 individuals Secondary prophylaxis Healthcare and indirect costs included Modeling undertaken to estimate lifetime costs and effects Treatment was assumed to be from the age of 3 years to 50 Costs discounted at 5% per annum Sensitivity analysis performed
Bohn *et al.*, 1998; US–Japan–European [7]; costing from a US perspective	Disability-related healthcare costs PPY: TC no prophylaxis: US$1600 TC partial prophylaxis: US$2200 TC full-time prophylaxis: US$800 Clotting factor costs PPY: TC no prophylaxis: US$30 800 TC partial prophylaxis: US$79 600 TC full-time prophylaxis: US$87 900	Cost analysis Utilized data from the Orthopaedic Outcomes Study [16] (*n* = 831) Prophylaxis defined as either "partial" or "full-time" On demand defined as no prophylaxis. Prophylaxis defined as treatment for >46 weeks in a year. Costs are per patient-year. Study based on the Orthopaedic Outcomes Study Healthcare and indirect costs included No modeling undertaken No sensitivity analysis performed
Miners *et al.*, 1998; UK	TC on demand: £27 800 TC prophylaxis: £76 900 ICER: £550 per bleed averted	Cost-effectiveness analysis Cost and effect data from a single source Only clotting factor costs included Included people with severe hemophilia A and B (*n* = 38) up to the age of 9 years Mostly secondary prophylaxis Treatment groups were not mutually exclusive No modeling undertaken Costs discounted at 6% per annum Limited sensitivity analysis performed
Miners *et al.*, 2003; UK	Healthcare costs accounted for 58–96% of TCs depending on the modeled treatment scenario TC on demand: £272 000 TC prophylaxis with FVIII every 56 h: £966 000 TC prophylaxis with FIX every 84 h: £407 000 ICER: FVIII £46 500 per QALY ICER: FIX £8600 per QALY	Cost–utility analysis Model-based evaluation Primary prophylaxis as specified in treatment guidelines Lifetime treatment costs and effects estimated Healthcare and indirect costs included Costs discounted at 6% per annum Sensitivity analysis performed Many scenarios modeled

PPY, per patient year; TC, total cost.

synthesize information on both the costs and benefits of treatment.

All five economic evaluations compared the costs and benefits associated with prophylaxis against treating on demand. The first to be published estimated the cost-effectiveness of using secondary prophylaxis to prevent bleeding episodes with severe hemophilia A in the USA [10]. Data were collected retrospectively from 11 treatment centers on 90 and 27 individuals who had been treated on demand and with secondary prophylaxis respectively. Modeling techniques were then used to extrapolate these findings. Prophylaxis was defined as treatment with FVIII at least three times per week for a minimum of 6.5 consecutive months, although this did not necessarily mean primary prophylactic therapy. The median observation period was 26 months (range 6.5–72 months) and all patients were under the age of 18 years at the time the data were collected. Future costs were extrapolated using a model whose detail was not well described. Medical resource (clotting factor use, hospital visits) use was abstracted from patient notes but indirect resource use was estimated. Clotting factor was valued at approximately £0.38/IU and charge data were used to value the remaining medical resources.

The results from this evaluation produced total lifetime net present treatment costs of US$870 000 (approximately £620 000), US$1 267 000 (approximately £900 000), and US$1 655 000 (approximately £1 200 000) for individuals treated on demand, with prophylaxis between the ages of 3 and 20 years, and with prophylaxis between the ages of 3 and 50 years respectively. The associated ICERs were US$1100–1380 (approximately £750–950) per bleed avoided.

The next study to be published evaluated the costs and effects of (secondary) prophylaxis over a 1-year time horizon [11]. The 50 individuals in the study were divided into those who had received treatment on demand ($n = 39$) and those who had received prophylaxis ($n = 11$). Nineteen individuals were known to be HIV seropositive. Prophylaxis was defined as prophylactic treatment with clotting factor 12–18 IU/kg three times per week but few other treatment details, such as duration of prophylaxis, were provided.

The reported total costs associated with treating on demand or with prophylaxis were DM17 200 (approximately £5700) and DM28 200 (approximately £9400) per patient-year (PPY) respectively. The associated ICER was DM2500 per averted joint bleed (approximately £800).

Despite the similarity of the ICER to that reported by Smith et al. [10], there are a number of limitations with this European analysis. First, no statistical tests were performed on the data and no consideration was given to the potentially confounding effects of HIV or HCV infection on treatment costs. Second, because participants were not randomized to receiving one or other of the treatments, and few details of their treatment histories were provided, observed differences in outcomes cannot be attributed to relative treatment effects. Finally, no attempt was made in the analysis to extrapolate the findings beyond the observed period (as was the case in Smith

et al.) or to assess the robustness of the ICER using sensitivity analysis.

The third analysis to be published compared the health care and indirect costs of treating individuals with hemophilia A with prophylaxis using data collected as part of the Orthopaedic Outcomes Study [7]. All individuals included in the original study were stratified according to one of three treatment groups according to how long they had received prophylaxis: 0–5 weeks (no prophylaxis), 6–45 weeks (partial prophylaxis), or greater than 46 weeks (full-time prophylaxis) per year. The study included resource data on inpatient days, surgery, and days lost from work or school.

The results of the analysis showed that the costs of clotting factor provision accounted for US$30 800 (approximately £20 000), US$79 600 (approximately £51 000), and US$87 900 (approximately £56 000) PPY for individuals receiving no, partial, or full-time prophylaxis respectively. However, no statistical tests were reported for these data and, as with the European study, no attempt was made to extrapolate these findings beyond the observed period to estimate the lifetime costs of treatment.

The next economic evaluation to be published was based on a cohort of children aged less than 10 years at a London-based comprehensive care center [12]. Data on clotting factor use and bleeding frequency were collected retrospectively for 38 children. The majority of individuals included in the analysis had severe (<1 IU/dL) hemophilia A (71%).

The net discounted costs of treating on demand and with prophylaxis over this period were approximately £27 800 and £76 900 per patient respectively. The ICER for prophylaxis compared with treatment on demand was £550 per bleed avoided. However, this result should be treated with caution because of a number of limitations with the study design. First, patients were not randomized to receive prophylaxis or treatment on demand, meaning that the estimates of treatment effect (and resource use) could be biased. Second, the evaluation only included the costs of clotting factor provision and excluded other items such as the costs of hospital visits. Lastly, and similarly to the studies by Szucs et al. [11] and Bohn et al. [7], the results were not extrapolated beyond the period of data collection.

Despite their usefulness, there a number of clear limitations with these studies. For example, none of the evaluations explicitly assesses the cost-effectiveness of prophylaxis for people with hemophilia B; nor do they include information on the progression of health-related QoL, when, arguably, the main aim of treatment is to modify QoL.

The strongest evaluation in terms of technical quality is undoubtedly the study by Smith et al. [10] because it makes an explicit attempt to model the long-term costs and effects of treatment. However, this analysis does not assess the cost-effectiveness of primary prophylaxis nor does it assess the cost-effectiveness of treatment for people with hemophilia B. A final criticism of this and the other evaluations surrounds the interpretability of the presented ICERs. While the results from these evaluations appear to suggest a cost per (joint) bleed prevented of no more than £1000, does this mean prophylaxis is cost-effective compared with treating on demand? It is arguable that this statistic is difficult to interpret compared with, say, a "cost per quality-adjusted life-year (QALY) gained."

A fifth economic evaluation was undertaken in an attempt to address some of the limitations with the existing evidence base and because of the desire to estimate the cost-effectiveness of primary prophylaxis using QALYs as the unit of health benefit [9]. The evaluation used a decision-analytic model to estimate the costs and effects of treatment on demand and primary prophylaxis for hypothetical cohorts of 100 people. Treatment was assumed to be from birth to either 70 years of age or death, whichever occurred first. However, the model was rerun several times so that a number of different scenarios could be represented in the analysis. For example, the time between prophylactic doses of clotting factor and the clotting factor acquisition costs were varied in some scenarios. It was assumed that the aim of primary prophylactic treatment was to prevent trough in vivo clotting factor activity levels from falling below 1 IU/dL at all times, in line with the Malmö protocol [13,14] and World Federation of Hemophilia treatment guidelines [15].

Information on the costs and benefits of treatment were taken from a number of different sources. However, perhaps the most pivotal assumption within the model, made in the absence of any better data, was that the people with severe hemophilia who are treated with primary prophylaxis experience levels of health that are equivalent to the levels experienced by people with more mild/moderate forms of the condition. The assumption was also made that people who were treated on demand experienced levels of health that were similar to those experienced by a cohort of individuals who had received treatment using a variety of regimens but had never been treated on demand. Again, this assumption was made in the absence of any more appropriate information.

The results from the analysis suggested that clotting factor provision alone accounted for the largest proportion of total costs: 58–96% depending on the clotting factor type (FVIII or FIX) and the time between prophylactic doses of clotting factor. The mean net present costs for major surgery for individuals receiving primary prophylaxis were £4000–5000 per patient or 1–4% of the total cost, whereas the mean costs of major surgery for individuals receiving treatment on demand were £8000–14 000 or 3–5% of the total cost. However, the productivity losses associated with either treatment method accounted for no more than 2% of the total costs in any scenario.

The mean lifetime net present discounted healthcare costs of treatment on demand were approximately £272 000 per person for people with severe hemophilia A or B. However, primary prophylaxis was considerably more costly. For example, the mean expected lifetime healthcare cost of infusing with FVIII every 56 h (three times a week) was £966 000. Similarly, the mean net present lifetime cost of providing primary prophylaxis with FIX every 84 h (twice a week) for individuals with hemophilia B was £407 000: 1.5 times greater than the cost of treating individuals with hemophilia B on demand.

The baseline analysis produced ICERs for individuals receiving FVIII and FIX of £46 500 per QALY gained and £8600 per QALY gained respectively. However, the scenario analysis showed that these results were very sensitive to the time between prophylactic doses and the unit clotting factor cost (Table 60.3). Indeed, in some scenarios, prophylaxis was less costly and more effective than treating on demand.

Sensitivity analysis showed that varying the unit cost of surgery did little to alter the ICER, as was also the case for increasing the cost per day of absenteeism from work. Increasing the unit cost of FVIII and FIX by 1% increased the corresponding ICERs by 0.5 and 0.8% respectively, which perhaps

Table 60.3 Scenario analysis on the unit clotting factor cost and the time between prophylactic clotting factor infusions.

	ICER*			
Clotting factor (p/IU)	22.5	32.5	52.9	70.0
Hemophilia A				
Infusing every 56 h	32 000	46 500	76 100	–
Infusing every 48 h	29 500	42 600	69 300	–
Infusing every 24 h	Dominant	Dominant	Dominant	–
Continuous infusion	Dominant	Dominant	Dominant	–
Hemophilia B				
Infusing every 84 h	5800	8600	–	19 500
Infusing every 56 h	385	829	–	2704
Infusing every 48 h	Dominant	Dominant	–	Dominant
Infusing every 24 h	Dominant	Dominant	–	Dominant
Continuous infusion	Dominant	Dominant	–	Dominant

*Incremental cost (£) per QALY (quality-adjusted life-year) gained.
"Dominant" indicates that primary prophylaxis is more effective and less costly than treatment on demand.
ICER, incremental cost-effectiveness ratio; P, UK pence, equivalent to approximately 0.6 US$.

indicates that this variable has a moderate role to play in terms of determining the cost-effectiveness of primary prophylaxis. The impact of changing the utility scores for primary prophylaxis on the cost-effectiveness of treatment was, however, much more dramatic. When these values were increased, the result was a 3% decrease in the ICER, which indicates that health-related quality-of-life has a large role to play in determining the cost-effectiveness of primary prophylaxis. The time between prophylactic doses of FVIII was also shown to be an important predictor of cost-effectiveness. The only other variable to exert a greater influence on the ICER than these two variables was the discount rate for the health benefits. If a 1% discount rate was applied to the health benefits in the baseline analysis, the ICERs for treatment with either FVIII or FIX increased to over £100 000 per QALY gained, which arguably indicates an inefficient use of resources.

The five economic evaluations of prophylaxis described in this section have a number of broad similarities. All five compared the outcomes associated with prophylaxis against treating on demand, four of the five appear to estimate the cost-effectiveness of secondary prophylaxis, and three assessed the cost of preventing an additional (joint) bleed. There are also a number of similarities in terms of their results. It is clear that clotting factor provision is by far the largest proportion of total costs — indeed the indirect costs associated with treatments are almost negligible in comparison. Also apparent is that prophylaxis as currently performed is more costly than treating on demand.

The question remains as to whether or not prophylaxis is cost-effective. As previously argued, this is difficult to determine using the results from the studies that reported a cost per additional (joint) bleed. However, the results from the single cost–utility analysis of primary prophylaxis using World Federation of Hemophilia guidelines suggests that it costs approximately £46 500 and £8600 per additional QALY to treat people with FVIII and FIX respectively. There is no absolute cut-off in terms of an acceptable cost per QALY; however, analysis suggests that in the UK it might be around £30 000. On this basis, therefore, it is at best marginal as to whether primary prophylaxis with FVIII is cost-effective, but treatment with FIX is probably a cost-effective use of resources.

Discussion

There is little doubt that treatments for people with severe hemophilia can be extremely costly. However, costly technologies can be considered cost-effective if they also produce sufficiently large improvements in health. The purpose of an economic evaluation is to quantify these costs and benefits relative to the next best course of action and to assess the level of certainty that can be attached to them.

What can be concluded from the economic evaluations of hemophilia treatments? With regards to treatments for high-responding inhibitors, the evidence suggests that treatment with rFVIIa when bleeds occur is cost-effective compared with other treatment options such as APCCs or pFVIII. There is also some evidence to suggest that ITT to remove high-responding inhibitors is more cost-effective than treating bleeds on demand with any of these agents. However, the evidence also suggests that this is not true for all ITT regimens, and no assessments have been made of the uncertainty surrounding these results. Finally, there is some evidence to suggest that treatment with rFVIIa is cost-effective in the treatment of minor bleeds compared with APCCs.

A central question in the management of hemophilia is the cost-effectiveness of increasing clotting factor purity. However, only one economic evaluation has addressed this question and it does so only indirectly. The reason for this paucity of economic evidence, however, is perhaps understandable if the information required to do such an evaluation is considered. One of the principal objectives of increasing clotting factor purity is to decrease the risk of iatrogenic infection, in terms of both known and unknown viruses. If the aim was restricted to the former, this would be relatively straightforward to model — the annual risk of (say) hepatitis C infection as reported in the literature for people who had received (say) high-purity FVIIIs could be compared with the same risk for people who have been treated with (say) recombinant FVIII. The costs of treating the sequelae of infection could then be included in the evaluation, as should the costs of the necessary clotting factors. However, this is almost impossible to do for as yet unknown viruses because the risk of future infection and the costs of treating such an infection should it occur are by definition unknown and are therefore unquantifiable. It is doubtful that a particularly useful economic evaluation of increasing clotting factor purity that considered this possibility could ever be performed (in terms of producing a robust ICER); thus, the cost-effectiveness of increasing clotting factor purity is likely to remain highly nebulous.

The evidence relating to prophylaxis is not particularly easy to interpret because most of the evaluations considered only short-term treatment costs and benefits, ICERs were expressed in terms of cost per (joint) bleed avoided (rather than QALYs), and definitions of prophylaxis were inconsistent across the studies. However, the results from a cost–utility analysis that did consider lifetime treatment benefits and costs suggest that primary prophylaxis with FVIII using a dosing schedule recommended by the WFH, and using a clotting factor cost of £0.33, is not particularly cost-effective. Methods of reducing amounts of clotting factor without reducing hemostatic activity need to be developed or the unit cost of clotting factor dropped considerably before it is likely to be cost-effective compared with treating on demand. This said, however, treatment with FIX is likely to be cost-effective without need of these changes.

In conclusion, despite the fact that collecting outcomes data for rare and lifelong conditions is difficult, the past 5 years has seen a significant increase in the number of publications that have attempted to use formal economic techniques to assess the cost-effectiveness of hemophilia treatments. Although arguably of variable quality, all have been useful contributions to the literature for a variety of reasons. However, it is imperative that authors of future evaluations critically evaluate these studies in an attempt to improve on them in terms of their methodologic rigor so that firmer conclusions can be drawn.

References

1 Drummond MF, O'Brien B, Stoddart GL, Torrance GW. *Methods for the Economic Evaluation of Health Care Programmes*, 2nd edn. Oxford: Oxford University Press, 1997.

2 Knight C, Paisley S, Wight J, Jones ML. Economic modelling of different treatment strategies for haemophilia A with high-responding inhibitors. *Haemophilia* 2003; **9**: 521–40.

3 Odeyemi IAO, Guest JF. Modelling the economic impact of recombinant activated Factor VII and activated prothrombin-complex concentrate in the treatment of a mild to moderate bleed in adults with inhibitors to clotting Factors VIII and IX at a comprehensive care centre in the UK. *J Med Econom* 2002; **5**: 51–64.

4 Colowick AB, Bohn RL, Avorn J, Ewenstein BM. Immune tolerance induction in hemophilia patients with inhibitors: costly can be cheaper. *Blood* 2000; **96**: 1698–702.

5 Ekert H, Brewin T, Boey W, *et al.* Cost-utility analysis of recombinant factor VIIa (NovoSeven) in six children with long-standing inhibitors to factor VIII or IX. *Haemophilia* 2001; **7**: 279–85.

6 Hay JW, Ernst RL, Kessler CM. Cost-effectiveness analysis of alternative factor VIII products in treatment of haemophilia A. *Haemophilia* 1999; **5**: 191–202.

7 Bohn RL, Avorn J, Glynn RJ, *et al.* Prophylactic use of factor VIII: an economic evaluation. *Thromb Haemost* 1998; **79**: 932–7.

8 Miners AH, Sabin CA, Tolley KH, Lee CA. Primary prophylaxis for individuals with severe haemophilia: how many hospital visits could treatment prevent? *J Intern Med* 2000; **247**: 493–9.

9 Miners AH, Sabin CA, Tolley KH, Lee CA. A cost-utility analysis of primary prophylaxis versus treatment on-demand for individuals with severe haemophilia. *Pharmacoeconomics* 2002; **20**: 759–74.

10 Smith PS, Teutsch SM, Shaffer PA, *et al.* Episodic versus prophylactic infusions for hemophilia A: a cost-effectiveness analysis. *J Pediatr* 1996; **129**: 424–31.

11 Szucs TD, Öffner A, Schramm W. Socioeconomic impact of haemophilia care: results of a pilot study. *Haemophilia* 1996; **2**: 211–17.

12 Miners AH, Sabin CA, Tolley KH, Lee CA. Assessing the effectiveness and cost-effectiveness of prophylaxis against bleeding in patients with severe haemophilia and severe von Willebrand's disease. *J Intern Med* 1998; **244**: 515–22.

13 Löfqvist T, Nilsson IM, Berntorp E, Pettersson H. Haemophilia prophylaxis in young patients — a long-term follow-up. *J Intern Med* 1997; **241**: 395–400.

14 Nilsson IM, Berntorp E, Lofqvist T, Pettersson H. Twenty-five years' experience of prophylactic treatment in severe haemophilia A and B. *J Intern Med* 1992; **23**: 25–32.

15 UK Haemophilia Centre Directors Organization Executive Committee. Guidelines on therapeutic products to treat haemophilia and other hereditary coagulation disorders. *Haemophilia* 1997; **3**: 63–77.

16 Aledort LM, Haschmeyer RH, Pettersson H. A longitudinal study of orthopaedic outcomes for severe factor-VIII-deficient haemophiliacs. The Orthopaedic Outcome Study Group. *J Intern Med* 1994; **236**: 391–9.

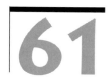

61 Comprehensive care and delivery of care: the developed world

Christopher A. Ludlam

Introduction

Historically, developments in hemophilia care have been entirely dependent on close collaboration between those who care directly for patients and their families and those from a wide range of professions and other organizations. Effective hemophilia therapy, until recently, was almost totally dependent on plasma-derived clotting factor concentrate, and in many countries this required detailed arrangements with national blood transfusion services and/or the purchase of concentrates from international plasma fractionators. Global issues have traumatized hemophilia like no other disease; the transmission of viral infections or sudden unpredictable shortages of therapeutic concentrates are but two examples. Those with responsibility for providing services, therefore, have to keep a very broad national and international perspective on factors that might influence the provision of therapy.

To collaborate with other organizations, e.g., blood transfusion services, hemophilia physicians have had to develop national organizations to negotiate provision for patients. In the UK, the Haemophilia Centre Doctors' Organisation (UKHCDO) is an example of an organization that has grown from a small beginning to a large and effective collaboration of doctors who have been able to lead effectively the developments in care and set standards to improve the lives of hemophiliacs. Similarly, patients have organized themselves into national societies, e.g., UK Haemophilia Society, and these have been very effective in patient advocacy. Many other countries have similar organizations, e.g., National Hemophilia Foundation (USA) (www.hemophilia.org). These national societies have been drawn together into the World Federation of Hemophilia (WFH), which has promoted hemophilia care particularly effectively in developing nations (www.wfh.org). It has encouraged international collaboration between designated specialist centers of expertise (WFH international training centers) and countries with developing services. This chapter is predominantly about how hemophilia care is organized in the UK as an example of a national system in the developed world, as the arrangements are well known to the author.

Development of hemophilia care in the UK

Since 1950, there has been a national UK approach to delivery of hemophilia care, and this was initially directed by the Medical Research Council (MRC), which recognized 19 centers where special facilities were available for diagnosis and treatment of hemophilia [1,2]. These centers issued hemophilia identity cards and kept a local list of patients as well as contributing names to a central register kept by the MRC. In the decade that followed, the early freeze-dried concentrates were developed from animal and human plasma but the major breakthrough was treatment with cryoprecipitate in 1965. In 1964, the responsibility for oversight of hemophilia passed to the Ministry of Health, which in 1968 issued a health memorandum [3] identifying 36 centers that would diagnose and treat patients, and three of these were designated special treatment centres that would undertake surgery. In October of that year, the directors of these hemophilia centers were invited to the opening of a new building at the Oxford Haemophilia Centre. At a party organized for the event by Dr Rosemary Biggs, it was agreed to have regular national meetings of directors and that annual treatment data would be sent to Oxford for collation. This was the beginning of what later formally became the UKHCDO. With further developments in the provision of hemophilia care, the Department of Health issued a further document in 1976 [4] setting out revised criteria for services that should be provided at the 52 hemophilia centers. Of these, seven were designated regional hemophilia centers and the others hemophilia centers and associate centers, although the facilities that should be provided at each of these three types of center were not specified. At this time, the collection of national data was extended to include all patients with hemophilia known to each center and, in addition, treated carriers. Subsequently, it was extended to include all patients with von Willebrand disease. Thus, over the past 50 years there has been national coordination of hemophilia care, with the arrangements having to change in response to advances in therapy as well as to the way the government has overall managed the state national health service.

The UK Haemophilia Doctors' Organisation (UKHCDO)

Current UKHCDO activities

The UKHCDO's structure had to change again in 1993 when the government abolished health regions and established more "independent" trust hospitals. This led to a further development in hemophilia care arrangements, with the recognition of comprehensive care hemophilia centers (CCCs). The 24 centers were so designated if they looked after at least 40 patients with severe hemophilia and offered a broad range of services as specified in a further government health circular [5]. In addition, there were 79 hemophilia centers with a responsibility to provide a more limited range of services. At this time the constitution of the organization was revised to extend the membership from directors of centers to all doctors working within the hemophilia environment and this was recognized by the "D" in UKHCDO changing from "director's" to "doctor's" thus allowing the abbreviation for the organization to remain unchanged! It is a three-tiered organization with an Executive, advisory group (of representatives of CCCs), and doctors working in hemophilia centers. The Executive, of office bearers, is elected by the entire membership, thus allowing more of those providing the service to be enfranchised. There is an annual meeting of all members, which often includes an educational symposium, and the advisory group meets about four times annually to take forward the business.

During the past 40 years in the UK, therefore, the benefits of advances in hemophilia care have extended from the small number of the original special treatment centers and many patients being treated in local district hospitals without ready access to comprehensive care, to a service with more large CCCs, and hemophilia centers able to offer a higher quality of service. The loss of associate centers and smaller hemophilia centers over the past 10 years has led to a gradual centralization of patient care in the UK. This has come with the loss of an association of individual patient with a local hematologist and hospital, a change that was possible with the development of freeze-dried concentrates and consequently home therapy. The centers at present vary greatly in the number of patients each treats annually; more than 30 treat less than 10, whilst a small number serving large metropolitan populations treat over 200 (Figure 61.1).

Over the past 20 years, Scotland, Wales, and Northern Ireland have developed a degree of devolution from the UK government in London. In Scotland, healthcare provision is now a different service from that in England, with its own funding and priori-

ties, and it is led by the Scottish Executive and the parliament in Edinburgh. To address this devolution, hemophilia directors in Scotland (along with those in Northern Ireland, for other historical reasons) meet regularly to promote and coordinate arrangements. This ensures that there is effective collaboration and participation by all hemophilia physicians and allows a coordinated approach to commissioners, particularly for concentrate procurement. These arrangements dovetail well with the national UKHCDO, and in the future it is likely that English regions (each of which has a population similar to that of Scotland) will have similar local networks.

Responsibilities of the UKHCDO

In Britain, the UKHCDO is formally defined as a charity and is subject in England to charity law and the Charity Commissioners. This offers some protection from taxation of its income but prevents it from "political campaigning." This does not prevent it, however, from offering firm guidance (wherever possible evidence-based) on matters related to provision of care for hemophiliacs, particularly in relation to therapy and blood product safety. The aims of the organization are formally set out in the constitution and are to promote care of those with hemophilia and related bleeding disorders, promote research, and advance education of medical and nursing staff and the general public.

The advisory group is the main forum for progressing the UKHCDO's professional remit to oversee the quality of hemophilia medical care throughout the UK. This includes all the responsibilities of CCCs directly (as set out below) as well as a general oversight of the large number of hemophilia centers and their activities. Although it is not managerially responsible directly for the service, this being the responsibility of the individual hospitals, it has a major commitment to inform those funding services and to work with the departments of health of the four countries in the UK. Over the years this has predominantly been with issues related to the quality of hemophilia care, the availability of therapeutic concentrates, and blood safety.

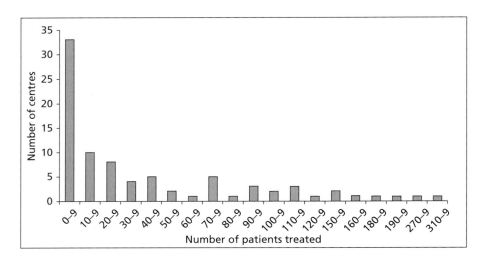

Figure 61.1 Total number of patients treated by UK hemophilia centers in 2000 (from UKHCDO, with kind permission).

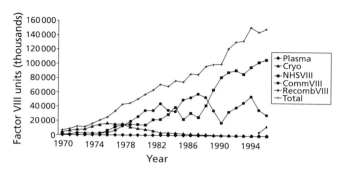

Figure 61.2 Total annual products used in the UK to treat hemophilia A (from ref. 13).

Table 61.1 UKHCDO current working parties.

Audit
Data Management Group
Inhibitor
Pediatrics
Transfusion transmitted infections
von Willebrand disease
Genetics
Rare hemostatic disorders

This has required a UK national approach partly because the issues are often technically complex (e.g., blood safety), costly, and require close collaboration with the blood transfusion services in each UK country.

National register of patients

Following on from the register of patients held by the MRC, the UKHCDO since 1969 has maintained a confidential national register of patients with heritable bleeding disorders (as well as acquired hemophilia and von Willebrand disease). Although initiated as a card index system, it has been computerized and is now held on a secure server that allows individual hemophilia centers to report new patients and review details of patients registered at their center. Oversight of the register is the responsibility of the UKHCDO Data Management Group, which is convened by the organization's vice-chairman and comprises the chairmen of the individual working parties, a representative of the Haemophilia Nurses Association (HNA), and two patient representatives. Under the Data Protection Act 1998, patients should give informed consent to being on the register and, to help the process of informing patients about the database, an information leaflet has been produced and widely distributed. Patients can request a copy of their own data on the register. Each year hemophilia centers inform the database which patients have been treated and the products received. It also records whether the patient has an inhibitor, the HIV status, and whether the genetic mutation is known (but not details — these being held at the hemophilia center that requested the investigation). At present, hemophilia centers report the total amounts of different treatments used annually, although in future it is likely that concentrate use for each individual patient will be recorded. This allows very accurate assessment of the national use of blood products, and Figure 60.2 illustrates the changes in hemophilia treatment in the period 1969–1996.

The UKHCDO database has been an essential resource for planning the healthcare needs, particularly in relation to knowing the total number of patients of each severity of hemophilia and the amount of concentrate used. Over the past 20 years, the increase in concentrate use has been recorded at 5–10% per annum and attempts have been made in some centers and in Scotland to assess the reasons for this [6,7].

Working parties

One of the other important responsibilities of the advisory group is to establish short-term working parties that develop guidelines to inform practice and set standards (against which the quality of the service can be audited). The trigger for establishment of a working party is either when new technology leads to a change in emphasis in clinical service — e.g., advances in ability to identify hemophilic mutations led to the establishment of a genetics working party [8] — or when existing guidelines require updating, e.g., Guidelines on Therapeutic Products [9]. While the membership of these working parties is predominantly those working directly in hemophilia care, they also offer an opportunity to include specialists in other fields, e.g., orthopedic surgery or hepatology, who offer stimulating contributions and different perspectives. As can be seen from the titles of the current working parties, listed in Table 61.1, they cover a broad range of topics that are all central to hemophilia.

Although the UKHCDO's remit is to promote hemophilia care in the UK, it does this also by active collaboration with other professional medical organizations, particularly the Royal Colleges of Physicians, Pathologists, and Paediatrics and Child Health, as well as the British Society of Hematology and the British Society for Haemostasis and Thrombosis. This is important to ensure appropriate dovetailing of hemophilia services with general healthcare arrangements and to enable the wider aspects of professional training and development to take place within the UK medical environment.

Haemophilia Society

The UK Haemophilia Society is an organization of patients and their families that provides support for those with heritable bleeding disorders (www.haemophilia.org.uk). It is a well-organized and effective pressure group, encouraging improvements in service provision. It has a major educational responsibility and publishes highly regarded information booklets. It is an active member of the WFH (www.wfh.org).

Haemophilia Nurses Association

In parallel with this development of the UKHCDO has been the emergence of organizations of other professions contributing to overall hemophilia care. Senior nurses now play a major role in both the organization of hemophilia activities and the day-to-day treatment of patients in hospital and at home. In the UK, the Haemophilia Nurses Association (HNA), led by an organizing committee, comprises about 100 members and is incorporated within the national Royal College of Nursing (www.rcn.org.uk). Nurses wishing to develop a career in hemophilia are now encouraged to take an advanced training course in hemophilia; these are run as part of a postgraduate studies program by several universities. Continuing professional development is through regular national educational meetings and the development of guidelines on various aspects of hemophilia care.

Haemophilia Chartered Physiotherapists Association

The Haemophilia Chartered Physiotherapists Association (HCPA) brings together those with skills in developing the musculoskeletal system, thus helping to prevent bleeds and minimizing their detrimental effects when they do occur (www.cps.org.uk). Although a much smaller group than the HNA, they have been well organized nationally and have recently developed and published a very useful guide.

Social work support

Social work support is critical both to help a family adjust to a new member with hemophilia and to assist those who develop relationship (and financial) difficulties as a result of their hemophilia or the consequences of its treatment, e.g., HIV. In the UK, hemophilia social workers collaborated nationally to sustain and develop their expertise and services. With the move from hospital-based social work services to the community it has been harder to maintain an active professional grouping and the amount of support overall that social workers can provide has regrettably declined.

Laboratory scientists

Laboratory scientists provide the critical diagnostic services essential for hemophilia centers. Those with an academic scientific background as clinical scientists are employed primarily in research and development activities and more recently in ensuring that the latest advances in genetic techniques are available to benefit hemophilia families. As this has become one of their primary responsibilities, they have collaborated to establish the UK Haemophilia Genetic Laboratory Network, and through this

grouping have developed effective guidelines and standards for hemophilia genetic services. Biomedical scientists, with a more technical focus on the laboratory service, are members of the Institute of Biomedical Scientists (IBMS), which is a large umbrella organization for scientists in all branches of pathology (www.ibms.org). Unfortunately, those biomedical scientists working in hemophilia center laboratories do not collaborate as a recognizable group nationally.

Hemophilia Alliance

One of the challenges of hemophilia care is to ensure that the multidisciplinary team works collaboratively within the hospital and community to provide as seamlessly as possible the range of appropriate services. To continue to develop this integrated service the professional organizations outlined above, along with the patients' Haemophilia Society, have come together to form the umbrella organization The UK Haemophilia Alliance (Table 61.2). This has developed and published models for comprehensive care for hemophilia in its Service Specification (www.haemophiliaalliance.org.uk). This is now accepted as the standard of service, which should be funded by commissioners and provided by hospitals with CCCs and hemophilia centers.

Comprehensive hemophilia care in the UK

One of the guiding principles in designing arrangements for providing care for those with hemophilia and their families is that all individuals, wherever they live, should have access to the full range of services and specialties that make up comprehensive care for hemophilia. While the majority who live near a CCC will be able to access these directly, those living more remotely who attend their local hemophilia center may need to be referred to the most convenient CCC for some of the more specialist aspects of clinical or laboratory service. For this to work well, there should be agreed arrangements for appropriate referral of patients between hemophilia centers and the local CCC as part of a collaborative network with agreed protocols.

The range of services that contribute to comprehensive care have been set out in the 1993 Health Circular [5] and more

Table 61.2 Professional organizations contributing to The Haemophilia Alliance.

UK Haemophilia Centre Doctors' Organisation
UK Haemophilia Society
UK RCN Haemophilia Nurses Association
Haemophilia Chartered Physiotherapists Association
Clinical Scientists Group
Institute of Biomedical Science
Haemophilia Social Workers Group

recently in greater detail in the Hemophilia Alliance Service Specification [10].

Hemophilia Alliance Service Specification

The Service Specification of standards for hemophilia care was compiled by a multidisciplinary team representing the Alliance's constituent professions and the Haemophilia Society. The standards were based on guidelines, which had been previously issued by the individual professional groups. It thus brought together into one document a description of the standards for a coordinated service for patients and their families, and in doing so provided an invaluable resource both for those funding services and those in the hospitals providing the care. The contents of the report are listed in Table 61.3.

Service standards and delivery

This section sets out in detail the provisions that need to be made to fulfill the requirements of the hemophilia health circulars issued by the departments of health for the constituent counties of the UK [3,4]. The importance of patients being able to choose at which CCC or hemophilia center they are registered is emphasized, as is their right of access to a CCC. The range of services that a CCC should provide are set out in Table 61.4. To provide these, it will often be necessary to have network arrangements with specialists, e.g., orthopedic surgery. The details of these networks will very much depend on how the other specialists provide their services locally and of the arrangements between CCC and the local hemophilia centers. Furthermore, hemophilia centers vary greatly in the range of services they provide, but as a minimum they must be able to provide an emergency 24-h treatment service, diagnose the commoner inherited bleeding disorders, provide advice, administer a home therapy program, and participate in appropriate audit and quality control. It cannot be emphasized too strongly that for these specialty networks of services to function effectively, investment must be made to ensure that there are good and effective communications between the providers of the individual specialist services.

The Service Specification also emphasizes the importance of the establishment of a regional hemophilia network that comprises those who commission and fund the service as well as those who provide and use it. This regional network should oversee the coordinated service provided by CCCs and hemophilia centers and promote strategic planning and implementation of the Service Specification. These regional networks are at different stages of evolution, with some areas having well-developed arrangements while others are still being established.

Table 61.3 National Service Specification for Haemophilia.

Topics covered in the specification
Target patient group
Methodology
Service objectives
Service standards and delivery
Quality standards
Treatment recommendations
Carrier detection, genetic counseling, and antenatal diagnosis
Outcomes
Service arrangements
Purchase of coagulation factor concentrates
Record keeping and data collection

Table 61.4 Functions of a comprehensive care center.

Coordination of the delivery of hemophilia services – both in hospital and in the community – while liaising with affiliated hemophilia centers and appropriate community agencies
A 24-h advisory and response service for hemophilia centers, general practitioners, dental surgeons, hospital doctors, patients, and families
Delivery of a comprehensive care program for patients with hemophilia; there must be at least 40 severely affected patients with hemophilia under the care of the center
A home therapy program for patients with severe hemophilia, including the administration of prophylactic therapy where appropriate
Home treatment training programs, including home and school visits where appropriate
Provision of coagulation factor concentrates, both for hospital treatment and home therapy programs
A diagnostic and reference laboratory service, performing a full range of laboratory tests for the diagnosis and monitoring of inherited and acquired disorders of hemostasis
Counseling for patients and their families
Social work support and welfare advice
Genetic counseling and diagnosis, in conjunction with specialized laboratories
Physiotherapy
Specialist operative and conservative dentistry
Specialist rheumatologic and orthopedic follow-up and intervention
Provision of obstetric and gynecological support for the clinical management of hemophilia carriers and women with von Willebrand disease
Specialized services for patients with HIV and hepatitis, including support groups
Family support groups
Participation in clinical trials
Participation in clinical and laboratory audit, external and internal quality control, with submission of results to commissioning authorities
Participation in research and development
Educational programs for medical and nursing staff, biomedical scientists and related paramedical personnel
Educational programs for patients and their families concerning all aspects of home therapy and community care

Quality standards

The service specification sets out standards for data collection, laboratory performance, and clinical protocols (as set out by the UKHCDO, HNA, and HCPA). Recommendations are set out for regular external audit of both CCC and hemophilia centers under the auspices of UKHCDO and HNA (see below).

Treatment recommendations

This section of the service specification covers in some detail the framework for treatment, prophylaxis and home therapy, arrangements for children, and clinical review, and includes the importance of patient participation in the care process and record keeping. Patient treatment is guided by Recommendations on Therapeutic Products as issued by the UKHCDO [9]. Advice is given on management of inhibitors, immune tolerance, acquired hemophilia, von Willebrand disease, and rarer coagulation defects including inherited platelet disorders.

Carrier detection, genetic counseling, and antenatal diagnosis

With the ability to relatively readily identify the individual mutation causing hemophilia in a family, this is now a recommended part of the assessment of hemophilic individuals. Knowledge of the mutation has made it much more straightforward to identify carriers directly rather than with the use of restriction fragment length polymorphisms (RFLPs) to track hemophilic genes within a family. As a result of this technical advance, there is a need now to offer to those who may be at risk knowledge of their carriership status. This has led in the UK to a re-examination of the arrangements for genetic counseling, establishment of local genetic registers, and genetic laboratory facilities at some CCCs as set out in the recent publication of detailed UKHCDO guidelines [8]. The guidelines considered in some detail issues related to consent to genetic diagnosis both in children and adults. A patient information sheet and consent form were developed.

Outcomes of hemophilia care

There is increasing interest in being able to assess the outcome of hemophilia therapy, particularly as treatment is difficult, potentially hazardous, and expensive. Relevant outcome measurements are difficult to quantify, particularly in the short term. One important aim of treatment is prevention of joint damage and its progression, but this needs to be assessed over many years. For this reason, a number of surrogate measures of effectiveness of treatment have been suggested, such as the number of breakthrough bleeds per year in those on prophylaxis and days missed from school or work. This is a developing area of hemophilia care and one in which socioeconomic evaluation is being increasingly applied [11].

Audit

Over the past 15 years in the UK, it has become increasingly important to objectively demonstrate, by external review, the quality of medical services. Hemophilia has been one of the specialties in the vanguard of medical audit [12]. The initial pilot scheme was developed in 1990 in Scotland and Northern Ireland, in which the service at each center was assessed and patients' access to comprehensive care audited. The CCCs (Belfast, Edinburgh, and Glasgow) and hemophilia centers (Aberdeen, Dundee, and Inverness) undertake this audit every 3 years. In 1994, the UKHCDO developed a triennial external audit of CCCs in the UK based on experience gained in Scotland and Northern Ireland, and more recently this has been extended to include the HNA. There is a comprehensive audit pro forma covering the topics listed in Table 61.5. Prior to the audit visit, a questionnaire is sent to a random selection of 30 patients registered at the center; the questionnaires are returned anonymously to the auditors. Two auditors, a hemophilia physician and a nurse, visit the center for a day and review the clinical and laboratory facilities. They also comment on whether recommendations in the previous audit have been implemented. Following their visit, a report is compiled and returned to the CCC. A copy is returned to the chairman of the UKCDO, to allow any unsafe arrangements or practices to be addressed urgently, but also to allow a national report to be compiled summarizing the national service and to highlight weaknesses and areas for development. While this UK audit is currently (in England and Wales) only for CCCs, there are plans to extend it to all hemophilia centers (as is current practice in Scotland and Northern Ireland).

Funding of hemophilia care

The funding arrangements for hemophilia have evolved with the development of both advances in treatment and the way the overall healthcare budget is managed nationally. The arrangements for England, Scotland, Wales, and Northern Ireland differ

Table 61.5 UKHCDO audit.

The audit includes a review of:
Recommendations of previous audit
Number of registered patients
Patient services at center
Coagulation factor stock control, storage, and issue
Treatment delivery
Availability of comprehensive care services
Patient medical records
Clinical governance, audit, lecture, teaching, continuing professional development, research
Pediatric care
Patient questionnaires/responses

in significant details. In the early days of UK plasma fractionation to provide concentrates, their manufacture was paid for directly by the government but latterly in England and Wales the cost of these concentrates has been "charged" to local commissioners or funders of care. Periodically, central government funds have been distributed to these local commissioners to pay for Department of Health directed changes in treatment, e.g., provision of recombinant factor VIII (FVIII) and factor IX to under-16-year-olds in 1998 and the current policy to make it available to all patients in the near future. Arrangements in Scotland and Northern Ireland have historically been more nationally coordinated and funded. In all countries of the UK, the cost of concentrate provision is recognized as being substantial and requires explicit identification by commissioners, whereas the cost of staffing and most other activities of CCCs and hemophilia centers is provided from local healthcare budgets. The Hemophilia Alliance Service Specification has been very helpful in both defining and agreeing what should be provided and it is therefore of great value for commissioners to see how the overall service is configured.

Future developments in provision of hemophilia care

Over the past 20 years, FVIII and other concentrate use has risen steadily at approximately 5% per annum, and there is no sign of this rate declining; it may in fact accelerate with increased use of prophylaxis. The cost is rising faster than the increase in use by FVIII unitage with the move from plasma-derived to the more expensive recombinant concentrates. This financial pressure will make more urgent the gathering of outcome data to justify the increased use of concentrates. There will be an increasing focus on treatment and immune tolerance of those with inhibitors and the outcome of the international immune tolerance induction study is awaited with great interest (www.itistudy.com). Patients are seeking increasing information about their condition, and with developments in reliable genetic diagnostic tests to identify carriers there is a need for more input of time for counseling both affected individuals and family members. The aspiration that all patients should have access to the full range of comprehensive care services, wherever they live, will best be brought about with networking arrangements between CCCs and hemophilia centers. To be effective these arrangements will need to be formalized. As ever, there will be a

need to be mindful of the potential side-effects of therapy, whether infectious pathogens in the concentrates or inhibitors arising secondary to their use. Those who provide hemophilia care have found the past challenging and in future it will be necessary to respond proactively to an unpredictably changing environment.

References

1 Spooner RJD, Rizza CR. *Development of a National Database to Provide Information for the Planning of Care of Patients with Congenital Blood Coagulation Defects in Haemophilia & Other Inherited Bleeding Disorders.* Rizza CR, Lowe G, eds. London: Saunders, 1997: 433–53.
2 Tansey WM, Christie DA. *Haemophilia: Recent History of Clinical Management,* Vol. 4. London: Wellcome Trust, 1999.
3 UK Ministry of Health. *Arrangements for the Care of Persons Suffering from Haemophilia and Related Disorders.* Health memorandum, 1968.
4 Department of Health. *Organisation of Haemophilia Centres.* Health Circular. HC (76) 4. London: HMSO.
5 Department of Health. *Provision of Haemophilia Treatment and Care.* Health Circular. HSG (93) 30. London: HMSO.
6 Ludlam CA, Lee RJ, Prescott RJ, *et al.* Haemophilia care in central Scotland 1980–94. Demograph characteristics, hospital admissions and causes of death. *Haemophilia* 2000; 6: 494–503.
7 Yee TT, Beeton K, Griffioen A, *et al.* Experience of prophylaxis treatment in children with severe haemophilia. *Haemophilia* 2002; 8: 76–82.
8 UKHCDO. Clinical Genetics Services for Haemophilia. *Haemophilia* 2004 (in press).
9 UKHCDO. Guidelines on the Selection and use of Therapeutic Products to Treat Haemophilia and Other Hereditary Bleeding Disorders. *Haemophilia* 2003; 9: 1–23.
10 Haemophilia Alliance. *A National Service Specification for Haemophilia and Related Conditions.* London: Haemophilia Alliance, 2001.
11 Schramm W, Royal S, Kroner B, *et al.,* for the European Haemophilia Economic Study Group. Clinical outcomes and resource utilisation associated with haemophilia in Europe. *Haemophilia* 2002; 8: 33–43.
12 Lowe GDO. *Clinical Audit of Haemophilia Care in Haemophilia & Other Inherited Bleeding Disorders,* Rizza CR, Lowe G, eds. London: Saunders, 1997: 433–53.
13 Rizza CR, Spooner RJ, Giangrande PL, UK Haemophilia Centre Doctors' Organisation (UKHCD). Treatment of Haemophilia in the United Kingdom 1981–1996. *Haemophilia* 2001; 3: 49–59.

62 Comprehensive care and delivery of care: the developing world

Alok Srivastava and Auro Viswabandya

Introduction

The management of patients with hemophilia, particularly those with severe disease (factor activity <1%), is more complex than replacement of factor concentrates alone. Since the clinical impact of the severely compromised hemostasis is felt from a very early age and the fact that optimal curative treatment still eludes this condition, these patients develop many complications that require involvement of a variety of healthcare personnel. These include the following:

- early recognition of the condition and accurate diagnosis by the primary physician before any serious complication occurs due to hemorrhage;
- consultation with a specialist physician/hematologist to plan the management for the individual, including a plan for factor replacement therapy and other supportive measures;
- counseling of the family on the implications of coping with this diagnosis and its socioeconomic impact (this usually involves a nurse or a social worker);
- involvement of a physical therapist, physiatrist, and an orthopedic specialist to manage the, currently inevitable, musculoskeletal complications;
- a dentist for dentition-related complications, which are not uncommon;
- an appropriate molecular genetics laboratory for carrier detection and prenatal diagnosis, if needed;
- infectious disease specialists and hepatologists to cope with the legacy of viral infection with HIV (human immunodeficiency virus) and HCV (hepatitis C virus) of many adult patients from factor concentrates used in the 1980s;
- inhibitors to factors VIII and IX develop in a proportion of these patients and require special management.

All of the above are collectively referred to as "comprehensive care" for people with hemophilia [1,2]. The actual delivery of such care to a person with hemophilia and his family requires a healthcare system and other supportive mechanisms that can make it possible. This chapter will describe the special considerations required in providing comprehensive care to people with hemophilia in developing countries.

The developing world and its problem with hemophilia care

Of the estimated 400 000 people with hemophilia in the world, about 80% live in developing countries [143 of the 191 member states of the World Health Organization (WHO)], reflecting the overall distribution of population in the world [3]. Compared with a per capita gross domestic product (GDP) of over $20 000 in developed countries, the per capita GDP in developing countries varies, from less than $1000 for about 40% of these people (low income), to $1000–3000 for another 40% (low-middle income) and $3000–7000 for the remaining 20% (middle income) [4]. The expenditure on health in these countries is usually between 1% and 3% of GDP, most of which goes toward maintaining infrastructure. The limited healthcare budget under these circumstances is therefore directed toward nutritional and infectious diseases (high-volume, low-cost conditions) rather than hemophilia or other hereditary bleeding disorders (low-volume, high-cost conditions). While there is no doubt that limited resources impacts very significantly on the ability of countries in the developing world to spend on hemophilia care, the other most important factor in this regard is the attitude of the people and their government toward healthcare in general and hemophilia in particular. Within the social and economic diversities of these countries, examples abound of countries with similar per capita GDP spending very differently on health [3].

Comprehensive care

Providing comprehensive care to people with hemophilia in developing countries requires a few core components to be established [5]:
1 appropriate medical infrastructure;
2 identification and registration of people with hemophilia;
3 selection of appropriate models of care — protocols and products;
4 educating patients and families about hemophilia care;
5 improving social awareness of hemophilia and promoting advocacy;
6 developing a program for delivery of care.

Establishing appropriate medical facilities

There must be at least one center in each country that can provide comprehensive care of international standards. It is essential therefore to identify and train physicians who are committed to the field of hemostasis. They can then help train others in the country. More emphasis should be placed on the management of bleeding disorders, indeed hematology in general, in the medical curriculum in developing countries. Annual workshops held in different regions, to emphasize various aspects of hemophilia care, can significantly improve the understanding and skills of the care providers. In this regard, various programs of the World Federation of Hemophilia (WFH), such as International Hemophilia Training Center fellowships, workshops, and the twinning program, have been very useful in rapid transfer of information and expertise [6,7].

The number of care centers required in each country will depend on the geographic distribution of the patient population.

The facilities at each center will vary according to the level of expertise and infrastructure available (Table 62.1). Detailed guidelines should be prepared for the management of these conditions in a way that is appropriate and practical for each country. It would be best to integrate these services with the existing healthcare system, if possible. The diagnostic and clinical facilities at these centers will be useful for patients with other bleeding disorders as well [5].

While the treatment of hemophilia is extremely expensive, prevention is not. This is an aspect of hemophilia care that needs particular emphasis in developing countries. Current techniques utilizing the knowledge of molecular genetics of hemophilia can be easily established in many of these countries in a cost-effective manner to provide highly accurate carrier detection and prenatal diagnosis [8].

It is also important that, together with help for establishing diagnostic and treatment facilities, concepts of quality management in all aspects of the work involved be emphasized. A

Table 62.1 Establishing facilities for different levels of care for people with hemophilia in developing countries.

Level of care	Facilities available
Level of clinical care	*Facilities available*
Primary care center	• Provision of basic care to patients with diagnosed bleeding disorders • Storage and administration of therapeutic products • Participation in appropriate clinical audit
Treatment center	All facilities mentioned above along with laboratory service for screening tests for the diagnosis of bleeding disorders. Facilities for assays and screening for inhibitors, if possible • Physiotherapy • Counseling and advisory services • Advice on home therapy, where appropriate
Comprehensive care center	All facilities mentioned above and 24-h clinical service capable of handling emergencies and advising other centers • Laboratory facilities for assays of factor levels and inhibitors • Specialist service for surgeries, infectious diseases and social issues • Rehabilitation services
Reference center	All facilities mentioned above and: • Reference laboratory for evaluation of atypical cases and rarer bleeding disorders • Genetic evaluation, carrier detection and antenatal diagnosis • Training of members of the comprehensive care team • Maintain national registry • Conduct data analysis programs and clinical audit • Formulation of national policies • Research appropriate for the country
Level of laboratory	*Tests available*
Coagulation laboratory	• Blood film, platelet count, clot retraction, bleeding time, prothrombin time (PT), activated partial thromboplastin time (aPTT), thrombin time (TT), correction studies with "control" and factor VIII- and factor IX-deficient plasma from appropriately screened patients and inhibitor screening, qualitative test for factor XIII
Comprehensisve coagulation laboratory	• All tests mentioned above and factor assays (VIII, IX, I, II, V, VII, X, XI), inhibitor assays, platelet function tests, von Willebrand factor (vWF) activity
Reference coagulation laboratory	• All tests mentioned above and vWF multimers, vWF antigen, factor IX antigen, genotypic analysis, carrier detection, prenatal diagnostic tests, and evaluation of rarer coagulation disorders • Coordinate external quality assessment program • Appropriate research

system of clinical audit should also be developed. All laboratories should be encouraged to participate in at least one external quality assessment program [9].

Identification and registration of people with hemophilia

The proportion of the estimated number of sufferers of hemophilia identified in developing countries from where data are available varies between 10 and 80% [10]. Overall, only about 30% of those with the disorder estimated to exist in these countries have been registered. Inadequacy of healthcare facilities, lack of adequate knowledge of bleeding disorders among primary-care physicians and poorly developed hematology services, particularly with respect to diagnosis of bleeding disorders, contribute to the fact that the majority of people with hemophilia in these countries remain undetected or inadequately diagnosed [10].

The challenge of detecting affected people and making an accurate diagnosis of hemophilia in developing countries needs to be met at different levels — educating healthcare personnel, increasing awareness in society, establishing laboratories capable of performing tests of hemostasis, quality control of these tests, and monitoring of these services and their long-term impact on hemophilia care.

The importance of creating a national registry cannot be overemphasized. This is the only way to chart out the demography of people with hemophilia in any country, document their clinical status, and monitor their progress over a period of time to assess the efficacy of the care program.

Selecting appropriate models of care

Much of factor replacement therapy in hemophilia is based on following convention and practice rather than on evidence for optimum protocols. In situations without significant constraints on resources, the guiding principle seems to be to use high doses that guarantee efficacy, albeit at an extremely high cost. In developing countries, this approach is mostly impractical and treatment requires a prudent selection of protocols that are most cost-efficient, since more than 90% of this cost is made up of factor concentrates. Therefore, selecting suitable protocols for use in each country becomes critical [11].

The three main indications for factor replacement in hemophilia are: (i) prevention/treatment of hemarthroses; (ii) surgery; and (iii) immune tolerance therapy.

Prevention/treatment of hemarthrosis

The predominant cause of morbidity in hemophilia is the damage resulting from repeated bleeding into joints. It has therefore been the aim of therapy to establish a standard where damage to the joints can be completely prevented, clinically and radiologically [2]. This has been achieved by prophylactic replacement of factor concentrates 2–3 times/week at 20–40 IU/dose. The effec-

tiveness of this approach in preserving *joint integrity* has been established with long-term follow-up data from Sweden [12]. Unfortunately, the annual cost of such therapy at $50–150 000 per person has been so high that it has been difficult even for countries with developed economies to adopt it universally. Since this is impractical in developing countries, the aim of replacement shifts from maintaining perfect joint integrity to reasonable joint function that will allow the person to remain functionally independent. This can be achieved with much smaller amounts of factor concentrates. Out of necessity and not out of choice, people with hemophilia in developing countries and their physicians have to accept this fact [13].

The actual amount of factor replacement for joint bleeding in developing countries is variable. The limited data available suggest that the total quantity of factor concentrate used varies from about 2–30 000 IU per person annually [14]. Some of these centers that use factor concentrates in the intermediate range have reported preservation of reasonable joint function and functional independence. However, this is not backed by carefully documented data on long-term orthopedic outcome at the different dosages being used in these countries. Therefore, it would be useful to study a large number of patients for orthopedic outcome with emphasis on the functional status. Such data could help establish the dose at which the cost–benefit ratio is the highest.

Surgery

Large quantities of factor concentrates are needed for hemophilic patients undergoing surgery. When factor concentrates are used at the usually recommended dosage for intermittent bolus infusions, most major surgical procedures require about 1000 IU/kg per procedure [15]. With continuous infusion of factor concentrates, this can be reduced to about 400–500 IU/kg per procedure [16]. In situations of extreme resource constraints, lower doses, aimed at maintaining 30–40% trough levels in the first 2–3 days, followed by 20–30% in the next 3–4 days and 10–20% levels during the subsequent days, can reduce factor usage to about 300 IU/kg per procedure even with intermittent infusion protocols for major surgical procedures, not including joint replacement surgery [17].

Immune tolerance therapy

Extremely large quantities of factor concentrates are required for immune tolerance therapy for people with hemophilia who develop persistent high-titer inhibitors. The optimal dose remains to be defined and varies; usually between about 50 and 200 IU per dose, 2–3 times per week, is administered for several months [18]. Very few data are available on such therapy from developing countries [19,20]. In Turkey, four out of seven patients underwent successful immune tolerance therapy with 25 IU/kg factor VIII three times weekly over 1–4 months. These are encouraging data, but the therapy needs to be attempted on larger numbers of patients. Unfortunately, most centers in developing countries are unable to offer such treatment for lack of resources.

Products for treatment

The greatest challenge for those attempting to provide care for people with hemophilia in developing countries is the provision of factor concentrates in adequate quantities for replacement therapy. Availability and cost determine the choice of products for factor replacement in developing countries, unlike in developed countries where safety and purity are the predominant considerations [21]. Different models and possibilities exist and each country needs to carefully choose its options.

Import of factor concentrates

Importing the required quantities of safe virus-inactivated factor concentrates of a suitable purity from the international market is an option. The advantage of this approach is that safe factor concentrates can be immediately made available to people with hemophilia. The problem is that even given the lower cost of plasma-derived concentrates at $0.20/IU, with increasing use of recombinant concentrates in developed countries, they remain out of reach of most hemophilic people in developing countries. The other important concern is that as more people with hemophilia are identified in developing countries, there will not be enough plasma-derived concentrates produced by the current manufacturers to meet the needs around the world. There is a need therefore for different levels of self-sufficiency in plasma and plasma products in developing countries.

Local self-sufficiency of plasma and factor concentrates

There are two separate issues here:
1 Self-sufficiency in plasma: this is certainly desirable, and requires improving and expanding blood transfusion services so that adequate quantities of safe plasma can be collected. Such plasma could be used as fresh-frozen plasma (FFP) or cryoprecipitate initially, with viral inactivation, if possible, until other options become available. If enough plasma can be collected, then fractionation can be considered.
2 Self-sufficiency in fractionation: this is a distinct issue. Two options exist for fractionation of locally collected plasma — contract fractionation outside the country at a suitable facility, or establishing the infrastructure for fractionation locally.

Though various factors need to be considered, including volume of plasma available, quantity and purity of factor concentrates required, and the resources available for it for choosing between these two options, it may be best for smaller countries to opt for contract fractionation and for those with larger population to choose the latter option.

Perhaps the best option is a combination of these two approaches. Initially, a country could import modest quantities of factor concentrates that can provide the existing people with hemophilia with a safe therapeutic option while trying to establish a good transfusion service for collecting large quantities of plasma. As plasma collection increases, fractionation could be done either locally or on contract at a distant site to different levels of purity as deemed appropriate, and factor replacement practices could change accordingly. Such an approach is also likely to be more acceptable for governments, which may prefer to use their resources to support local industry rather than on import of factor concentrates alone [21].

There are a few examples of plasma fractionation facilities in developing countries. Brazil, Cuba, Thailand, and South Africa have been able to produce small quantities of low/intermediate-purity virus-inactivated products in modest plasma fractionation plants that have served their needs well. [21]. In South Africa, the needs of about 1500 people with hemophilia, using about 12 000 IU each annually, have been almost entirely met from these manufacturing units. Large quantities of factor concentrates and other plasma products are fractionated at multiple facilities in China. [22]. While developing countries attempt to establish facilities for fractionation, the overriding principle should be attention to good manufacturing prcactices with regard to quality of plasma and viral inactivation.

Educating patients and families about hemophilia

While this is extremely important everywhere, it is even more so in situations where care is inadequate. A knowledgeable patient can actually help prevent iatrogenic complications of hemophilia, which are not uncommon in these conditions. Facilities should be established for adequate counseling and education about the disease for families with individuals diagnosed to have hemophilia. Apart from information related to the principles of managing this condition, they should also be made aware of the support systems available to cope with it socially and financially. Written information should also be provided to them. It would be very useful if, at the time of diagnosis and registration, a standardized information booklet in the local language is given to each patient and his family. This would not only provide essential information immediately, but would also compensate to some extent for lack of proper counseling facilities at the center where the diagnosis was made. It could later be supplemented by discussions regarding specific problems.

Improving social awareness and providing advocacy

Increasing social awareness of hemophilia is important for two reasons. First, it helps identify more people affected by the conditions as families with individuals who may have hemophilia seek medical attention. Second, it also helps in creating social support for the cause of hemophilia, which can play a crucial role in improving care for people with hemophilia. Both the print and visual media can be used to achieve this.

Experience in the world has shown that getting support from government for hemophilia care requires strong advocacy groups. Patient groups and their well-wishers need to get organized and seek support for their cause. The World Federation of Hemophilia also has major programs to assist in this process.

Developing a program for delivery of care

Two models currently exist in many developing countries. The first involves support from the government and a program of care integrated with national healthcare facilities. The level of support from government and insurance agencies varies in different countries. The second is a situation in which there is no significant support from the government for people with hemophilia and where most of the care is provided by a parallel system of healthcare involving private hospitals and other nongovernmental organizations.

The data collected by the WFH through its global survey confirm that countries with the lowest gross national product (GNP) have inadequate or absent organized care for hemophilia. Thus, public health officials in countries of low economic capacity often choose to utilize their resources on programs directed toward more common conditions of greater public health importance, with little or no consideration for rarer diseases such as hemophilia [23]. It should be noted that, in nearly all the countries where hemophilia care has significantly improved over the last decade, governmental support of their program has been significant. Lobbying for support from the health budget of the country therefore becomes crucial for successful implementation of such programs.

Conclusion

The majority of people with hemophilia in the world continue to suffer inadequate care due to paucity of resources and lack of knowledge. Varying conditions that prevail in developing countries make it difficult to recommend an ideal model for the delivery of hemophilia care. It is possible, though, to define the basic requirements that are necessary to achieve this, as described in this chapter. The details will depend upon local circumstances and each country will need to choose the model best suited for its purpose. However, in the last decade, mainly due to the efforts of the WFH and the cooperation of many governments, significant progress has been made in improving hemophilia care in developing countries. If this momentum is sustained, indeed accelerated, then the quality of life of people with hemophilia in developing countries could vastly improve over the next decade.

References

1 Kasper CK, Mannucci PM, Boulyzenkov V, *et al*. Haemophilia in the 1990s: principles of treatment and improved access to care. *Semin Thrombosis Haemost* 1992; **18**: 1–10.
2 Berntorp E, Boulyzenkov V, Brettler D, *et al*. Modern treatment of haemophilia. *Bull WHO* 1995; **73**: 691–701.
3 Human Development Report, 2003. United Nations Development Program, Geneva.
4 World Bank. World Bank Report, 2000.
5 Srivastava A. Delivery of haemophilia care in the developing world. *Haemophilia* 1998; **4** (Suppl. 2): 33–40.
6 Giangrande PL, Mariani G, Black C. The WFH Hemophilia Center Twinning program: 10 years of growth, 1993–2003. *Haemophilia* 2003; **9**: 240–4.
7 Carman CJ. Developing and maintaining of hemophilia programs in developing countries. *Southeast Asian J Trop Med Public Health* 1993; **24** (Suppl. 1): 46.
8 Jayandharan G, Shaji RV, Chandy M, Srivastava A. Identification of factor IX gene defects using a multiplex PCR and CSGE strategy — a first report. *J Thromb Haemost* 2003; **1**: 2051–4.
9 Preston FE. Laboratory diagnosis of hereditary bleeding disorders: external quality assessment. *Haemophilia* 1998; **4** (Suppl. 2): 12–18.
10 World Federation Hemophilia. Global Survey, 2001.
11 Srivastava A. Factor replacement therapy in haemophilia — Are there models for developing countries? *Haemophilia* 2003; **9**: 391–7.
12 Nilsson IM, Berntorp E, Lofqvist T, Pettersson H. Twenty-five years' experience of prophylactic treatment in severe haemophilia A and B. *J Intern Med* 1992; **232**: 25–32.
13 Srivastava A. Choice of factor concentrates for haemophilia: a developing country perspective. *Haemophilia* 2001; **7**: 117–22.
14 Srivastava A, Chuansumrit A, Chandy M, *et al*. Management of haemophilia in the developing world. *Haemophilia* 1998; **4**: 474–80.
15 Rickard KA. Guidelines for therapy and optimal dosages of coagulation factors for treatment of bleeding and surgery in haemophilia. *Haemophilia* 1995; **1** (Suppl. 1): 8–13.
16 Martinowitz U, Schulman S, Gitel S, *et al*. Adjusted dose continuous infusion of factor VIII in patients with haemophilia A. *Br J Haematol* 1992; **82**: 729–34.
17 Srivastava A, Chandy M, Sunderaraj GD, *et al*. Low-dose intermittent factor replacement for post-operative haemostasis in haemophilia. *Haemophilia* 1998; **4**: 799–801.
18 DiMichele D. Immune tolerance therapy dose as an outcome predictor. *Haemophilia* 2003; **9**: 382–6.
19 Kavakli K, Gringeri A, Bader R, *et al*. Inhibitor development and subsititution therapy in a developing country: Turkey. *Haemophilia* 1998; **4**: 104–8.
20 Chuansumrit A, Pakakasama S, Kuharthong R, *et al*. Immune tolerance in a patient with haemophilia A and high titre inhibitors using locally prepared lyophilized cryoprecipitate. *Haemophilia* 2000; **6**: 523–5.
21 Bird A, Isarangkura P, Almagro D, *et al*. Factor concentrates for haemophilia in the developing world. *Haemophilia* 1998; **4**: 481–5.
22 The World Federation of Hemophilia's third global forum on the safety and supply of hemophilia treatment products, 22–23 September, 2003, Budapest, Hungary. *Haemophilia* 2004; **10**: 290–4.
23 Evatt BL, Robillard, L. Establishing haemophilia care in developing countries: using data to overcome the barrier of pessimism. *Haemophilia* 2000; **6**: 131–4.

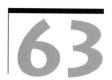

Comprehensive care and delivery of care: the global perspective

Bruce L. Evatt and Claudia Black

Comprehensive care in the developed world

A discussion of global comprehensive care must include consideration of at least two different cycles of healthcare development, one for developed countries and one for countries with emerging economies. Prior to the 1960s, no comprehensive care was available and individuals with hemophilia suffered much the same fate throughout the world. Life expectancy was less than 20 years and severe disabilities due to joint disease developed by early teens [1]. In the developed countries, hemophilia associations were established for the purpose of recruiting the donors needed to supply blood to be used for hemophilia patients. The discovery of cryoprecipitate in 1964 and subsequent development of clotting factor concentrates dramatically increased the options of clinical management for patients [2]. Concentrates could be easily stored, administered at home, and carried with patients during travel. These qualities allowed early treatment of bleeding episodes before extensive joint damage occurred, and home therapy quickly evolved as a management option. The increasing popularity of home therapy necessitated the training and education of patients about disease management. Soon specialized centers began to emerge that delivered a number of services including home care and patient education [3–5]. Studies conducted by these centers demonstrated that these approaches had a profound effect on patient survival and general health. As a result, patient associations and physicians requested and received government support for national programs (predominantly in countries of Europe, North America and Australia, New Zealand, and Japan) consisting of networks of hemophilia treatment centers (HTCs). These centers, made possible by the advanced economic condition of these countries, provided comprehensive services consisting of hemophilia care, orthopedic and dental services, and education and psychosocial support [6–8].

Today, the comprehensive care model in developed countries continues to prove itself superior to unorganized care for both survival and effective utilization of healthcare resources [6]. Recent studies on over 3000 patients with hemophilia in the USA examined mortality rates and hospitalization rates of patients receiving care in comprehensive care centers or alternatively by private physicians. Both patient groups had similar access to clotting factor and healthcare resources. Although the most severely affected patients with the most complications were those cared for by the comprehensive care centers, they had lower mortality rates and lower hospitalization rates than those cared for by private physicians (Figure 63.1) [6,7]. Important elements of this effect were the availability of expertise for serious complications, home therapy, and consistent education of patients about their diseases — all standard services at the comprehensive centers.

The net effect is that the comprehensive care model has normalized life for patients with hemophilia in countries of the developed world. Life expectancy is approximately 65 years, serious blood-borne infections have not been transmitted by concentrates since 1990, and joint disease produced by bleeding episodes is nonexistent in children under the age of 15 [6,9–11]. Individuals with hemophilia pursue life with the vigor of any normal population.

As a result, the success of HTCs in improving healthcare has had a secondary effect of reducing the need for the services provided in a number of countries. Surveys of HTCs in the USA have shown that currently the average number of patient visits/week to HTCs has dropped to 5.2, only 69% of the staff time is spent on hemophilia care, and physicians in the clinics are spending only 20% of their time taking care of hemophilia patients [12,13]. As a result, training of young physicians to take care of patients with hemophilia has decreased and an impending crisis is beginning as HTCs try to replace retiring physicians with unavailable trained personnel. Therefore, the nature of HTCs is changing. Services are expanding to include women with bleeding and clotting disorders as well as a rapidly expanding population of persons with newly diagnosed thrombophilia. In some HTCs, these patients already make up as much as 80% or more of the clinic population, but have the result of justifying and maintaining services for hemophilia patients [Centers for Disease Control and Prevention (CDC), unpublished data].

Comprehensive care in the developing world

Current status of comprehensive care in developing countries

Developing comprehensive care in the developing world has often remained an elusive dream.

Extensive information concerning the status of comprehensive care does not exist for countries outside Europe, North America, Australia, and New Zealand. To be sure, excellent

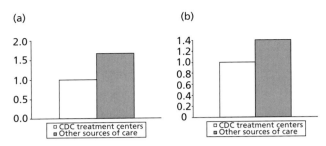

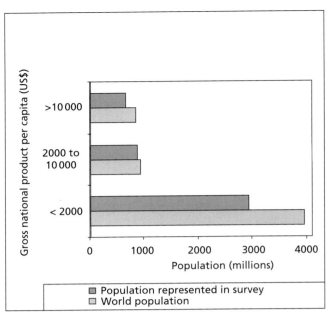

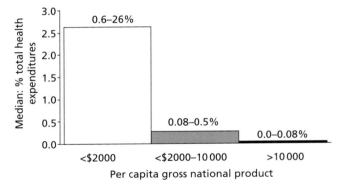

Figure 63.1 Outcomes for hemophilia treatment centers, 1993–1995. Patients receiving hemophilia care outside the hemophilia treatment centers have 67% higher mortality rates (a) and 40% higher hospitalizations (b) for a bleeding complication [6,7]. CDC, Centers for Disease Control and Prevention.

HTCs have been developed in a number of countries, but few countries have developed national networks of centers. Information has been recently published on a few countries that are developing or completing successful hemophilia programs, but in most of the developing countries, standards of care similar to those in developed countries are generally lacking and services vary widely, depending upon availability of resources [14–18].

The World Federation of Hemophilia (WFH) maintains a database containing information on the status of care in a large number of countries throughout the world. In 1998, WFH began collecting demographic information and health outcome data for hemophilia patients living in its member countries. These data are collected annually from more than 70 of its 101 member countries and the information is used to determine priorities and assist in directing the WFH's developing country programs. Termed the World Federation of Hemophilia's Global Survey, the database is one of the tools used to evaluate the level of care in various countries targeted for program development [19–22].

According to these data, the levels of services available among the different countries vary widely, and are usually related to the economic capacity of the country as reflected by the per capita gross national product (GNP) [23]. Countries may be grouped into three categories of GNP: <$2000, $2000–10 000, and >$10 000. Developed countries generally have GNPs > $10 000 per capita per annum and almost always have fully fledged comprehensive care programs. Some of the countries in the $2000–10 000 per capita per annum group have established or are developing comprehensive care programs; however, the third group, <$2000 per capita per annum, contains the largest number of countries [22] (Figure 63.2). The relationship of GNP to available health resources is dramatic. In the typical country with the highest GNP, adequate care requires approximately 2–3 times the health resources available to the average inhabitant (based on the assumption that 30 000 units per year per inhabitant are needed for adequate care). In many countries with the lowest GNP, adequate care would require 500–700 times or more of the health resources available to the average inhabitant. Graphically, this can be expressed as the amount of a countries'

Figure 63.2 World population compared with hemophilia populations in countries with different levels of economic development [21].

Figure 63.3 Percent of countries' total health expenditures needed to provide minimal standardized care.

total health expenditures that would be needed to provide what the developed countries consider as adequate healthcare (Figure 63.3).

The impact of available comprehensive care greatly affects survival. Existing data suggest that the incidence of hemophilia is constant for a number of races and ethnic groups [8]. Under these circumstances, the prevalence of hemophilia in a country might be considered a crude measurement of the overall hemophilia care because, historically, inadequate care results in premature death, shortened life expectancy, and few patients at a moment in time. When countries are grouped by GNP and examined for prevalence of hemophilia and availability of clotting factor concentrate, we see the wide gap between available care between the developed and developing world (Figure 63.4). As a

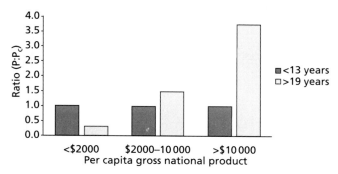

Figure 63.4 Relationship of economic capacity to the number of children with hemophilia (less than 13 years of age) and adult hemophilia patients (above the age of 19) [23]. P: Pc, ratio of adult hemophilia patients to children with hemophilia.

result of the shortened life expectancy, the populations in the lowest level of per capita GNP have hemophilia populations that are composed primarily of children (Figure 63.4). In addition, in these countries, the majority of patients will be affected by severe joint disease by their teenage years, a truly rare occurrence for patients living in developed countries. Although most countries report that specific laboratory diagnostic testing is used to diagnose patients with hemophilia, 18–30% of the countries still use nonspecific tests or clinical symptoms only to make the diagnosis of hemophilia [19–22].

Developing care in countries with emerging economies

Prior to 1990, WFH development programs struggled for lack of resources. Development of the International Hemophilia Training Centers (IHTCs) by the WFH to train healthcare professionals began in 1969 and IHTC fellowships were instrumental in providing trained physicians and other health professionals to developing countries. As a result, a number of excellent centers were established [14–17,23,24]. The WFH conducted periodic workshops on hemophilia management in selected developing countries whenever funding was obtained, and the WFH Congresses, held on an annual or biannual basis, provided a forum for an interchange of ideas that stimulated interest in management of hemophilia throughout the world. A new WFH strategic plan, entitled the "Decade Plan," was published in 1992 and generated motivational energy to initiate new programs and set the goals for the WFH to make effective treatment available to patients with hemophilia throughout the world [25].

Several new, very successful programs were started between 1994 and 1997, such as the Hemophilia Center Twinning Program, which pairs emerging hemophilia treatment centers with well-established and experienced centers, to improve diagnosis and clinical care through coaching and training. The Hemophilia Organization Twinning Program enables emerging national hemophilia associations to develop partnerships with well-established patient organizations to share knowledge and experience in areas such as patient education, advocacy, and outreach.

Integrated, individualized country projects were soon created to target specific aspects of hemophilia care in a country. Intensive efforts at country-specific program development soon began. Successful programs to develop hemophilia care in countries such as Chile (Operation Access), Uruguay, and Venezuela (Operation Improvement) provided experience and increasing optimism on achieving long-term success [26]. By working with the clinicians, healthcare teams, hemophilia societies, and governments to put together national programs, the WFH developed sustainable progress in hemophilia care with limited resources. These country-based programs have led to significant and measurable outcomes in the management of hemophilia. They prove that the efficient use of limited resources can make a significant difference in reducing mortality and improving life expectancy among people with hemophilia.

In 2003, elements of these programs were combined into an ambitious new plan, the Global Alliance for Progress in Hemophilia (GAP). GAP aims to introduce or expand national hemophilia care programs in up to 30 or 40 developing/emerging countries over the next 10 years and double the number of people diagnosed with hemophilia in these countries. The WFH goal is to diagnose 50 000 new people with hemophilia and improve access to care for these 50 000 and others who are currently diagnosed but untreated. This will be achieved through the implementation of sustainable national comprehensive hemophilia care programs integrated in the public health system and involving government support.

The WFH model for improving care through these programs consists of first conducting an evaluation and careful assessment of each member country in the five major areas of hemophilia care based on a series of development steps. Countries are classified based on levels of hemophilia care achieved in each of the five categories: (i) level of government support; (ii) care delivery structure; (iii) level of medical expertise and diagnosis; (iv) quality and availability of treatment products; and (v) strength and organization of the hemophilia association (Table 63.1). Next, the goals and objectives are set with each country, directed toward raising the level of care by a number of realistic and sustainable steps in each area of care. Attempts are made to make these goals and objectives realistic by basing them on a careful assessment of the resources available and the chances of success in the environment of the country setting. These national programs can dramatically increase the life expectancy of people with hemophilia following this step-by-step approach.

Overcoming barriers to comprehensive care

Preconceptions about the cost of care have been one of the primary barriers to expanding hemophilia services to developing countries [27]. Publications concerning the high cost of hemophilia care in developed countries often generate an impression by public health planners that hemophilia care is too expensive for a country with an emerging economy, especially if faced with

Table 63.1 Steps for developing national hemophilia care programs.

		Medical expertise			
Government support	Care delivery	Laboratory diagnosis	Medical treatment	Treatment products	Patient organization
Objectives					
To obtain government support for national hemophilia care program within the health system	To set up a national hemophilia care program (national plan defined with key treaters and NMO); To make the organization of hemophilia treatment more efficient	To provide accurate diagnosis and appropriate treatment		To obtain the best quality blood products in sufficient quantity at an affordable cost; Develop and improve regulatory knowledge	To develop a strong patient organization for advocacy and education
Development steps					
No government support or interest in hemophilia care	Isolated doctor in major city works with no resources	Basic laboratory diagnostic ability	Basic medical knowledge in hematology (includes pediatricians and general practitioners)	Local production of: whole blood, plasma, fresh-frozen plasma (FFP), cryoprecipitate, freeze-dried cryoprecipitate. Combination of local production of cryo and/or FFP and some purchase of plasma-derived factor concentrates: (1) less than 0.2 IU per capita of concentrates; (2) between 0.2 and 0.5 IU; (3) between 0.5 and 1 IU; (4) between 1 and 2 IU	Organization formed by a nucleus of patients; Organization structured, recognized/registered with a constitution
Government recognition of main HTC as a reference center	Basic treatment is possible in hospital(s) in major city	Basic screening tests (bleeding time, platelet count, coagulation test): PT, aPTT, TT	Doctor specialized in hematology. Hematologist(s) assigned to hemophilia care	Proper national tender system in place	Organization holds regular meetings with a core group of volunteers and educates patients and families in major city
Some level of government involvement in hemophilia care (e.g., hemophilia committee or task force)	Regular hematology outpatient clinic with follow-up offered	Internal quality control; Factor assays	Key hematologist(s) trained in hemophilia	Examine feasibility of contract fractionation of plasma-derived concentrates	NMO patient registry

Limited central or regional government resources allocated for hemophilia care	Creation of a core team within hospital that forms the basis of a full hemophilia treatment center (HTC) Core team within hospital (HTC) has a medical patient registry and treatment guidelines/protocols	Participation in EQASVWD assays and inhibitor detection	Specialized hemophilia core team (hematologist, nurse, physiotherapist, orthopedist, lab technologist)	Examine feasibility of local fractionation of plasma-derived concentrates	Organizes activities including: educational services, fundraising, training, membership, volunteer recruitment, advocacy, budgeting
Official government commitment to hemophilia care	Additional hemophilia treatment centers with core teams for children and/or adults in major cities	Molecular genetic detection/DNA mutation detection and carrier detection/prenatal diagnosis	Education provided to patients Home care available for patients Specialized comprehensive care team (social worker, dentist, psychologist, infectious diseases specialist, genetic counselor)	Purchase of plasma-derived concentrates (>2 IU per capita)	Outreach to other regions of the country to identify new patients Regional chapters are formed
Government contributes substantial financial support for hemophilia care	Coordinated network of designated HTCs with national treatment protocols		Education offered to general medical community	Examine feasibility of combined purchase of plasma-derived and recombinant concentrates	National organization follows a strategic plan
Hemophilia is a line item in a country's annual healthcare budget	Full comprehensive hemophilia care team is formed in the major HTC(s)				National organization is a partner in national hemophilia care program
Government is a key partner in sustainable national hemophilia care program	Basic teams formed in other areas/regions				
	Established national medical patient registry				
	Established sustainable national hemophilia care program				

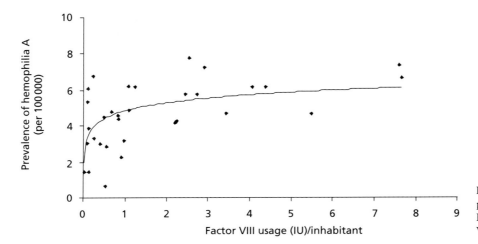

Figure 63.5 The observed prevalence of hemophilia A patients compared with the amount of FVIII used in 32 countries reporting to the World Federation Global Survey [35].

a number of high health priorities that affect large numbers of the population. It is not surprising then, that the conclusion is drawn that the only option is to ignore hemophilia as a health problem.

The financing of hemophilia care is complex, however, and conclusions based on this reasoning do disservice to persons with hemophilia living in those countries because it delays low-cost elements of healthcare that would greatly improve survival and decrease morbidity. For example, in the developed countries, the most significant cost element to the healthcare system can be attributed to the cost of clotting factor. Health services used by patients consist of only 5% or less of the cost [28–30]. A wide variation in healthcare costs produced by individual patients has been found to be related to the severity of the hemophilia and the presence or absence of inhibitors [29]. Likewise, in any given year, as many as 24% of the patients living in a country may use no clotting factor because they do not bleed. If we look at the use of clotting factor by the approximately 17 000 patients with hemophilia A and B in the USA, we see that, of the 75% that use clotting factor, half the factor usage is for prophylaxis and immune tolerance regimens for only 15% of the population. This has important implications for developing countries making decisions based on these data about undertaking national programs of hemophilia care [31,32]. This issue is complicated by the fact there is wide variation between countries of the developed world as to the appropriate quantity of clotting factor to use (Figure 63.5). The majority of developed countries use 2–4 international units (IU) of factor VIII per inhabitant living in the country for their patients with hemophilia. In some countries, the quantity reaches almost 2–3 times these figures [33]. The level of clotting factor use appears to have insignificant effect on survival (if we assume that survival is reflected in the prevalence of hemophilia in the country) in the range of 1 IU to 6 or more IU per inhabitant (Figure 63.5). The higher usage then must accrue other benefits, such as reducing joint disease, making possible corrective surgery for pre-existing deformities, desensitizing inhibitors, and using prophylaxis [34,35]. As we

have noted, these benefits affect a decreasing percentage of the hemophilia population and are achieved at large increases in cost of products, not at the expense of utilizing other healthcare resources. Healthcare planners deciding to provide comprehensive care and on-demand therapy face an entirely different cost liability than those that plan to supply these services, including prophylaxis for everyone and inhibitor desensitization therapy for all patients with inhibitors. A stepwise approach to health services (Table 63.1), beginning with the organization of healthcare and blood banking services and provision of small amounts of concentrate supplemented by cryoprecipitate, can achieve much benefit; developing no program because resources do not permit everything needed leaves much to be desired.

In conclusion, a wide discrepancy exists between hemophilia care availability in the developed and the developing world. Although the availability of resources is a major contributor to this discrepancy, a significant amount of improvement can be achieved by reorganization of resources, education and training. The World Federation of Hemophilia is working with governmental agencies, healthcare providers, patient organizations and industry to achieve this improvement and has had a significant measurable impact on the status of hemophilia care.

References

1 Smith PS, Levine PH. The benefits of comprehensive care of hemophilia: a five-year study of outcomes. *Am J Publ Hlth* 1984; **74**: 616–17.

2 Pool J, Hershgold E, Pappenhagen A. High-potency antihemophilic factor concentrates from cryoglobulin precipitate. *Nature* 1964; **203**: 312.

3 Levine PH, McVerry BA, Segelman AE, *et al.* Comprehensive health care clinic for hemophiliacs. *Arch Intern Med* 1976; **136**: 792–4.

4 Smith PS, Keyes NC, Forman EN. Socioeconomic evaluation of a state-funded comprehensive hemophilia-care program. *N Engl J Med* 1982; **306**: 575–9.

5 Jones P. Hemophilia home therapy. *Homeostasis* 1992; **22**: 247–50.

6 Soucie JM, Nuss R, Evatt B, *et al.* and the Hemophilia Surveillance System Project Investigators. Mortality among males with hemophilia: relations with source of medical care. *Blood* 2000, **96**: 437–42.

7 Soucie JM, Symons J 4th, Evatt B, *et al.* and the Hemophilia Surveillance System Project Investigators. Home-based factor infusion therapy and hospitalization for bleeding complications among males with haemophilia. *Haemophilia* 2001; **7**: 198–206.

8 Soucie JM, Evatt BE, Jackson D, and the Hemophilia Surveillance System Project Investigators. Occurrence of Hemophilia in the United States. *Am J Hematol* 1998, **59**: 288–94.

9 Manco-Johnson MJ, Riske B, Kasper CK. Advances in care of children with hemophilia. *Semin Thromb Haemost* 2003; **29**: 585–94.

10 Soucie JM, Cianfrini C, Janco RL, *et al.* Joint range of motion limitations among young males with hemophilia: prevalence and risk factors. *Blood* 2004; **103**: 2467–73.

11 Steen Carlsson K, Hojgard S, Glomstein A, *et al.* On demand vs. prophylactic treatment for severe hemophilia in Norway and Sweden: differences in treatment characteristics and outcome. *Hemophilia* 2003; **9**: 555–66.

12 Isarangkura P, Chuansumrit A. Developing and maintaining the hemophilia program in Thailand. *Southeast Asian J Trop Med Public Health*. 1993; **24** (Suppl. 1): 61–5.

13 CDC Unpublished HSS Data, 1996–1998.

14 National Hemophilia Survey of United States Hemophilia Treatment Centers, 2000.

15 Antunes SV. Hemophilia in the developing world: the Brazilian experience. *Hemophilia* 2002; **8**: 199–204.

16 Kim KY. Development and maintenance of hemophilia care program in Korea. *Southeast Asian J Trop Med Public Health* 1993; **24** (Suppl. 1): 52–60.

17 Fontes EM, Amorim L, Carvalho SM, Farah MB. Hemophilia care in the state of Rio de Janeiro, Brazil. *Rev Panam Salud Publica* 2003; **13**: 124–8.

18 Srivastava A, Chauansumrit A, Chandy M, *et al.* Management of hemophilia in the developing world. *Hemophilia* 1998; **4**: 474–80.

19 WFH. *Global Survey on Hemophilia*. Montreal, Canada, July 2000.

20 WFH. *Global Survey on Hemophilia*. WFH: Montreal, 2001.

21 WFH. *Global Survey on Hemophilia*. WFH: Montreal, 2002.

22 WFH. *Global Survey on Hemophilia*. WFH: Montreal, 2003.

23 Evatt BL, Robillard L. Establishing hemophilia care in developing countries: using data to overcome the barrier of pessimism. *Hemophilia* 2000; **6**: 131–4.

24 Rickard KA. Development and maintenance of hemophilia programs in developing countries. *Southeast Asian J Trop Med Public Health* 1993; **24** (Suppl. 1): 47–51.

25 Rickard KA. The International Hemophilia Training Centres of the World Federation of Hemophilia: 30-year review. *Hemophilia* 2000 Sep; **6**: 471–3.

26 Lee CA. Towards achieving global haemophilia care – World federation of Hemophilia Programs. *Haemophilia* 1998; **4**: 463–73.

27 Smith PS, Teutsch SM, Shaffer PA, *et al.* Episodic versus prophylactic infusions for hemophilia A: a cost-effectiveness analysis. *J Pediatr* 1996; **129**: 424–31.

28 Evatt BL. Public health and international health-care development for persons with haemophilia. Operation Improvement and Operation Access *Haemophilia* 1998; **4**: 491–7.

29 Santiago-Borrero PJ, Ortiz I, Rivera-Caragol E, Maldonado NI. Financial aspects of hemophilia care in Puerto Rico and other Latin American countries. *Hemophilia* 1999; **5**: 386–91.

30 Globe DR, Cunningham WE, Andersen R, *et al.* Hemophilia Utilization Group Study. *Hemophilia* 2003; **9**: 325–31.

31 Schramm W, Royal S, Kroner B, *et al.* for the European hemophilia economic study group. *Hemophilia* 2002; **8**: 33–43.

32 Srivastava A. Factor replacement therapy in hemophilia – are there models for developing countries? *Hemophilia* 2003; **9**: 391–6.

33 Srivastava A, Chuansumrit Am Chandy M, Duraiswamy G, Karagus C. Management of hemophilia in the developing world. *Hemophilia* 1998; **4**: 474–80.

34 Evatt BL. Observations from Global Survey 2001: an emerging database for progress. *Hemophilia* 2002; **8**: 153–6.

35 Miners AH, Sabin CA, Tolley KH, Lee CA. The changing patterns of factor VIII (FVIII) and factor IX (FIX) clotting factor usage in a comprehensive care centre between 1980 and 1994. *Hemophilia* 1998; **4**: 4–9.

Index

Note: page numbers in *italics* refer to figures, those in **bold** refer to tables. Coagulation factors are abbreviated to 'F' in subentries and von Willebrand disease and von Willebrand factor to VWD and VWF respectively.

uremia 14
urinary calculus
    bleeding 156
    immune tolerance induction 99–100

vaccinations 123
vacuum extraction 253, 254
vaginal delivery 253–4
valgus deformity 179, *180*
Van Creveld regimen 72, 76
vascular diseases 342
venous thromboembolism
    FXI deficiency 323
    VWF-containing concentrates 291, 294
VHP-VWF 291, **292**
viral infections 303
    transmission in blood products 158, **159**, 160
    see also named viruses
vitamin K
    intramuscular 125, 127
    neonates 254
vitamin K deficiency
    FX deficiency 317
    neonates 128, 316
vitamin K-dependent enzyme complexes 1, 2
    blood coagulation 5
    disulfide bond formation 7
volume of distribution 106–7
von Willebrand disease (VWD) 13
    ABO blood group 281
    acquired 276, 280
        VWF concentrate use 294
    antifibrinolytics in menorrhagia treatment 299
    bleeding
        history evaluation 280–1
        mucocutaneous criteria 113
        score 280–1, **282**
        symptoms 282–3
    carriers 268
    classification **17**, **116**, 259, 260, 265–6, 279, **280**
    clinical definition of severe/mild disease 279–80
    clinical features 282–3
    desmopressin 279
        menorrhagia treatment 298–9
        therapy 285–7
    diagnosis 17, 265, 270–1
        biological 272–6, **277**
        children 116–17
        examination 280
        false 296
        flow chart *276*
        history 280
        mild bleeding symptoms 270
        strategy 275–6, **277**
    epidemiology 265–71
    family assessment 266–7
    family history 281–2
    FVIII concentrate treatment 143
    FXI deficiency association 323
    groups 265–6, 267–8
    gynecological disorders 249
    inheritance 114, 281–2

intermediate 265, **266**, 267
laboratory tests 272–5
menorrhagia 114
    clinical characteristics 297–8
    management 298–9
    mild 265–6, 267–8, 279–80
        desmopressin use 132
    Mirena in menorrhagia treatment 299
    moderate 280
    molecular aspects 257–63
    Normandy type 300
    oral contraceptives in menorrhagia treatment 299
    partial deficiency 259–60
    patient register 361
    PFA-100® 115
    phenotypic characterization **277**
    platelet-type 117
    postpartum hemorrhage 299
    practical implications 269–71
    pregnancy 299–300
    presurgical screening 269
    prevalence 265, 268
        developing countries 268–9
    qualitative defects 260–3
    quantitative defects 257, **258–9**, 259–60
    ristocetin-induced platelet agglutination test (RIPA) 262, 274, 275
    severe 265, **266**, 267–8, 279–80
    therapeutic concentrates 289–94
    treatment cost–utility study 41–2
    type 1 116–17, 259–60, 265
        assays 274
        clinical expression 282
        desmopressin response 285
        frequency 268
        inheritance 281
        menorrhagia 297
        mutations 259–60
        phenotypic characterization **277**
        severe disease 279
        VWF-containing concentrates 289, 294
    type 2 116, 265
        assays 275
        clinical expression 282
        desmopressin response 285
        frequency 268
        inheritance 281
        menorrhagia 297
        pregnancy 300
    type 2A 260–1, 265
        mutations 261
        phenotypic characterization **277**
        severe disease 279
        VWF-containing concentrates 289, 294
    type 2B 261–2, 265
        assays 274
        mutations 262
        phenotypic characterization **277**
        pregnancy 300
        VWF-containing concentrates 289, 294
    type 2M 262
        assays 274